HEMATOLOGY

HEMATOLOGY

edited by William S. Beck

fifth edition

The MIT Press
Cambridge, Massachusetts
London, England

This book was set in Times Roman by Asco Trade Typesetting Ltd., Hong Kong, and printed and bound by Halliday Lithograph in the United States of America

Library of Congress Cataloging-in-Publication Data
Hematology / edited by William S. Beck. —5th ed.
p. cm.
Includes bibliographical references and index.
ISBN 0-262-02316-4 (hard). —ISBN 0-262-52157-1 (pbk.)
1. Blood—Diseases. 2. Hematology. I. Beck. William Samson, 1923–
[DNLM: 1. Hematologic Diseases. WH 100 H486]
RC633.H433 1991
616.1′5—dc20
DNLM/DLC
for Library of Congress 90-13588
CIP

Contents

Preface to the Fifth Edition

Since the first edition of this book appeared in 1973, revisions have emerged at four-year intervals—the second edition in 1977, the third in 1983, and the fourth in 1985. A web of circumstance kept this edition, the fifth, from appearing in 1989. But here it is—a year late and all the better.

In previous revisions, the need for renewal was always clear and compelling. This time, it was overwhelming. Among the additions are discussions of the myeloid growth factors, erythropoietin, the red cell cytoskeleton, oncogenes, and newer aspects of immunology, hemato-oncology, and clotting. Indeed, the percentage of text replaced or updated was far higher than in any previous revision—a clear sign of the pace and sweep of contemporary research in hematology and allied fields.

To make the fifth edition something of a special event, we have introduced the following changes and new features:

- Although this syllabus was written orginally for first and second year medical students, it found many readers among house officers and practicing physicians. To better serve them (and medical students in their clinical years), we have included more tables, charts, and text on diagnosis and approach to the patient. It has been said in jest that practicing hematologists face seven major clinical problems: too few and too many red cells; too few and too many white cells; too few and too many platelets; and bleeding. To an extent, it is possible to construct binary logic trees outlining optimal approaches to each of these problems, indicating among other things what tests are to be done when. We urge those confronting such clinical problems to think in large categories before delving into the minutiae of individual diseases. Thus, in the analysis of anemia, one wants to know early whether there is premature red cell destruction (or hemorrhage), or failure of production. The reticulocyte count helps to distinguish these categories and should be considered before other tests—and so on. The flow sheets in this edition suggest rational approaches to several of the hematologist's major problems. They are not written in stone. Other approaches could be described. These are the ones we use and recommend.
- Reference lists and bibliographies are more extensive than in previous editions. As a service to the reader, we have segregated references under the headings Reviews and Original Papers.
- A new lecture has been added on general principles of malignant disease, an acknowledgement that hematology today in many institutions has been converted to hematology-oncology—in practice, if not in course

design and teaching. This lecture covers a number of general points that we felt were not covered elsewhere in the medical curriculum and would provide useful background to the lectures that follow on the aspects of hematologic oncology.

- There is a new appendix containing laboratory methods that should be useful to students in taking hematology or clinical pathology courses as well as to physicians performing such tests in their own laboratories, if such there be.
- The fifth edition is being published in combination with *HEMAVID*, a comprehensive computer program for the teaching of blood and bone marrow morphology. That program, as noted elsewhere, includes an extensive menu that permits users to examine multiple examples of all of the major hematologic disorders discussed in the text. It also includes some hematologic cases in which blood and bone marrow morphology are presented as unknowns as well as a collection of examination questions. The *HEMAVID* program makes extensive references to text in this volume, and we hope our readers will have an opportunity to study both the book and the computer program in tandem.
- The lectures are again in outline form. This seems to help with the organization of ideas and to facilitate note-taking. However, we have tried to make the text even more readable. As before, there is a wide margin and outline headings and their ranks are indicated by labels and font styles. We have made these clearer in this edition and have, in addition, for the first time in the text used bulleted lists, which should add further clarity to the material.
- Finally, to mark this edition I have included on the first page of each lecture brief Editor's Comments, which incorporate remarks of the kind one might offer in the classroom when introducing a new lecturer or topic. These, in effect, set the stage for the material to be covered and in some cases celebrate some of the major advances that have taken place since the first edition of 1973.

The book's general concept remains unchanged. These are lectures—we resolutely call them that rather than chapters—that may be read by students in their own time, both as preparation for and reminder of discussions in lecture hall and laboratory. There is no intention here to preempt lectures and lecturers. Long experience in the hematology courses of Harvard Medical School and the Harvard-MIT Division of Health Sciences and Technology suggests that the lecture hour is now best used for illustration and expansion.

Emphasis remains on physiology and pathophysiology. Discussions of therapy are still framed in terms of principles. We refer readers elsewhere for dosage schedules and other details. Topics are treated in a traditional sequence—red cells, then white cells, then clotting—and we assume that lectures will be read in that sequence. However, cross-references are offered for those who prefer to read the lectures in another sequence.

Reluctantly, we deleted a lecture, which appeared in the first four editions, on histiocytoses and lipidoses. These, of course, have relevance to hematology because the storage cells they display are often found in bone marrow and need to be recognized. Also, these disorders are part of the differential diagnosis of hepatosplenomegaly. However, in the current scheme of things, we felt that if something had to go, it would be a topic that is adequately covered in other courses.

I note again that authors of many of these lectures are indebted to those who lectured in former years and who contributed to earlier editions. Rather than adopt complex rules of authorship, we have chosen to acknowledge these fine predecessors in this preface. I acknowledge with thanks the stimulating past contributions of N. Abramson, A. Aisenberg, C. A. Alper, R. H. Aster, R. W. Colman, R. A. Cooper, A. C. Crocker, D. Deykin, L. K. Diamond, B. G. Forget, B. Glader, H. A. Godwin, R. I. Handin, S. E. Lux, W. C. Moloney, P. R. Reich, G. K. Sherwood, J. T. Truman, and I. Umansky. I also wish to recognize the efforts of Carol Sparling, who assisted in the preparation of the manuscript.

William S. Beck
September 1990

From the Introduction to the First Edition

In the present Harvard Medical School curriculum, hematology is one of a dozen blocks within the large one-year Pathophysiology course, which begins in the middle of the first year. For many years we have furnished our students in this course with syllabus materials and lecture notes. These notes have long been known as "the camel," which, as everyone knows, is an animal that looks as though it had been put together by a committee. When responsibility for the course came to me, the scanty lecture notes took the form of severe and often uninformative outlines. Students complained of the burdens of note taking, and some brought tape recorders. Accordingly lecturers were asked to flesh out their outlines, and our camel grew. It became apparent in time that the value of the syllabus would be enhanced by careful editing. The result is the present volume. The vast expansion of knowledge in the various branches of pathophysiology poses an increasingly difficult problem for those who would define the content of a core curriculum and establish standards and priorities for what is to be taught. It is my view that this difficult cause can be furthered only by the thoughtful preparation of texts such as this, for the very act of editing such a volume necessitates choices and permits correlations and overviews that are never quite possible when many and diverse individuals are responsible for a course of instruction.

The major goal of this endeavor is to improve the quality and usefulness of these notes as teaching instruments. It is our intention to revise this small volume frequently so it will retain the freshness and currency that characterized the informal syllabus materials of previous years.

Some believe it would now be appropriate to abandon formal lectures. I see much merit in that proposal. Surely medical students are capable of handling reading assignments. Surely they deserve exemption from having read to them lectures that they could as well read themselves. Still there is cause for regret about a step that would deny students an hour or two with colleagues who rate high as teachers, scientists, and personalities. How to make the best use of these hours will be the subject of experimentation and innovation in the years ahead.

In a sense, this volume is a successor to Ham's famous *Syllabus* and its revision by Page and Culver. Unlike the present book, however, the earlier syllabuses placed major emphasis on laboratory diagnosis. We hope that this volume will be useful to our students, both in the first- and second-year hematology courses and in later clinical years. We hope too that students and physicians beyond Harvard Medical School may find this a helpful review of hematology, one that may serve as a compendium and guide to the several large new textbooks of hematology.

William S. Beck
February 1973

Contributors

William S. Beck
Professor of Medicine, Harvard Medical School and Massachusetts General Hospital; Professor of Health Sciences and Technology, Massachusetts Institute of Technology; Tutor in Biochemical Sciences, Harvard College

H. Franklin Bunn
Professor of Medicine, Harvard Medical School and Brigham and Women's Hospital

William B. Castle
Late Francis Weld Peabody Faculty Professor of Medicine, Emeritus, Harvard Medical School

W. Hallowell Churchill, Jr.
Associate Professor of Medicine, Harvard Medical School and Brigham and Women's Hospital

Alice Weaver Flaherty
M.D.-Ph.D. candidate, Harvard Medical School and Massachusetts Institute of Technology

David C. Harmon
Assistant Professor of Medicine, Harvard Medical School and Massachusetts General Hospital

Nancy L. Harris
Associate Professor of Pathology, Harvard Medical School and Massachusetts General Hospital

James H. Jandl
George Richards Minot Professor of Medicine, Harvard Medical School

David J. Kuter
Instructor in Medicine, Harvard Medical School and Massachusetts General Hospital

Stuart E. Lind
Assistant Professor of Medicine, Harvard Medical School and Massachussetts general Hospital

David G. Nathan
Robert A. Stranahan Professor of Pediatrics, Harvard Medical School, the Children's Hospital, and Dana-Farber Cancer Institute

Stephen H. Robinson
George C. Reisman Professor of Medicine, Harvard Medical School and Beth Israel Hospital

Robert D. Rosenberg
Professor of Medicine, Harvard Medical School, and Professor of Biology, Massachusetts Institute of Technology

David S. Rosenthal
Henry K. Oliver Professor of Hygiene and Director of the University Health Services; Associate Professor of Medicine, Harvard Medical School and Brigham and Women's Hospital

Thomas P. Stossel
American Cancer Society Professor of Clinical Research; Professor of Medicine, Harvard Medical School and Massachusetts General Hospital

Robert I. Tepper
Instructor in Medicine, Harvard Medical School and Massachusetts General Hospital

HEMATOLOGY

LECTURE 1

Hematopoiesis

William S. Beck

EDITOR'S COMMENT

Of all the topics in this book, those in this important lecture have required the most revision in successive editions, with some sort of climax occurring in this one. Studies of hematopoiesis have surged in recent years owing to tissue culture techniques for various colony-forming units (CFUs) and progress (much of it in industrial laboratories) in the identification, purification and cloning of the cytokines, lymphokines, and monokines that regulate blood cell production. Knowledge of these factors has both simplified and complicated the field. Certainly, it has opened large new doors in its promise of revolutionary clinical applications. Some have already been realized. The prospect of being able to control cell proliferation and differentiation pushes at the frontiers of clinical hematology: the refractory anemias, bone marrow failure, leukemia, and lymphoma. It is worth noting that these advances were directly attributable to the dogged persistence of some investigators through long years of tedious assays and discouraging results. A case in point: Metcalf's discovery of GM-CSF and related factors. In its auspicious outcome, hematologic research again yielded important insights into basic biologic mechanisms.

I. BIOLOGY OF HEMATOPOIESIS

Hematopoiesis consists in a series of events wherein the hematopoietic stem cells mature into functional blood cells. Its locus changes in the course of development.

A. Ontogeny

In the third week of human embryogenesis, mesenchymal cells in the yolk sac from clusters called **blood islands**. Peripheral cells of the islands join to form a primitive vascular system. Simultaneously central cells of the islands differentiate into elements that become detached and are carried off by the mounting stream of primitive plasma. These are the **yolk sac stem cells**. Some differentiate into **primitive erythroblasts**, the earliest hemoglobin-synthesizing cells. Unlike pronormoblasts of adult bone marrow, they do not mature into erythrocytes.

In the third month of embryonic life, yolk sac stem cells migrate to the liver, which then becomes the chief site of blood cell formation. Additional contributions are then made by the spleen, lympth nodes, and thymus. Hematopoiesis may continue in the liver unitl after birth. However, bone marrow hematopoiesis begins in the fourth lunar month and by the end of gestation is the major source of blood cells. The terms **medullary** and **extramedullary hematopoiesis** denote blood cell production by bone marrow and by tissues other than bone marrow, respectively.

At birth, medullary hematopoiesis occurs in almost every bone. Flat bones (sternum, ribs, skull, vertebrae, and innominates) retain most of their hematopoietic activity throughout life, but hematopoiesis progessively diminishes within the shafts of long bones. In the adult, it is limited to the ends of these bones. At times of increased demand for blood cells, active marrow reappears in these sites. Hematopoiesis in the adult occurs exclusively in bone marrow. As noted below, even lymphocytes derive from medullary precursors. Some extramedullary hematopoiesis persists at birth, but it rapidly diminishes, to resume only under abnormal circumstances. In such instances, liver and spleen are the major loci of extramedullary hematopoiesis.

B. Phylogeny

Much has been learned of the physiology of blood from studies of the evolution of the hematopoietic system. Amphioxus and other primitive chordates lack blood cells. In some invertebrates, hemoglobin occurs in solution in plasma. The mature red cells of reptiles, birds, and fish contain nuclei, mitochondria, and ribosomes that are actively engaged in hemoglobin synthesis. The locus of adult blood-forming tissue varies in different speices. For example, it is the kidney in amphibia and teleosts; the gonads in some fishes; the liver in turtles; and tissues around the heart in sturgeon and paddlefish.

C. Mammalian bone marrow

Nutrient arteries enter marrow cavities through bone foramina. Arteries branch into distributing arterioles that give rise to an endosteal bed of **sinusoids**. From the bed, sinuses travel in a radial direction toward the central longitudinal veins lying in the long axis of the bone. Hematopoietic tissue lies between the sinuses. **(Erythropoiesis, granulopoiesis** (or **myelopoiesis**), and **thromobopoiesis** take place extravascularly in the marrow **stroma**.

Sinusoidal walls have three layers: **endothelial cells**, **basement membrane**, and **adventitial cells**. Endothelial and adventitial cells are both mononulcear reticulum cells that are capable of phagocytosis (see lecture 2). Blood is present within the sinusoids, but intrasinusoidal materials (both diffusible and particulate) have free access to extrasinusoidal areas through gaps in the walls. Hematopoietic cells, having undergone maturation outside the sinusoids, enter the sinusoid at a critical moment in the maturation sequence. This critical event is termed the **release** of blood cells from marrow into blood. Its mechanism is still poorly understood.

II. STEM CELLS

The marrow of adult mammals contains pluripotent **stem cells** that give rise to the several lines of differentiated blood cells—erythrocytes (red cells), granulocytes-monocytes (white cells), thrombocytes (platelets), and probably lymphocytes of various kinds (T- and B-lymphocytes, plamsa cells). The term *stem cell* has been used in three different ways.

A. Definitions

1. Morphologic definition

In one definition, the stem cell is a **morphologic** entity. However, stem cells are few in number and they have still not been identified to everyone's satisfaction. Present evidence suggests that they are small mononuclear cells resembling lymphocytes. They are mobile cells, and many are normally present in the blood (about 1–5 per 10^5 nucleated cells). At certain times (e.g., after whole-body irradiation, during antigenic stimulation), the number in blood increases. As noted above, waves of migration also occur during embryonic life.

2. Kinetic definition

The stem cell is also definable as a **kinetic** entity. A stem cell pool is characterized by its ability (1) to be self-renewing and (2) to give rise to further differentiated cells. Our knowledge of bone marrow function implies that such cells must exist. In kinetic terms, any cell with these properties is a stem cell, even if it is already partially differentiated.

To obviate confusion between kinetic and morphologic definitions, the noncommittal term **α cell** has been used in kinetic discussions in place of stem cells. An α cell is any cell that can replace itself *and* give rise to a more differentiated cell. The latter is termed an **n cell**. Discussions of bone marrow kinetics ordinarily deal with the behavior of **compartments** of cells. A compartment is defined as any distinct class of cells, whether the distinction is based on function, morphology, developmental stage, or other properties. The definition of the α cell just given is perhaps more accurately applied to the α cell compartment, for it is the compartment that renews itself and gives rise to further differentiated cells. This is the case because indeterminacy surrounds the behavior of individual α cells, which may behave *asymmetrically* ($\alpha \rightarrow \alpha$, n) or *symmetrically* ($\alpha \rightarrow 2\alpha$ or $\alpha \rightarrow 2n$). Thus, descriptions of the net behavior of a population of α cells must rest on statistical considerations since experimental difficulties obscure the behavior of any single stem cell.

3. Operational definition: CFU

This definition regards the stem cell as a **colony-forming unit** (CFU) in the various laboratory systems that make it possible to *assay* stem cells. In the first of these, devised by Till and McCulloch, suspensions of marrow cells are injected intravenously into heavily irradiated mice in which the spleen and marrow are reduced to stroma and are hematologically empty. In 8–10 days, discrete macroscopic colonies are observed in the animal's *spleen*, which has become a "home" for the wandering injected stem cells. Hence, the stem cell progenitors of these colonies were termed **CFU-S** (S for spleen).

a. CFU-S (CFU-GEMM)

Single stem cells (CFU-Ss) lodge in the spleen stroma and there, under the peculiarly specific influence of the **hematopoietic inductive microenviroment** (HIM), proliferate and differentiate into large colonies. At first, stem cells proliferate actively and produce minute clonal colonies of undifferentiated stem cells. After 5 days, specific differentiation takes place, and discrete colonies are seen macroscopically on the surface of the spleen and within its parenchyma.

Chromosome studies indicate that each colony is derived from a single stem cell, Colony enumeration permits a valid quantitative assay of the number of injected CFU-Ss. In this method, stem cells are detected indirectly by observing the results of their proliferation and differentiation; hence CFU is a noncommittal or operational term applicable to colony-forming units from injected suspensions of marrow, spleen, or diverse materials.

Table 1.1
Evidence Indicating Existence of Hematopoietic Inductive Environment

1. Transfused stem cells "home" to marrow and spleen of irradiated mice.
2. Occasional failure of "take" after marrow transplantation between identical twins. This suggests defect in receptiveness of stroma.
3. Delay of aplasia (termination of hematopoiesis) after heavy local irradiation and delay of resumption of hematopoiesis after ectopic implantation of hematopoietic tissue. This suggests that HIM must be destroyed or regenerated before permanent aplasia or resumption of hematopoiesis can occur—and that sustained stem cell proliferation requires intact stroma.
4. Studies in two genetically anemic strains of mice. $S1/S1^d$ and W/W^v, show dichotomy between stroma and stem cells. In $S1/S1^d$ mice, stroma cannot make stem cell factor (SCF) needed for stem cell proliferation. In W/W^v mice, stem cells are defective and incapable of proliferating in normal stroma.
5. Regional difference in ratio of erythroid and myeloid colonies in the spleens of irradiated mice infused with allogeneic stem cells. Presumably stroma has compartments, each supporting differentiation of stem cells in one or the other cell lines.
6. Marrow-derived "fibroblasts" supposedly arising from stromal cells lack markers of hematopoietic stem cells. Fibroblasts and adipose cells or fat-filled macrophages may be instrumental in sustaining hematopoiesis in vitro.
7. Ultrastructural evidence of close association between developing hematopoietic cells and stromal cells. The latter appear different for different cell lines.

Table 1.2
Some Hematopoietic Progenitor Cells

Term	Required stimulus	Detected by	Postulated role
CFU-LM	Multiple growth factors	Spleen colony assay	Pluripotent stem cell
CFU-GEMM (CFU-S)	GM-CSF, G-CSF, M-CSF, IL-3	Spleen colony assay	Pluripotent stem cell
CFU-GM (CFU-C)	GM-CSF, G-CSF, M-CSF, IL-3	Colony formation in conditioned agar medium	Committed progenitor of granulopoiesis
BFU-E	Erythropoietin, helper T lymphocytes (IL-1, GM-CSF, IL-3, IL4)	Colony formation in plasma clot culture	Committed progenitor of erythropoiesis (early)
CFU-E	Erythropoietin	Colony formation in plasma clot culture	Committed progenitor of erythropoiesis (late)
CFU-Meg	IL-3, GM-CSF, G-GSF, thrombopoietin	Colony formation in plasma clot culture	Committed progenitor of thrombopoiesis

The majority of spleen colonies (60–70%) contain only erythriod cells. Most of these are on the spleen surface. About 15% are megakaryocytic. These grow beneath the capsule. About 20% contain only granulocytic (myeloid) cells. These grow within the spleen. Presumably these differences in colony position reflect effects of the HIM. After 10 days, colonies may include more than one cell line—and more CFUs. This is evidence that the marrow stem cell is pluripotent, giving rise to each of the principal cell lines: granulocytic, erythrocytic, macrophages, and megakaryocytes. (This had led to replacement of the term **CFU-S** with **CFU-GEMM**.) Some believe this cell also gives rise to other marrow elements, including lipocytes, fibrocytes, chrondrocytes, and osteocytes.

The relation of CFU-GEMM to **lymphopoiesis** (production of lymphocytes) was long debated, Since (1) spleen colonies lack lymphocytes, and (2) a stem cell chromosome marker can be found in spleen colony cells *and* in lymphoid cells repopulating lymphoid organs, it appears that CFU-GEMM and lymphoid cells both derive from a common precursor. This more primitive pluripotent stem cell was termed **CFU-LM** (colony-forming unit–lymphoid-myeloid). This concept is illustrated in the model in figure 1.1 (see also figure 24.2).

The HIM, currently under active study, exists in bone marrow as well as spleen. It is defined as an environment that (1) favors extensive expression of restricted cell functions, (2) permits exchange of information or molecules between stem cells and environment, (3) produces a newly discovered multipotent **stem cell factor**, and (4) permits necessary interactions among important cell types. Evidence for the existence of the HIM is summarized in table 1.1. Some major progenitor cells are listed in table 1.2.

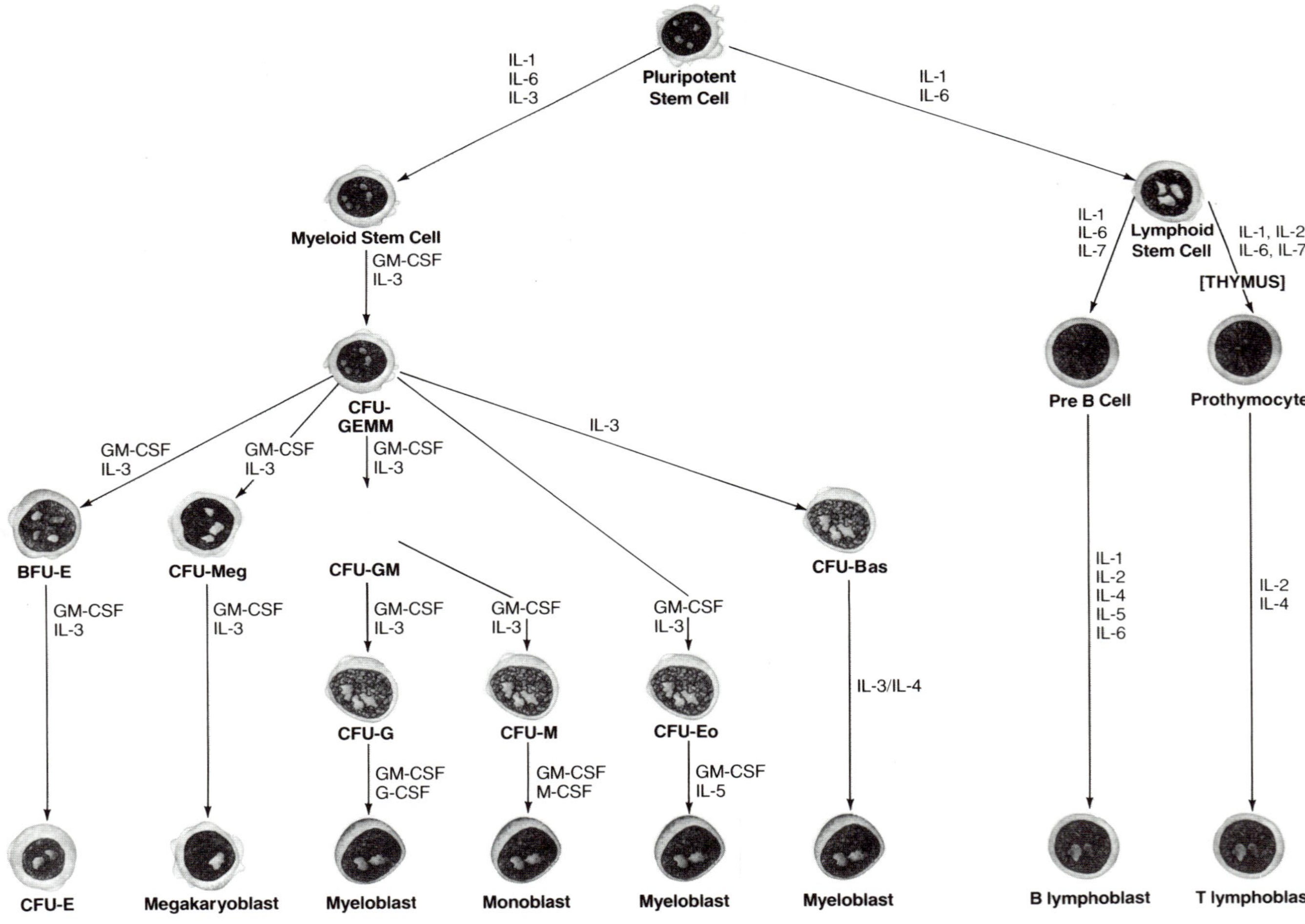
Pluripotent Stem Cell
IL-1 IL-6 IL-3
IL-1 IL-6
Myeloid Stem Cell
GM-CSF IL-3
Lymphoid Stem Cell
IL-1 IL-6 IL-7
IL-1, IL-2 IL-6, IL-7
[THYMUS]
Pre B Cell
Prothymocyte
CFU-GEMM
GM-CSF IL-3
GM-CSF IL-3
GM-CSF IL-3
IL-3
BFU-E
CFU-Meg
CFU-GM
CFU-Bas
GM-CSF IL-3
GM-CSF IL-3
GM-CSF IL-3
GM-CSF IL-3
GM-CSF IL-3
IL-3/IL-4
IL-1 IL-2 IL-4 IL-5 IL-6
IL-2 IL-4
CFU-G
CFU-M
CFU-Eo
GM-CSF G-CSF
GM-CSF M-CSF
GM-CSF IL-5
CFU-E
Megakaryoblast
Myeloblast
Monoblast
Myeloblast
Myeloblast
B lymphoblast
T lymphoblast

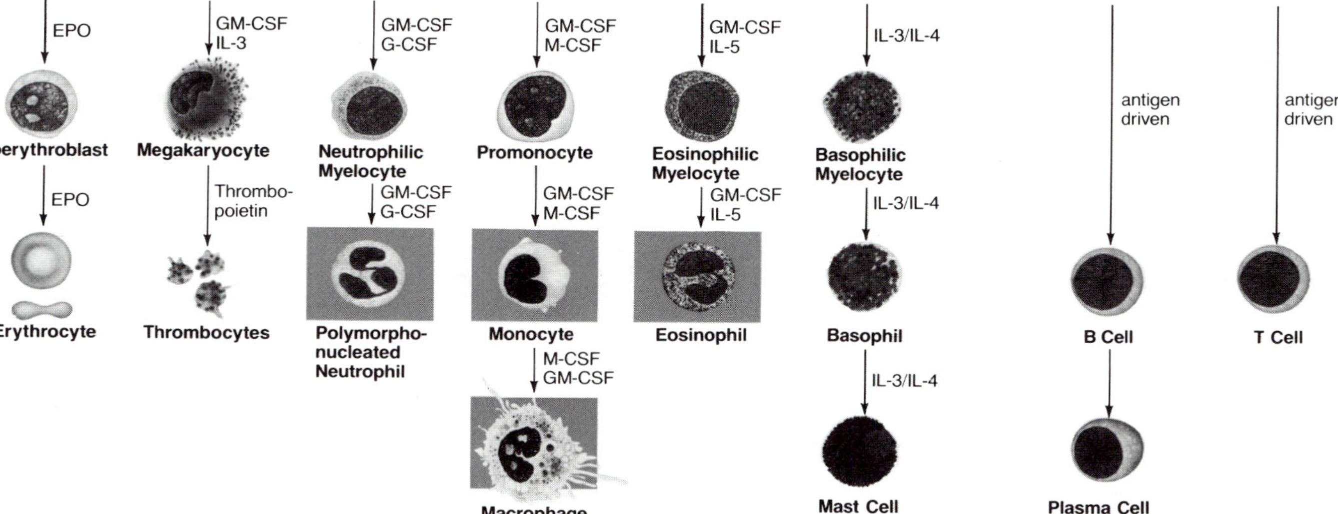

Fig. 1.1
A model of hematopoiesis. The system consists in a series of steps that begins with a pluripotent stem cell, which gives rise to lymphoid as well as myeloid elements and ultimately to all differentiated blood cells. Stem cells with restricted potential (committed stem cells) include erythroid burst-forming units (BFU-E), megakaryocytic colony-forming units (CFU-Meg), eosinophilic colony-forming units (CFU-Eos), granulocyte/macrophage colony-forming units (CFU-GM), and many others. These colony-forming units are to be distinguished from their more mature descendants (myeloblasts, pronormoblasts, etc.), which represent the earliest visible stages of each maturation series. A complex network of hormones, growth factors, or cytokines regulates the system, stimulating hematopoietic cells to undergo differentiation that is coupled with progressive loss of the capacity for self-renewal. Some growth factors induce resting stem cells in the dormant G_0 phase to enter the cell mitotic cycle. Others act to move the cell through the G_1 phase and into the S phase (DNA synthesis). Note that many of these factors affect multiple steps in the system, many steps are affected by multiple factors, and many factors influence cells in both early and late stages of maturation. Further details are given in the text. (Photograph © Sandoz Pharmaceuticals.)

b. CFU-C (CFU-GM)

Tissue culture assay systems for stem cells were soon developed. Such techniques were unreliable until it was found that media must be semisolid and contain **stimulating factors** or **growth factors**. The first colonies obtained in culture consisted of myeloid cells and macrophages and depended on material called **colony-simulating factor** (CSF), or **colony-stimulating activity** (CSA) which is provided by "feeder cells" or by addition of extracts of various cell types (macrophages, monocytes, activated lymphocytes, endothelial cells, certain fetal tissues, etc.). The presence of CSF disposes marrow stem cells to form clones of granulocytes and/or macrophages in 7–10 days. Two important cellular sources of CSF are mononuclear leukocytes and stimulated T cells. When leukocytes are fractionated, the richest subcellular source of CSF is the cell membrane fraction. In recent years, many CSFs (now called **hematopoietic growth factors** or **cytokines**) have been purified to apparent homogeneity and cloned. They are discussed further below.

c. CFU-F AND BFU-E

Culture methodology employing plasma clots (or methylcellulose plates) soon led to the discovery of **CFU-E**, a colony-forming unit committed to erythropoiesis, which forms tiny erythroid colonies of 8–64 cells, and the more primitive **BFU-E** (burst-forming unit–erythroid), also committed to erythropoiesis and precursor of the **CFU-E** (colony-forming unit–erythroid), which forms irregular macroscopic erythroid clusters containing thousands of cells. Both are dependent on the hematopoietic growth factor **erythropoietin**. BFU-Es respond to erythropoietin by differentiating into CFU-Es. The ability of BFU-Es to proliferate and differentiate in culture also depends on helper effects of added T lymphocytes and monocytes, which are mediated by various growth factors (see below).

d. CFU-Meg

The progenitor of megakaryocytes, the **CFU-Meg**, also derives from the CFU-GEMM. Its further differentiation is also influenced by the HIM. A putative hematopoietic hormone **thrombopoietin** is believed to control platelet production.

Figure 1.1 schematically summarizes the role of the major progenitor cells of hematopoiesis.

B. Hematopoietic growth factors: myeloid

The hematopoietic growth factors are glycoprotein hormones that regulate the proliferation and differentiation of hematopoietic progenitor cells and the function of mature blood cells. Indeed, they interact with blood cells at many different levels in the maturation sequence—from pluripotent progenitor stem cells to circulating mature cells. Each growth factor is encoded by a single gene. The cellular sources of all but erythropoietin are monocytes or macrophages, T lymphocytes, fibroblasts, and endothelial cells. Their biologic effects, as measured by the stimulation of cell growth in vitro, was the basis for the isolation of these factors and the genes that encode them. Many have been cloned and made available for clinical use. Discussions of their therapeutic uses appear in later lectures.

Table 1.3 summarizes some of their common features and Table 1.4 lists presently known factors and their widely accepted abbreviations. In the current convention for naming CFUs, letters after the hyphen indicate which cell lines arise from the CFU.

The following remarks deal briefly with the major myeloid hematopoietic growth factors. The term **myeloid** means related to bone marrow; these factors promote the differentiation of the blood arising in bone marrow. Their physiologic roles are discussed in context in later lectures (as noted).

1. Erythropoietin (Epo)

Epo regulates the growth of erythroid cells. It is formed mainly, but not exclusively, in the kidney, probably by a peritubular cell. The first human hematopoietic growth factor to be identified, it was originally purified from the urine of patients with aplastic anemia. Later it was cloned using a complementary DNA (cDNA) based on its amino acid sequence. Its activity is affected by the degree of glycosylation. Hence, recombinant products used clinically are derived from mammalian-cell rather than bacterial systems. (see lecture 2.)

2. GM-CSF

Human GM-CSF affects cells of the **granulocyte**, **macrophage**, and **eosinophil** series. Recombinant human GM-CSF is produced by mammalian

Table 1.3
Common General Features of the Hematopoietic Growth Factors

1. All are glycoproteins.
2. Regulators of blood cell development and maturation and enhancers of mature cell functions, which are active at very low concentrations.
3. Active both in vitro and in vivo.
4. Produced by cells of many types.
5. Usually have both unique and overlapping specificities (i.e., affect one primary target cell as well as multiple cell lineages).
6. Active on both stem (progenitor) cells and end cells (see table 1.4).
7. Biologic affects are mediated after binding to a small number of specific high-affinity receptors on the surfaces of target cells.
8. Also bind to receptors on some nonhematopoietic cells. The significance of this is unknown.
9. Display synergy or additive effects with other growth factors.
10. Also act on neoplastic counterparts of normal cell types.

Table 1.4
Myeloid Hematopoietic Growth Factors

Factor	CFU and Colony Formation Stimulated in vitro	Mature Cell Targets in vitro	Major Biological Activities in vivo
Erythropoietin (Epo)	BFU-E (with other factors) CFU-E	None	Stimulates erythropoiesis Mediates its feedback control
GM-CSF	Granulocyte colonies Macrophage colonies Megakaryocyte, BFU-E (with Epo) Blast cells	Mature neutrophils Mature eosinophils	Stimulates granulopiesis Stimulates macrophage production
G-CSF	Granulocyte colonies Megakaryocyte, blast cells (with IL-3) Granulocyte-macrophage colonies (with GM-CSF)	Mature neutrophils	Stimulates granulopoiesis Stimulates proliferation of some leukemic cells (not all)
M-CSF	Macrophage colonies	Mature macrophages	
IL-3 (Multi-CSF)	Granulocyte, macrophage, eosinophil, mast cell colonies BFU-E (with Epo) Induces (CFU-GEMM and leukemic blasts into cell cycle		Stimulates granulocyte, monocyte, eosinophil, and mast cell production

Abbreviations used in this table and elsewhere in lecture 1:
BFU-E, burst-forming unit–erythroid
BFU-Meg, burst-forming unit–megakaryocyte
CFU-Baso, colony-forming unit–basophil
CFU-Blast, colony-forming unit–blast
CFU-E, colony-forming unit–erythroid
CFU-G, colony forming unit–granulocyte
CFU-GEMM, colony-forming unit–granulocyte, erythroid, macrophage, megakaryocyte
CFU-GM, colony-forming unit–granulocyte, macrophage
CFU-LM, colony-forming unit–lymphoid, myeloid (multipotent stem cell)
CFU-Meg, colony-forming unit–megakaryocyte
Epo, erythropoietin
G-CSF, granulocyte colony-stimulating factor
GM-CSF, granulocyte-macrophage colony-stimulating factor
IL-3, interleukin-3
M-CSF, macrophage colony-stimulating factor
Multi-CSF, multipotent colony-stimulating factor

cells, yeast, and bacteria, each system yielding a protein with a different glycosylation pattern. The importance of the sugar residues in biological activity, immunoreactivity, and toxicity remains unclear.

3. G-CSF

Human G-CSF has been cloned and expressed in bacterial and mammalian cells. The nonglycosylated, bacterially synthesized recombinant molecule is the main product used in clinical trials. Unlike most of the other hematopoietic growth factors, G-CSF is selective in its action, inducing formation of only **granulocytes**.

4. M-CSF

M-CSF was purified from urine and a pancreatic carcinoma cell line. Like G-CSF, it has limited specificity, influencing only **macrophage** production.

5. Multi-CSF

Multi-CSF, also called interleukin-3, potentiates the growth of multiple cell lineages, including megakaryocytic, erythroid, and myeloid precursor, as well as multipotent progenitor cells. An unusual strategy involving direct functional analysis of the products of a cDNA library led to its identification.

C. Hematopoietic growth factors: lymphoid

To obviate growing nomenclatural confusion, investigators decided at a 1979 meeting in Ermatingen, Switzerland to give factors the generic name **interleukin** (IL) with a defining number, a name intended to reflect their role as communication links between leukocytes.

IL-3 (multi-CSF) was discussed above. Most of the other interleukins are concerned with the differentiation of B and T lymphocytes (see lecture 3). However, investigators are rapidly assigning them new roles. Note that they also affect myeloid cells. This accounts for the intimate connections between B and T lymphopoiesis, their growth factors, and myeloid hematopoiesis. There is no apparent homology between the myeloid growth factors and all but one the lymphoid-active factors (IL-6). Some of the roles of these factors are summarized in figure 1.1. Highlights are as follows:

- **IL-1** has many diverse effects on the activation, proliferation, and differentiation of B and T lymphocytes, but many other cells (macrophages, connective tissue, and endothelial cells) have IL-1 receptors and respond to IL-1, which thus is a major inducer of many of the myeloid growth factors. For example, it stimulates myeloid leukemia cells by stimulating GM-CSF release.
- **IL-2** (or T cell growth factor) is produced by T cells and is of immunologic importance (see lectures 3 and 24). It acts on T cells, B cells, and

monocytes. It also induces blast formation in some cases of leukemia.

- **IL-4** is produced by T cells, natural killer cells, and mast cells. It is a growth factor for both B and T cells; it supports proliferation of CFU-GM (in the presence of G-CSF) and of CFU-E (in the presence of Epo); and it has eosinophil and basophil growth-promoting activities. Many hematopoietic and nonhematopoietic cells have IL-4 receptors.
- **IL-5** is produced only by T cells. It regulates production of eosinophils in culture and activates mature eosinophils (see lecture 19).
- **IL-6** synergizes with M-CSF in promoting macrophage formation and with GM-CSF in promoting granulocyte production; interacts with other growth factors in promoting megakaryocytopoiesis in vitro and thrombopoiesis in vivo (in mice); and stimulates mature B cells to produce IgG. It affects many target cells and has some homology with G-CSF.
- **IL-7** is a constitutive product of a stromal cell line derived from bone marrow. It supports long-term survival of B and T cells in vitro. It has no effect on mature B cells.
- **IL-8** is a recently described neutrophil-activating peptide.

D. Functional states

Studies of stem cells by "suicide" techniques (in which only actively dividing cells take up enough [^{3}H]thymidine to cause radiation-induced cell death) revealed that many multipotent stem cells are spared. These were said to be in the **G_0 phase** of the cell cycle (see below).

Such data indicted that progenitor cells exist in two functional states: quiescent and actively proliferating. The former, a large majority of the cells, can exchange reversibly with the latter. Hence, quiescent nondividing cells compromise a dormant bone marrow reserve. A major factor activating dormant CFU-GEMM, for example, is depopulation of the bone marrow.

E. Summary of current model

Three aspects of the current model of hematopoiesis merit emphasis: (1) progenitor cells (the various CFUs) range from pluripotent to unipotent; (2) hematopoietic cell development is regulated by multiple growth factors of overlapping specificities that are progressively restricted in their biological activities and target cells (figure 1.2); and (3) there is a hierarchical series of hematopoietic cell populations (figure 1.3) as follows:

- **Stage 1.** Under the influence of the HIM, pluripotent stem cells are irreversibly transformed to unipotent committed or determined progenitors of erythropoiesis of granulopoiesis (or other cell lines).
- **Stage 2.** A pool of committed progenitor cells undergoes further differentiation and commitment. Like the pluripotent stem cells of stage 1,

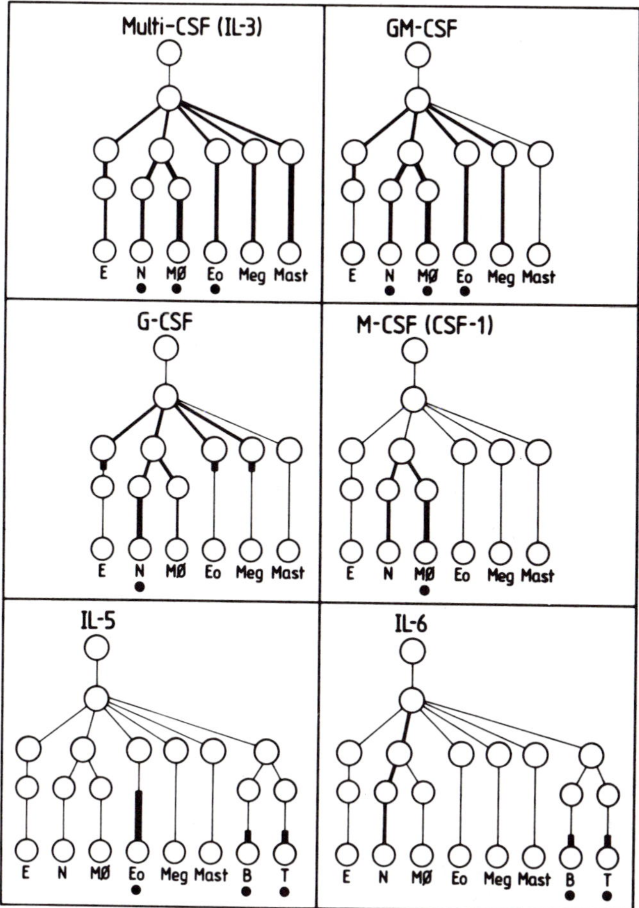

Fig. 1.2
Biologic specificities of the hematopoietic growth factors. The hematopoietic tree in each panel represents the self-renewing pluripotent stem cell at the top with successive restriction to individual cell lineages going down the diagram. Heavy lines indicate a proliferative effect of the factor even at low concentrations, medium lines a proliferative effect at high concentrations only, and light lines indicate no effect. (E, erythroid; N, neutrophil; MØ, monocyte/macrophage; Eo, eosinophil; Meg, megakaryocyte; Mast, mast cells. Dots under the abbreviation indicate the ability of the factor to stimulate functional activities of the mature cells.) (From N. A. Nicola: Hemopoietic cell growth factors and their receptors. *Annu. Rev. Biochem.* 59[1989]:45.)

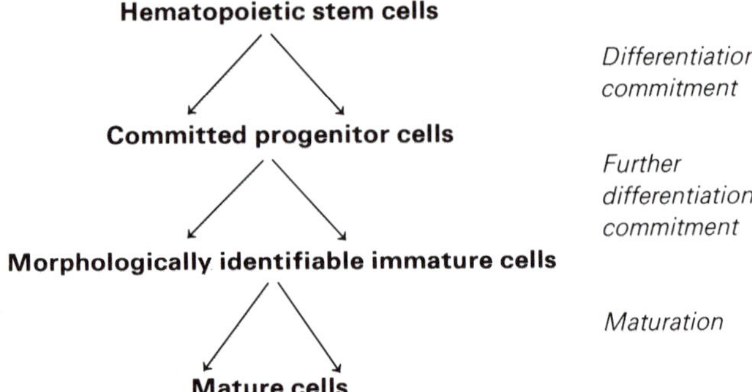

Fig. 1.3
The hierarchy of hematopoietic populations. Hematopoiesis proceeds by the clonal proliferation of three successively larger classes of cells. This pattern is common to all the eight blood cell lineages. Maturation proceeds in parallel with the final clonal proliferation; the most mature cells, which enter the blood, are postmitotic and incapable of further division in some but not all lineages. (Reprinted with permission from Metcalf, D. The molecular control of cell division, differentiation commitment and maturation in haemopoietic cells. *Nature* 339[1989]: 27–30.)

unipotent committed cells are partitioned between resting and proliferating compartments; however, many more of them are actively proliferating. Their further differentiation is induced by growth factors.

- **Stage 3.** There arises a series of morphologically identifiable immature precursor cells. These are the well-known stages of the the maturation series which populate marrow.
- **Stage 4.** Mature postmitotic cells enter the blood where their functions are influenced by the same growth factors.

These arrangements with their diverse controls have obvious survivial value. Pluripotent stem cells essential for continuing hematopoietic function respond mainly to local factors that influence their numbers and are elegantly protected from external influences that might lead to their depletion. Committed progenitor cells, on the other hand, are capable (as they must be) of responding to external humoral influences, which convey essential regulatory information. For example, anoxia stimulates Epo production, which increases erythropoiesis (see lecture 2). Infection increases GM-CSF levels, which stimulate granulopoiesis (see lecture 20).

III. CYTOKINETICS

Cytokinetics is the study of the kinetics of proliferating cell populations. It is concerned with the behavior of cell compartments, each of which can be charecterized in terms of its kinetic parameters: size (the numbers or mass of cells), transit time, and flux.

A. Modes of proliferative behavior

1. Constantly proliferating

Some cells (e.g., germinative cells of epidermis, cryptepithelial cells of intestinal mucosa, and stem cells of bone marrow) are constantly proliferating. Metabolic activities in these cells are devoted primarily to replication. Derangements of these cells or their regulators can lead to serious illnesses.

Constantly proliferating cells serve to replace the mature cells of a *maturation series* that are continuously being lost to attrition.

2. Nonproliferating

Nonproliferating cells, that is, cells that cannot divide, are typified by neurons and muscle cells. In humans most tissues consist largely of differentiated cells in this category. Metabolic activities in such cells are devoted primarily to specialized functions. Mature blood cells are nonproliferating.

3. Proliferating on demand

Some cells proliferate only when called upon to do so, e.g., in wound healing, the regeneration occurring after partial extirpation of an organ, or repletion of nutritional deficiency. Many cells (e.g., parenchymal cells of liver, kidney, exocrine glands, and other organs) have a proliferative potential that may seem surprising in view of their specialized functions.

B. Patterns of proliferation

The cytokinetics of bone marrow cells may be divided into **erythrokinetics**, **granulokinetics**, and **thrombokinetics**. Bone marrow cells, like other proliferating cells, may have two patterns of behavior.

1. Steady-state pattern

In the steady state, proliferation is at a constant rate. Bone marrow cells in the steady state proliferate at a rate equaling the rate at which cells in the peripheral blood are removed. The proliferation population thereby keeps the population of mature blood cells constant. The existence of such steady-state kinetics implies the existence of a feedback control loop. Elements of the loop will be described later.

2. Non-steady-state pattern

Under physiologic or pathologic conditions to be described, proliferative behavior may be altered so that cell production rates rise or fall. It is not possible to predict the consequences of a change in the number of cells in a proliferating cell compartment unless the new proliferation rate is specified. Thus, a compartment of proliferating bone marrow cells containing twice the normal number will provide new cells at the normal rate if the enlarged cell population proliferates at half the normal rate.

C. Biologic mechanisms

1. Definitions

The term **proliferation** is often used loosely in discussions of bone marrow function. It should refer to cell division alone; however, it sometimes implies cell division plus differentiation and maturation. It signifies a change in numbers and thus is not a property of the steady state.

- **Differentiation** is the process whereby a dividing cell gives rise to progency that differ from it qualitatively. A differentiating cell has a higher **potentiality** level than the differentiated cell. Some genes of pluripotent parent cells are repressed in the course of differentiation. Thus differentiation, which occurs only in dividing cells, represents a change in gene expression that is attributable to reprogramming of the genome.
- **Maturation** refers to the specialization that is associated with **accumulation of gene products** (e.g., hemoglobin in erythroid cells, immunoglobulins in plasma cells) and **refinement of structure** (e.g., loss of erythrocyte nucleus, segmentation of granulocyte nucleus). In a sense, it is a quantitative change. It is initiated by differentiation but does not require cell division; in fact, it is accompanied by loss of the ability to divide.

2. Cell division cycle

Studies of synchronized cells in culture have shown that the life cycle of a cell has four phases, as shown in figure 1.4: phase **M**, the period of mitosis (about 0.5–1 hr); phase $\mathbf{G_1}$, the postmitotic or presynthetic gap (about 10 hr); phase **S**, the period of DNA synthesis and chromosome replication (about 9 hr); and phase $\mathbf{G_2}$, the postsynthetic or premitotic gap (about 4 hr). The total **generation time**, or **time of cycle** (T_c), of a typical proliferating bone marrow cells is about 24 hr (though T_c varies with stage of maturation). As noted, a resting or nonproliferating cell is in phase $\mathbf{G_0}$. Knowledge of the cell cycle provides useful insights into the interpreation of cytokinetic techniques and the planning of chemotherapy for leukemia and other proliferative disorders (see lecture 22).

D. Techniques for studying marrow

As in other areas of hematology, available techniques may be roughly divided into simple methods that can be employed in a clinical setting and elaborate methods that require the research laboratory or some other special facility. Almost every patient with a hematologic disease raises problems of cytokinetics. Is bone marrow function active, hypoactive, or hyperactive? Is marrow activity effective in the sense that it leads to delivery of cells into the blood? The following are methods for judging the level of bone marrow activity. Techniques for assessing specific aspects of marrow function (e.g., erythrokinetics, granulokinetics, thrombokinetics) will be

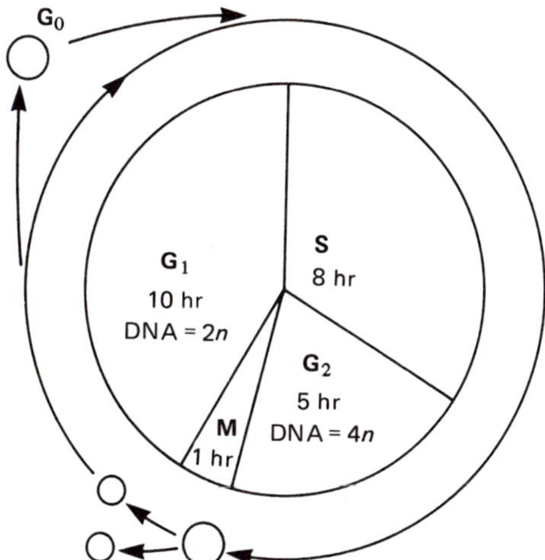

Fig. 1.4
Diagrammatic representation of the eukaryotic cell cycle. Details are given in the text.

discussed later. Table 1.5 summarizes the kinds of information obtainable from examination of the bone marrow.

1. Examination of bone marrow

a. BY ASPIRATION

Bone marrow is most commonly removed by aspiration from the posterior iliac spine, sternum, or vertebral spine (figure 1.5). Aspiration disturbs marrow architecture. Hence, this technique is employed primarily to determine types of cells present and their relative numbers. Smears are ordinarily stained with Wright's stain or Wright plus Giemsa's stain. Excess aspirated marrow in the clotted specimen may then be sectioned, stained with H&E (hematoxylin and eosin), and examined for tumor cells or otherwise studied. Stained smears of bone marrow aspirates are subjected to the following studies:

- Determination of the E/M ratio, that is, the ratio of the erythroid cell total to the myeloid cell total (normal ratio is 1:3)
- Differential count
- Search for abnormal cells
- Evaluation of iron stores in reticulum cells (see lecture 7)
- Special stains and immunochemical studies

b. BY BIOPSY

Alternatively, marrow may be sampled in a coherent piece with a biopsy needle. When decalcified, sectioned, and stained with H&E, this specimen

Table 1.5
Kinds of Information Obtainable from Examination of Bone Marrow

Procedure	Property	Examples of abnormal states
Bone marrow aspiration	Degree of cellularity	Decreased in hypoplastic or aplastic anemia Increased in reactive states (leukocytosis, erythrocytosis) and proliferative disorders (leukemia, myeloma, etc.)
	Relative preponderance of erythroid and myeloid precursors (E/M ratio)	Increased when erythropoiesis increased (polycythemia) or when myelopoiesis decreased (hypoplastic neutropenia) Decreased when erythropoiesis decreased (hypoplastic anemia, pure red cell aplasia) or when myelopoiesis increased (leukemia, leukocytosis)
	Presence of megakaryocytes	Present in normal marrow and in immune-mediated thrombocyopenia (ITP)
	Morphology of erythrocyte precursors	Abnormal in megaloblastic and hypochromic anemias
	Morphology of granulocyte precursors	Abnormal in leukemia, myeloid metaplasia
	Presence of foreign cells:	
	Nests of cancer cells	Metastatic cancer
	Granulomas	Tuberculosis, sarcoidosis etc.
	Lymphocytes and lymphoblasts	Lymphoma and lymphocytic leukemia
	Plasma cells	Multiple myeloma and severe infection
	Storage cells	Gaucher's disease and other lipidoses
	Evaluation of iron stores	Decreased in iron deficiency Increased in iron-loading disorders and defective iron reutilization
	Other procedures:	
	Bacteriologic culture	Positive in tuberculosis, brucellosis, other infections
	Chromosome studies	Abnormal in chronic myelocytic leukemia, etc.
	Special stains	Useful in usual proliferative and metabolic disorders
Bone marrow biopsy	Detects all of the above, although morphology of individual cells not as clearly delineated as in aspirate. However, *architecture is preserved.*	
	Therefore, biopsy more accurately detects:	
	Marrow/fat ratio	Increased in marrow hyperplasia Decreased in aplastic anemia
	Fibrosis	Present in myelofibrosis
	Vasculitis	Present in lupus erythematosus, acute vasculitis, etc.
	Plasma cells	See above
	Granulomas and cancer cells	See above

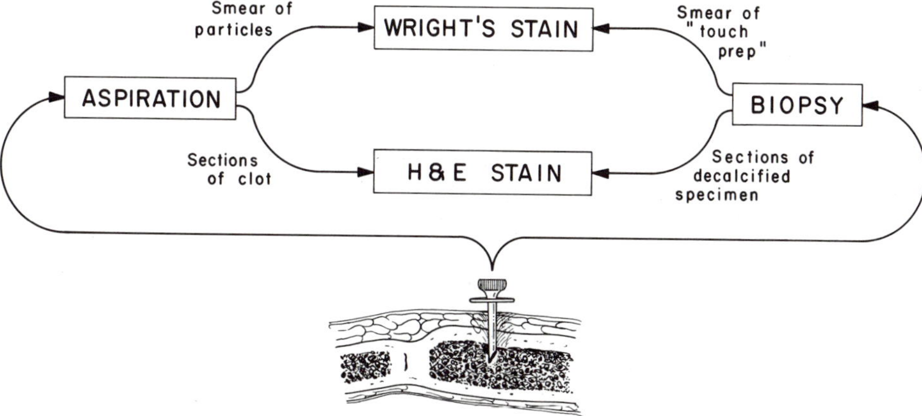

Fig. 1.5
Summary of two main methods for examination of bone marrow. The sketch shows a sternal marrow examination. Most studies today are done in the posterior iliac crest. See Appendix.

reveals the undisturbed marrow architecture. Since marrow cells stained with H&E are often difficult to identify, it is customary to smear a biopsy specimen on a cover slip before placing it in formalin. The Wright's stained "touch prep" or "imprint" is useful in facilitating cell identification.

2. *Activity of marrow*

a. CELLULARITY

A marrow aspirate that is richly cellular implies normal or increased marrow activity. However, the degree of cellularity does not indicate whether marrow activity is effective.

b. AVERAGE MATURITY

Marrow is studied for a shift in average maturity of a cell line using morphologic criteria. By inference, a "shift to left" signifies a rising ratio of dividing to nondividing cells.

c. MITOTIC INDEX

The **mitotic index** (MI) is the percentage of cells in mitosis relative to the total number of cells in a closed compartment. It is affected by duration of mitosis and duration of resting stage (G_0). An elevated MI usually implies increased proliferation, though when mitosis is prolonged, as in megaloblastic anemia, its significance needs careful interpretation. When bone marrow is examined in a clinical setting, the MI is usually only roughly approximated. Normally, it is 1–2%.

d. RATE OF DNA SYNTHESIS

This determination requires techniques for assaying the incorporation of [^{3}H]dThd into cellular DNA. This method is based on assumptions that the ^{3}H of [^{3}H]dThd is nonexchangeable after DNA is labeled, DNA turnover is due solely to cell division and cell death, and [^{3}H]dThd is not diluted unpredictably by varying pools of endogenous unlabeled dThd. Application of the technique is difficult in vivo. However, if a cell culture is exposed to a brief pulse of [^{3}H]dThd and the percentage of labeled mitotic figures followed, it is found that none is labeled initially since only cells in the S phase incorporate [^{3}H]dThd. As these cells move into mitosis, the percentage increases sharply. A second wave of mitosis in 20–24 hr permits assessment of T_c. The duration of S (**T_s**) divided by generation time (time of cycle, **T_c**) equals the **labeling index**, which is the percentage of cells labeled if all the cells are proliferating. The extent to which the labeling index falls short of expectation (**T_s/T_c**) is a measure of nonproliferating cells in G_0.

SELECTED REFERENCES

Reviews

Cannistra, S. A., and Griffin, J. D. Regulation of the production and function of granulocytes and monocytes. *Semin. Hematol.* 25(1988): 173–188.

Cronkite, E. P. Analytical review of structure and regulation of hemopoiesis. *Blood Cells* 14(1988): 313–328.

Dexter, T. M. Haemopoietic growth factors. *Br. Med. Bull.* 45(1989): 337–349.

Dorshkind, K. Regulation of hemopoiesis by bone marrow stromal cells and their products. *Annu. Rev. Immunol.* 8(1990): 111–137.

Feldmann, M., Londei, M., and Haworth, C. T cells and lymphokines. *Br. Med. Bull.* 45(1989): 361–370.

Johnson, G. R. Erythropoietin. *Br Med. Bull.* 45(1989): 506–514.

Kelos, A., and Metcalf, D. T lymphocyte-derived colony-stimulating factors. *Adv. Immunol.* 48(1990): 69–106.

Metcalf, D. Haemopoietic growth factors 1. *Lancet* 1(1989): 825–827.

Metcalf, D. Haemopoietic growth factors 2: clinical applications. *Lancet* 1(1989): 885–887.

Metcalf, D. The molecular control of cell division, differentiation commitment and maturation in haemopoietic cells. *Nature* 339(1989): 27–30.

Metcalf, D. Some of what you need to know about the molecular control of blood cell formation. *Cell* 61(1990): 756–758.

Metcalf, D. The colony stimulating factors: discovery, development, and clinical applications. *Cancer* 65(1990): 2185–2195.

Mizel, S. B. The interleukins. *FASEB J.* 3(1989): 2379–2388.

Nicola, N. A. Hemopoietic cell growth factors and their receptors. *Annu. Rev. Biochem.* 58(1989): 45–77.

Owen, J. J. T., and Jenkinson, F. J. Regulatory factors in lymphoid development. *Br. Med. Bull.* 45(1989): 350–360.

Quesenberry, P. J. Hemopoietic stem cells, progenitor cells, and growth factors. Im Williams, W. J., et al., eds. *Hematology*, 4th ed. New York: McGraw-Hill, 1990, pp. 129–147.

Sherr, C. J. Colony-stimulating factor-1 receptor. *Blood* 75(1990): 1–12.

Sieff, C. A. Biology and clinical aspects of the hematopoietic growth factors. *Annu. Rev. Med.* 41(1990): 483–496.

Waterfield, M. D. (ed.) Growth factors (Special issue). *Br. Med. Bull.* 45(1989): 317–604.

Witte, O. N. Steel locus defines multipotent new growth factor. *Cell* 63(1990): 5–6.

Original articles

Andreesen, R., Brugger, W., et al. Surface phenotype analysis of human monocyte to macrophage maturation. *J. Leukocyte Biol.*

Choudhury, C. Role of the microenvironment on hematopoiesis. I. Stem cell differentiation into granulocytic and megakaryocytic cell lineage. *J. Lab. Clin. Med.* 114(1989): 378–381.

Choudhury, C., and Sparks, R. Role of the microenvironment on hematopoiesis. II. Regulation of cell kinetics in vitro during granulopoiesis and megakaryocytopoiesis. *J. Lab. Clin. Med.* 114(1989): 382–388.

Flanagan, J. G., and Leder, P. The kit ligand: a cell surface molecule altered in steel mutant fibroblasts. *Cell* 63(1990): 185–194.

Graham, G. J., Wright, E. G., et al. Identification and characterization of an inhibitor of haemopoietic stem cell proliferation. *Nature* 334(1990): 442–444.

Jordan, C. T., McKearn, J. P., and Lemischka, I. R. Cellular and developmental properties of fetal hematopoietic stem cells. *Cell* 61(1990): 953–963.

Martin, D. I. K., Zon, L. I., ed al. Expression of an erythroid transcription factor in megakaryocytic and mast cell lineages. *Nature* 344(1990): 444–447.

Romeo, P.-H., Prandini, M.-H., et al. Megakaryocytic and erythrocytic lineages share specific transcription factors. *Nature* 344(1990): 447–449.

LECTURE 2

Erythropoiesis and Introduction to the Anemias

William S. Beck

EDITOR'S COMMENT

Progress in the study of erythropoiesis consisted mainly in the advances in the study of erythropoietic colony-forming units and the dissection of their sequence, regulation, and interactions with various other cells. Perhaps the most dramatic development was the revelation of the complexity of humoral controls and the long delayed purification, cloning, and commercial production of an erythropoietin identical to the human hormone. As discussed here and in later lectures, erythropoietin has now entered the therapeutic armamentarium for the treatment of certain anemias.

I. OVERVIEW

Erythropoiesis is the segment of hematopoiesis concerned with the production of **erythrocytes**, and **red cells** (terms used interchangeably). In essence, it is a system for the production and packaging of hemoglobin moleucles.

The sequence of maturation stages begins with the **pronormoblast** (also termed **proerythroblast**), which derives from a pool of more primitive stem cells and is the first cell committed to erythropoiesis (see figure 1.1). Hence, it is unipotent. Nonetheless, it satisfies the kinetic definition of a stem cell, since it is capable of self-renewal and further differentiation.

II. PHYSIOLOGY OF ERYTHROPOIESIS

A. The erythron

1. Definition

The term **erythron** refers to the combined population of erythrocytes, their precursors, and progenitors, whether in blood or bone marrow. By suggesting that these components constitute an organ, the term erythron emphasizes that erythrocytes and their precursors, however dispersed, have a functional unity.

2. Quantitative aspects

The erythron has three cell compartments: (1) a pool of early progenitor cells, which can form erythroid colonies in vitro; (2) a pool of maturing erythroid precursors in bone marrow; and (3) the mature erythrocytes of blood.

Table 2.1
Components of the Erythron in a Normal Human Adult

Cell type	Cell number/kg ($\times 10^9$)	Relative number	Estimated volume of each cell (μm^3)	Total volume of cell compartment (ml)		Approximate transit time (days)
Marrow						
Nucleated cells	5.0	1.7	250	88	6% in marrow	5.0
Reticulocytes	8.2	2.7	120	44		2.8
Blood						
Reticulocytes	3.1	1.0	100	23	94% in blood	1.0
Erythrocytes	307	100	90	2,000		120

Adapted from C. A. Finch, *Blood* 50(1977): 699.

Data on the numbers of cells in fixed and circulating components of the erythron are summarized in table 2.1. Of the **pool of nucleated erythroid precursors** in marrow, about 2% are pronormoblasts, about 18% are basophilic normoblasts, 54% are polychromatophilic normoblasts, and 26% are orthochromatic normoblasts. Of the **total pool of hematopoietic precursors** in marrow, about 0.2% are pronormoblasts, 2% are basophilic normoblasts, 6% are polychromatophilic normoblasts, and 3% are orthochromatic normoblasts (see table A.3). Note in table 2.1 that the circulating adult erythocyte compartment is by far the largest. The pool of reticulocytes in bone marrow is slightly larger than the pool of reticulocytes in blood.

B. Erythrocyte maturation

The stem cell pool of the marrow continually generates a supply of cells committed to erythropoiesis, which yield, in turn, a series of nucleated erythroid precursors. These undergo four divisions in about 4 days, during which nuclear and cytoplasmic maturation take place (figure 2.1). Thus they are called **maturational divisions**. Each division yields a smaller cell. Size reduction—from about 25 μm to about 9 μm—is due largely to reduction in absolute nuclear size.

1. Cytoplasmic maturation

The **pronormoblast** is a large cell, rich in polyribosomes and actively engaged in the synthesis of protein (mainly hemoglobin). A Golgi apparatus and mitochondria are present. Wright's stain reveals marked cytoplasmic basophilia and one or more nucleoli. With maturation, the hemoglobin content of the cytoplasm increases and the content of ribosomes (and RNA) decreases in linear fashion. The staining reaction changes from the blue of the **basophilic normoblast** to the lavender of the **polychromatophilic normoblast** to the orange-pink of the **orthochromatic normoblast**. Electron micrographs of these cells reveal bundles of **microtubules**, clumps and

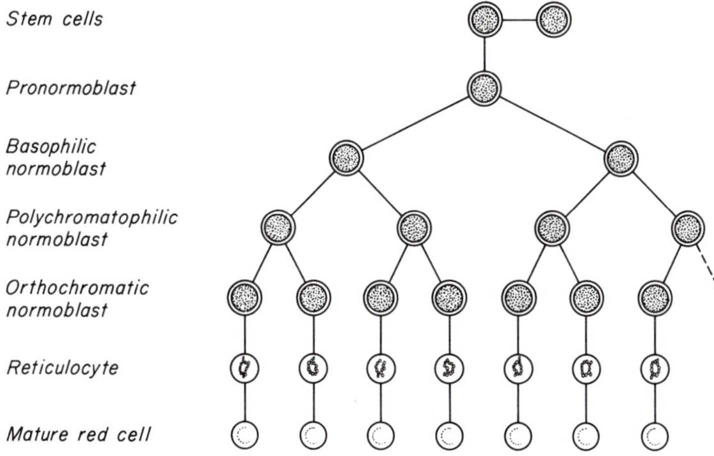

Fig. 2.1
Scheme of erythropoiesis. Number of divisions may be larger or smaller. Dotted line indicates intramedullary cell death (i.e., ineffective erythropoiesis).

individually dispersed **ferritin** molecules (see lecture 7), and occasional membrane-bound aggregates of ferritin celled **siderosomes**. Cells containing ferritin aggregates are called **normal sideroblasts**.

2. *Nuclear maturation*

In the early stages, nuclear chromatin is loosely arranged in fine aggregates. As maturation progresses, nuclear chromatin becomes clumped, condensed, and more basophilic by a process called **pyknosis**, and the nucleolus disappears. Following the fourth maturational division, pyknosis accelerates and nuclear chromatin becomes maximally compressed. The nucleus is then ejected from the cell by poorly understood mechanisms. The expelled nucleus is ingested by a macrophage.

3. *The reticulocyte*

The **reticulocyte** is the cell that remains after ejection of the nucleus from the orthochromatic normoblast. Although anucleate, it contains polyribosomes and later monoribosomes (hence, it actively synthesizes globin), mitochondria (hence, it synthesizes heme and utilizes oxygen), and Golgi remnants. In a Wright's stained smear, the reticulocyte is slightly larger than a mature erythrocyte and is identifiable by a diffuse basophilia (bluish color) that is termed **polychromatophilia**. The reticulocyte is so named because exposure to a supravital stain (brilliant cresyl blue or new methylene blue) causes cytoplasmic organelles to clump into an easily recognized artefactual aggregate of blue-staining reticulum. Although reticulocytes can be recognized by their polychromatophilia (especially when their numbers are increased) in a routine blood smear, supravital staining is necessary if reticulocytes are to be counted accurately.

Maturation of a reticulocyte to an adult erythrocyte takes 24–48 hr. In the course of maturation, mitochondria, ribosomes, and other organelles disappear—and the cell thereby loses the capacity for hemoglobin synthesis and oxidative metabolism. Ribosomal RNA is degraded ultimately to extracellular ribonucleosides.

Most maturing erythrocytes enter the blood as reticulocytes. Release of the reticuloctyes from the marrow involves a poorly understood process of physical extrusion through gaps in the walls of marrow sinusoids.

The reticulocyte level of blood is the most commonly used clinical index of erythropoietic activity (see below). About 1% of the circulating erythrocyte mass is generated by normal marrow each day. Hence, the normal **reticulocyte count** is 1%—that is, 1% of circulating red cells are reticulocytes. Note the difference between the reticulocyte count, expressed as a percentage of the erythrocyte count (the usual mode), the absolute reticulocyte count per cubic millimeter, and the **reticulocyte index**, which corrects the reticulocyte percentage for abnormalities in the hematocrit (assuming that the normal hematocrit is 45%).

4. *The erythrocyte*

The mature erythrocyte is a biconcave disk with a diameter of 7.5–8.5 μm, a normal volume of about 90 μm^3, and a hemoglobin concentration of about 33%. Further descriptions appear in later lectures. Abnormal red cells are described in the appendix.

5. *Ineffective erythropoiesis*

As indicated in figure 2.1, cell death may occur within the marrow during the maturation sequence. Normally about 10% of the maturing cells die in this way, though some say the number is smaller. To the extent that erythropoiesis fails to deliver cells to the blood, it is termed **ineffective**. In certain diseases (e.g., megaloblastic anemia), the extent of ineffective erythropoiesis is abnormally great, and relatively few red cells reach the blood despite intense erythropoietic activity.

C. Regulation

The rate of erythropoiesis is governed by the rate by oxygen transport to the tissues, which can be expressed as the product of oxyhemoglobin concentration and cardiac output. (This relation and the effects on it of blood viscosity and blood volume are discussed further in lecture 21). When oxygen transport decreases, erythropoiesis generally increases.

The existence of a feedback loop between erythropoietic marrow and tissues was postulated by Paul Bert in 1878, who found that survival of Andean natives at high altitudes was dependent on increased erythropoiesis. Later work revealed that low tissue PO_2 stimulated erythropoiesis. Since anemia leads to a decrease in tissue PO_2, this discovery explained both the compensatory increase in erythropoiesis in most anemias and the homeostatic balance between red cell production and destruction.

1. Erythropoietin

Early in the twentieth century, Carnot and DeFlandre postulated that a humoral agent adjusts erythropoiesis in response to tissue PO_2 level. The suggestion received experimental support in 1950 when Reissmann showed that inducing hypoxia in one of a pair of parabiotic rats increases red cell production in both rats. The agent, named **erythropoietin**, was finally demonstrated in 1953 by Erslev in the serum of anemic rats.

a. PROPERTIES

Erythropoietin (Epo) is a heavily glycosylated α-globulin (carbohydrate content 50–60%, sialic acid content 10–15%) with a molecular weight of 38,000. Desialation results in total loss of biologic activity when assayed in vivo but not when assayed in vitro. The discrepancy is due to the fact that asialoerythropoietin (like other asialoglycoproteins) is rapidly cleared from blood by hepatic cells. The carbohydrate portion of the molecule may convey specificity in the recognition of target cell receptors. The human Epo gene on chromosome 7 has more than 80% homology with the mouse gene.

b. SOURCE

Epo is found in both plasma and urine. Early studies on nephrectomized rats showed that it is produced in the kidneys, but later work revealed that small amounts (5–10% of total Epo production) arise in extrarenal tissues. Extrarenal (mainly hepatic) production in anephric animals and patients rises in response to tissue hypoxia. Thus the renal oxygen sensor, recently shown to be a novel hemoprotein, and the renal Epo-producing cell both have extrarenal alternatives. After long controversy over which renal cells or structures synthesize Epo, mRNA probes showed its sources to be cortical (and outer medullary) interstitial and endothelial cells, lining the peritubular capillaries, with possible participation by tubular cells.

c. LOCUS OF ACTION

Epo selectively stimulates erythropoiesis in bone marrow by stimulating early committed cells (BFU-E and CFU-E) to differentiate into pronormoblasts. Its mechanism depends on selective gene activators. Epo binds to specific receptors on cell surfaces and thereby stimulates synthesis of messenger RNA and perhaps cyclic AMP and cyclic GMP in Epo-responsive cells. The Epo receptor is currently under intense study.

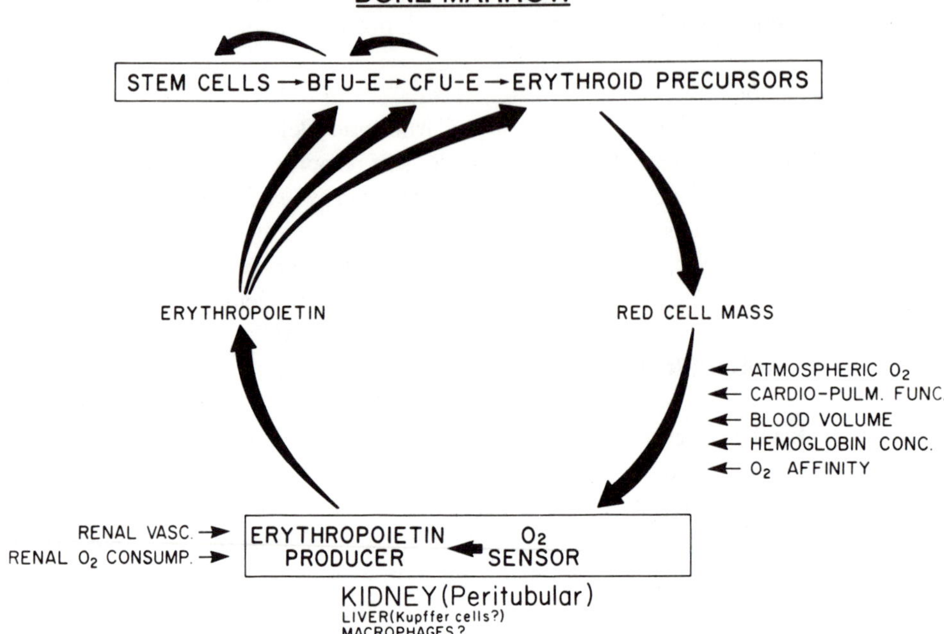

Fig. 2.2
Current model of the feedback circuit that regulates the rate of red blood cell production to the need for oxygen in the peripheral tissues. (From A. J. Erslev. In W. J. Williams et al., eds. *Hematology*, 4th ed. New York: McGraw-Hill, 1990.)

d. PHYSIOLOGIC ROLE

Early workers were uncertain whether Epo is a "panic mechansim" that is called into play only when anemia is present, or whether there is a slow, constant baseline Epo effect in normal subjects. The following evidence suggests that the latter view is correct: (1) elevation of the red cell mass to supranormal levels by hypertransfusion decreases erythropoiesis; (2) anti-Epo antibodies lead to aplasia of marrow erythroid elements; (3) some Epo is found in normal urine; and (4) Epo levels rise in serum and urine in most anemias—but not in most patients with the anemia of renal disease (see lecture 4). A reliable erythropoietin assay suitable for routine clinical use has only recently become available. Figure 2.2 summarizes the elements of the feedback loop that normally regulates red cell production. Elements of this loop are discussed further in lectures 3 and 26. The promising and actively expanding use of recombinant Epo in the therapy of anemias is discussed in later lectures.

2. *Erythropoietic response to anoxia*

a. EARLY EVENTS

When anoxia is brought about by sudden anemia (as after a hemorrhage), there occurs first a premature release of marrow reticulocytes (see table 2.1). These so-called **shift reticulocytes** are recognizable in the blood as large polychromatophilic cells. They take longer to mature than the ordinary reticulocytes of normal blood. The accelerated release of reticulocytes from marrow under hypoxic conditions may be mediated by Epo, but a separate **reticulocyte releasing factor** (comparable to granulocyte release factors) has been postulated. Such factors are still hypothetical.

b. LATER EVENTS

Epo secretion leads to increased activity of erythroid marrow, which may lead to compensation of the anemia (i.e., to a normal hemoglobin level despite continued blood loss). If it does, there is a new steady state at a higher level of marrow activity. The marrow can increase its activity in this way to about 10 times the normal level. There is a corresponding rise in the blood reticulocyte count (table 2.2). A few normoblasts may enter the blood when the marrow is stressed further. If marrow cannot keep up with rate of blood loss, the hemoglobin level decreases. Sustained anoxia leads to centrifugal expansion of erythroid marrow throughout the skeleton and somtimes to extramedullary erythropoiesis. The signals leading to the expansion of erythroid marrow at the expense of fatty marrow are not known.

D. Erythrokinetics

Diagnosis of the underlying cause of anemia requires an appraisal of the patient's "erythrokinetics"—that is, the kinetics of red cell production. The following methods are employed in the clinical evaluation of erythrokinetics.

Table 2.2
Expected Reticulocyte Responses in Anemias of Varying Severity in the Presence of Normal Bone Marrow Function*

Hematocrit (%)	45	40	35	30	25	20	15
Hemoglobin (g/dl)	15.0	13.3	11.7	10.0	8.3	6.6	5.0
Reticulocyte count (%)	1.0	2.0	5.0	10.0	15.0	20.0	30.0
Reticulocyte index	1.0	1.8	4.0	7.0	8.3	9.0	10.0

*These data are intended only as rough guides. Considerable variations may occur among different patients. Note that reticulocyte counts would be lower if bone marrow function were impaired.

1. Red cell production

Effective red cell production may be judged by (1) the **reticulocyte count**, perhaps the single most useful piece of information in the analysis of anemia; (2) the **erythroid/granulocytic (E/G)** or **erythroid/myeloid (E/M) ratio** in bone marrow smears, a useful substitute for the unavailable data on the total number of erythroid cells in marrow, which is meaningful only when granulocyte production is normal; and (3) the study of **ferrokinetics**, quantitative data on the traffic of iron, which are rarely available in the clinic. This methodology will be discussed in lecture 7.

2. Red cell destruction

Red cell destruction may be judged from (1) measurements of **red cell life span** and (2) studies of the **rate of hemoglobin catabolism**. These techniques will be discussed in lectures 8 and 12.

V. THE ANEMIAS

A. Definition

Anemia must be defined circumspectly. Ordinarily it refers to a decrease in the total number of circulating erythrocytes, a decrease in the concentration of hemoglobin in blood, or a decrease in the hematocrit compared to a normal group. But the normal population must be relevant. A hemoglobin level that is normal at sea level is relatively low at high altitudes. The hematocrit may also be a deceptive parameter. In hypovolemia (decreased blood volume), red cell mass may be decreased, but plasma volume is also decreased. Thus, the hematocrit may remain normal. In physiologic hypervolemia (as occurs in pregnancy), blood volume is increased and hematocrit decreased, but red cell mass is actually increased. Hence, a defintion of anemia must encompass the functional competence of blood to deliver oxygen to tissues.

B. Clinical features

1. Significance of adaptation

Signs and symptoms depend significantly on the rate of onset of anemia. In anemia due to acute hemorrhage, a 30% decrease in red cell mass may lead rapidly to circulatory collapse and death. In slowly developing anemia of equal severity, symptoms may be few. This means that the body adapts to anemia and that the process of adaptation takes time. Adaptation consists of a combination of mechanisms that increase the oxygen-delivering capacity of a decreased amount of hemoglobin. It includes (1) acceleration of the heart rate and respiratory rate; (2) increased cardiac output; and (3) a "shift to the right" in the oxygen saturation curve that is now known to be mediated by an increase in red cell 2,3-diphosphoglycerate (see lecture

9). As a result of these adaptations, a patient can tolerate without symptoms a slowly developing 50% decrease in red cell mass.

2. *Signs and symptoms*

Signs and symptoms in a patient with anemia are those of the underlying disorder (if one is present) *and* those due to anemia per se. The latter may be classified into three groups: (1) those due to decreased oxygen transport (e.g., fatigue, syncope, dyspnea, angina pectoris, widespread impairment of organ function in GI, GU, and other body system); (2) those due to decreased blood volume (e.g., pallor, postural hypotension); and (3) those due to increased cardiac output (e.g., palpitation, with pulse pressure, "hemic" heart murmurs, onset of congestive heart failure).

C. Classification

Anemias have been classified in many ways. The two most useful ways are based on (1) the size and other characteristics of the average red cell and (2) the pathophysiologic mechanism responsible for the red cell deficit. Neither scheme is wholly satisfactory. In the following lists, references are given to lectures in which disorders are discussed.

1. *By red cell morphology*

This classification is useful because it leads from the initial laboratory data on a patient's mean red cell *size* and *chromicity* (i.e., mean hemoglobin concentration in red cells) to a consideration of disease categories most likely responsible. Classification is based on three **red cell indexes**, of which the first two mentioned are most useful.

- **MCV** denotes the mean corpuscular volume of red cells (normal = 80–96 μm^3). It is calculated by the formula

$$MCV = \frac{\text{volume (in ml) of packed RBC/l}}{\text{red count/mm}^3\text{ (in millions)}} \text{ or } \frac{\text{hematocrit (\%)} \times 10}{\text{red count/mm}^3\text{ (in millions)}}$$

  For example, a normal individual with 420 ml of red cells per liter and a red count of 4.6 million per mm^3 would have an MCV of 420/4.6 or 91 mm^3. Alternatively, the MCV may be calculated by dividing the actual hematocrit percentage by the red count per mm^3 (in millions), and multiplying by 10.
- **MCHC** denotes mean corpuscular hemoglobin concentration (normal = 33–35 g/dl):

$$MCHC = \frac{\text{hemoglobin (g/dl)} \times 100}{\text{hematocrit (\%)}}$$

- **MCH** a third red cell index, represents the mean cell hemoglobin (normal = 27–33 pg/red cell). It is noted here although it is less useful in the classification of anemias than the MCHC:

$$\text{MCH} = \frac{\text{hemoglobin (g/dl)} \times 10}{\text{red count/l} \, (\times 10^{-12})} \text{ or } \frac{\text{hemoglobin (g/dl)} \times 10}{\text{red count/mm}^3}$$

Alternatively, the MCH may be calculated by dividing the hemoglobin (g/dl) by the red count per mm^3.

Note: MCV measures volume; MCHC concentration; MCH mass.

a. NORMOCYTIC-NORMOCHROMIC ANEMIAS:

MCV = 80–96
MCHC = 33–35

1. Acute bleeding
2. Hemolytic anemias (lectures 12–15)
   a. Extracorpuscular defects, immune and nonimmune
   b. Intracorpuscular defects, membrane, metabolic, and hemoglobinopathic
   c. Combined defects
3. Marrow failure associated with hypoproliferation of hematopoietic cells (lecture 4)
   a. Aplastic anemia
   b. Pure red cell aplasia
   c. Anemia of chronic renal failure
   d. Anemia of endocrine disease
   e. Toxic depression of bone marrow
   f. Myelophthisic anemia
   g. Myelodysplastic syndrome

b. MICROCYTIC-HYPOCHROMIC ANEMIAS:

MCV < 80
MCHC < 33

1. Iron deficiency (lecture 7)
2. Sideroblastic anemias
   a. Refractory
   b. Reversible
   c. Pyridoxine-responsive
3. Thalassemia

c. MACROCYTIC-NORMOCHROMIC ANEMIAS:

MCV > 96
MCHC = 33–35

1. Megaloblastic anemias (lectures 5, 6)
   a. Cobalamin deficiency
   b. Folic acid deficiency
   c. Others
2. Nonmegaloblastic macrocytic anemias (see lecture 6)

2. *By pathophysiologic mechanism*

This classification fosters understanding of the disease process in kinetic terms. Its major shortcoming is the fact that some anemias are due to more than one pathophysiologic mechanism. Often one mechanism predominates early in the course but another supervenes. In practice these complications should be borne in mind.

a. INCREASED RED CELL LOSS

1. Bleeding, acute and chronic
2. Hemolytic anemias (see lectures 12–15)

b. DECREASED RED CELL PRODUCTION

1. Marrow failure associated with hypoproliferation of hematopoietic cells (see lecture 4)
2. Marrow failure associated with ineffective erythropoiesis
   a. Impaired hemoglobin synthesis: the hypochromic anemias (see lecture 7)
   b. Impaired DNA synthesis: the megaloblastic anemias (lectures 5, 6)

D. Approach to the patient

The diagnosis of anemia, like the diagnosis of any other disease, rests on the data derived from a careful history, physical examination, and laboratory evaluation. A history of drug ingestion or exposure to other toxic substances must be recorded in detail. A family history of anemia makes a genetic disorder likely, and a history of previous anemia in the patient suggests either an inherited disorder or persisting cause (e.g., menorrhagia in the female). Racial and geographic derivations are pertinent in certain hemoglobinopathies (hemoglobin S or C) and red cell metabolic disorders (G-6-PD deficiency). Signs or symptoms of inflammation, evidence of a bleeding tendency, splenic enlargement, and lymphadenopathy provide important diagnostic clues. Chronic leg ulcers are sometimes seen in hemolytic disease, Epithelial changes including flattening of the nails and glossitis occur in iron deficiency. A depapillated tongue and neurologic signs of posterior and lateral column disease are found with cobalamin deficiency. As indicated above, the basic approach to the differential diagnosis of anemia depends on the laboratory. After anemia has been detected by a hematocrit or hemoglobin determination, a blood film should be carefully examined and red cell indexes (MCV and MCHC) obtained. A reticulocyte count should be obtained early, along with the plasma iron concentration and iron-binding capacity. These usually permit the physician to characterize the functional abnormality of the erythron and indicate what other information is needed for a more specific diagnosis.

SELECTED REFERENCES

Reviews

Bull, B. S, Breton-Gorius, J., et al. Morphology of the erythron. In Williams, W. J., Beutler, E., et al., eds. *Hematology*, 4th ed. New York: McGraw-Hill, 1990, pp. 297–316.

Erslev, A. J. Production of erythrocytes. In Williams, W. J., Beutler, E., et al., eds. *Hematology*, 4th ed. New York: McGraw-Hill, 1990, pp. 389–398.

Fried, W. Factors that affect the rate of erythropoietin production by extrarenal sites. *Ann. HY Acad. Sci.* 554 (1989): 1–8.

Johnson, G. R. Erythropoietin. *Br. Med. Bull.* 45(1989): 506–514.

Keown, P. A. Recombinant human erythropoietin: from concept to clinic. *Transplant. Proc.* 21 Suppl. 2 (1989): 49–53.

Spivak, J. L. Erythropoietin: a brief review. *Nephron* 52 (1989): 289–294.

Original articles

Beru, N., McDonald, J., et al. Studies of the constitutive expression of the mouse erythropoietin gene. *Ann. NY Acad. Sci.* 554 (1989): 29–35.

Boussios, T., Bertles, J. F., et al. Erythropoietin. Receptor characteristics during the ontogeny of hamster yolk sac erythroid cells. *J. Biol. Chem.* 264 (1989): 16017–16021.

Burstein, S. A. and Ishibashi, T. Erythropoietin and megakaryocytopoiesis. *Blood cells* 15 (1989): 193–201.

Dubé, S., Fisher, J. W., et al. Glycosylation at specific sites of erythropoietin is essential for biosynthesis, secretion, and biological function. *J. Biol. Chem.* 263 (1988): 17516–17521.

Fukuda, M. N., Sasaki, H., et al. Survival of recombinant erythropoietin in the circulation: the role of carbohydrates. *Blood* 73 (1989): 84–89.

Goldberg, M. A., Dunning, S. P., et al. Regulation of the erythropoietin gene: evidence that the oxygen sensor is a heme protein. *Science* 242 (1988): 1412–1415.

Grossi, A., Vannucchi, A. M., et al. Recombinant human erythropoietin has little influence on megakaryocytopoiesis in mice. *Br. J. Haematol.* 71 (1989): 463–468.

Im, J. H., Lee, S. J., et al. Partial purification and characterization of erythropoietin receptors from erythroid progenitor cells. *Arch. Biochem. Biophys.* 278 (1990): 486–491.

Jelkmann, W. and Wiedemann, G. Serum erythropoietin level: relationships to blood hemoglobin concentration and erythrocytic activity of the bone marrow. *Klin. Wochenschr.* 68 (1990): 403–407.

Kurtz, A. and Eckardt, K.-U. Assays for erythropoietin. *Nephron* 51 Suppl. S1 (1989): 11–14.

Meyer, F. From authentic to recombinant human erythropoietin. Biotechnological production of recombinant human erythropoietin. *Nephron* 51 Suppl. S1 (1989): 20–25.

Noble, N. A., Xu, Q.-P., et al. Reticulocytes II: reexamination of the in vivo survival of stress reticulocytes. *Blood* 75 (1990): 1877–1882.

Rhyner, K., Egli, F., et al. Serum erythropoietin levels in various diseases. *Nephron* 51 Suppl. S1 (1989): 39–46.

Sawyer, S. T. The two proteins of the erythropoietin receptor are structurally similar. *J. Biol. Chem.* 264 (1989): 13343–13347.

Sawyer, S. T., Krantz, S. B., et al. Receptors for erythropoietin in mouse and human erythroid cells and placenta. *Blood* 74 (1989): 103–109.

Schuster, S. J., Badiavas, E. V., et al. Stimulation of erythropoietin gene transcription during hypoxia and cobalt exposure. *Blood* 73 (1989): 13–16.

Smith, K. A. Interleukin-2. *Sci. Am.* 262 (1990): 50–57.

Trainor, C. D., Evans, T., et al. Structure and evolution of a human erythroid transcription factor. *Nature* 343 (1990): 92–96.

LECTURE 3

Reticuloendothelial (Mononuclear Phagocyte) System, Lymphatic System, and Spleen

William S. Beck

EDITOR'S COMMENT

Studies of the mononuclear-phagocyte system, or reticuloendothelial system, and the lymphatic system have been part of the current revolution in immunology. As noted in this lecture, these scientific developments have been animated by the discovery and practical exploitation of cell surface markers that are detected by specific monoclonal antibodies, the resolution of the many humoral growth factors regulating the ontogeny and function of T and B cells, and the recognition of the surprisingly complex functions of macrophages, which are prodigious producers of cytokines.

I. INTRODUCTION

The **reticuloendothelial system** (RES), the **lymphatic system**, and the **spleen** have certain features in common:

- They are of major hematologic importance in health and disease.
- They are complex and many faceted, with shared or overlapping functions.
- They are objects of extraordinarily intense research interest.
- They still pose many unsolved basic problems.

The following discussion gives emphasis to hematologic aspects and is intended only as an introductory guide. The text will call attention to later lectures that deal with immunologic and other aspects of these systems.

II. RETICULOENDOTHELIAL SYSTEM

A. Definitions

The term **reticuloendothelial system**, or **RES**, was introduced in 1924 by Aschoff to designate those scattered body cells that avidly take up vital dyes. The definition later came to include cells taking up injected particulate matter (e.g., India ink, iron). Anatomically the system consists of the (1) **fixed macrophages**, or **reticulum cells**, of spleen, lymph nodes, bone marrow, and liver (Kupffer cells); (2) **free macrophages**, or **histiocytes**, in spleen, lymph nodes, lung, serous cavities, and other tissues; (3) **endothelial cells** lining **sinusoids** (or **sinuses**) in liver, bone marrow, spleen, and lymph nodes (plus similar cells in the adrenal and pituitary glands); (4) marrow **monoblasts** and **promonocytes**; and (5) circulating blood **monocytes**.

Because later work showed that most of these cell types arise from the blood **monocyte**, which in turn derives from precursors in the bone marrow, the system was renamed **mononuclear phagocyte system**, or **MPS**. The terms **RES** and **MPS** are now used interchangeably, although some authorities restrict the RES to fixed cells and exclude free macrophages and monocytes. This text retains the older term, RES, and defines its component cells as above.

Functionally, RES cells are distinguished by their ability to ingest particulate matter by the process of *phagocytosis*. In addition, they play significant roles in *humoral defense* and *metabolism*. (The physiology and pathophysiology of phagocytosis are discussed in detail in lecture 19.)

B. Distribution and size

Its component cells are so widely distributed that investigators have facetiously suggested that the body is simply an inert matrix designated to support the RES. Its size is not precisely known. In the rat, each of the three major organs of the RES (spleen, liver, and bone marrow) has been estimated to contain 10^9 RES cells. A normal human spleen contains about 1.4×10^{11} cells. If it is assumed that half the cells in the human spleen are RES cells (as in the rat) and that liver and bone marrow contain an equal number of RES cells, the RES of a normal person must then consist of 2×10^{11} cells. Thus it is of substantial size.

C. Major cell types

As noted above, the major cell types are reticulum cells, free macrophages or histiocytes, endothelial cells, and monocytes and their precursors. In tissues these cells are usually associated with **lymphocytes** and **plasma cells** (or **plasmacytes**). Properties of RES cells are investigated by three methods: (1) study of morphology by techniques of histology, cytochemistry, phase microscopy, and electron microscopy; (2) study of structural transitions in health and diseases; and (3) study of functional properties in health and disease. The following is a brief description of the major cell types.

1. Fixed macrophages (reticulum cells)

A typical inactive fixed macrophage is a large cell, with a diameter of more than 20 μm. In stained imprints, the abundant cytoplasm is pale blue and homogeneous in appearance. The relatively small nucleus is usually round. Blue nucleoli are usually present. They are capable of phagocytosis and may be sites of abnormal accumulations of proteins, lipids, and other materials.

Fixed macrophages apparently are in dynamic equilibrium with free mobile macrophages. They occur in so-called **lymphoreticular tissues** (lymph nodes and spleen, where they are called **littoral cells**) and in bone marrow (where they are often called **reticulum cells**). Such tissues are interlaced with

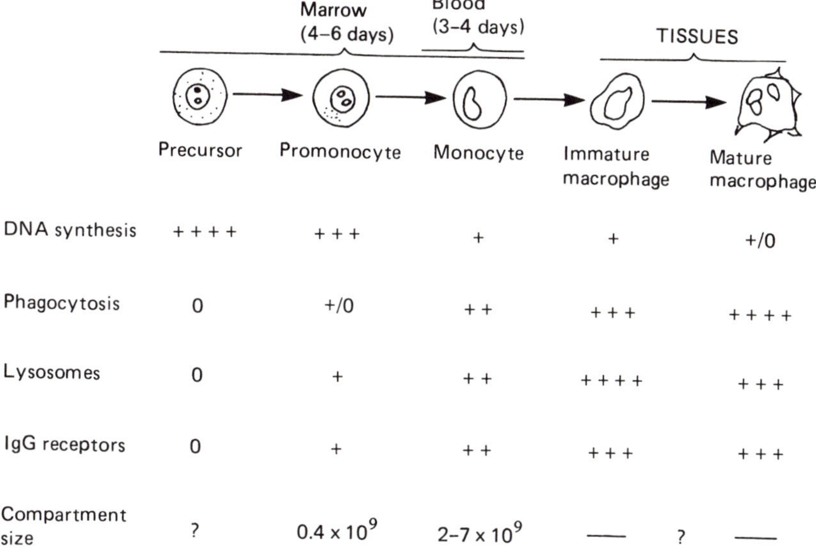

	Precursor	Promonocyte	Monocyte	Immature macrophage	Mature macrophage
DNA synthesis	+ + + +	+ + +	+	+	+/0
Phagocytosis	0	+/0	+ +	+ + +	+ + + +
Lysosomes	0	+	+ +	+ + + +	+ + +
IgG receptors	0	+	+ +	+ + +	+ + +
Compartment size	?	0.4×10^9	$2\text{–}7 \times 10^9$	—— ?	——

Fig. 3.1
The mononuclear phagocyte system. Monocytes, promonocytes, and more primitive precursors are found in the marrow. Monocytes circulate in the blood and enter the tissues to differentiate into macrophages. Normally only promonocytes and earlier cells actively proliferate, although cells are capable of division through the immature macrophage stage. The development of phagocytic activity, lysosomes, and IgG receptors is illustrated. Figures for compartment size are estimates for a normal adult. There are approximately 7.3×10^9 monocytes in the marrow compartment and 1.7×10^9 monocytes in the blood. (Modified from W. J. Williams et al., eds., *Hematology*, 4th ed. New York: McGraw-Hill, 1990.)

a reticular fibrillary network that ramifies throughout the tissue. They also include: the macrophages of the liver (Kupffer cells), which have a characteristic stellate appearance; the macrophages of pulmonary alveoli; the lamina propria of the gastrointestinal tract; perivascular microglial cells of the central nervous system; and osteoclasts.

A comment is in order on the relation between these cells and pluripotent stem cells (see lecture 1) in the light of past claims that reticulum cells (or other RES cells) can undergo transition into lymphocyte precursors and other cell types. Neither the reticulum cell nor the sinusoidal endothelial cell is identical with the pluripotent stem cell—labeling data having shown that these cells lack the kinetic and migratory properties required of a competent hematopoietic stem cell. Rather, as shown in figures 1.1 and 3.1, fixed and free macrophages arise from the following maturation sequence: pluripotent stem cell (CFU-GEMM) → CFU-GM → CFU-M → promonocyte → monocyte → macrophage.

2. *Free macrophages*

Free macrophages are largely lysosome-filled wandering cells (diameter up to 80 μm) with functions resembling those of primarily fixed macrophages.

Direct evidence of their bone marrow origin is suggested by chromosome studies of pulmonary macrophages in patients transplanted with marrow from donors of the opposite sex.

3. Endothelial cells

The endothelial cell component of the RES was originally thought to include only the sinusoid-lining cells of lymph nodes and spleen and the endothelial cells of the capillaries of liver, bone marrow, adrenals, and pituitary. Later models included the endothelial cells of all blood vessels. These cells are now enjoying intense scientific scrutiny after years of neglect, especially in connection with blood coagulation (see lectures 27 and 28).

Endothelial cells are connected with one another (and with surrounding reticulum cells) by a fiber lattice. Thus they resemble specialized reticulum cells. The loose arrangement of the cells in spleen, bone marrow, and lymph nodes differs from that of the endothelium in ordinary blood vessels in that they rest upon a basement membrane distinctive for its defective strandlike character. In a normal adult, their collective mass exceeds 100 gm and surface area 1000 m^2.

Electron microscopic study of cells lining sinusoids reveals **clefts** between and among extensions of these cells. These surrond **pores** that begin at the sinusoid surface and become continuous with similar clefts between adjacent reticulum cells. The presence of these intercellular clefts (and the absence of obturating basement membranes) is characteristic of sinuses and helps to explain their high permeability.

4. Monocytes

As noted above, the blood monocyte is the precursor of fixed and free macrophages in tissues. The mature monocyte is a large motile cell (diameter 12–20 μm) with a characteristic indented nucleus, lacy chromatin, grayish-blue cytoplasm in Wright's stained smears, and very fine pinkish granules. Living monocytes adhere avidly to glass surfaces and display cytoplasmic spreading. Electron microscopy reveals a well-developed Golgi complex and numerous mitochondria, lysosomes, and microtubules. Monocytes are discussed further in lecture 18.

D. Functions of RES

The major functions of the RES are phagocytic, immunologic, and secretory. In spleen and lymph nodes, RES cells are in close proximity to immunologically reactive cells. In liver and bone marrow, however, RES cells are adjacent to hepatocytes and hematopoietic cells, respectively. This may mean that the functions of RES cells differ in different locations.

1. Clearing function

The capacity of the RES for engulfing particulate material, denatured plasma proteins, and effete or damaged red cells is called its **clearing function**. Such ingestion can lead to rapid killing and destruction of bacteria or red cells or to indefinite storage of particles such as silica, carbon, and thorium dioxide. This RES function is a fundamental body defense mechanism. Its impairment by disease can have disastrous consequences.

2. Immunologic functions

Tissue macrophages play a key role in the antigen-induced blastic transformation of lymphocytes. This involves:

- A preliminary processing of foreign or pathogenic antigens by macrophages
- Enhancement of lymphocyte proliferation by secretion of mitogenic protein, T and T cell differentiation factors, T cell activating factor, and other products
- Secretion of multiple substances involved in tissue organization and repair
- Subsequent regulation by the activated lymphocyte of microbicidal and cytocidal functions of the macrophage

3. Secretory functions

In addition to the products just mentioned, macrophages secrete enzymes that hydrolyze tissue components (e.g., lysosomal proteases, collagenase, nucleases), products involved in body defense (muramidase, complement components, interferon, etc.), products that modulate other cells (e.g., angiogenesis factors, low-molecular-weight chemotactic factor, CSF), and various other products (e.g., pyrogen, transferrin, transcobalamin II, thromboplastin).

E. Techniques for studying the RES

1. Measurement of clearing capacity

The **clearing capacity** of the RES can be quantified in animals by injecting increasing doses of particulate materials such as carbon, saccharated iron oxide, colloidal gold, or thorium dioxide. Such experiments show that (1) with increasing doses, the rate of particle clearance approaches a maximal clearance rate asymptotically; (2) maximal clearance rates of different colloids are not the same; and (3) the maximal clearance rates (expressed as milligrams cleared per 100 g body weight) differ from species to species. This variation is a function of spleen and liver weight.

2. Blockade of the RES

The clearing function of the RES can be blocked to a variable extent by injection of suspensions of particulate matter such as carbon. There is some blockade specificity in that clearance of one substance by the RES (e.g., carbon) may not be blocked by prior injections of another substance (e.g., thorotrast). The mechanism of blockade specificity is unknown. It may reflect saturation of phagocytes (or a specific population of them) or depletion of serum factors needed to facilitate phagocytosis (**opsonins**). The actual site of particle clearance in RES is influenced by many factors—rate of blood flow, possible presence of local tissue damage, nature of the particles, and so forth. As we shall see, the spleen has a special capacity to clear mildly damaged red cells from the circulation. More severely damaged red cells are removed mainly by the liver. More will be said of these RES functions in later discussions of red cell destruction (lectures 12 and 13) and phagocytosis (lecture 19).

3. Visualization of the RES

Since cells of the RES are identifiable by their ability to ingest particulate matter, many early workers studied tissue distributions of radioactive colloidal particles. Such particles when injected intravenously are rapidly cleared from the blood and trapped by the RES in the liver, spleen, and bone marrow. These observations led to the development of external scanning techniques that employ radioactive colloids to delineate the structure and functional integrity of organs rich in RES cells. The use of short-lived radionuclides greatly reduces the radiation dose. Use of radionuclides that decay rapidly increases the yield of emitted photons and improves the spatial resolution of scanning procedures without increasing the radiation dose. Finally, advances in radiation detection methods have permitted both visualization of a specific organ system and its functional evaluation.

a. SCANNING LIVER AND SPLEEN

Nuclear medicine services currently scan the liver and spleen by injecting technetium-99m sulfur colloid. The usual dose of 2 mCi gives a whole-body radiation dose of only 0.008–0.03 cGy and a critical organ dose of 0.3–0.6 cGy to the liver. An image of liver and spleen is thus readily obtained (figure 3.2). Focal defects due to neoplasm, cysts, abscesses, and so forth appear as circumscribed areas of decreased uptake. Diffuse diseases cause mottling. With increasing severity of hepatocellular disease, more colloid is shunted to other parts of the RES.

b. SPECIAL METHODS FOR SCANNING SPLEEN

A second method used in scanning the spleen exploits a physiologic process peculiar to that organ—the sequestering of damaged red cells (i.e., heat-damaged red cells, labeled with a suitable gamma-emitting nuclide such as ribidium-81). The type of red cell damage is not the critical factor in producing sequestration; the degree of damage is. If damage is too great,

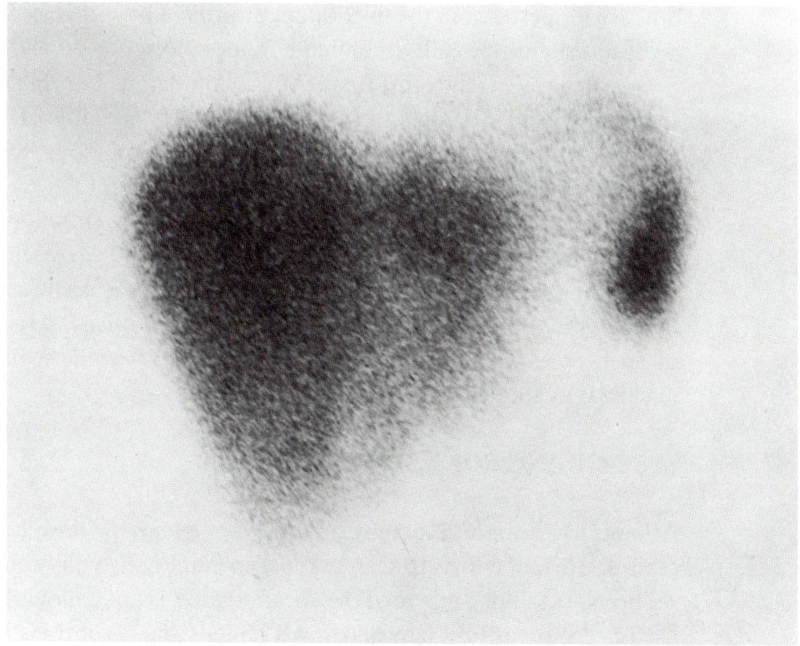

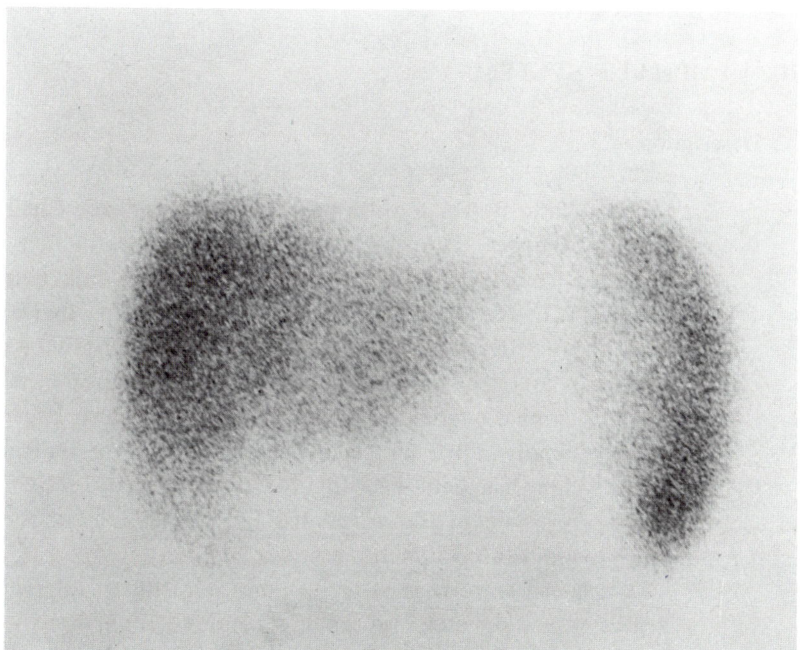

Fig. 3.2
Image of liver and spleen scan. Patients were previously injected with 6 mCi of technetium-99m sulfer colloid. *A*. Normal Subject. *B*. Patient with splenomegaly associated with hepatic cirrhosis. (Courtesy of Dr. D. A. McKusick.)

cells are sequestered in the liver or are destroyed by intravascular hemolysis; if too slight, the cells accumulate in the spleen too slowly.

Splenomegaly is the most frequently encountered abnormality in spleen scanning. Space-occupying lesions are also demonstrable. These include abscess, lymphomatous involvement, and granulomatous lesions of sarcoid. Evidence of splenic infarction may also be seen.

The term **functional asplenia** refers to failure of the spleen to develop on image. This is usually due to failure of the radionuclide to reach the spleen's macrophages because of reduced perfusion to the spleen (as may result from elevated blood viscosity during a sickle cell crisis). After resolution of such crisis with resulting improvement in arterial perfusion, radionuclide is again delivered in sufficient quantity.

c. SCANNING BONE MARROW

Attempts to scan and thereby quantify bone marrow have been less successful. Current efforts to scan that organ employ two physiologic processes peculiar to bone marrow: the accumulation (1) of colloids labeled with ^{99m}Tc, ^{113m}In, or ^{198}Au by marrow RES cells and (2) of transferrin-bound ^{59}Fe by marrow erythroid cells—a process that is discussed in lecture 7.

III. LYMPHATIC SYSTEM

A. Description

The **lymphatic system** consists principally of **lymphatic capillaries**, **ducts**, and **lymph nodes**. The small lymphatic capillaries in body tissues are separated from the capillaries carrying blood. They make up a complex network of fragile distensible vessels, resembling veins, that collect **lymph**, the watery extravascular fluid of tissues, and conveys it to the blood. Their function is drainage, not perfusion or circulation; thus they end blindly in tissues. Lymphatic capillaries unite to form progressively larger vessels that converge finally in two main channels, the **thoracic**, or **left lymphatic duct**, and the **right lymphatic duct** (figure 3.3). Lymphatic vessels, like blood vessels, are present in nearly every tissue. An exception is the bone marrow, which contains no lymphatic vessels.

Lymph nodes are bean-shaped bodies occuring at intervals along the larger lymphatic vessels and ranging from 1 to about 15 mm in diameter. Despite an occasional solitary node, most nodes occur in groups or chains that are known by regional names, for example, **inguinal**, **axillary**, **supratrochlear**, and **cervical** groups, which are superficial; and **mesenteric** and **retroperitoneal** groups, which are deep. Each group receives the lymph draining from a particular body area.

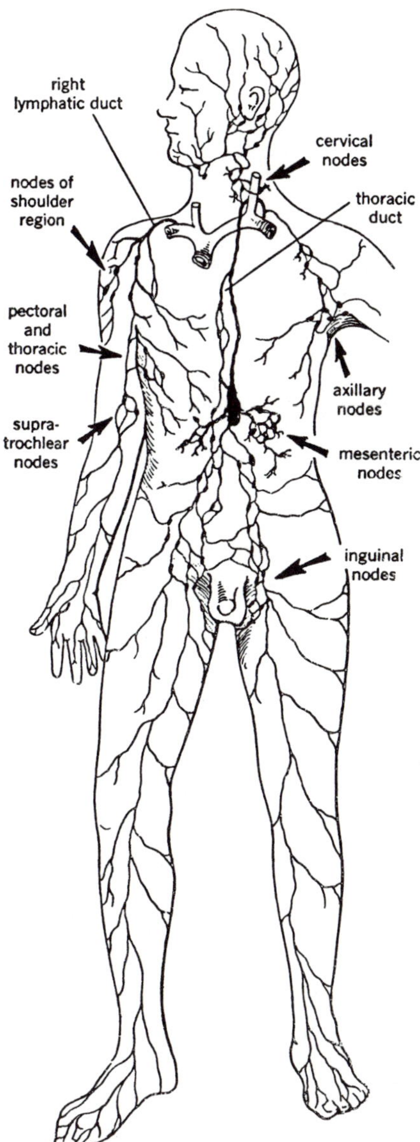

Fig. 3.3.
Human lymphatic system. (From W. S. Beck, *Human Design: Molecular, Cellular, and Systematic Physiology*. New York: Harcourt Brace Jovanovich, 1971.)

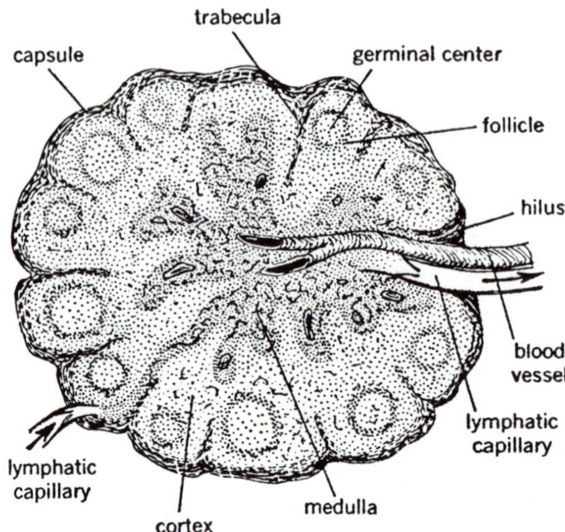

Fig. 3.4
Gross structure of a lymph node. (Compare with figure 24.1.) (From W. S. Beck, Human Design: *Molecular, Cellular, and Systematic Physiology*. New York: Harcourt Brace Jovanovich, 1971.)

B. Lymph node structure

The gross internal structure of a typical lymph nodes is shown in figure 3.4. The **hilus** is a slight depression through which pass blood and lymphatic vessels. The outer covering is a **capsule** of connective tissue from which fibrous **trabeculae** proceed into the substance of the node, dividing it into irregular, freely communicating spaces. Suspended within this framework is the **reticular framework**. Its most loosely meshed areas are the **sinusoids**, through which the lymph percolates. RES cells line the sinusoids. The cut section of a node shows an outer **cortex** and an inner **medulla**. Both consist of **lymphoid tissue**. However, the cortex contains lymphatic **follicles**, or **nodules**, structures whose appearance varies with their state of activity. (Similar follicle occur in the spleen and throughout the body in regions of **diffuse** lymphoid tissue, as in the walls of the intestine and respiratory passages.)

- Follicles consist of masses of lymphocytes (mainly B lymphocytes) of various ages, plasma cells, and macrophages, in a characteristic structural pattern. When appropriately stimulated, proliferating cells in the central portions of the follicles produce new lymphocytes. Hence, these regions are **germinal centers**. Germinal centers also contain large lymphocytes and macrophages.
- The deep cortex (paracortex) consists mainly of T lymphocytes (T : B ratio about 3 : 1).
- The medulla consists mainly of B lymphocytes.

Lymph enters a node via an afferent lymphatic vessel at the hilus, circulates through the sinusoids, and leaves by efferent vessels. In passing through the node, it picks up the lymphocytes arising in germinal centers.

C. Lymphoid cells

1. Lymphocytes

The familiar lymphocyte in stained blood smears is a small round cell with a characteristic dark nucleus and a thin, pale, or blue rim of cytoplasm lacking distinct granules. Similar cells are found in the lymph nodes, spleen, bone marrow, and other tissues—indeed, more than a kilogram of lymphocytes are found outside blood, lymph nodes, and bone marrow. All of these cells are called lymphocytes because they have similar morphology, but we now recognize this group to be functionally heterogeneous.

Lymphocyte precursors arise from CFU-LM, the pluripotent hematopoietic stem cell shown in figure 1.1.

- The earliest recognizable lymphocyte precursor is the **lymphoblast**, a larger mononuclear cell with basophilic cytoplasm.
- This cell matures into a smaller **prolymphocyte**, which has coarse, clumped chromatin with distinct open spaces.
- The prolymphocyte then evolves into a **mature lymphocyte**, which may be large, intermediate, or small in size. These are the most numerous cells in lymphoid tissues, which contain all three sizes. Most blood lymphocytes are intermediate or small.

As discussed in more detail later (see lectures 18, 23, and 24), the morphologically homogeneous population of small lymphocytes consists of two major types, **T lymphocytes**, or **T cells** (thymus derived) and **B lymphocytes**, or **B cells** (bursa or bursa-equivalent derived). About 75% of blood lymphocytes are T cells, 10% are B cells. About 15% are **null cells**, which lack T or B markers.

These cells play key roles in the immune system and thus are said to be **immunocompetent**.

- T cells are the primary effectors of cellular immunity and immunoregulation.
- B cells are the antibody-forming cells of the lymphoid system.

a. T LYMPHOCYTES

The undifferentiated precursors of T cells migrate from the bone marrow during fetal life (and perhaps throughout life) to the cortex of the thymus, where a high rate of cellular proliferation and turnover prevails. The maturation and differentiation of T cells is profoundly influenced by early interactions with the stromal (epithelial) cells of the thymus.

Intrathymic differentiation of T lymphocytes requires cell-to-cell interaction between lymphoid cells and thymic epithelial cells, which produce the various hormones (thymopoietin, thymosine, thymic humoral factor, etc.) that promote maturation. The effects of these hormones are augmented by lymphokines produced by mature T cells in the medulla. The final result is a selection of T cells that recognize, but do not react with, cells identical in surface molecules of the major histocompatibility complex (MHC) genes. It is their stay in the thymus that makes T lymphocytes immunocompetent.

Immunocompetent T lymphocytes leave the thymus and settle in distinct loci in lymphoid tissues, spleen, and lymph nodes (figure 3.5). Some T cells travel constantly from lymph nodes and spleen back into efferent lymphatics and from there into the venous and arterial circulation. They leave the circulation in postcapillary venules, percolate through tissues, and eventually reenter the lymphatics. When a T cell encounters the specific antigen with which it can interact, it may then undergo **blastic transformation**, proliferate, and develop into a clone of cells, some of which beocme the effector cells that mediate specific cellular immunity. Other clone members may persist as "memory cells" for subsequent encounters with the same antigen.

T lymphocytes are recognized in the laboratory by their ability to form "rosettes" with sheep red cells and by the presence of certain surface markers—for example, CD2 (T11), the sheep red cell binding protein, or CD3, a part of the T cell antigen receptor complex, which appears late in maturation.

(1) Classification

There are three major T cell categories.

- **Helper T cells** regulate—or help—other cells. For example, they help B cells to secrete antibody, T cytolytic cells to become functional, and macrophages to become activated.
- **Suppressor T cells** act to limit or terminate the immune response. The intensity of their influence reflects the balance existing between helper and suppressor functions. Extreme shifts in this balance may result in abnormalities of immune function, such as occur in AIDS.
- **Cytolytic** (or **killer**) **T cells** recognize specific antigens in the surfaces of abnormal cells (e.g., tumor cells, cells infected with viruses), attach to them and destroy them. Null cells, a lymphocyte subset lacking T and B markers, also display cell-mediated cytotoxicity. They include natural killer (NK) cells and antibody-mediated killer (K) cells. When the cytotoxicity of these cells is activated by IL-2, the resulting lymphokine-activated killer (LAK) cells actively attack some tumor cells.

(2) Functions

The immune response is dependent on T cells, which have the following functions:

- They regulate (modulate) the activities of B cells (and other T cells). This is the function of helper T cells and suppressor T cells.

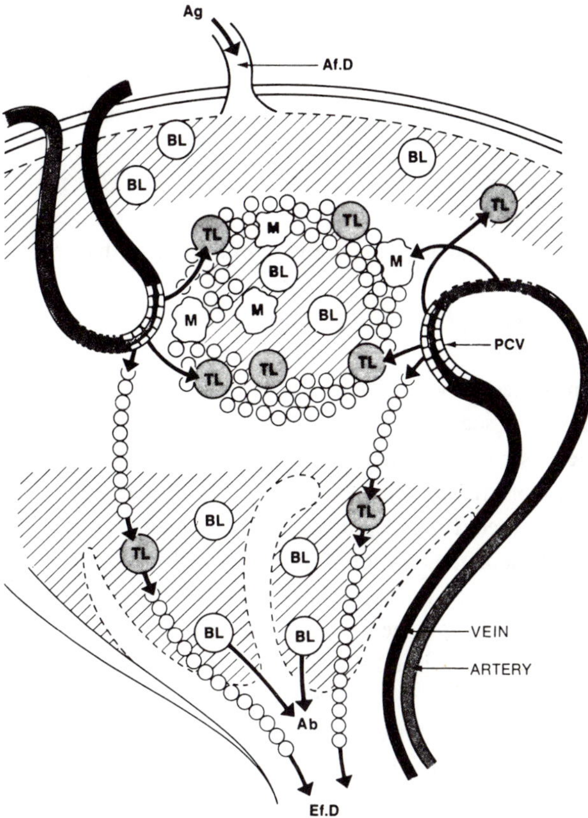

Fig. 3.5
Diagram of lymph node showing characteristic loci of various cells. TL, T lymphocyte; BL, B lymphocyte; M, macrophage; Ag, antigen; Ab, antibody; Af. D, afferent lymphatic duct; Ef. D, efferent lymphatic duct; PVC, postcapillary venule. The crosshatched zones represent areas populated by B lymphocytes. Areas containing open circles represent T lymphocyte regions.) T lymphocytes circulate in close proximity to macrophages, allowing interaction between these cells and specific antigen. (From C. G. Craddock et al., *N. Engl. J. Med.* 285[1971]: 380, reprinted by permission.)

- They are involved in cellular immunity (e.g., delayed hypersensivity, immunity to certain bacterial infections). T cells do these chores by elaborating specific proteins called **lymphokines**, which influence the behavior of macrophages and other cells of the inflammatory reaction (see below).
- They are killers of certain viruses and tumors. This is the function of cytotoxic T cells.
- They are major participants in the immunology of tissue transplantation.

(3) Lymphokines

T cells influence other cells in two ways: by cell contact and by the production and secretion of potent mediation molecules called **lymphokines**. The existence of such factors was inferred from experiments showing that media from tissue cultures of antigen-stimulated T cells contain factors—then termed T-cell replacing factor(s)—that could substitute for T cells in T cell–depleted lymphoid tissues by restoring production of specific antibodies. Within a short time, many factors were discovered in similar experiments. Only after the development of a reliably specific monoclonal antibody to each individual factor was it possible to sort them out.

The major currently recognized lymphokines are summarized in table 3.1. They include the interleukins and a number of other factors, including GM-CSF (not listed in the table). Several generalizations can be made about these factors.

- They are numerous and their effects are diverse.
- They are generally soluble proteins of low molecular weight.
- Most are produced only transiently after T cell activation. CD4 cells are the most prolific lymphokine producers.
- Some have multiple functions, including possible anticancer effects. Many mediate inflammation and may be beneficial as well as harmful.
- Some have turned out to be identical (e.g., lymphotoxin and TNF, perforin and cytolysin).
- Many have been cloned and are being tested as therapeutic agents.

b. B LYMPHOCYTES

The lymphoid cell line that eventually gives rise to plasma cells develops differently. In birds the precursors of plasma cells migrate from the bone marrow to the **bursa of Fabricius**, a lymphoepithelial organ, where they become immunocompetent. The anatomic equivalent of the bursa in mammals is not yet definitely identified. It is probably fetal liver and later marrow. Immunocompetent B cells migrate to spleen and lymph nodes where they occupy distinct sites in the cortex and germinal centers of lymphoid follicles, the superficial cortex of the lymph node, and the medullary cords.

Table 3.1
The Major Lymphokines

Name	Source	Molecular Weight ($\times 10^{-3}$)	Functions
IL-1 (interleukin 1)	Macrophages; T and B cells; fibroblasts	15	Stimulates growth of B and T cells; mediates inflammation; inhibits growth of some cancer cells
IL-2 (interleukin 2)	Helper T cells	15	Binds to receptors on cytoxic T cells, promotes their growth; stimulates growth of helper T
IL-4 (interleukin 4)	Helper T cells; natural killer cells; mast cells	15	Stimulates and regulates growth and differentiation of B and T cells, eosinophils and basophils
IL-5 (interleukin 5)	Helper T cells	15	Regulates production of eosinophils. Activates mature eosinophils
IL-6 (interleukin 6)	Lymphocytes; fibroblasts	21	Promotes macrophage formation. Stimulates IgG production by B cells
Tumor necrosis factor (TNFα, cachectin)	Macrophages; lymphocytes	17	Extensive regulatory effects. Affects immunity, inflammation. Promotes cachexia
LT (lymphotoxin)	Lymphocytes	17	Kills tumor cells; promotes B cell proliferation
MCF (macrophage chemotactic factor)	Lymphocytes	—	Attracts macrophages and monocytes
MIF (macrophage inhibitory factor)	T cells	20–40	Inhibits macrophage motility
Cytolysin	Cytoxic T cells	65–70	Makes holes (pores) in cell membranes that kill target cells

T cells interact with MHC determinants on B cells and macrophages to stimulate the differentiation of B cells into active antibody-forming cells called **plasma cells**. Plasma cells secrete antibody with the same antigen specificity as that of the surface receptor of the B cell from which it is derived.

2. *Plasma cells*

Plasma cells (plasmacytes) originate in two ways (see figure 24.2):

- By a **maturation pathway** (B-immunoblast → plasmacytoid lymphocyte → plasmacyte) that derives from the stem cell (see figure 1.1)
- Through **blastic transformation of B lymphocytes** following antigenic stimulation

The product of both pathways is an enlarged cell with cytoplasmic basophilia (due to RNA in the endoplasmic reticulum so prominent in electron micrographs), eccentric positioning of the nucleus in the cell, and characteristic coarsening of the chromatin masses.

D. Functions

1. *Filtration of lymph*

Lymph nodes remove foreign particles from lymph before it enters the blood. All lymph passes through at least one node. In its tortuous course through a node, it is cleansed of bacteria, dead cells, and other foreign particles by simple mechanical filtration and by phagocytic RES cells. This function is especially important when lymph is infected. Unless infection is severe, it is eliminated by the first node or group of nodes in the pathway of the lymph.

2. *Production of lymphocytes*

As noted, lymph nodes are centers for the proliferation of lymphocytes and other immunocompetent cells, sometimes termed **immunocytes**. Antigens arriving at a node stimulate such cell production.

IV. SPLEEN

A. Structure

The **spleen** is a discrete organ with both lymphoid and RES elements. Indeed, it comprises the largest collection of lymphocytes and RES cells in the body. It is beneath the diaphragm, behind and to the left to the stomach. It is covered by peritoneum and held in positiion by peritoneal folds. Like a lymph node, it has a connective tissue capsule from which trabeculae extend inward. Both capsule and trabeculae contain a few smooth muscle fibers. They are less prominent in humans than in dogs and other animals, in which the capsule is contractile.

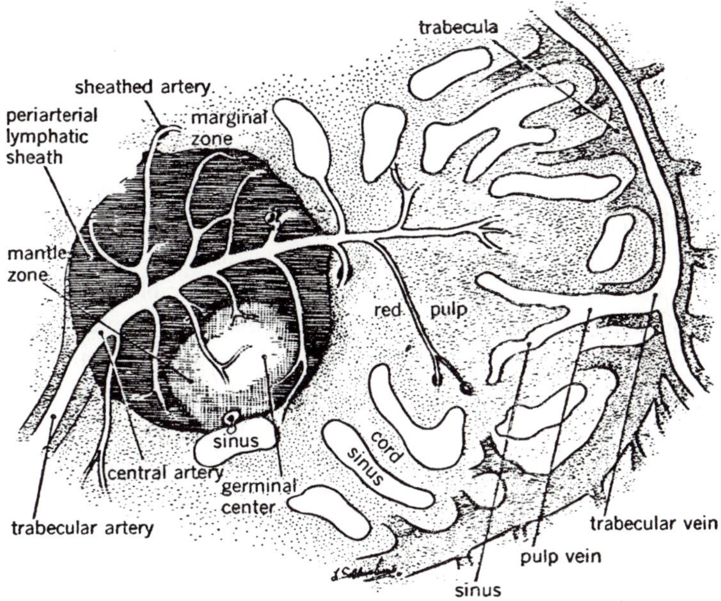

Fig. 3.6
Diagram of organization of blood vessels in spleen. (From L. Weiss, in R. Greep, ed., *Histology*. New York: McGraw-Hill, 1965, used by permission.)

The spaces between trabeculae contain three types of splenic pulp: **white pulp**, **red pulp**, and **marginal zone** (figure 3.6). All are distinguishable to the naked eye on cut section.

White pulp consist of scattered **follicles** with germinal centers and the **periarterial lymphatic sheaths**, sleeves of loose reticular connective tissue that is packed with lymphocytes and free macrophages. The sheaths surround arteries as they enter the splenic parenchyma.

Sheaths are surrouned by a poorly defined region between white and red pulp called the marginal zone. It is made up of a reticular meshwork with narrow interstices, blood vessels, and free cells. Many arteries terminate within it.

Red pulp consists primarily of **vascular sinusoids** (or **sinuses**) that are separated by **cords**. Both are vascular spaces lined by RES cells arrayed upon a lattice-like reticular framework. Sinuses are thin-walled, cucumber-shaped, venous vessels that anastomose freely and form the first stage of the efferent circulation. Cords are bands or septums of reticular fibers that separate sinuses. Many arterial vessels terminate in them.

B. Pathway of circulation

Arterial blood entering the spleen follows a complex pathway before emerging as venous blood. The main **splenic artery** has many branches, called **trabecular arteries**. These enter the white pulp as the **central arteries**, which also have many branches. Some terminate in th white pulp; later branches terminate in the marginal zone; still later branches terminate in the red pulp. Those that acquire lymphatic sheaths before terminating in the white pulp are termed **sheathed arteries**. A few arteries communicate directly with sinuses. Two routes are taken by blood passing through the spleen. A small portion of it passes directly into the sinusoids—or into the cords at a point that affords free and immediate transfer into the sinuses. Blood taking this pathway has a virtually unobstructed route to the venous collecting system and out of the spleen via the **splenic veins**. This is the **rapid transit pathway** or closed portion of the splenic blood flow. Essentially it bypasses the cords. A larger portion of the blood empties into the cords of the red pulp. (The substantial amount that empties into the white pulp and marginal zone finds it way into the cords.) Blood in the cords must navigate the circuitous and macrophage-lined cordal compartmens before penetrating the narrow holes through which it gains access to the sinuses. This is the **slow transit pathway** or open portion of the splenic blood flow. In traversing this pathway through the spleen, blood is brought into intimate contact with the phagocytic RES cells of white pulp, marginal zone, and red pulp.

C. Functions

The spleen is not essential for life, and serious disturbances do not usually follow splenectomy. However, some of the events occurring after splenectomy have yielded clues to the spleen's functions.

1. Hematopoietic functions

The spleen's hematopoietic functions in the embryo were mentioned in lecture 1. The spleen retains the ability to reinitiate broad hematopoietic functions into adult life, namely, erythropoiesis, myelopoiesis, and thrombopoiesis. Extramedullary hematopoiesis in the spleen occurs in several circumstances.

- When there is excessive demand for blood cell production, as in severe chronic hemolytic anemia. Here splenic hematopoiesis is reactive.
- In the poorly understood disorder agnogenic myeloid metaplasia (see lecture 20). Here splenic hematopoiesis is autonomous or proliferative.

Lymphocyte production does occur normally in the spleen.

2. Culling function

The culling function (also termed **hemoclastic function**) refers to the spleen's ability to destroy by phagocytosis aged or imperfect red blood cells. In this role, the spleen acts as an inspector, scurtinizing circulating red cells and removing the few that, so to speak, fail to meet specifications. Such selective destructions are facilitated by the unique splenic circulation. As blood passes through the white pulp, plasma tends to be skimmed off, and the cells are concentrated. This phenomenon, coupled with the slow transit open circulation pathway, leads to stasis of flow, so that opportunities for phagocytosis of old or damaged red cells by RES cells increase. Even after passage through the cords, red cells may remain for some time in the sinusoids. There the glucose supply is rapidly diminished and the oldest cells fail to survive. The red cells are thereby subjected to additional culling. In sum, the materials removed by the spleen in normal subjects include senescent red cells, acanthocytes, and those particles or bodies removed by "pitting" (see below). Materials removed in disease include spherocytes, sickled red cell, hemoglobin C red cells, antibody-coated red cells, white cells, platelets, and microorganisms.

3. *"Pitting" function and reticulocyte conditioning*

The "pitting" function of the spleen refers to its ability to remove particles from intact red cells without destroying them. Such particles include the siderotic granules of siderocytes (see lecture 7), Howell-Jolly bodies, Pappenheimer bodies, Heinz bodies (see lecture 14), and so forth. This function results from the pinching off of particle-containing portions of red cells that are having difficulty squeezing through the pores between cords and sinusoids. The pinched-off red cell reseals itself but, because its membrane surface ares is reduced, it becomes a **spherocyte** (see lectures 12, 14). Some of these cells appear thereafter to have had a bite taken from them.

The intricate splenic filter, which receives 5% of the blood volume each minute, makes the spleen a "training camp" for reticulocytes. Reticulocytes that have excess membrane or weak surface charges are preferentially retained by the spleen. During their sojourn, they are molded, pitted, or if beyond repair culled out.

4. *Immunologic functions*

As noted above, lymphocytes leave the thymus in early life and colonize the spleen and lymph nodes. Lymphocytes found in the adult spleen are partly sequestered blood-borne lymphocytes. The spleen is rich in lymphocytes and RES cells and is an active immunoreative organ. When blood enters the spleen, soluble antigens are skimmed off with the plasma and enter the right-angled arterioles supplying the germinal centers of the white pulp. Particulate antigens lodge first in the red pulp and are transported across the marginal zone into the germinal center, where IgM antibody response begins. Captured antigens are processed and eventually concentrated in the white pulp, where T and B cell interventions lead to antibody synthesis. Splenic macrophages produce many components of the complement system.

When the splenic microcirculation is impaired, as in sickle cell anemia, or when the spleen has been removed, the antibody response to intravenous antigen is blunted. **Tuftsin** and **properdin**, two plasma proteins that serve as opsonins (see lecture 19) and that fall in concentration after splenectomy, are synthesized in the spleen.

5. *Clearance function*

Because of its unique circulation, the spleen is the major site of clearance of poorly opsonized microorganisms. (The liver clears the bulk of well-opsonized bacteria from the blood.) Ninety percent of the blood entering the spleen is dumped into the "open circulation" of the red pulp, and the blood is then forced into the sinuses. This means the blood cells and other particles contained in the blood are required to percolate along the fine meshwork of the splenic cords until they can squeeze through tiny 0.5 μm to 2.5 μm pores between endothelial cells lining the walls of the venous sinuses to enter the venous circulation and leave the spleen. This meandering microcirculation allows time for splenic phagocytes to remove even poorly opsonized bacteria.

6. *Reservoir functions*

The spleen serves as a store or reservoir of platelets, lymphocytes, and reticulocytes. When autologous platelets are transfused, about 30% are pooled in the spleen and can be mobilized by epinephrine.

In dogs, cats, and guinea pigs, the spleen also serves as a reservoir of red blood cells, which tend to accumulate in the sinuses during sleep. The cells are ejected back into the blood under stress or under the influence of epinephrine. Recent studies have cast doubt on the importance of this function in normal humans. A healthy adult human spleen contains only 20–30 ml of blood. Although pooling of red cells does not normally occur in the spleen, with massive splenomegaly up to 30% of the red cell mass and 80–90% of the platelet mass may be pooled in the spleen. There is no evidence that the spleen serves as a reservoir for granuloctyes.

D. Pathophysiology

1. *Hyposplenism: consequences of splenectomy*

Asplenia (i.e., absence of the spleen) may be due to surgical removal perfomed in an otherwise normal individual who has suffered traumatic rupture in the therapy of various hematologic disorders. In sickle cell anemia repeated spontaneous splenic infarction of the spleen may lead to "autosplenectomy" in childhood (see lecture 10).

Functional asplenia or "hyposplenism" may also occur in newborn infants, in old age, and in various conditions leading to RES blockade (e.g., chronic hemolysis in which erythrophagocytosis blocks the splenic RES cells).

A wide variety of conditions are associated with hyposplenism. These can be associated with spleens of all sizes. Atrophic spleens are noted in ulcerative colitis, celiac disease, dermatitis herpetiformis, thyrotoxicosis (Graves' disease), and hemorrhagic thrombocytopenia and as a result of therapeutic irradiation and after radiocontrast studies with thorium dioxide (Thorotrast®). The spleen may be normal sized or large in sickle cell anemia, sarcoidosis, and amyloidosis and with the use of high-dose corticosteroids.

Clinically the diagnosis confirmed by spleen scan. Splenectomy, or "hyposplenism," usually leads to typical changes in the blood:

- A rise in platelet and granulocyte counts, sometimes reaching alarming levels in 10 days and then subsiding to nearly normal values
- Absolute lymphocytosis and monocytosis
- Appearance of Howell-Jolly bodies and other red cell inclusions (see appendix)
- Appearance of many target cells and spiculated red cells ("burr" cells)
- Slight increase in reticulocyte count
- Appearance of giant platelets

In about 10% of normal individuals, small **accessory spleens** occur in the mesentery in the region of the splenic hilum or elsewhere. They may enlarge after splenectomy and rarely may cause relapse of the hematologic condition for which the spleen was originally removed.

Hyposplenic (or splenectomized) children are vulnerable to overwhelming, often fatal, pneumococcal infection. Older patients are more likely to have acquired immunity to the different types of pneumococcus.

2. *Splenomegaly*

A small number (3–5%) of normal subjects have palpable spleens. The major systemic causes of splenic enlargement are summarized in table 3.2. In addition, splenomegaly is rarely due to an intrinsic abnormality such as splenic cyst. The pattern obtained on scanning an enlarged spleen is shown in figure 3.2B. Table 3.3 summarizes the major medical indications for splenectomy.

3. *Hypersplenism*

The term **hypersplenism** is noted for its imprecision. Classically the clinical state given this name is characterized by (1) reduction in the blood of red cells, platelets, granulocytes, or any combination thereof; (2) splenomegaly of any cause; (3) adequately cellular bone marrow (i.e., marrow is compensating adequately in response to cytopenia); and (4) correction of this picture by splenectomy. Since this picture is not always complete, a better definition might be a situation in which the spleen is better out than in. Much evidence suggests that the major cause of blood cytopenias is splenic hypersequestration of blood cells.

SELECTED REFERENCES

Reviews

Balkwill, F. R. Tumour necrosis factor. *Br. Med. Bull.* 45 (1989): 389–400.

Bohnsack, J. F., and Brown, E. J. The role of the spleen in resistance to infection. *Annu. Rev. Med.* 37 (1986): 49–59.

Table 3.2
Major Causes of Splenomegaly

Disorders of the lymphatic system
Viral infections (e.g., infectious mononucleosis, infectious hepatitis.)
Connective tissue disorders (e.g., systemic lupus erythematosus, Felty's syndrome.)
Lymphoproliferative disorders (lymphocytic leukemia, lymphoma)

Infiltrative disorders
Myeloproliferative disorders (myeloid metaplasia, polycythemia vera)
Chronic myelocytic leukemia*
Amyloidosis
Sarcoidosis
Gaucher's disease*
Metastatic cancer

Macrophage disorders
Bacterial infections (e.g., subacute bacterial endocarditis, miliary tuberculosis.)
Chronic hemolysis (e.g., hereditary spherocytosis, thalassemia.* See lecture 14)
Immunocytopenias (immunothrombocytopenia, immunoneutropenia, immunohemolysis)
Parasitic diseases (e.g., malaria,* schistosomiasis, kala-azar*)
Lipidoses (e.g., Gaucher's disease. See lecture 26)
Histiocytoses (e.g., Letterer-Siwe disease. See lecture 26)
Hairy cell leukemia*

Vascular congestion
Splenic or portal vein thrombosis
Hepatic cirrhosis
Budd-Chiari syndrome

*These disorders are often associated with massive splenomegaly, with the spleen extending into the lower quadrants of the abdomen.

Table 3.3
Major Indications for Splenectomy

To control (or stage) basic disease
Hereditary spherocytosis
Immunothrombocytopenia
Immunohemolysis
Hodgkin's disease

To correct chronic or severe hypersplenic symptoms
Hairy cell leukemia
Felty's syndrome
Myeloid metaplasia
Thalassemia major
Gaucher's disease
Hemodialysis splenomegaly
Splenic vein thrombosis

Callard, R. E. Cytokine regulation of B-cell growth and differentiation. *Br. Med. Bull.* 45 (1989): 371–388.

Dinarello, C. A. Interleukin-1 and its biologically related cytokines. *Adv. Immunol.* 44 (1989): 153–206.

Dinarello, C. A., and Savage, N. Interleukin-1 and its receptor. *CRC Crit. Rev. Immunol.* 9 (1989): 1–20.

Feldmann, M., Londei, M., et al. T cells and lymphokines. *Br. Med. Bull.* 45 (1989): 361–370.

Fowlkes, B. J., and Pardoll, D. M. Molecular and cellular events of T cell development. *Adv. Immunol.* 44 (1989): 207–264.

Kelos, A., and Metcalf, D. T lymphocyte-derived colony-stimulating factors. *Adv. Immunol.* 48 (1990): 69–106.

Kincade, P. W. The lymphopoietic microenvironment in bone marrow. *Adv. Cancer Res.* 54 (1990): 235–272.

Mizel, S. B. The interleukins. *FASEB J.* 3 (1989): 2379–2388.

Mosmann, T. R., and Coffman, R. L. Heterogeneity of cytokine secretion patterns and functions of helper T cells. *Adv. Immunol.* 46 (1989): 111–148.

Owen, J. J. T. and Jenkinson, E. J. Regulatory factors in lymphoid development. *Br. Med. Bull.* 45 (1989): 350–360.

Paige, C. J., and Wu, G. E. The B cell repertoire. *FASEB J.* 3 (1989): 1818–1824.

Wadenvik, H., and Kutti, J. The spleen and pooling of blood cells. *Eur. J. Haematol.* 41 (1988): 1–5.

Young, L. H. Y., Liu, C.-C., et al. How lymphocytes kill. *Annu. Rev. Med.* 41 (1990): 45–54.

Young, M., and Geha, R. S. Human regulatory T-cell subsets. *Annu. Rev. Med.* 37 (1986): 165–172.

Original articles

Aster, R. H. Pooling of platelets in the spleen: role in the pathogenesis of "hypersplenic" thrombocytopenia. *J. Clin. Invest.* 45 (1966): 645.

Chen, L.-T. Microcirculation of the spleen: an open or closed circulation? *Science* 201 (1978): 157.

Eichner, E. R. Splenic function: Normal, too much, too little. *Am. J. Med.* 66 (1979): 311.

Najar, H. M., Ruhl, S., et al. Adenosine and its derivatives control human monocyte differentiation into highly accessory cells versus macrophages. *J. Leukocyte Biol.* 47 (1990): 429–439.

Otten, U., Ehrhard, P., et al. Nerve growth factor induces growth and differentiation of human B lymphocytes. *Proc. Natl. Acad. Sci. USA* 86 (1989): 10059–10063.

Weiss, L. A scanning electron microscopic study of the spleen. *Blood* 43 (1974): 665–691.

LECTURE 4

Normocytic Anemias

William S. Beck

EDITOR'S COMMENT

The normocytic anemias were once a wasteland of hematology, including in their disparate numbers many poorly understood disorders that were generally beyond clinical correction. The most familiar examples, of course, were aplastic anemia and the anemia of renal disease. The recent revolution discussed in the preceding lectures has completely changed this picture: the anemia of renal disease has responded dramatically to therapy with erythropoietin, and aplastic anemia has yielded in many cases to therapy with antithymocyte globulin, bone marrow transplantation, and androgens. While it has been known for years that androgens are sometimes helpful in marrow hypoplasia, newer work shows them to be valuable in modulating immunity and in disorders of cells involved in immunologic processes, including autoimmunity and cancer.

I. INTRODUCTION

A normal MCV and MCHC is a feature of many anemias. In these normocytic-normochromic anemias, as in all anemias, the reticulocyte count is critically important (figure 4.1)

- When **elevated**, it suggests normal or adequate bone marrow function (at least as regards erythropoiesis), and thus suggests hemolysis or hemorrhage as a causal mechanism.
- When **normal** or **depressed**, it suggests the presence of bone marrow failure.

This lecture is concerned with normocytic anemias in the absence of reticulocytosis. Hemolytic anemias are considered in lectures 12–15.

The term **bone marrow failure** signifies failure of the marrow to deliver blood cells into the blood, that is, failure of effective hematopoiesis. A patient with marrow failure may have a hypocellular marrow, which is empty or nearly empty of hematopoietic cells, or a normocellular or hypercellular marrow, which is full of hematopoietic cells. In the latter case, erythropoiesis is taking place, but it is ineffective. Experienced hematologists can usually predict whether the marrow of a patient with marrow failure is hypocellular or hypercellular, but they are sometimes surprised. In many of these disorders, bone marrow aspiration or biopsy is necessary for precise diagnosis.

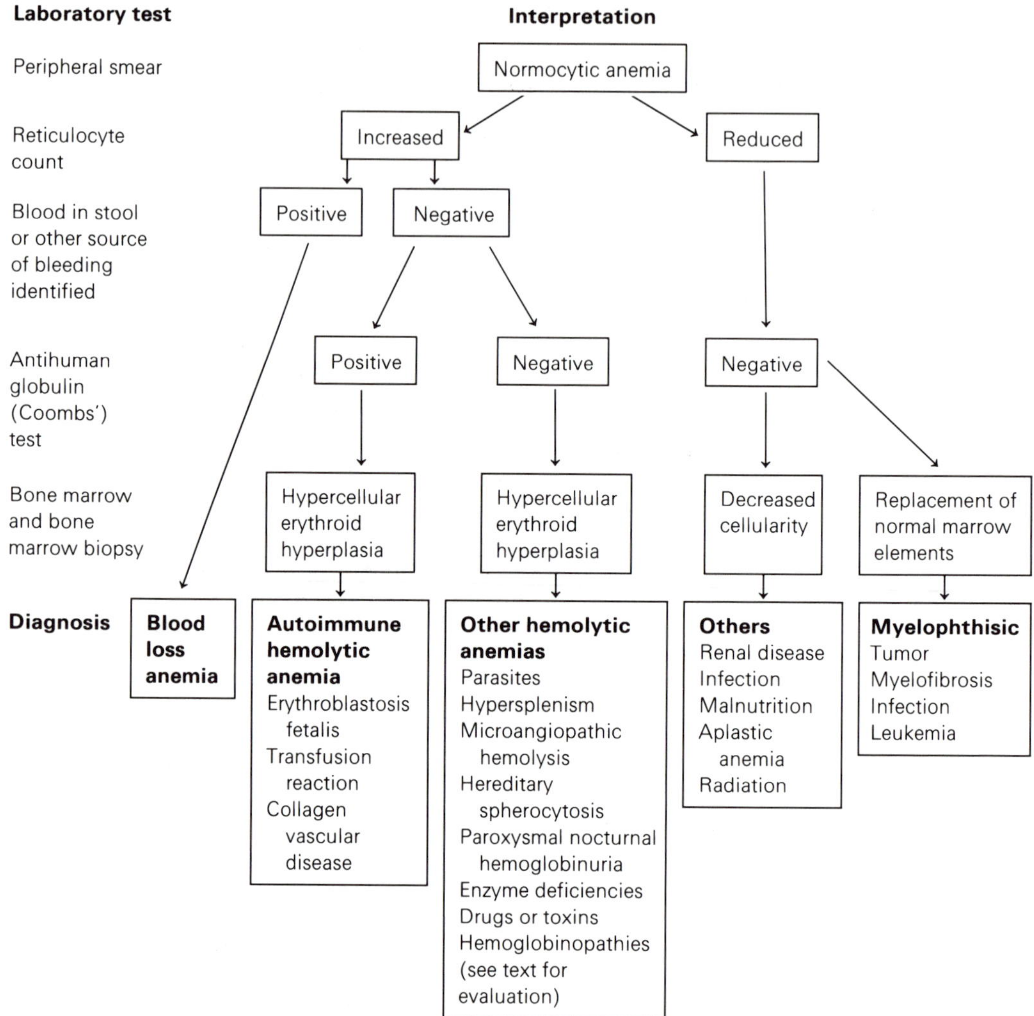

Fig. 4.1
Scheme for investigation of patients with normocytic anemia. This figure represents a convenient approach to diagnosis that is intended only as a general guide.

A classification of the anemias of bone marrow failure appears in table 4.1. Note that some forms of bone marrow failure lead to microcytic-hypochromic anemias while others lead to macrocytic anemias. These two categories are discussed in later lectures. This lecture summarizes the major normocytic anemias of bone marrow failure. Although of diverse cause, they share certain features:

- They are extremely common.
- Many of them are not well understood.
- Often, but not always, they have a poor prognosis. Even so, therapy is often beneficial, especially since the advent of bone marrow transplantation and therapy with recombinant erythropoietin.

A classification of the normocytic anemias without reticulocytosis appears in table 4.2.

II. APLASTIC ANEMIA

Aplastic anemia is a disorder (or group of disorders) characterized by the diagnostic triad:

- Cellular depletion and fatty replacement of bone marrow
- Pancytopenia
- Delayed plasma iron clearance

The second and third elements of the triad are sequelae of the first. It is due to toxic or unknown factors that injure stem cells and impair their capacity to renew themselves. Some evidence suggests that in some cases the microenvironment necessary for stem cell proliferation may be amiss.

A. Terminology

Until the 1930s, physicians were not aware that anemia has many causes. In that decade, they learned that liver extract and iron benefits some anemias and not others, and they began to classify anemias as **responsive** or **refractory**—or alternatively, **regenerative** or **aregenerative**. The classification went no further because until the late 1930s bone marrow was almost never examined ante mortem. It was customary in those days to apply the term aplastic anemia to all instances of refractory anemia with pancytopenia. Thus the term was applied to a functional rather than a morphologic state of the bone marrow.

In 1941, Bomford and Rhoads attempted to classify the refractory anemias on the basis of bone marrow architecture and cellularity observed post mortem. Interestingly, some cases of refractory anemia were found to be associated with a full bone marrow that was normocellular or hypercellular; others were associated with an empty or hypocellular (or aplastic) marrow. Despite the diversity of associated marrow pictures, the imprecise terms **refractory anemia** and **aplastic anemia** have continued in

Table 4.1
Three Bone Marrow Failure Syndromes

Type of anemia	Stage of erythropoiesis principally affected	Functional defect	Marrow morphology	Pattern of cell indices	Causes
Aplastic (this lecture)	Early	Marrow hypoproliferation due to defect of stem cell, or HIM	Hypocellular, normoblastic	Normocytic, normochromic	Chemical agents, drugs, radiation, infection, uremia, idiopathic
Megaloblastic (see lectures 5, 6)	Middle	Ineffective erythropoiesis due to impaired DNA synthesis	Hypercellular, megaloblastic	Macrocytic, normochromic	Cobalamin deficiency, folic acid deficiency, cytoxic drugs, erythroleukemia, inborn errors
Hypochromic (see lectures 7, 8)	Late	Ineffective erythropoiesis due to impaired hemoglobin synthesis	Hypercellular, under-hemoglobinized erythroid precursors	Microcytic, hypochromic	Iron deficiency, thalassemia, lead poisoning, sideroblastic anemias

Table 4.2
Classification of the Normocytic Anemias (Without Reticulocytosis)

Aplastic anemia
Drug (chemical)-induced
Radiation-induced
Viral
Idiopathic
Associated with other diseases (e.g., paroxysmal nocturnal hemoglobinuria)
Red cell aplasia
Acute type
Chronic type
Constitutional type (Diamond-Blackfan syndrome)
Aplastic crisis of hemolytic disease (see lecture 12)
Myelophthisis (marrow replacement)
Metastatic cancer
Granulomatous disease
Hematologic malignancies
Decreased erythropoietin (and other factors)
Chronic renal disease
Endocrine disorders
Protein malnutrition
Myelodysplastic syndromes

vogue, as synonyms of each other and of pancytopenia. This usage has complicated the scientific literature. In the present discussion, the term *aplastic anemia* will be reserved for **pancytopenia** due to morphologic and functional **hypoplasia** of the marrow. Indeed **hypoplastic anemia** is a more appropriate term than *aplastic anemia* since the marrow is never totally aplastic (total aplasia would probably be incompatible with life) and since the pathologic process is often patchy, with island-like foci of normocellular or even hypercellular marrow present.

Although aplastic anemia must always be considered as a possible diagnosis in a patient with normocytic anemia without reticulocytosis, pancytopenia more commonly triggers consideration of this diagnosis. The common causes of pancytopenia are listed in table 4.3.

B. Etiologic classification

1. Drugs and chemicals

Many chemical agents are known to cause aplastic anemia. Many more are suspected to do so from circumstantial evidence, but proof is lacking. Agents capable of depressing bone marrow can be divided roughly into two groups (table 4.4): those that regularly produce marrow hypoplasia if the dose is sufficiently large; and those that occasionally (frequently or infrequently) produce hypoplasia.

Table 4.3
Major Causes of Pancytopenia

Aplastic anemia
Marrow replacement
Myelofibrosis
Metastatic carcinoma
Acute leukemia
Multiple myeloma
Hodgkin's disease
Malignant lymphoma
Lipid storage diseases
Myelodysplastic syndromes
Hypersplenism
Leukemia
Lymphoma
Congestive splenomegaly
Splenic infiltration
Lipid storage diseases
Sarcoidosis
Malaria
Leishmaniasis (kala-azar)
Infection
Miliary tuberculosis
Disseminated fungal disease
Fulminating septicemia
Megaloblastic anemia
Disseminated intravascular coagulation

a. BENZENE

Benzene exposure is a well-known cause of marrow suppression, aplasia, and occasionally leukemia. It was the first clear-cut specific causal agent, having been identified in the rubber tire industry after many workers had been fatally exposed. Benzene has since been incriminated in many hematologic abnormalities, sometimes uncritically, and it remains a serious problem for industrial medicine. Benzene is also present in tobacco smoke. It has been claimed that pancytopenia may occur years after actual exposure to benzene. Many benzene-related chemicals (e.g., toluene, trinitrotoluene, DDT) are also suspected of causing aplastic anemia.

b. CHLORAMPHENICOL

Today the agents causing aplastic anemia are more commonly pharmacologic than industrial. Chloramphenicol is a widely used antibiotic that is the best studied of the agents causing aplastic anemia. The drug is nitrobenzene derivative that commonly causes a brief, reversible suppression of the bone marrow in many (perhaps all) exposed patients. Patients

Table 4.4
Agents Associated with Aplastic Anemia

Those regularly producing marrow hypoplasia if dose is sufficient		
Ionizing radiation		
Benzene and derivatives (e.g., toluene)		
Cytostatic agents (e.g., 6-mercaptopurine, busulfan, melphalan, vincristine)		
Other poisons (inorganic arsenic)		
Those occasionally associated with marrow hypoplasia		
Class	Relatively frequent	Infrequent
Antimicrobial	Chloramphenicol	Streptomycin
	Organic arsenicals	Amphotericin B
	Penicillin, tetracycline	Sulfisoxazole (Gantrisin®)
		Sulfonamides
Anticonvulsant	Methylphenylethylhydantoin (Mesantoin®)	Methylphenylhydantoin
	Trimethadione (Tridione®)	Diphenylhydantoin (Dilantin®)
		Primidone
Anti-inflammatory	Phenylbutazone	Aspirin®
		Acetophenetidin
		Naproxen®
		Gold salts
Antithyroid	$KClO_4$	Carbamizole
		Methimazole (Tapazole®)
Hypoglycemic		Tolbutamide (Orinase®)
		Chlorpropamide (Diabinese®)
Anti-anxiety		Chlorpromazine (Thorazine®)
		Chlordiazepoxide (Librium®)
		Lithium
Insecticide		DDT
		Parathion
Cardiovascular		Quinidine
		Acetazolamide (Diamox®)
		Captopril
		Tocainide
Miscellaneous		Colchicine
		Allopurinol
		Chloroquine
		Quinacrine
		Cimetidine®
		Hair dyes
		CCl_4, Bi, SCN

with this dose-related disorder exhibit anemia and sometimes thrombocytopenia, decrease in reticulocytes, increase in serum iron, and vacuolization of bone marrow cells. Rarely (in 1 of every 25,000 treated subjects) chloramphenicol causes prolonged, self-sustaining, often fatal marrow aplasia. This disorder seems dose-independent. Many of its victims have had previous exposure to the drug. There is now evidence that reversible marrow suppression is due to the ability of chloramphenicol to inhibit mitochondrial protein synthesis. The irreversible suppression, like certain other forms of aplastic anemia, is due to a defect of the stem cells that renders them incapable of dividing and differentiating (see below). Study of this serious medical problem has been limited by the lack of an animal model.

c. OTHER AGENTS

Many agents (see table 4.4) are suspected of causing aplastic anemia because patients with the disease have been previously exposed to them. Some of these are common household chemicals. In most cases, it is possible to do no more than guess at their importance, especially in cases of commonly used drugs such as aspirin. Since the incidence of aplastic anemia with these agents is low, it is assumed that the patient is in some way sensitive or otherwise abnormal.

Despite the pitfalls inherent in any effort to incriminate a specific agent, a serious search should always be attempted. The history should cover the patient's work, hobbies, cosmetics, and daily activities, as well as medications.

2. *Radiation*

High radiant energies (x-rays, γ-rays, and neutrons), from laboratory or reactor accidents or from deliberate therapeutic exposure affect all tissues in which cell turnover is rapid. These include the germinal epithelium of the gonads, bone marrow hematopoietic cells, and intestinal epithelium. Intensive radiation kills cells in each of these tissues, and death of the patient may follow acute marrow aplasia or intestinal ulceration. If the patient survives a critical 3- to 6-week period, surviving stem cells slowly induce marrow regeneration. If stem cells are damaged, regeneration may be incomplete, and permanent marrow hypoplasia with pancytopenia may result. Injury to the microvasculature of marrow may be the fundamental defect in this situation. This injury is believed to alter the stromal microenvironment and thereby interfere with marrow regeneration.

3. *Infection and immunologic rejection*

Aplastic anemia is a complication of several infections, especially **viral hepatitis** and **miliary tuberculosis**. This suggests that an immunologic mechanism may be responsible for marrow aplasia in these cases. This is supported by occasional cases of aplastic anemia following transfusion of whole blood or bone marrow into immunologically deficient children.

Presumably, the mechanism is graft-versus-host rejection of marrow stem cells. In such cases treatment with immunosuppressive drugs might be justified.

Viruses may directly attach or suppress stem cells. Such a mechanism was observed in marrow culture systems in recent cases in which a parvovirus was implicated as the causal agent of aplastic anemia. HIV and Epstein-Barr virus can also cause aplastic anemia.

4. *Constitutional factors*

The term **constitutional aplastic anemia** is applied to poorly understood group of congenital disorders or syndromes. **Fanconi's anemia** is a familial marrow hypoplasia that appears in the first decade of life and is accompanied by multiple congenital abnormalities in other tissues—bone, kidney, spleen, and skin. There is a high incidence of later leukemia and other neoplasms.

5. *Idiopathic*

In about half of the patients with aplastic anemia, an etiologic agent cannot be implicated. These are termed **idiopathic**, though it is likely that many are due to exposure to occult pollutants that have not yet been identified. Occasional cases develop during or immediately after pregnancy. The cause is unknown.

6. *Paroxysmal nocturnal hemoglobinuria (PNH)*

PNH is a rare disease in which red cell membranes and perhaps membranes of other formed elements are abnormal, with resulting hemolytic anemia and other phenomena. It frequently develops as a complication of marrow aplasia and, like other aplastic disorders, may terminate in acute leukemia. Conversely, aplastic anemia can develop in the course of PNH. PNH is discussed in lectures 14 and 22.

C. Pathophysiologic mechanisms

1. *Defects of stem cells, HIM, and suppressor T cells*

Although the pathogenesis of bone marrow failure in aplastic anemia remains unclear, there seems little doubt that it is a result of defective function of pluripotent stem cells. Some of the data from marrow culture studies (see lecture 1) have been confusing. For example:

- CFU-GM counts are low in some aplastic marrows.
- There is suppression of CFU-GM formation of normal marrow when co-cultured with some aplastic marrows.
- Other aplastic marrows do not suppress CFU-GM formation.
- CFU-GM counts are normal in some aplastic marrows.

In some individuals, pluripotent stem cells probably have a genetic or acquired vulnerability. In others, disorders such as myelodysplastic syndrome can cause such chromosomal abnormalities as $5q^-$, which suppress stem cell growth.

Other possible mechanisms include a defective HIM or some immunologic mechanism, perhaps involving suppressor T cells. Recent work in severe aplastic anemia revealed high levels of lymphokines, which (like interferon-γ and TNF) may be cell suppressors. Presumably, therapy with antithymocyte globulin (see below) is more likely to be successful when abnormal T cell activity is involved. Presumably, only bone marrow transplantation could be effective when CFU-GM formation is limited by a defective HIM.

2. *Defects of DNA or DNA repair*

Abnormal DNA (multiple strand breaks) has been observed in lymphocytes of some aplastic anemia patients. This pattern, which may be due to defective DNA repair enzymes, may be responsible for observed maturation defects (e.g., some macrocytic red cells, increased levels of fetal hemoglobin).

D. Clinical features

The onset is often insidious but it may be acute. In the following list of clinical manifestations, the first three are sequelae of pancytopenia:

- Clinical signs of anemia (see lecture 1).
- Susceptibility to infection as a result of neutropenia (see lecture 20).
- Thrombocytopenia and resulting bleeding (especially when infection is present), though it is often not severe.
- Low reticulocyte count.
- Hemolysis is not prominent, but as in other normocytic-normochromic anemias, red cells are somewhat short-lived. Often there is moderate anisocytosis and poikilocytosis.
- In some patients, especially children, red cells may contain increased levels of fetal hemoglobin.
- Hypocellular bone marrow. A biopsy is needed as well as an aspirate. In severe cases, the marrow consists of strands of reticulum with small clusters of lymphocytes, reticulum cells, and plasma cells scattered throughout large areas of acellular stroma and fat.
- Elevated serum iron, sometimes to the point of 100% saturation of transferrin. (The characteristic "ferrokinetics" of aplastic anemia are described in lecture 7.) Iron disappears from the plasma slowly, does not reappear in the red cells as it should, and does not localize in the marrow but is taken up instead by the parenchymal cells of the liver.
- Splenomegaly is usually absent. When it is present, one should seek a specific cause such as leukemia, lymphoma, miliary tuberculosis, lupus erythematosus, or metastatic carcinoma.
- Erythropoietin levels are high. This may account for occasional macrocytosis in aplastic anemia.

E. Therapy

Until recently, the therapeutic mainstays for aplastic anemia were merely supportive. Therapy improved considerably the advent of immunosuppressive agents and bone marrow transplantation.

1. Supportive therapy

Supportive measures include the following:

- Avoidance of suspected offending chemical agent.
- Careful hygiene (e.g., use of soft toothbrush, avoidance of needles) to minimize minor bleeding.
- Transfusion with red cells. The purpose is to buy time until a remission occurs. Unfortunately this happens rarely in adults. Transfusions should be kept to a minimum in order to avoid hepatitis, hemosiderosis, and isoimmunization. Chronic anemia is well tolerated, and it is rarely necessary to raise hemoglobin above 8–9 g/dl. In severe aplastic anemia, this goal can be met with about 2 units of blood every 2 weeks. Careful cross-matching is necessary to avoid immunization with minor blood groups. Washed or frozen red cells are used to avoid immunization to transfused white cells and platelets. Total body iron is about 3500 mg, and the body has no way of eliminating excess iron. Since 1 unit of blood contains about 250 mg of iron, 15 transfusions more than double body iron.
- Transfused platelets are used when necessary, but they inevitably lead to alloimmunization. They are best reserved for life-threatening thrombocytopenic bleeding (see lectures 17 and 28). Leukocyte transfusions have not yet proved reliable. All transfusions should be avoided when bone marrow transplantation is contemplated.
- Corticosteroids are used primarily for their "capillary-tightening" effect in minimizing capillary bleeding. They do not stimulate hematopoiesis. The rise in white count is more likely due to the effect of steroids in blocking egress of white cells from blood to tissues (see lecture 20). High doses of corticosteroids may have a beneficial immunosuppressive effect.

2. Marrow stimulants

Since the work of Shahidi and Diamond in 1959, androgens in high doses have been widely used in aplastic anemia. Somehow androgens stimulate erythropoiesis and sometimes leukopoiesis and thrombopoiesis. The erythropoietic effect of androgen is mediated in other disorders at least in part by an increase in erythopoietin activity. This seems curious since in aplastic anemia plasma erythropoietin levels are already high. When favorable results are obtained with testosterone, they may appear only after several months. Prolongation of therapy (up to 20 months) improves results. Good remissions are obtained in a number of cases. Some responses have been short-lived. Another androgen, oxymetholone, is more effective when given in large doses. Striking remissions are obtained in occasional testosterone-resistant cases. $CoCl_2$ and phytohemagglutinin have been tried as marrow stimulants with unimpressive results.

3. *Immunosuppressive therapy*

In as many as 50% of cases, antithymocyte globulin (ATG), derived from horses immunized against thymocytes, has produced excellent and prolonged remission. The failure of ATG therapy in many cases may be evidence that not all cases of aplastic anemia are immunologically mediated. Although ATG inevitably causes serum sickness, it is often used as initial therapy.

4. *Bone marrow transplantation*

Marrow transplantation would be ideal therapy if it could always be done successfully. In fact, **syngeneic transplantation** (i.e., donor and recipient are identical twins) almost always leads to prompt engraftment.

Allogeneic transplantation of marrow (i.e., donor and recipient genetically dissimilar but matched in major histocompatibility antigens, or HLAs) has presented great difficulties, but improved technique has steadily brought the rate of improvement or cure (in an ideal untransfused recipient) to about 75%. When multiple transfusions have been given, there is rejection in 50–60% of cases.

Before the recognition in the mid-1960s of the importance of HLA matching, allogeneic transplant invariably failed. It was regularly found that when bone marrow cells from a nonidentical donor were infused into a recipient, problems arose not only from graft rejection but also from the reaction of immunocompetent cells in the marrow grafts against recipient's tissues (i.e., "graft-versus-host disease," or GVHD), manifested by skin rash, diarrhea, increased susceptibility to infection, and, ultimately, destruction of engrafted marrow. Even when HLAs matched, half the patients developed GVHD of varying severity. This indicates the probable existence of other histocompatibility loci of importance in tissue tolerance. A higher rate of success has recently been achieved by employing vigorous methods of abolishing the patient's immune response in order to prevent graft rejection, and continuing immunosuppression after the transplant to modify or prevent GVHD. Methods used included total body irradiation, high doses of immunosuppressive drugs such as cyclophosphamide, and antilymphocyte serum. In addition, massive supportive therapy (including a sterile environment) are employed. By such methods, as well as by careful matching of the donor recipient, recent results have been much more encouraging, although the proportion of patients responding varies from series to series.

5. *Splenectomy*

Splenectomy is indicated if active hemolysis is present (i.e., if the transfusion requirement is increasing and red cell sequestration in the spleen can be shown by scanning methods). Some have held that splenectomy has an ill-defined beneficial effect in aplastic anemia even in the absence of hemolysis. The claim is controversial. Splenectomy does lead to better responses to platelet transfusions, especially after the appearance of platelet isoantibodies.

6. *Hematopoietic growth factors*

The use of recombinant Epo. GM-CSF, and G-CSF is currently being evaluated. In view of the basic marrow defect and the already high plasma Epo level, it seems unlikely that Epo therapy will prove useful.

F. Prognosis

Useful statistics are difficult to obtain. Many large series have been reported but with frequent changes in supportive therapy, some involving methods of red cell or platelet transfusion, it is difficult to apply published survival data to cases at hand. Only about a quarter of the patients with idiopathic aplastic anemia survive 5 years. These may be the less severely affected patients. Some live only a few months. Severe anemia is a bad prognostic sign. Most patients die of infection and hemorrhage. A few develop acute leukemia.

III. PURE RED CELL APLASIA

A. Terminology

Pure red cell aplasia (PRCA) is an interesting uncommon disorder characterized by isolated loss of erythroid precursors in the bone marrow. Synonyms include red cell agenesis, erythroblastic hypoplasia, erythroblastopenia, erythroid hypoplasia, and Diamond-Blackfan syndrome. PRCA was recognized as an entity distinguishable from aplastic anemia in 1922. It has received increasing attention because of the appearance of specific erthropoietic failure in association with autoimmunity and thymic tumors. However, it is observed both in association with and in the absence of other diseases. The disorder may be acute or chronic. Both groups include hereditary and acquired cases.

B. Acute type

A self-limited form of erythroid aplasia occurs in both hematologically normal and abnormal individuals. Typically pallor develops rapidly in a patient with preexisting hemolytic anemia (e.g., hereditary spherocytosis, drug-induced hemolytic anemia). The episode is usually introduced by a mild febrile illness.

Laboratory examination reveals a sometimes severe anemia, low reticulocyte count, normal or low serum bilirubin, and normal white count and platelet count. The bone marrow early shows depletion of all erythroid elements. During the early stage of spontaneous recovery, bone marrow displays many early erythroid cells. A brisk reticulocytosis ensues. The recovery phase may be associated with bone pain resulting from bone marrow expansion. In patients who were previously splenectomized for hemolytic anemia, the recovery phase may be associated with an outpouring of nucleated red cells. This "erythroblastic crisis" may reflect the lack of an essential extramedullary site for final maturation of immature erythroid cells.

The cause of such acute crises of red cell production is unknown in some cases. In other cases, they are related to virus infections such as infectious mononucleosis, primary atypical pneumonia, influenza, and parvovirus infections. They are also related to certain drugs, especially diphenylhydantoin (Dilantin®), chloramphenicol (Chloromycetin®), and others.

C. Chronic type

1. Constitutional

In this disorder, chronic isolated erythroid hypoplasia occurs early in childhood. Presumably, it is congenital or hereditary. This is the disorder described in 1938 by Diamond and Blackfan.

Recent studies of BFU-E and CFU-E formation in these conditions point to an inherited stem cell defect of unknown nature. These committed stem cells are diminished in number and Epo-resistant.

Anemia is first observed at age 2 weeks to 2 years. Later signs, including congestive heart failure, hepatomegaly, and splenomegaly, are reversed by transfusion. Subsequently liver damage may be induced by transfusion hemosiderosis, serum hepatitis, and cardiac cirrhosis. Irreversible hepatomegaly and splenomegaly may come to dominate the clinical picture.

Normochromic-normocytic anemia with absolute reticulocytopenia is the rule. White count and platelet count are normal or slightly decreased. Secondary hypersplenism may cause pancytopenia, but examination of the bone marrow distinguishes that condition from the pancytopenia of marrow aplasia. The marrow is cellular, but there is erythroid hypoplasia and a low E/M ratio. Remaining erythroid cells are immature. Myeloid cells and megakaryocytes appear normal.

Transfusions and corticosteroid therapy have been useful in the management of many patients. Some develop prolonged remissions, but many later need further therapy. Of the reported deaths many are due to complications of therapy.

2. Acquired

PRCA arising for the first time in an adult is assumed to be acquired, though this conclusion may be questionable. It is an uncommon and fascinating disease of adults over age 50, characterized by isolated erythroid hypoplasia and an association in half the cases with thymic tumors. Females predominate over males (2:1) in the group with pure red cell aplasia and thymoma; males dominate in the group without thymoma. Association with thymoma (usually a noninvasive spindle cell thymoma) suggests that an immunologic mechanism is involved in the etiology or pathogenesis. Thymic hyperplasia or thymoma is found in association with seemingly unrelated "immunologic" diseases such as myasthenia gravis, hypogammaglobulinemia, and rheumatoid arthritis. The possibility that red cell aplasia is caused by immunologic rejection of erythroid tissue is supported by striking erythropoietic responses to therapy with corticosteroids and immunosuppressive agents and by direct demonstration of autoantibodies against mature red cells (i.e., immunohemolytic anemia), immature erythropoietic cells, and unrelated tissue components. Krantz and coworkers have demonstrated an IgG antibody in the serum of patients with PRCA and with and without a thymoma against bone marrow erythrocyte precursors. A patient of the author's had an IgG antibody that prevented BFU-E formation by circulating stem cells. Her own rate of BFU-E formation was restored to normal in vitro when her serum is replaced by normal serum.

When a thymic tumor is present, thymectomy is useful in preventing possible malignant extension and promoting reactivation of the bone marrow, though it is sometimes difficult to judge its benefits. Remissions occur in 25%, both with and without thymomas, but half of these are sustained without further therapy. Exploratory thoracotomy is undertaken only when x-ray or CT-scan evidence of thymic enlargement is found.

The role of a thymoma in PRCA is unclear. Some evidence suggests that the tumor secretes the antierythroblast antibody, disappearance of the antibody having been demonstrated after thymectomy in one case. However, thymoma may be only one manifestation of a generalized immunodeficiency syndrome.

IV. ANEMIA OF CHRONIC RENAL FAILURE

A. Introduction

Chronic renal failure, whatever its cause, is invariably associated with anemia, the extent of which is roughly proportional to the severity of the uremia, though exceptions are observed. The anemia of renal failure is attributable to several diverse mechanisms that affect red cell production and destruction.

B. Underlying mechanisms

The anemia of chronic renal failure has a diversity of causes. The first three are of primary importance.

1. Erythropoietin deficiency

The role of the kidney in Epo synthesis was discussed in lecture 1. More than 90% of Epo synthesis occurs in the endothelial cells lining the peritubular capillaries in the cortex and outer medulla of the kidneys (the liver synthesizes about 10% in adults). Chronic renal disease usually (but not always) results in decreased Epo production, despite the hypoxia of anemia, which normally enhances Epo synthesis. The decrease in Epo release and the degree of bone marrow compensation vary widely. In some cases, red cell production is well maintained, possibly because of extrarenal Epo secretion. In severe cases, Epo production ceases almost completely. Intensive dialysis does not restore production.

That this is one of the few anemias associated with low Epo levels is confirmed by recently developed radioimmunoassays of serum Epo levels. Indeed, it is now apparent that Epo deficiency is a primary cause of the anemia of chronic renal failure.

2. Hemolysis

Red cell life span in chronic renal failure is shortened. The defect is evidently extracorpuscular since patients' red cells survive normally when injected into healthy recipients and normal red cells have a shortened life span in uremic recipients (see lecture 12). There is a linear relation between blood urea nitrogen levels and red cell life span. Normalization of red cell life span often follows intensive dialysis. Even a mild shortening of red cell survival can have serious consequences when red cell production is depressed.

Changes in red cell membrane ATPase and glutathione stability have been described in red cells suspended in uremic plasma. The burring of red cells in uremia is caused by a nondialyzable, heat-labile plasma factor. By causing metabolic impairment, these factors may promote hemolysis. Another factor is mechanical disruption of metabolically fragile red cells by an abnormal renal microvasculature.

3. Bleeding

Purpura and gastrointestinal and gynecologic bleeding occur in a third of all uremic patients. This contributes significantly to the development of anemia. The basis of the bleeding tendency is not wholly understood. Thrombocytopenia, when present, is rarely of a magnitude to explain spontaneous blood loss. However, platelet function, as evaluated from bleeding time, platelet aggregation, and other platelet function tests, is commonly abnormal (see lecture 28). Since these patients are often closely monitored, iatrogenic blood loss may also be significant.

4. Inhibitors of erythropoiesis

Although nephrectomized uremic animals can respond to administered Epo with increased erythroid activity, the response in uremic human subjects is subnormal and inversely proportional to the degree of anemia.

This suggests circulating toxic materials blunt or block the actions of Epo and interfere with red cell production.

Support for this mechanism in found in in vitro studies with murine marrow cells showing that uremic serum inhibits red cell production in the presence of Epo. Parathyroid hormone, spermine, and ribonuclease are also inhibitors of erythropoiesis. Support for the inhibitor theory is found in data showing that some hemodialysis patients remain anemic even though their serum Epo levels are 3–4 times normal levels. This finding suggests that inhibitors suppress the normal response to elevated Epo levels. However, most of these patients have decreased Epo levels during progressive renal failure and dialysis treatment.

5. *Other factors*

Other factors contributing the anemia of renal failure are:

- Hydremia, which may complicate the hematocrit data
- Nutritional deficiencies (of iron, folic acid, and other vitamins) and defective reutilization of iron (see lecture 7)
- Toxic effects of aluminum and vitamin A

C. Clinical features

Manifestations of renal failure depend on the underlying disorder. However, pallor and anemia are universally present. The anemia is normocytic-normochromic, and usually slightly reticulocytopenic. A few red cells are deformed, some with multiple tiny spicules and others with gross shape changes and loss of volume. These cells have been called, respectively, **schistocytes** (or **burr cells**) and **helmet cells** (or **triangular cells**). The total and differential leukocyte count and platelet count are usually normal, but the underlying disorder may modify the picture. The bone marrow may appear somewhat hypoplastic, but characteristically it is nearly normal in appearance. The normality is deceptive because, in the context of a reduced hemoglobin concentration, a normal bone marrow should display a compensatory increase in erythroid activity.

D. Therapy

Recent progress in the therapy of the anemia of chronic renal failure is a prime example of the successful use of recombinant growth factors.

1. *Supportive therapy*

Until recently, the only therapy available was dialysis. When the anemia was mild to moderate, it was generally tolerated without further therapeutic intervention. In some cases, androgens were tried. In many cases, repeated blood transfusions was mandatory, despite its risks, such as iron loading and viral infections (see lecture 17), and high cost.

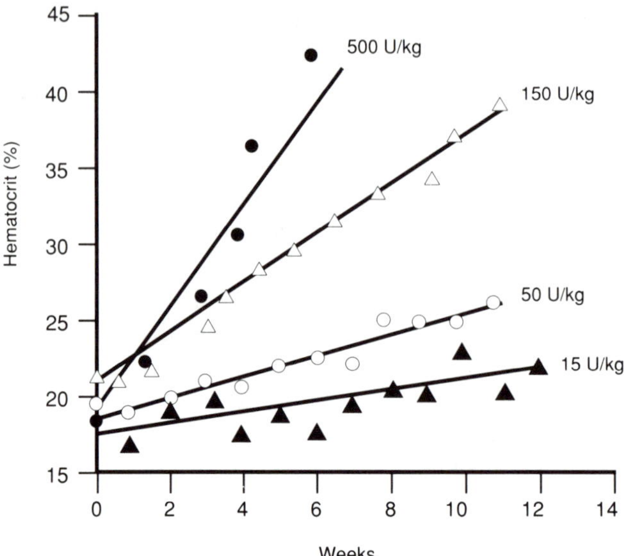

Fig. 4.2
Slopes of the rates at which the hematocrit values (%) rose following various dosages of recombinant human erythropoietin. Mean weekly values for all evaluable patients. (From *Anemia Associated with Chronic Renal Failure* with permission. Copyright Healthmark, New York, NY.)

2. *Erythropoietin*

The advent of recombinant Epo therapy was a major advance in the management of this anemia, which is uniquely associated with low serum Epo levels. In a sense, Epo therapy in these patients is replacement therapy. At this time, intensive investigation is still in progress. Present reports show excellent responses, with dramatic elevations of hemoglobin and hematocrit that obviate transfusions (figure 4.2). Epo is given several times per week (IV or SC) for 12 or more weeks, with repeated cycles as necessary. Exercise tolerance is uniformly increased, but renal function is not improved.

The major adverse event is elevated blood pressure, which occurs in a third of the patients and is manageable with antihypertensive therapy. This probably reflects reversal of the hemodynamic adaptation to anemia. Another adverse effect is financial. At present, Epo therapy is extremely costly.

V. ANEMIA OF ENDOCRINE DISEASE

Many hormones (in addition to erythropoietin) participate in the regulation of erythropoiesis, and patients lacking such hormones often develop hypoplastic anemia. Hormones that affect enzymes and protein synthesis also affect synthesis of hemoglobin and production of red cells. The hormones most often involved in the development of hypoplastic anemia are those of the pituitary, thyroid, adrenal cortex, and gonads.

A. Anemia of pituitary deficiency

Hypophysectomy in an experimental animal leads to the development of a moderate hypoplastic anemia owing to loss of adenohypophyseal hormones. Of these, the thyroid-stimulating hormone seems most important since the anemia of hypophysectomy resembles the anemia of thyroidectomy. In human subject, pituitary dysfunction or pituitary ablation leads to normochromic-normocytic anemia. Red cell life span is normal, but bone marrow examination and ferrokinetic studies disclose relative bone marrow failure and moderate hypoplastic anemia. Replacement therapy with combination of thyroid, adrenal, and gonadal hormones usually reverse the anemia.

B. Anemia of thyroid disease

1. Hypothyroidism

The mechanism of anemia observed in patients with myxedema or other hypothyroid disorders is not always clear-cut since the conditions may be complicated by nutritional deficiencies. However, many hypothyroid patients have hypoplastic anemia that is unresponsive to therapy with iron, cobalamin, or folic acid and that is similar to the normochromic-normocytic, reticulocytopenic anemia of thyroidectomized animals. In this disorder, red cell life span is normal, and ferrokinetics indicates hypoactive but effective marrow function. The anemia in hypothyroid subjects is mild to moderate with a hemoglobin concentration rarely less than 8–9 g/dl. The hematocrit may not accurately reflect the reduction of bone marrow activity and red cell mass since plasma volume is decreased in hypothyroidism. This may result in temporary aggravation of "anemia" after thyroid replacement therapy since plasma volume is restored to normal before red cell mass. Although the characteristic anemia of hypothyroidism is normochromic-normocytic, the anemia observed may be microcytic-hypochromic due to iron deficiency resulting from (1) menorrhagia, a frequent complication; (2) achlorhydria, present in half the anemic patients; or (3) intestinal malabsorption of iron. The anemia may also be macrocytic. Occasionally hypothyroidism coexists with true pernicious anemia (see lecture 5).

2. Hyperthyroidism

Despite the erythropoietic effect of thyroid hormones in experimental animals, patients with hyperthyroidism or thyrotoxicosis rarely have elevated hemoglobin concentration. However, since the erythroid activity of the marrow and the turnover of plasma and red cell iron are above normal, an increase in plasma volume may keep the hematocrit within normal limits. Red cell life span is moderately shortened in patients with thyrotoxicosis. In a few severe cases, iron utilization is subnormal.

C. Anemia of adrenal disease

Adrenalectomy in animals causes a mild anemia responsive to therapy with corticosteroids or erythropoietin. A similar normochromic-normocytic anemia occurs in Addison's disease, but becasue of the concomitant reduction in plasma volume, the hemoglobin and hematocrit do not reflect the true red cell mass. The basis of this anemia and the erythropoietic effect of ACTH and cortical hormones (in physiologic amounts) is not known.

D. Anemia of gonadal disease

The erythropoietic effect of androgen is well known and extensively utilized in the treatment of patients with various types of refractory anemia.Castration of the male animal causes a decrease in the rate of red cell production until hemoglobin concentration and red cell mass become stabilized at levels approximating those of the normal female. In pharmacologic doses, androgens are potent stimulators of red cell production. They act by enhancing either the production of erythropoietin or its effect on the bone marrow.

VI. MYELOPHTHISIS

A. Definition

The archaic, tongue-twisting term **myelophthisis** denotes a situation in which bone marrow has been replaced by nonmarrow elements. Common invaders of the bone marrow cavity are leukemic cells, tumor cells, infectious granulomas, fibrous tissue, and lipid storage cells. It is commonly said that the resulting anemia is due to simple mechanical replacement of bone marrow. However, the pathophysiology is probably more complex. For example, the anemia may be due in part to local competition between invading cells and hematopoietic cells for essential nutrients. There is also evidence that metastatic tumor lesions or granulomas may secrete substances that are inhibitory to surrounding marrow cells. It is of interest in this regard to note that some of the same peripheral blood alterations found in patients with metastases to the bone marrow are also observed in patients who have metastatic cancer without marrow involvement.

B. Clinical features

Typical clinical features of myelophthisis include:

- Normocytic-normochromic anemia with reticulocytopenia
- **Leukoerythroblastic reaction**: elevated white count with immature white cells and nucleated red cells in the blood (see lecture 21)
- Anisocytosis, poikilocytosis, and teardrop forms of red cells
- Low, normal, or high platelet count, often with bizarre or giant platelets

Table 4.5
Common Causes of Anemia in Cancer Patients

Secondary to the cancer
A. Inhibition of erythrocyte production
  1. Myelophthisis (see text)
  2. Folate deficiency (see lecture 6)
  3. Iron deficiency (due to bleeding) (see lecture 7)
  4. Anemia of chronic disease (see lecture 7)
B. Hemolysis
  1. Immunohemolytic anemia (see lecture 13)
  2. Microangiopathic hemolytic anemia (see lecture 14)
Secondary to treatment
A. Marrow suppression, hypoplasia (see text)
B. Hemolysis
  1. Immunohemolytic anemia (see lecture 13)
  2. Microangiopathic hemolytic anemia (see lecture 14)
  3. Oxidative hemolysis (see lecture 14)
  4. Transfusion reactions (see lecture 17)
C. Bleeding (see lectures 2, 29)

The diagnosis rests on histologic demonstration of invading cells in a bone marrow biopsy.

C. On the anemia of cancer

Anemia is common in cancer patients (see lecture 21), but myelophthisic involvement of bone marrow by tumor cells is only one of its many possible causes. As shown in table 4.5, these causes are usefully grouped into those secondary to the cancer and those secondary to therapy. Many of these disorders are discussed in later lectures.

VII. MYELODYSPLASTIC SYNDROMES

This now widely used term replaces **preleukemia**, **sideroachrestic anemia**, and a cluster of other vague terms that dot the literature. This marrow disorder, which often antedates acute myelocytic leukemia, is discussed in lecture 22. We list it here as a common cause of marrow failure with normochromic-normocytic anemia, though in some cases red cells are macrocytic. Red cells are often misshapen, with teardrop forms, elliptocytes, and other odd shapes.

SELECTED REFERENCES

Reviews

Adamson, J. W. and Erslev, A. J. Aplastic anemia. In Williams, W. J., Beutler, E., et al., ed. *Hematology*, 4th ed. New York: McGraw-Hill, 1990, pp. 158–747.

Adamson, J. W. and Eschbach, J. W. Management of the anaemia of chronic renal failure with recombinant erythropoietin. *Q. J. Med.* 73(1989): 1093–1101.

Adamson, J. W. and Eschbach, J. W. Treatment of the anemia of chronic renal failure with recombinant human erythropoietin. *Annu. Rev. Med.* 41(1990): 349–360.

Aitchison, R. G. M., Marsh. J. C. W., et al. Pregnancy associated aplastic anaemia: a report of five cases and review of current management. *Br. J. Haematol.* 73(1989): 551–545.

Bacigalupo, A., Piaggio, G., et al. T cells and myeloid progenitors in patients with severe aplastic anemia (SAA). *Blood Cells* 14(1988): 485–496.

Rotbart, H. A. Human parvovirus infections. *Annu. Rev. Med.* 41(1990): 25–34.

Original articles

Bacigalupo, A., Hows, J., et al. Bone marrow transplantation (BMT) versus immunosuppression for the treatment of severe aplastic anaemia (SAA): a report of the European Group for Bone Marrow Transplantation (EMBT) SAA working party. *Br. J. Haematol.* 70(1988): 177–182.

Chandra, M., Clemons, G. K., et al. Relation of serum erythropoietin levels to renal excretory function: evidence for lowered set point for erythropoietin production in chronic renal failure. *J. Pediatr.* 113(1988): 1015–1021.

Cotes, P. M., Pippard, M. J., et al. Characterization of the anaemia of chronic renal failure and the mode of its correction by a preparation of human erythropoietin (r-HuEPO). An investigation of the pharmacokinetics of intravenous erythropoietin and its effects on erythrokinetics. *Q. J. Med.* 70(1989): 113–137.

Eshbach, J. W., Kelly, M. R., et al. Treatment of the anemia of progressive renal failure with recombinant human erythropoietin. *N. Engl. J. Med.* 321(1989): 158–163.

Koeffler, H. P. Myelodysplastic syndromes. *Semin. Hematol.* 23(1988): 284–295.

Mary, J. Y., Baumelou, E., et al. Epidemiology of aplastic anemia in France: a prospective multicentric study. *Blood* 75(1990): 1646–1653.

Means, R. T., Jr., Olsen, N. J., et al. Treatment of the anemia of rheumatoid arthritis with recombinant human erythropoietin: clinical and in vitro studies. *Arthritis Rheum.* 32(1989): 638–642.

Miller, C. B., Jones, R. J., et al. Decreased erythropoietin response in patients with the anemia of cancer. *N. Engl. J. Med.* 322(1990): 1689–1692.

Ríos, A., Cañizo, M. C., et al. Bone marrow biopsy in myelodysplastic syndromes: morphological characteristics and contribution to the study of prognostic factors. *Br. J. Haematol.* 75(1990): 26–33.

Van der Weide, M., Sizoo, W., et al. Myelodysplastic syndromes: analysis of morphological features related to the FAB-classification. *Eur. J. Haematol.* 41 (1988): 58–61.

Young, N., Griffith, P., et al. A multicenter trial of antithymocyte globulin in aplastic anemia and related diseases. *Blood* 72(1988): 1861–1869.

LECTURE 5

Megaloblastic Anemias I. Cobalamin Deficiency

William S. Beck

EDITOR'S COMMENT

The study of megaloblastic anemia has always been a special branch of hematology, in part because of its rich history and in part because it is one of the categories of hematologic disease that is often correctable. It also has great appeal for its many significant interfaces with biochemistry, biology, and immunology. Historically, many of the discoveries in this field—the liver treatment of pernicious anemia, cobalamin, intrinsic factor, and so forth—had implications far beyond hematology, as they energized and recreated the whole field of clinical investigation. They also changed the character of hematology from a microscope-bound discipline to a dynamic one. The study of cobalamin continues to reveal important new insights, the most recent of which have been the presence of cobalamin analogues in plasma and the discovery of newer, more sensitive methods of diagnosis that have extended the perimeter of the clinical syndrome.

I. INTRODUCTION

Previous lectures pointed out that the major categories of anemia due to bone marrow failure include (1) microcytic-hypochromic anemias (discussed in lecture 7); (2) normocytic-normochromic anemias (lecture 4), and (3) megaloblastic anemias. This lecture considers the megaloblastic anemias.

Macrocytic anemias (anemias in which the MCV exceeds $\sim$97) can be nonmegaloblastic or megaloblastic. The former group includes disorders (e.g., alcoholism, certain hemolytic anemias) in which red cell size is increased but marrow and blood do not display megaloblastic changes. Such changes are found in marrow and blood in the latter group. Megaloblastic anemias are divisible into (1) those due to vitamin B_{12} (better termed *cobalamin*) deficiency; (2) those due to folate deficiency; and (3) those unresponsive to cobalamin or folic acid. Cobalamin and folate deficiency, in turn, have many specific causes. Pernicious anemia, for example, is but one cause of cobalamin deficiency. Care should be taken not to employ "megaloblastic anemia," "cobalamin deficiency," and "pernicious anemia" as interchangeable synonyms as many writers do.

This lecture first discusses the features of megaloblastic anemias in general terms applicable to all cases irrespective of cause. We shall then discuss cobalamin dificiency (first in general terms and then in the context of specific causes) and folate deficiency. This sequence parallels a physi-

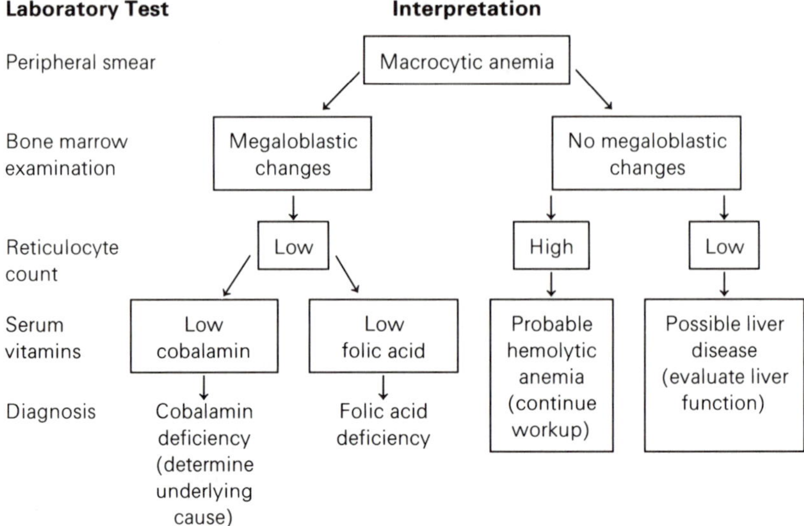

Fig. 5.1
Scheme for investigating patients with macrocytic anemia.

cian's approach to a patient (figure 5.1), which should include the following steps:

- Recognize the presence of anemia (blood count).
- Determine whether it is caused by bone marrow failure (reticulocyte count).
- Determine whether it is megaloblastic anemia (examination of blood smear and bone marrow).
- Elucidate the broad etiologic category (i.e., cobalamin deficiency, folate deficiency), as outlined in table 5.1 (e.g., serum vitamin assays).
- Elucidate the specific etiologic mechanisms (e.g., Schilling test).
- Administer specific therapy and observe the response to treatment.

II. MEGALOBLASTIC ANEMIA PER SE

A. Terminology

Megaloblastic anemia is a widely used though imprecise term for a group of disorders having in common a characteristic pattern of morphologic and functional abnormalities in blood and bone marrow. The pattern is due to impairment of DNA synthesis by any of several causes. The term is imprecise because (1) the condition may be unassociated with anemia and (2) through usage the adjective **megaloblastic** and the noun **megaloblast** have acquired different connotations. "Megaloblastic" denotes an abnormal morphologic pattern in *any* cell line, in and out of the bone marrow. In the marrow, its normal antithesis is "normoblastic." Thus, one speaks

Table 5.1
Etiologic Classification of the Megaloblastic Anemias

Category	Etiologic mechanisms
Cobalamin deficiency	
A. Decreased intake	Poor diet, lack of animal products, strict vegetarianism
	Impaired absorption
	Pernicious anemia
	Gastrectomy (total and partial)
	Destruction of gastric mucosa by caustics
	Other types of gastric dysfuncton
	Anti-IF antibody in gastric juice
	Abnormal intrinsic factor molecule
	Intrinsic intestinal disease
	Familial selective malabsorption (Imerslund's syndrome)
	Illeal resection, ileitis
	Sprue, celiac disease
	Infiltrative intestinal disease (e.g., lymphoma, scleroderma)
	Drug-induced malabsorption
	Competitive parasites
	Fish tapeworm infestations (*Diphyllobothrium latum*)
	Bacteria in diverticula of bowel, blind loops
	Chronic pancreatic disease
B. Increased requirement	Pregnancy
	Neoplastic disease
	Hyperthyroidism
C. Impaired utilization	Enzyme deficiencies
	Abnormal serum cobalamin-binding protein
	Lack of TC II
	Nitrous oxide administration
Folate deficiency	
A. Decreased intake	Poor diet, lack of vegetables
	Alcoholism
	Infancy
	Hemodialysis
	Impaired absorption
	Intestinal short circuits
	Steatorrhea
	Sprue, celiac disease
	Intrinsic intestinal disease
	Anticonvulsants, oral contraceptives, other drugs
B. Increased requirement	Pregnancy; infancy
	Hyperthyroidism
	Hyperactive hematopoiesis
	Neoplastic disease; exfoliative skin disease

Table 5.1 (continued)

Category	Etiologic mechanisms
C. Impaired utilization	Folic acid antagonists: MTX, triamterene, trimethoprim
	Enzyme deficiencies
Unresponsive to cobalamin or folate therapy	Metabolic inhibitors
	Purine synthesis: 6-mercaptopurine, 6-thioguanine, azathioprine
	Pyrimidine synthesis: 6-azauridine
	Thymidylate synthesis: 5-fluorouracil
	Deoxyribonucleotide synthesis: hydroxyurea, cytosine arabinoside, severe iron deficiency
	Inborn errors
	Lesch-Nyhan syndrome
	Hereditary orotic aciduria
	Deficiency of formininotransferase, methyltransferase, etc.
	Unexplained disorders
	Pyridoxine-responsive megaloblastic anemia
	Thiamine-responsive megaloblastic anemia
	Erythremic myelosis (Di Guglielmo's syndrome)

of megaloblastic erythropoiesis, granulopoiesis, or thrombopoiesis. In contrast, "megaloblast" through usage refers only to cells of the erythroid series. In 1880, Ehrlich gave the name **megaloblast** to the abnormal erythroid precursors found in pernicious anemia. He thought these cells belonged to a cell series separate and distinct from that of normal erythroid precursors, which were termed **normoblasts**. Now we regard megaloblasts as functionally and morphologically abnormal normoblasts. The abnormality of an individual cell is usually irreversible, but the overall megaloblastic character of the blood and bone marrow is rapidly reversible in most cases.

In this lecture, "megaloblast" denotes any maturation stage of a megaloblastic erthroid series (the series is: promegaloblast → basophilic megaloblast → polychromatophilic megaloblast → orthochromatic megaloblast → adult macrocyte). Specific maturation stages are referred to by their full names.

B. Megaloblastic transformation

1. Morphology

The following descriptions deal with the morphology of individual megaloblastic cells in Wright's stained smears of bone marrow aspirates (figure 5.2A)

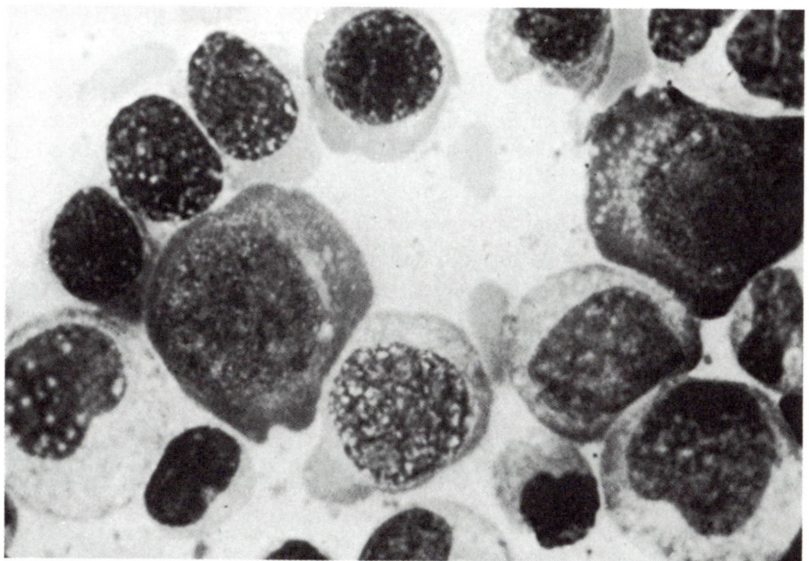

A

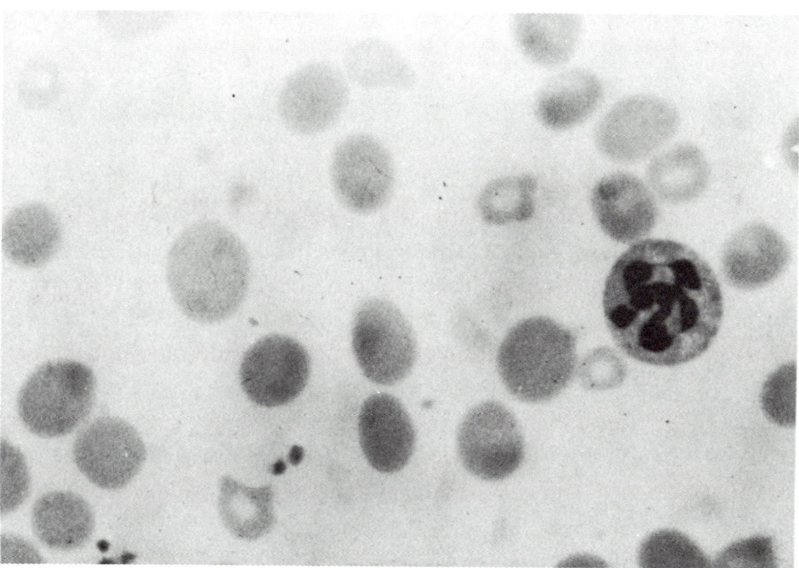

B

Fig. 5.2
Appearance of megaloblastic bone marrow (*A*) and blood (*B*).

a. MEGALOBLASTIC RED CELL PRECURSORS

Megaloblastic erythroid cells at all stages of development are larger than corresponding cells of the normoblastic series and often have a higher than normal ratio of cytoplasmic area to nuclear area. Promegaloblasts, the most immature of the series and the most easily recognized, display a brilliantly colored, deeply basophilic, granule-free cytoplasm and a lavender-tinted chromatin with a characteristic open and fine-grained, or particulate, texture that contrasts with the ground-glass texture of the fibrous or strandlike pronormoblast chromatin. Large blue nucleoli and a prominent perinuclear halo may be present.

As the cell matures, the chromatin retains its granular texture and is slow to form coarse, deeply basophilic clumps. Development of a dense pyknotic nucleus like that of an orthochromatic normoblast either fails to occur or is delayed. With the appearance of hemoglobin, the apparent maturity of the cytoplasm contrasts with the apparent immaturity of the nucleus—a feature termed **nuclear-cytoplasmic asynchronism** or **dissociation**. In mild or incipient megaloblastic anemias, or in megaloblastic anemias associated with iron deficiency and other conditions, the bone marrow may contain partially developed or intermediate megaloblasts.

b. MEGALOBLASTIC WHITE CELL PRECURSORS

Such cells also display nuclear-cytoplasmic asynchronism and apparent enlargement, the most striking enlargement occurring at the metamyelocyte stage. A **giant metamyelocyte** has a relatively large nucleus, sometimes bizarre in shape, with a characteristic ragged or uneven chromatin pattern. The nucleus takes stain poorly and may be pinched off in several places, in apparent anticipation of the hypersegmentation of the mature neutrophil. The cytoplasm appears more immature (i.e., more basophilic and freer of granules) than that of a normal metamyelocyte. Comparable changes may be found in myelocytes and in band forms. The characteristic hypersegmented neutrophil of the peripheral blood will be described below.

c. MEGALOBLASTIC MEGAKARYOCYTES

These cells may be abnormally large. Granulation of the cytoplasm may be deficient. The nucleus is sometimes bizarre, showing numerous distinct and unattached lobes that give the cell an exploded appearance. It should be noted that megakaryocytes are often not distinctly abnormal in appearance.

2. Mechanism

Megaloblasts contain a substantially increased amount of RNA and a normal or slightly increased amount of DNA per cell, the former presumably accounting for the cytoplasmic basophilia; and (2) tritiated thymidine ([^{3}H]dThd) is readily incorporated into the DNA of megaloblasts and, thus, DNA synthesis can occur. These results suggested that the megaloblast is in a state of "unbalanced growth" owing to impaired synthesis of one or more deoxyribonucleotides, the precursors of DNA. As in the unbalanced growth pattern observed in other species, DNA replication and cell division are blocked while synthesis of cytoplasm (RNA and protein) proceeds normally; hence the RNA/DNA ratio rises.

a. PATHWAY OF DNA SYNTHESIS

It had been anticipated that cells in which DNA synthesis is impaired by cobalamin deficiency would contain a cobalamin-dependent ribonucleotide reductase resembling that of lactobacilli inasmuch as the metabolic and growth behavior of cobalamin-deficient lactobacilli closely resembles that of cobalamin-deficient marrow cells (elevated RNA/DNA ratios, unbalanced growth, etc.). However, the scheme of RNA and DNA synthesis in animal cells (figure 5.3), like that in *E. coli*, includes a cobalamin-independent reductase containing a tyrosyl free radical that is stabilized by nonheme iron. As discussed below, the actual role of cobalamin in DNA synthesis is described by the "methylfolate trap theory" according to which cobalamin deficiency results in sequestration of tetrahydrofolate in the form of N^5-methyltetrahydrofolate, which cannot be utilized in the critical thymidylate synthetase reaction (see figure 5.8).

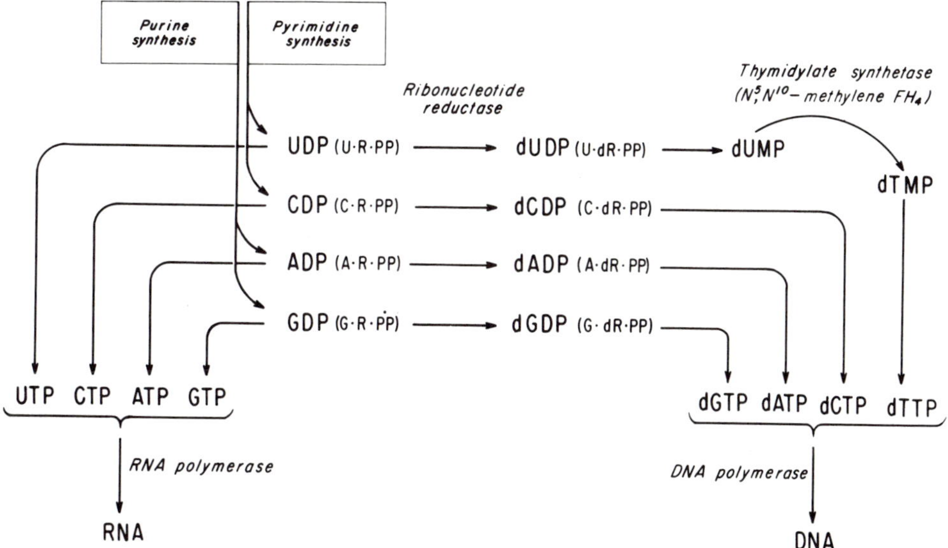

Fig. 5.3
Pathways of nucleotide and nucleic acid synthesis in *Escherichia coli* and animal cells. (From W. S. Beck, *Vitamins and Hormones* 26[1968]: 395.)

b. THE "THYMINELESS" STATE

Until recently, it was believed that the only major consequence of cobalamin deficiency, folate deficiency, and other disorders causing megaloblastosis is impairment of dTTP biosynthesis, with resulting impairment of DNA synthesis. This, it was held, was the critical defect that led to the unbalanced growth state, whether in bacteria or animal cells, and to loss in the capacity for cell division, with eventual cell death. This phenomenon is still an important mechanism in the megaloblastic state, but it is not the whole story.

c. URACIL MISINCORPORATION INTO DNA

In view of data showing extensive DNA fragmentation in megaloblastic cells, a phenomenon that would be difficult to explain entirely on the basis of thyminelessness, a new view of megaloblastic transformation held that there is an increase in dUMP (and dUTP) levels in cells unable to convert dUMP to dTMP (figure 5.4). As a result, there is sharp increase in the dUTP/dTTP ratio. Since DNA polymerase does not distinguish between dUTP and dTTP, uracil is incorporated into DNA in place of thymine. An editorial enzyme, uracil-DNA-glycosylase, detects misincorporated uracils and excises them. Since there is insufficient dTTP for satisfactory repair, DNA is fragmented, with resulting impairment in cell division and cell death. This theory, which is now amply supported, has interesting biologic implications.

First, it suggests that a cell's level of dUTPase, the enzyme normally responsible for preventing accumulation of dUTP, may in part explain the fact that the degree of impairment of DNA synthesis varies from cell line to cell line in megaloblastic anemia. Usually it is more severe among erythrocyte precursors than among granulocyte precursors.

Second, it is clear that the role of uracil-DNA-glycosylase in normal cells is to excise the uracils arising from an occasional deamination of cytosine in DNA. Such an event would be mutagenic since it would alter the genetic

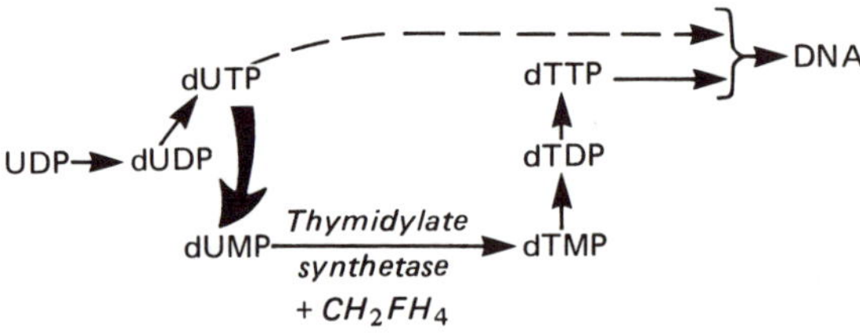

Fig. 5.4
Enzymatic machinery for exclusion of uracil from DNA. The pyrophosphatase, *dUTPase*, destroys dUTP (by converting it do dUMP) before it can serve as substrate for DNA polymerase. *Uracil-DNA-glycosylase* removes uracil from DNA that was misincorporated in place of thymine, or that arose from cytosine by deamination.

code. If DNA were synthesized with a substantial amount of misincorporated uracil in place of thymine (which does not alter the genetic code), the glycosylase would be overwhelmed and play a harmful role since repair would be inadequate.

C. Clinical features

1. General symptoms

The following description includes manifestations that are common to all of the megaloblastic anemias. (Features associated with specific syndromes will be given later.) The anemia is often severe but because it develops slowly may produce few symptoms until the hematocrit reaches a low level. When symptoms appear, they are the usual symptoms of anemia: weakness, palpitation, ease of fatigue, light-headedness, and shortness of breath. Congestive heart failure may supervene. Patients characteristically demonstrate pallor, slight jaundice, glossitis, and stomatitis.

2. Blood picture

a. RED CELLS

Red cells display striking variations in size and shape and are normochromic (unless iron deficiency coexists) and macrocytic with MCVs ranging from 100 μm^3 to more than 140 μm^3. **Macroovalocytes**, oval-shaped red cells up to 14 μm in diameter, are characteristically present (see figure 5.2B). The reticulocyte count is lower than normal, in both absolute terms and terms of percentage. Red cell changes become more severe as the anemia worsens. When the hematocrit is low (i.e., $<20\%$), nucleated red cells may appear in the blood. Such cells show typical megaloblastic features—indeed, frank promegaloblasts are occasionally found.

b. NEUTROPHILS

Many have more than four segments (see figure 5.2B). Some have up to 16 segments. These *macropolycytes* may be very large. Typically, more than 5% of the neutrophils have five or more segments. Hypersegmentation of neutrophils is probably due to an abnormality of nuclear division or of the chromatin itself.

3. Bone marrow

Aspirated bone marrow is cellular. The megaloblastic changes described above may be seen in erythrocyte, granulocyte, and platelet precursors, though frequently major changes are only in the erythroid series. The E/M ratio typically rises from 1:3 to 1:1. Megaloblastic granulopoiesis is more evident in situations such as infection, in which increased granulocyte production is called forth. In typical severe megaloblastic anemia, most of the erythroid cells are promegaloblasts. Many mitotic figures (i.e. cells in metaphase) are found among them. Unless iron deficiency is present, iron in reticulum cells is commonly increased.

4. Chemical changes

Changes secondary to megaloblastic anemia per se include the following:

- Slight to moderate increases in serum bilirubin and iron
- Marked elevation in serum lactic dehydrogenase (isoenzymes 1 and 2) and muramidase
- Occasional decrease in serum potassium that may worsen dangerously in the early stages of repletion therapy
- Decreased serum uric acid

Changes specific to the underlying cause (e.g., cobalamin deficiency, folate deficiency) are discussed below.

D. Cytokinetics

1. Erythrokinetics

Whatever its cause, megaloblastic anemia is associated with two pathophysiologic abnormalities: **ineffective erythropoiesis** and moderate **hemolysis** of circulating erythrocytes.

a. INEFFECTIVE ERYTHROPOIESIS

The following phenomena suggest the presence of ineffective erythropoiesis:

- Marked increase in the number of erythroid precursors in bone marrow and in the ratio of erythroid precursors to released erythrocytes
- Increase in plasma iron turnover to 3–5 times the normal level, with normal iron uptake by individual erythroid precursors (see figure 7.3)
- Increased rate of reappearance of labeled plasma iron in peripheral blood erythrocytes
- Indirect evidence of intramedullary destruction of megaloblasts, which includes: (1) the high serum levels of lactic dehydrogenase (isoenzymes typical of erythroid precusors) and muramidase (from leukocyte precursors); (2) increase in production of "early-labeled peak" bilirubin (see lecture 8) and endogenous carbon monoxide; (3) the ease with which megaloblasts undergo autohemolysis in vitro compared to normoblasts; and (4) the fact, noted above, that marrow reticulum cells phagocytize megaloblastic erythroid precursors

b. HEMOLYSIS

Ineffective erythropoiesis is usually associated with intramedullary cell destruction or hemolysis. A degree of extramedullary hemolysis also occurs, as is indicated by decreased red cell life-span (to one-half to one-third normal), owing mainly to intracorpuscular defect.

2. *Ferrokinetics*

Ferrokinetic abnormalities are:

- Elevated plasma iron
- Elevated plasma iron turnover
- Decreased incorporation of plasma iron into circulating hemoglobin
- Accumulation of iron in marrow reticulum cells
- Increased iron stores in the liver (hepatic siderosis) and other tissues

Unlike the situation in uncomplicated iron overload, radioiron moves rapidly in megaloblastic anemia from the plasma to the marrow. After a period of retention there, it is slowly released, most of it moving to the liver.

3. *Leukokinetics*

Inadequate bone marrow production or delivery of myeloid cells accounts for their decreased numbers in the blood. The elevated serum muramidase in megaloblastic anemia is due to an increased rate of myeloid cell destruction in the marrow; thus, the mechanism of leukopenia is "ineffective granulopoiesis."

4. *Thrombokinetics*

"Ineffective thrombopoiesis" is characterized by an increased megakaryocyte mass in the bone marrow with a decreased rate of platelet production. According to Harker and Finch, the term "ineffective thrombopoiesis" should be restricted to situations in which daily platelet production per nuclear megakaryocyte unit is less than half of that expected. Their data showed that in subjects with megaloblastic anemia, mean daily platelet production averaged 6 (platelets per nuclear unit) compared with a normal rate of 49. Megakaryocyte mass was 4 times normal, but platelet production was 40% of normal. Hence, platelet production was only 10% of that expected from the megakaryocyte mass.

E. Etiology

Table 5.1 summarizes the major categories of megaloblastic anemia according to etiologic mechanism. Cobalamin deficiency and folic acid deficiency are the most common causes, each having many possible causes. Both deficiencies result in a tissue coenzyme deficiency that is correctable by repletion of the lacking vitamin. Repletion is followed by reversion of megaloblastic hematopoiesis to normal. The table also lists megaloblastic anemias that are unresponsive to therapy with cobalamin and folic acid. This group and the megaloblastic anemias of folic acid deficiency will be discussed in lecture 6.

III. COBALAMIN VITAMINOLOGY

A. Historical notes

Classic studies of pernicious anemia (PA) have led to much of our present knowledge of both cobalamin and folic acid. Until the demonstration by Minot and Murphy (1926) of the successful treatment of PA by liver feeding, the disease was frequently fatal. The efficacy of liver treatment implied that the disease is a deficiency state, but its appearance in individuals taking normal diets was unexplained until Castle discovered in 1929 that intestinal absorption of the anti-PA principle of liver—a dietary and therefore "extrinsic factor"—requires prior binding to an "intrinsic factor" secreted in the stomach. An individual with PA synthesizes little or no intrinsic factor; therefore, the resulting vitamin deficiency is a conditioned one caused by impairment of an absorptive mechanism whose biologic novelty sets cobalamin apart from other vitamins. Potent liver extracts soon replaced liver feeding in the treatment of PA, but difficulties plagued investigators attempting to purify the anti-PA principle of liver.

After the unsuccessful attempts of two decades to purify liver principle by E. J. Cohn and coworkers, discoveries of the following factors by workers in the fields of bacterial and animal nutrition led to the discovery of cobalamin; (1) **LLD factor**, a factor in yeast and liver extracts that is essential in the nutrition of *Lactobacillus lactis* Dorner and other microorganisms; (2) **animal protein factor**, a factor obtained from tissue extracts and animal feces that promotes growth of pigs and poultry receiving only vegetable rations; and (3) a **ruminant factor**, lack of which causes a wasting disease of ruminants grazing in cobalt-poor pastures and replacement of which can be effected by oral feeding of cobalt salts (or by dusting cobalt on pastures), parenteral cobalt being ineffective. The discovery and crystallization of cobalamin by E. L. Rickes and associates (1948) of Merck Laboratories followed the astute observation by Shorb of proportionality between the nutrient activity of liver extracts in cultures of *L. lactis* Dorner and their therapeutic activity in PA. The resulting simple microbiologic assay facilitated purification and identification of the vitamin. Animal protein factor and cobalt-dependent ruminant factor were then identified with cobalamin.

B. Nutritional aspects

1. Sources

Cobalamin is synthesized only by certain microorganisms. Whenever it is found in nature, it can be traced to microorganisms growing in soil, sewage, water, intestine, or rumen. Animals depend ultimately upon microbial synthesis for their cobalamin supply. Foods in the human diet that contain cobalamin are essentially those of animal origin—meat, liver, fish, eggs, and milk. Although nitrogen-fixing bacteria associated with leguminous plants are cobalamin-dependent, cobalamin is not found in plant tissues.

The most intensive natural synthesis of cobalamin occurs in rumen bacteria. Of the microorganisms that synthesize the vitamin, many do so in quantities just sufficient for their needs. However, organisms such as the rumen organism *Propionibacterium shermannii* and the antibiotic-producing molds *Streptomyces griseus* and *Streptomyces aureofaciens* synthesize amounts sufficient to make them feasible commercial sources. Some microorganisms that cannot synthesize cobalamin (e.g., *L. lactis, L. leichmannii*) require an exogenous supply and hence are useful in the microbiologic assay of cobalamin. Other microorganisms cannot synthesize cobalamin and appear not to require it (e.g., *Escherichia coli*).

2. *Daily requirements*

The average daily diet in Western countries contains 5–30 μg of cobalamin. Of this, 2–5 μg is absorbed. Total body content is 1–5 mg in an adult man. Of this, approximately 1 mg is in the liver. Kidneys are also rich in the vitamin. Cobalamin has a daily rate of obligatory loss approximating 0.1% of the total body pool.

The daily dietary requirement is 2–5 μg; hence, a deficiency state will not develop for several years after cessation of cobalamin ingestion. Because of the buffering effects of body stores, it has been difficult to obtain precise data on the normal daily requirement.

C. Chemical aspects

1. *Structure*

The chemical structure of cobalamin was elucidated in 1955 by Hodgkin following skillful x-ray crystallographic analysis. The structure displays several unique features (figure 5.5, formula I). The cyanocobalamin molecule (mol. wt. 1335) has two major portions: (1) a planar group, which bears a close but imperfect resemblance to the porphyrin macro-ring (shown in figure 8.1); and (2) a nucleotide, which lies nearly perpendicular to the planar group (formula II). The porphyrin-like moiety contains four reduced pyrrole rings (designated A–D) that link to a central cobalt atom whose two remaining coordination positions are occupied by a cyano group (above) and a 5,6-dimethylbenzimidazolyl moiety (below the planar group). With one exception, the pyrrole rings are connected to one another by methene carbon bridges similar to those found in porphyrins. The exception is the direct linkage between the α-carbons of rings A and D. The macro-ring of cobalamin and related compounds is termed **corrin**; the major corrin derivatives are known generically as **corrinoid** compounds. Both corrin and porphin macro-rings are synthesized from δ-aminolevulinic acid.

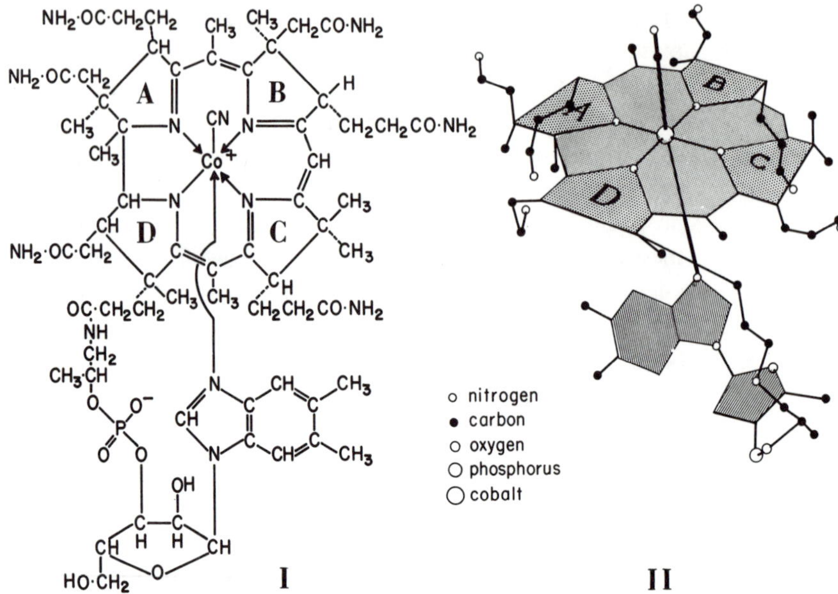

Fig. 5.5
Chemical structure of cyanocobalamin. *Formula I*, molecular structure; *Formula II*, semidiagrammatic representation of three-dimensional structure showing relations of planar and nucleotide moieties. Hydrogen atoms and a number of oxygen atoms are omitted. (From W. S. Beck, *N. Engl. J. Med.* 266[1962]: 708.)

2. *Nomenclature*

Many corrinoid compounds are known. Some occur naturally; others have been prepared synthetically. Compounds were early given trivial names (e.g., cobalamin). Even the semisystematic term **cobalamin** was introduced before chemical structure was known. After much confusion, approval was given in 1973 to a system of names and abbreviations. Table 5.2 lists these terms for the four compounds found in the human body. In this system cobalamin becomes cyanocobalamin. In other compounds, the cyano-ligand is replaced by another moiety.

The four compounds of importance in animal cell metabolism are the vitamin **cyanocobalamin** (CN-Cbl) and its analogue **hydroxocobalamin** (OH-Cbl) and the two coenzyme forms **adenosylcobalamin** (AdoCbl) and **methylcobalamin** (MeCbl). In AdoCbl, a 5′-deoxyadenosyl moiety is the ligand of cobalt above the plane (figure 5.6). This coenzyme, discovered by H. A. Barker in studies of the isomerization of glutamate by bacterial extracts, was soon identified as the main storage form of cobalamin in liver.

- In AdoCbl the 5′-methylene carbon atom of the 5′-deoxyadenosyl moiety is linked directly to the cobalt atom.
- In MeCbl, the ligand of cobalt is a methyl group. MeCbl cobalamin occurs in small amounts in liver. Yet it is the major cobalamin in blood plasma.

Table 5.2
Names of Cobalamins Found in Human Body

Semisystematic name	Abbreviation	Systematic name
Cyanocobalamin*	CN-Cbl	α-(5,6-dimethylbenzimidazolyl)-cyanocobamide
Hydroxocobalamin	OH-Cbl	α-(5,6-dimethylbenzimidazolyl)-hydroxocobamide
Adenosylcobalamin	AdoCbl	α-(5,6-dimethylbenzimidazolyl)-adenosylcobamide
Methylcobalamin	MeCbl	α-(5,6-dimethylbenzimidazolyl)-methylcobamide

*Also called vitamin B_{12}.

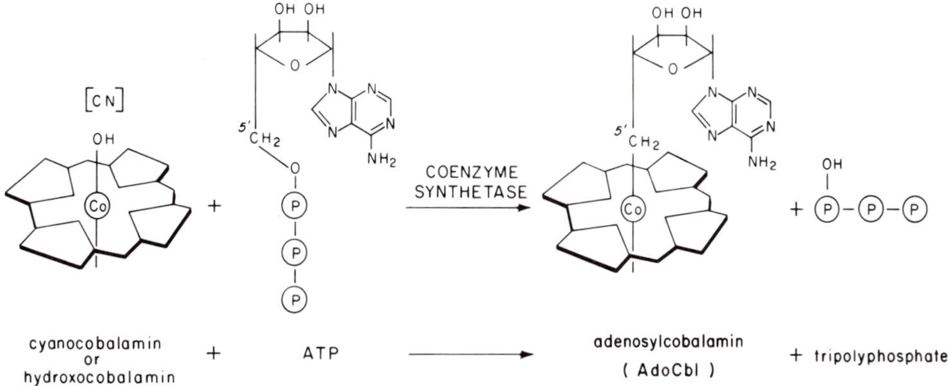

Fig. 5.6
The coenzyme synthetase system in which ATP adenosylates cobalamin to form adenosylcobalamin. The reaction requires a thiol and a reduced flavin or ferredoxin. Reducing agents are required in a preliminary step that converts tervalent cobalt of cobalamin (termed cob(III)alamin) through the bivalent state (cob(II)alamin) to the univalent state (cob(I)alamin), which has nucleophilic properties. (From W. S. Beck, in W. J. Williams et al., *Hematology*, 3d ed. New York: McGraw-Hill, 1983.)

- CN-Cbl occurs only from the attack by cyanide on coenzyme forms and other cobalamins.

In both coenzyme forms the carbon-cobalt bond is labile to light, cyanide, and acid. The fragility of this bond makes cobalamin an excellent free radical former. This property accounts for its metabolic functions.

D. Metabolic functions

Only two cobalamin-dependent enzymes are found in human tissues. (Many more occur in bacteria.)

1. AdoCbl-dependent methylmalonyl CoA mutase

AdoCbl functions as an acceptor-donor of hydrogen. On the coenzyme, hydrogen is carried by C-5′ of the adenosyl group. The only AdoCbl-dependent enzyme in animal tissues is **methylmalonl CoA mutase**:

$$\underset{\text{methylmalonyl CoA}}{CH_3{-}\overset{\overset{\displaystyle COCoA}{|}}{C}H{-}COOH} \underset{}{\overset{\text{AdoCbl}}{\rightleftharpoons}} \underset{\text{succinyl CoA}}{\overset{\overset{\displaystyle COCoA}{|}}{C}H_2{-}CH_2{-}COOH}$$

This reaction is a step in the pathway of propionic acid catabolism (figure 5.7). Propionic acid is metabolized in animal tissues by a biotin-dependent carboxylation of propionyl CoA to methylmalonyl CoA, an α-carboxy derivative of propionyl CoA. After a racemization step, methylmalonyl CoA mutase catalyzes the reversible conversion of methylmalonyl CoA to its β-carboxy isomer, succinyl CoA, which after deacylation enters the tricarboxylic acid cycle.

2. MeCbl-dependent methyltransferase

MeCbl participates in the cobalamin-dependent synthesis of methionine in bacteria and animal cells according to the scheme in figure 5.7. This pathway, one of several pathways of methionine synthesis, serves primarily as a means for converting N^5-methyltetrahydrofolate to tetrahydrofolate (see lecture 6). Interestingly, nitrous oxide (N_2O), an anesthetic gas, impairs this enzyme by promoting the oxidation of cob(I)alamin to cob(III)alamin, thereby depleting the level of MeCbl and producing a state resembling cobalamin deficiency. N_2O thus offers a useful research tool.

3. Cobalamin deficiency in metabolism

As noted above, an explanation for the role of cobalamin in animal cell DNA synthesis finally won acceptance after long controversy. According to the so-called "methylfolate trap" theory, cobalamin deficiency slows the cobalamin-dependent pathway of methionine synthesis (figure 5.8). As a result, folate is sequestered as N^5-methyltetrahydrofolate, a form that is unavailable to the critical thymidylate synthetase reaction (see figure 5.2).

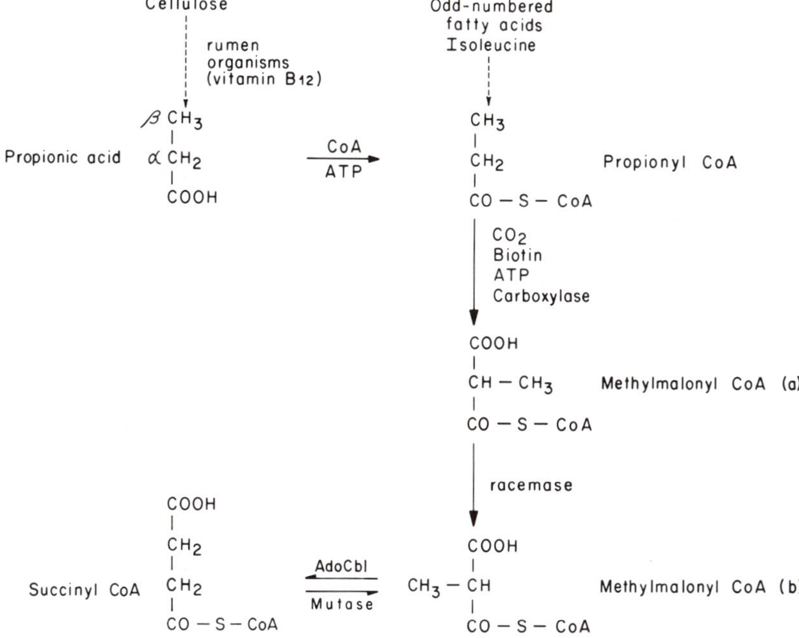

Fig. 5.7
Pathway of propionic acid metabolism.

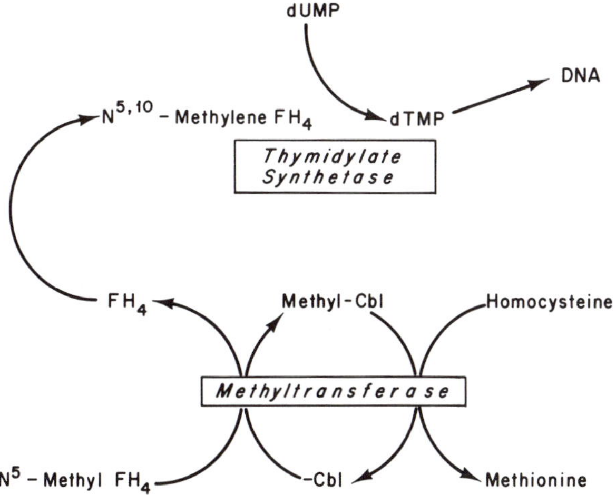

Fig. 5.8
Diagram of relation between N^5-methyltetrahydrofolate: homocysteine methyltransferase and thymidylate synthetase. In cobalamin deficiency, folate is sequestered as N^5-methyltetrahydrofolate. This ultimately deprives thymidylate synthetase of its folate coenzyme (N^5, N^{10}-methylene FH_4) and thereby impairs DNA synthesis.

Evidence favoring this theory includes the following abnormalities in cobalamin deficiency: (1) altered partitioning of tissue folate compounds; (2) elevated serum N^5-methyltetrahydrofolate levels; and (3) increased excretion of formiminoglutamic acid after histidine loading in some subjects. Other supporting evidence is discussed in lecture 6.

In summary, the two metabolic systems impaired in cobalamin deficiency are (1) methylmalonyl CoA isomerization, and thus propionate catabolism; and (2) methionine methyl synthesis, and thus tetrahydrofolate regeneration. Impairment of DNA synthesis accounts for megaloblastic erythropoiesis and related phenomena. Trapping of folate as N^5-methyltetrahydrofolate impairs thymidylate synthesis, which depresses DNA synthesis, and causes accumulation of dUTP, which causes uracil misincorporation into DNA. This mechanism may also underlie the neurologic damage of human cobalamin deficiency. However, impairment of methylmalonyl CoA metabolism is probably more important. (see below) since nondividing nerve cells are not engaged in DNA synthesis.

E. Physiologic aspects

1. Intestinal absorption: the intrinsic factor mechanism

Intrinsic factor (IF), a protein normally present in human gastric juice, is necessary for the absorption in the ileum of ingested cobalamins. Following discovery of IF by Castle in 1929, efforts to purify it were complicated by the need before the advent of radioactive cobalamin to use a patient in relapse as an assay system. Substantial purifications were finally achieved in 1973 by the use of affinity chromatographic methods. This elegant work opened a new era in the study of IF and other cobalamin-binding proteins.

a. STRUCTURE OF IF

Human IF is an alkali-stable glycoprotein that binds a molecule of cobalamin (cyano-, hydroxo-, or adenosyl-derivative) with high affinity. The mol. wt. is about 44,000 (human IF) and 50,000–59,000 (hog IF). IF contains about 15% carbohydrate. When bound to cobalamin, IF forms dimers. Bound vitamin alters the conformation of IF, producing a more compact form that is more resistant to proteolytic digestion (although free IF is more resistant to proteolysis than once believed).

b. COBALAMIN-BINDING PROTEINS OF GASTRIC JUICE

Gastric juice contains several cobalamin-binding proteins (table 5.3). Only one possesses IF activity (such activity being defined as the capacity to promote intestinal absorption of cobalamin).

Electrophoresis reveals two immunologically nonidentical binders or classes of binders, one with slow and one with rapid mobility, that have

Table 5.3
Major Cobalamin-Binding Proteins

Protein(s)	Occurrence (source)	Function
Intrinsic factor (IF)	Gastric juice (gastric parietal cells)	Promotes absorption of cobalamin in ileum
Haptocorrins (R proteins)	Gastric juice (gastric mucosal cells)	May participate in formation of IF-Cbl; binds cobalamin analogues
Haptocorrin I (TC 1; R proteins)	Plasma (macrophages, other cells)	Plasma transport of cobalamin
Transcobalamin II (TC II)	Plasma (many body cells)	Promotes entry of cobalamin into cells

been designated, respectively, **S-protein** and **R-protein**(s). IF activity resides in the S-protein.

IF is secreted by the parietal cells of the fundic mucosa in the human, guinea pig, cat, rabbit, and monkey, by the chief cells in the rat and by glandular cells of the pylorus and duodenum in the hog. Its secretion is enhanced by histamine, metacholine, and gastrin. IF secretion usually parallels HCl secretion.

c. HAPTOCORRINS (R-PROTEINS)

R-proteins, now preferably termed **haptocorrins**, are a class of immunologically related proteins that are found in serum, leukocytes, saliva, gastric juice, milk, and virtually all body cells. Other names for R-proteins have included cobalophilin, transcobalamin I (TC I) and III (TC III); and granulocyte binder. Genetic evidence suggests that these are all one protein with one structural gene. We shall return to them in discussions of plasma cobalamin transport proteins and serum cobalamin assays.

2. *Locus and mechanism of cobalamin absorption*

Cobalamins in food are liberated by peptic digestion in the stomach and bound there by IF. The stable IF-Cbl complex encounters specific mucosal receptors in the microvilli of the ileum. A specific site on the IF molecule (other than the cobalamin binding site) attaches to a receptor. Attachment requires neutral pH, Ca^{2+}, or other divalent cations, but no energy. Mucosal receptors accept IF-Cbl in preference to free IF and are readily saturated. The IF receptor has been isolated and purified. It contains two subunits, and the similarity of its amino acid sequence to that of IF suggests that it arose by gene duplication.

The model in figure 5.9 has been proposed for the attachment of IF-Cbl complex to IF receptor. As the IF-Cbl complex has a tendency to form oligomers, the binding of complex to receptor may be analogous to the formation of an IF oligomer. Cobalamin (without IF) is taken into the cell by endocytosis and ultimately transferred to portal vein blood.

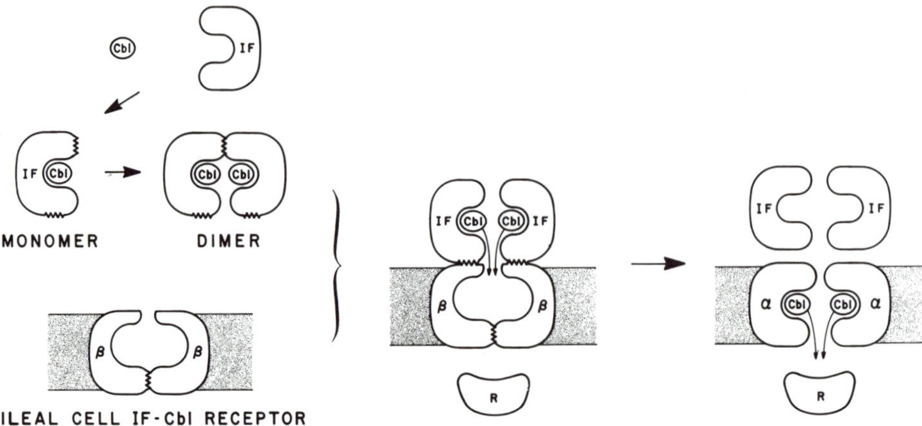

Fig. 5.9
A hypothetical model for the binding of IF-Cbl complex to IF receptor. The complex forms a pseudooligomer with its "relative," the IF receptor. It probably attaches to the β subunit of the receptor, which then undergoes conformational change to α. Intracellular R-proteins then accept Cbl from α. (Adapted from R. Gräsbeck, in B. Zagalak and W. Friedrich, eds., *cobalamin: Proceedings of the Third European Symposium on cobalamin and Intrinsic Factor*, New York: Walter de Gruyter, 1979, p. 743.)

3. *Antibodies to IF*

Two types of anti-IF antibodies occur. **Blocking antibodies** prevent binding of cobalamin by IF and show little species specificity. Antibodies of this type occur in some individuals receiving hog IF by mouth. **Binding antibodies** combine with IF-Cbl complex but also with free IF without impairing its ability to bind cobalamin. Both types of antibodies occur in sera of some patients with PA.

4. *Assay of cobalamin absorption*

After observing that increasing the dose of parenteral cobalamin leads to excretion of increasing percentages of the dose in the urine, Schilling showed that a large parenteral dose (1 mg) of nonradioactive cobalamin given 2 hr after oral administration of radioactive cobalamin increases excretion of radioactive cobalamin, presumably by blocking cobalamin binding sites in plasma and liver. Thus, cobalamin absorption can be assayed by studies of urinary excretion following oral administration—an advance over methods requiring stool analysis.

a. STANDARD SCHILLING TEST

In the **Schilling test** (part I), a fasting patient is given 0.5 μCi (0.5–1.0 μg) ^{57}Co-cyanocobalamin by mouth at time zero. A 24 hr urine collection is begun. At 2 hr, 1 mg of nonradioactive cyanocobalamin is administered intramuscularly. This is the "flushing" dose. An adequate sample of pooled urine is assayed for radioactivity. If excretion of radioactivity is low

(<7%), the Schilling test (part II) is performed (in no less than 5 days) by the same procedure except that 60 mg of hog IF is given orally with the radioactive cobalamin. If poor excretion in part I was due to IF deficiency, the result in part II should be normal. If excretion is again abnormal, other explanations must be found for cobalamin malabsorption.

Note that the kidneys excrete CN-Cbl and inulin in a similar manner. Indeed, radioactaive cobalamin can be used to measure glomerular filtration rate. Renal disease with impaired glomerular filtration may delay excretion of radioactivity in the Schilling test.

b. FOOD SCHILLING TEST

Recent recognition of a fairly common pattern—unexplained low serum cobalamin levels with normal Schilling test results—has stimulated increasing use of a "food Schilling test" (or egg-yolk cobalamin absorption test), in which the ingested labeled cobalamin derives from eggs produced by hens injected with labeled cobalamin. In many such patients, egg test results are significantly low, while standard Schilling test results are normal.

5. *Plasma transport of cobalamin*

Normal plasma contains 150–650 pg/ml of cobalamin (normal range varying with method and laboratory), all of which is protein bound. The two major cobalamin-binding proteins of plasma are usually designated **haptocorrin**, or **transcobalamin I** (TC I), and **transcobalamin II** (TC II). A third protein, **transcobalamin III** (TC III), may appear in disease states associated with elevated white counts. Probably TC III is an isoprotein of TC I that is unsaturated with cobalamin and therefore less charged. The properties of haptocorrin are summarized in table 5.4. Their known functions are two:

- Prevention of loss of cobalamins in urine, sweat, and other body secretions
- Transport of cobalamins through cell membranes

As noted below, they probably have other functions as well.

a. HAPTOCORRIN

The R-protein **haptocorrin** arises from granulocytes, but also from salivary and gastric glands. All R-proteins possess the same acid sequence, differences among them being attributable to variations in carbohydrate moieties. (Much of the plasma TC III appears to arise from granulocytes in vitro after blood has been collected—that is, during clotting. Thus, the content of R-proteins differs in plasma and serum.) Haptocorrin levels rise in myeloproliferative and malignant diseases (e.g., hepatoma, metastatic breast cancer).

Table 5.4
Properties of Cobalamin-Binding Proteins of Plasma

Property	TC I	TC II
Electrophoretic mobility (pH 8.6)	α_1	$\alpha_2\beta$
Molecular weight	120,000[a]	38,000[b]
Cobalamin-binding capacity (μg/mg)	12.2	28.6
Protein type (R or S)	R	S
Salic acid, residues/mole	18	0
Portion of plasma cobalamin bound (approx.)	75%	25%
Portion of binder unsaturated (approx.)	50%	98%
Half-life of TC-Cbl complex	9–12 days	12 hr
Reacts with:		
Anti-TC II	No	Yes
Anti-TC I	Yes	No
Anti-saliva R-protein	Yes	No

a. Isolated R-proteins have a "true" mol. wt. of 63,000–72,000, but in gel filtration and gel electrophoresis values of approximately 120,000 are obtained due to high (~40%) carbohydrate content.
b. Some evidence has suggested that TC II consists of two peptides of mol. wt. 38,000 and 27,000.

Within cells, R-proteins promote uptake of cobalamin by mitochondria and other organelles.

R-proteins differ from TC II and IF in the specificity of their binding sites. This property, which is discussed below, may give them a role in the binding and disposition of biologically inert and potentially harmful cobalamin analogues and corrins.

b. TC II

When a small amount of cobalamin enters the blood (portal and systemic), it is taken up first by TC II. Indeed, more than 90% of *recently* absorbed cobalamin is carried by TC II. TC II-Cbl complex is then cleared from plasma rapidly (in hours); vitamin and protein moiety disappear at comparable rates.

Haptocorrin, in contrast, carries most of the cobalamin in plasma and is cleared from plasma slowly (half-life of 9–12 days). Nevertheless, a quarter of the circulating cobalamin continues to be carried by TC II long after its intestinal absorption.

The nonessentiality of haptocorrin as a transport protein is puzzling. Congenital absence of haptocorrin is harmless, but severe megaloblastic anemia occurs in infants lacking TC II. Only TC II can promote cellular uptake of cobalamin. Cobalamin is taken up by many cells, which possess specific surface receptors for TC II-bound cobalamin that are analogous to the IF-Cbl receptors of ileal cells. Uptake involves pinocytosis followed by lysosomal degradation of TC II. Hepatic cells have an especially high affinity for TC II–bound cobalamin.

TC II levels decrease in chronic myeloproliferative disorders and occasionally in pernicious anemia. The sum of the levels of unsaturated haptocorrin and TC II—sometimes called serum **unsaturated cobalamin binding capacity** and largely contributed by TC II—may be decreased in cirrhosis and hepatitis.

6. *Assay of serum cobalamin*

The microbiologic assay of serum cobalamin (using such cobalamin-dependent organisms as *Lactobacillus leichmannii* and *Euglena gracilis*) was largely supplanted in the 1960s by a radioisotope dilution assay (RIDA) employing a cobalamin-binding protein. The fact that this assay gave higher results than the microbiologic assay was finally explained by the discovery in serum (and then in tissue) of a class of cobalamin **analogues** that are not recognized as cobalamin by microorganisms but are assayed as cobalamin by RIDA procedures when the binder is R-protein but not when it is IF. In other words, the relatively low binding specificity of R-proteins produces a misleading, falsely high value in serum cobalamin assays. This discovery led to RIDA methods using IF as binder that yield results in agreement with those of microbiologic assays. In addition, it raised several interesting questions that still lack answers: (1) What is the source and fate of these analogues? (2) Do they have pathophysiologic significance? (3) Is it the role of R-proteins in gastric juice to bind these compounds, which may be of dietary origin, in order to minimize their absorption in the intestine? (4) Is it the role of granulocyte R-protein (TC III) to prevent the dissemination of these analogues, which may escape exclusion in the intestine, by binding them and delivering them to hepatocytes, which retain and eventually excrete them? These matters are now under study.

IV. COBALAMIN DEFICIENCY

A. Clinical features

The clinical picture of cobalamin deficiency includes the nonspecific manifestations of megaloblastic anemia and its sequelae—glossitis, elevated serum LDH, weight loss, and so forth—that occur as well in folic acid deficiency *plus* the following specific features that make possible the diagnosis of cobalamin deficiency, irrespective of the underlying cause:

- Neurologic abnormalities
- Decreased serum cobalamin level
- Methylmalonic aciduria and elevated serum methylmalonate
- Elevated serum homocysteine
- Characteristic response to cobalamin therapy and lack of response to therapy with physiologic doses of folic acid

1. Neurologic syndrome

The neurologic syndrome of cobalamin deficiency is classically said to consist of symmetric paresthesias in feet and fingers with associated disturbances of vibratory sense and proprioception, progressing to spastic ataxia with "subacute combined system" disease of spinal cord, that is, degenerative changes of the dorsal and lateral columns. In fact, the picture is more often chronic than subacute and more varied and complex. Indeed, recent studies employing the newer, more sensitive diagnostic tests described below (serum methylmalonate and homocysteine) suggest that many common neuropsychiatric symptoms (e.g., anxiety, mood changes, forgetfulness) may be due to cobalamin deficiency that would be overlooked if the only diagnostic criterion of cobalamin deficiency were a lowered serum cobalamin level.

The classic neuropathy typically develops late in untreated PA, and if not treated it becomes irreversible. Significantly, both the classic syndrome and the recently described syndrome can occur in the absence of megaloblastosis. In the classic syndome, early pathologic changes in the cord consist of focal swelling of individual myelinated nerve fibers. Lesions later coalesce into larger foci involving many fiber systems. As noted, clinical signs can include a variety of cerebral abnormalities, irritability, somnolence, "megaloblastic madness," and perversion of taste, smell, and vision with central scotomata and occasional optic atrophy. Tobacco amblyopia, a curious visual disorder in cobalamin-deficient smokers, has been attributed to the tendency of cyanide in tobacco smoke to convert a limited supply of cobalamin coenzyme to metabolically inert cyanocobalamin.

As noted earlier, the mechanisms of neurologic involvement is unknown. Proposed theories include:

- Chronic cyanide intoxication
- Synthesis and incorporation into myelin of "funny fatty acids" owing to competition between acetyl CoA or malonyl CoA and accumulated methylmalonyl CoA in the biosynthetic pathway of fatty acids
- Depression of the methionine synthetase system in nervous tissue with consequent impairment of myelin synthesis

2. Decreased serum cobalamin level

Decreased serum cobalamin level is a decisive diagnostic datum. As noted above, the normal range is 200–850 pg/ml. Clinical signs generally begin to appear when the serum level is below 150. Serum folate is usually elevated when serum cobalamin is depressed unless there is a coexisting folate deficiency.

Note that serum cobalamin is often not a valid measure of total body cobalamin or intracellular levels of cobalamin enzymes. Depression of the latter, the ultimate cause of clinical signs and symptoms, can occur in the presence of a normal serum cobalamin level.

3. *Elevated urine and serum methylmalonate*

Methylmalonic aciduria was long ago shown to be a sensitive index of cobalamin deficiency, except in rare cases in which it is due to inborn error. Normal subjects excrete only trace amounts of methylmalonate, that is, 0–3.5 mg/24 hr. Levels are variably elevated in cobalamin deficiency, sometimes to 300 mg/24 hr or more. Cobalamin therapy restores excretion patterns to normal. In practice, the assay of urinary methylmalonate has been difficult to perform and thus has not been performed in many cases.

In 1989, Allen, Lindenbaum, and coworkers developed an assay for serum methylmalonate that is still beyond the scope of many laboratories. Nonetheless, they showed in careful studies that this test is more sensitive than serum cobalamin and becomes abnormal much earlier in cobalamin deficiency.

4. *Elevated serum homocysteine*

The rationale for this assay for cobalamin deficiency, developed by the same workers, is seen in figure 5.8, which shows that homocysteine accumulates in cobalamin deficiencies. The assay is also more sensitive than the serum cobalamin level, but is still not generally available. Serum homocysteine (N^5-methyltetrahydrofolate) is also elevated in folate deficiency (see figure 5.8).

5. *Response to cobalamin therapy*

Cobalamin therapy of cobalamin deficiency produces an abrupt reticulocyte crisis that begins several days after the start of therapy (figure 5.10). Reversal of clinical abnormalities then ensues. A partial response follows large (i.e., pharmacologic) doses of folic acid (i.e., 5 mg/day), though the hematocrit is not fully restored to normal and patients previously without neurologic symptoms may suffer an acute onset of such symptoms. However, small (i.e., physiologic) doses of folic acid (i.e., 200–400 μg/day), produce no response in cobalamin deficiency, whereas they produce good responses in folic acid deficiency.

B. Specific syndromes

1. *Introduction*

Deficiency of cobalamin, as of all other vitamins, may result from inadequate dietary intake, defective intestinal absorption, abnormally increased requirements, or impaired utilization in the tissues (see table 5.1).

Deficiency of cobalamin results from **poor diet** only rarely. Reported instances have occurred mainly in vegetarians who also avoid all dairy products and eggs. Occasionally it is associated with severe general malnutrition.

Cobalamin deficiency is most often the result of **diminished intestinal absorption** of various etiologies. The most common cause is pernicious anemia, to be discussed below, in which a gastric mucosal defect decreases

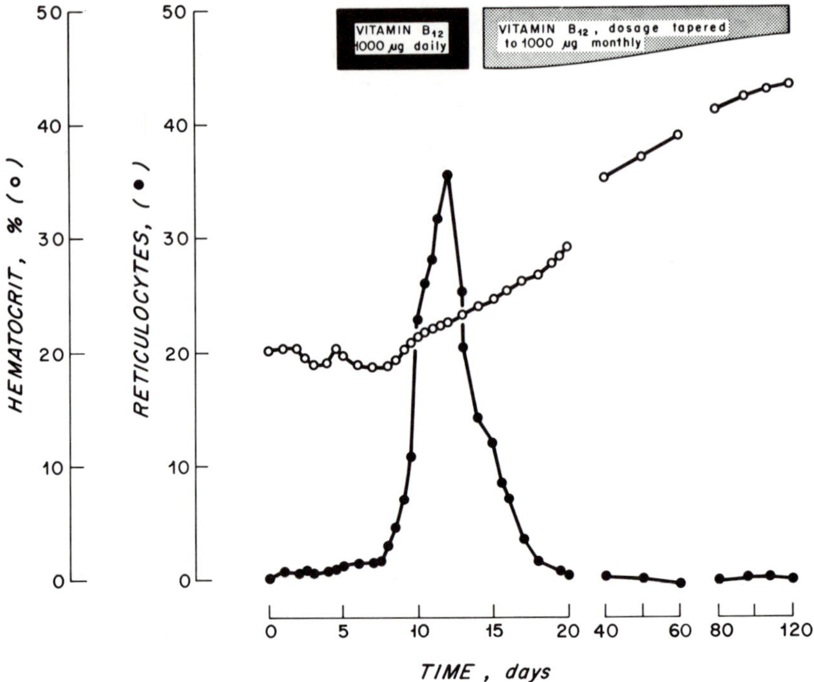

Fig. 5.10
Time course of reticulocyte count and hematocrit level during treatment of pernicious anemia with cobalamin. (From W. S. Beck and M. Goulian. In J. R. DiPalma, ed., *Drill's Pharmacology in Medical Practice*, 4th ed. New York: McGraw-Hill, 1971, chapter 51.)

IF synthesis. Other and less common causes include:

- Total (occasionally subtotal) gastrectomy
- Various types of gastric dysfunctions that impair absorption of food cobalamin but not crystalline cobalamin, and detectable only by the food Schilling test
- Pancreatic disease, in which lack of proteases in the duodenum appears to interfere with formation of the IF-Cbl complex
- Overgrowth of intestinal bacteria that occurs in the "blind loop" syndrome, strictures, anastomoses, diverticula, and other conditions producing intestinal stasis
- Parasitic infestation with the cobalamin-utilizing fish tapeworm *Diphyllobothrium latum*, a common condition in Scandinavian countries
- Organic disease (or absence) of the ileum that impairs cobalamin absorption despite the presence of adequate IF

The body's large cobalamin reserve must be largely depleted before development of a deficiency of intracellular cobalamin coenzymes and thus of clinical symptoms. Hence, several years may pass before the appearance of deficiency symptoms after total gastrectomy or cessation of treatment in pernicious anemia.

Cobalamin deficiency due to **increased requirements** occurs mainly in pregnancy, presumably arising from the superimposition of fetal demands upon a backgroud of poor nutrition. No examples are known in which a tissue deficiency of cobalamin arises from failure of activation or antimetabolites.

2. *Pernicious anemia*

a. TERMINOLOGY

The old name "pernicious anemia" (PA) is now reserved for the once fatal condition resulting from defective secretion of IF by cells in the fundus and upper part of the body or the stomach. Cobalamin therapy makes it quite unpernicious. The term **pernicious anemia** is often wrongly used as a synonym for cobalamin deficiency, of which PA is but one cause, or of megaloblastic anemia, of which cobalamin deficiency is one cause. In recognition of the fact that PA was first described in 1855 at Guy's Hospital by Thomas Addison, the term **Addisonian pernicious anemia** is sometimes used to distinguish true PA from "non-Addisonian pernicious anemia" (i.e., cobalamin deficiency arising from other causes).

b. ETIOLOGY

A genetic basis for PA is suggested by the high incidence of the disease in Scandinavians, a relatively inbred population. Also, minor abnormalities (e.g., achlorhydria) are reported in relatives of patients. The disorder is basically a chronic atrophic gastritis that eventually compromises IF (and HCl) secretion. The discovery that 55–70% of the patients have binding or blocking anti-IF antibodies in serum and gastric juice suggests an underlying autoimmune process. But although such antibodies can block IF function (if they enter the intestine), there is no evidence that they are responsible for cessation of IF synthesis. Also, anti-IF antibodies occur in the serum of patients with diabetes mellitus, thyroid disease, and other diseases in the absence of PA. It is of interest that serum from PA patients often contains antibodies against gastric parietal cell cytoplasm and thyroid acinar cell cytoplasm. Both antibodies also occur in Hashimoto's thyroidities and rarely in normals. In sum, evidence is still lacking that these phenomena are related to the initiation or perpetuation of the basic gastropathy of PA. Nor is it clear how the process is instigated by genetic determinants.

c. CLINICAL FEATURES

PA occurs typically in 40- to 70-year-old north Europeans of fair complexion, with one notable exception: there is an unusually early onset of PA in black American (and South African) women, 21% of whom are under age 40.

Typically in PA, there is a slow onset of the following phenomena:

- Megaloblastic anemia and related phenomena
- Neurologic changes (in some but not all patients)
- Other specific signs of cobalamin deficiency (low serum cobalamin, elevated serum and urine methylmalonate, elevated serum homocysteine)
- A striking response of reticulocytes and hematocrit to therapy with cobalamin
- Partial response to high doses of folic acid (5 mg) but not to "physiologic" doses (200–400) μg)

The following features are diagnostically important:

- Achlorhydria after histamine stimulation
- Decreased cobalamin absorption in the first part of the Schilling test which is corrected in the second part by oral IF
- Increased incidence of associated gastric carcinoma, myxedema, and rheumatoid arthritis

d. THERAPY

Patients with PA require the life-long administration of cobalamin. Ordinarily it is given parenterally at monthly intervals after reserves have been repleted.

3. *"Juvenile pernicious anemia"*

So-called juvenile pernicious anemia includes four entities:

- True PA with failure of IF secretion, which is extremely rare in children.
- Congenital IF lack, with no other associated abnormality of gastric secretion.
- Production of a biologically inert IF.
- Familial selective malabsorption of cobalamin (i.e., absorption of other nutrients is normal) with normal secretion of IF and HCl in the stomach. Presumably there is a defect of specific mucosal receptors for the IF-Cbl complex. The disorder is familial (recessive) and is associated with proteinuria. The Schilling test indicates decreased absorption of cobalamin uncorrected by IF.

SELECTED REFERENCES

Reviews

Allen, R. H., Stabler, S. P., et al. Diagnosis of cobalamin deficiency I. Usefulness of serum methylmalonic acid and total homocysteine concentrations. *Am. J. Hematol.* 34(1990): 90–98.

Babior, B. M., ed. *Cobalamin: Biochemistry and Pathophysiology*. New York: John Wiley & Sons, 1975.

Beck, W. S. Cobalamin as coenzyme: a twisting trail of research. *Am. J. Hematol.* 34(1990): 83–89.

Beck, W. S. Metabolic aspects of cobalamin and folic acid. In Williams, W. J., Beutler, E., et al., eds. *Hematology*, 3rd ed. New York: McGraw-Hill Book Co. (Blakiston Division), 1983, pp. 311–331.

Beck, W. S. Megaloblastic anemias. In Wyngaarden, J. B., and Smith, L. H., Jr., eds. *Cecil's Textbood of Medicine*, 18th ed. Philadelphia: W. B. Saunders Co., 1988, pp. 900–907.

Beck, W. S. Neuropsychiatric consequences of cobalamin deficiency. *Adv. Intern. Med.* 36(1990): 33–56.

Dolphin, D., ed. B_{12}. *Vol. 1: Chemistry. Vol. 2: Biochemistry and Medicine*. New York: John Wiley & Sons, 1982.

Beck, W. S. The assay of serum cobalamin by *Lactobacillus leichmannii* and the interpretation of serum cobalamin levels. In Hall, C. A., ed. *The Cobalamins. Methods in Hematology Vol. 10*. New York: Churchill Livingstone, 1983, pp. 31–50.

Lindenbaum, J. Status of laboratory testing in the diagnosis of megaloblastic anemia. *Blood* 61(1983): 624–627.

Lindenbaum, J., Savage, D. G., et al. Diagnosis of cobalamin deficiency II. Relative sensitivities of serum cobalamin, methylmalonic acid, and total homocysteine concentrations. *Am. J. Hematol.* 34(1990): 99–107.

Rosenberg, L. E., and Fenton, W. A. Disorders of propionate and methylmalonate metabolism. In Scriver, C. R., Beaudet, A. L., et al, eds. *The Metabolic Basis of Inherited Disease*, 6th ed. New York: McGraw-Hill, 1989, pp. 821–844.

Victor, M., and Lear, A. A. Subacute combined degeneration of the spinal cord. Current concepts of the disease process. Value of serum cobalamin determinations in clarifying some of the common clinical problems. *Am. J. Med.* 20(1956): 896–911.

Zagalak, B., Friedrich, W., et al. *Cobalamin. Proceedings of the Third European Symposium on Cobalamin and Intrinsic Factor. University of Zürich, March 5–8, 1979, Zürich, Switzerland.* New York: Walter de Gruyter, 1979.

Original articles

Carmel, R., Sinow, R. M., et al. Food cobalamin malabsorption occurs frequently in patients with unexplained low serum cobalamin levels. *Arch. Intern. Med.* 148(1988): 1715–1719.

Cox, E. V., and White, A. M. Methylmalonic acid excretion: an index of cobalamin deficiency. *Lancet* 2(1962): 853–856.

Gimsing, P., and Beck, W. S. Cobalamin analogues in plasma. An in vitro phenomenon. *Scand. J. Clin. Lab. Invest.* 49 Suppl. 194(1989): 37–40.

Goodman, A. M., Harris, J. W., et al. Studies in B_{12}-deficient monkeys with combined system disease. I. B_{12}-deficient patterns in bone marrow deoxyuridine suppression tests without morphologic or functional abnormalities. *J. Lab. Clin. Med.* 96(1980): 722–733.

Kolhouse, J. F., Kondo, H., et al. Cobalamin analogues are present in human plasma and can mask cobalamin deficiency because current radioisotope dilution assays are not specific for true cobalamin. *N. Engl. J. Med.* 299(1978): 785–792.

Lindenbaum, J., Healton, E. B., et al. Neuropsychiatric disorders caused by cobalamin deficiency in the absence of anemia or macrocytosis. *N. Engl. J. Med.* 318 (1988): 1720–1928.

Pelliniemi, T.-T., and Beck, W. S. Biochemical mechanisms in the Killmann experiment. Critique of the deoxyuridine suppression test. *J. Clin. Invest.* 65(1980): 449–460.

Schilling, R. Intrinsic factor studies. II. The effect of gastric juice on the urinary excretion of radioactivity after the oral administration of radioactive cobalamin. *J. Lab. Clin. Med.* 42(1953): 860–865.

Stabler, S. P., Marcell, P. D., et al. Assay of methylmalonic acid in the serum of patients with cobalamin deficiency using capillary gas chromatography-mass spectrometry. *J. Clin. Invest.* 77(1986): 1606–1612.

Stabler, S. P., Marcell, P. D., et al. Elevation of total homocysteine in the serum of patients with cobalamin or folate deficiency detected by capillary gas chromatography-mass spectrometry. *J. Clin. Invest.* 81(1988): 466–474.

LECTURE 6

Megaloblastic Anemias II. Folic Acid Deficiency

William S. Beck

EDITOR'S COMMENT

Studies of folic acid and its deficiency syndrome cover a wide spectrum of topics, including clinical features of one of the world's most common clinical disorders (i.e., folate deficiency), scientific issues surrounding the roles of folate as cofactor of several critical metabolic systems, including thymine synthesis, purine synthesis, and others, and aspects of its role as a factor in many ecosystems. One of the most interesting outgrowths of our knowledge of folate metabolism was the development of antifolate drugs, which from the beginning were among the most effective of all antileukemic and anticancer drugs. Their development continues actively.

I. FOLIC ACID VITAMINOLOGY

A. Historical notes

In 1891 Sir Frederick Gowland Hopkins's classic studies of the pigments of butterfly wings led to the isolation of xanthopterin and leucopterin, yellow and white pigments that were not characterized until 1940 when Wieland showed them to be members of a novel group of heterobicyclic compounds, the **pterins** or **pteridines**. Many pteridines are found in nature as free compounds; the metabolic role of some of them was recognized only recently. Their most important roles was appreciated only after the discovery of folic acid.

Converging lines of nutritional research led to the recognition of folic acid and its related derivatives in the mid-1940s. The first began in 1931 with the description of the "Wills factor," an antianemia principle of yeast. Subsequently reported unidentified factors included "vitamin M," an antianemia principle of liver, yeast, and brain; "vitamin B_c" a liver factor that prevents macrocytic anemia in chicks; "Norit eluate factor," a factor that supports the growth of *Lactobacillus casei*; and finally "folic acid," the name given to a substance from spinach leaves that promotes growth of *Lactobacillus casei* and *Streptococcus lactis R*, later renamed *Streptococcus fecalis R*. Each factor was subsequently identified as pteroylmonoglutamic acid or one of its derivatives. In 1948 crystalline folic acid was obtained from liver and its structure confirmed by organic synthesis.

Although experimental folic acid deficiency was known to produce megaloblastic anemia, it was early recognized that folic acid is not the antipernicious anemia principle of liver. Confusion arose early when folic acid therapy was found to provide notable reticulocyte responses in PA. Hemoglobin regeneration was incomplete, however, and relapses and neurologic complications occurred during treatment. Liver extracts active in PA were then found by direct assay to contain little or no folic acid. Thus, it was recognized that cobalamin deficiency is the basis of the megaloblastic anemia of PA and that folic acid deficiency is a distinctive cause of megaloblastic anemia.

B. Chemical aspects

1. Structure and nomenclature

Folic acid is the trivial name for **pteroylmonoglutamic acid** (figure 6.1), parent compound of the large family of compounds known collectively as "folate" or "folates." The molecule contains three moieties: (1) a pteridine derivative; (2) a *p*-aminobenzoic acid residue; and (3) an L-glutamic acid residue. The combination of the first two comprises pteroic acid, the systematic name of which is *N*-(2-amino-4-hydroxypteridin-6-ylmethyl)-*p*-aminobenzoic acid. The corresponding acyl radical is termed pteroyl; hence, folates are pteroylglutamates.

2. Classification of derivatives

a. BY NUMBER OF GLUTAMATE RESIDUES

Folic acid occurs in nature largely in the form of **pteroylpolyglutamates**, in which multiple glutamic acid residues are attached by peptide linkage to the γ-carboxyl group of the preceding glutamic acid residue. Folic acid supplied by pharmacies is pteroylmonoglutamate. Higher forms are termed **pteroyldiglutamate**, **pteroyltriglutamate**, and so forth. Pteroylmonoglutamate is designated by the symbols **PteGlu** or **F** (folic acid). For simplicity, we shall use the latter except in referring to polyglutamates, which are abbreviated $PteGlu_2$, $PteGlu_3$, and so forth.

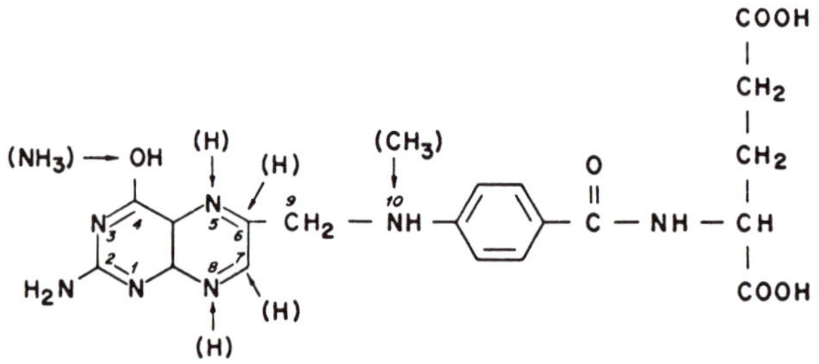

Fig. 6.1
Chemical structure of folic acid (pteroylmonoglutamic acid.) Substituents in parentheses are attached to molecules in the several chemical derivatives described in the text.

b. BY LEVEL OF OXIDATION

Folic acid occurs at three levels of oxidation: (1) folic acid (F); (2) 7, 8-dihydrofolic acid (FH_2); and (3) 5, 6, 7, 8-tetrahydrofolic acid (FH_4). The reduction of F to FH_4 is a necessary prerequisite to participation of folic acid in enzyme reactions. In this reduction, F is reduced first to FH_2, which is then reduced to FH_4. In animal cells, both reactions are catalyzed by a single NADPH-linked enzyme, **dihydrofolate reductase**. A notable property of dihydrofolate reductase is its extreme sensitivity to folate analogues containing a 4-amino group (figure 6.1) such as aminopterin and amethopterin, later renamed methotrexate (MTX), which are avidly bound and inhibitory at concentrations as low as 10^{-9} M. Indeed, MTX binds 10,000–50,000 times more tightly to the reductase than does its natural substrate. This is the major basis for their cytotoxic action as antileukemic agents.

c. BY IDENTITY OF ONE-CARBON GROUP

The folate family consists largely of FH_4 derivatives bearing a "one-carbon" substituent. Such a compound may be symbolized as "C-FH_4." The varieties of "C-FH" differ in the identity of the one-carbon substituents of FH_4 (figure 6.2). Known one-carbon substituents of FH_4 are the following:

formyl	—CHO	methylene	$—CH_2—$
hydroxymethyl	$—CH_2OH$	methenyl	—CH=
methyl	$—CH_3$	formimino	—CHNH

Note that three oxidation levels of carbon are represented among the one-carbon units (formyl, hydroxymethyl, and methyl) and that only one type (formimino) contains nitrogen.

d. BY LOCUS OF ONE-CARBON GROUP

It is seen in figure 6.2 that one-carbon units attach to N^5 or N^{10} or both and that specific enzymes interconvert many of these compounds.

e. BY CHEMICAL STABILITY

Most reduced derivatives of folic acid are sensitive to oxidation in air and hence are unstable, especially under autoclave conditions. A notable exception is N^5-formyl FH_4, a compound isolated from liver and yeast soon after the discovery of folic acid. It was first recognized as a growth factor for *Leuconostoc citrovorum* (later renamed *Pediococcus cerevisiae*) and thus was named "citrovorum factor." (Other of its trivial names are "leucovorin" and "folinic acid.") Prior to the identification of its structure, a relation to folic acid was established by the observation that citrovorum factor levels, low in the urine of folate-deficient rats, are increased by folic acid.

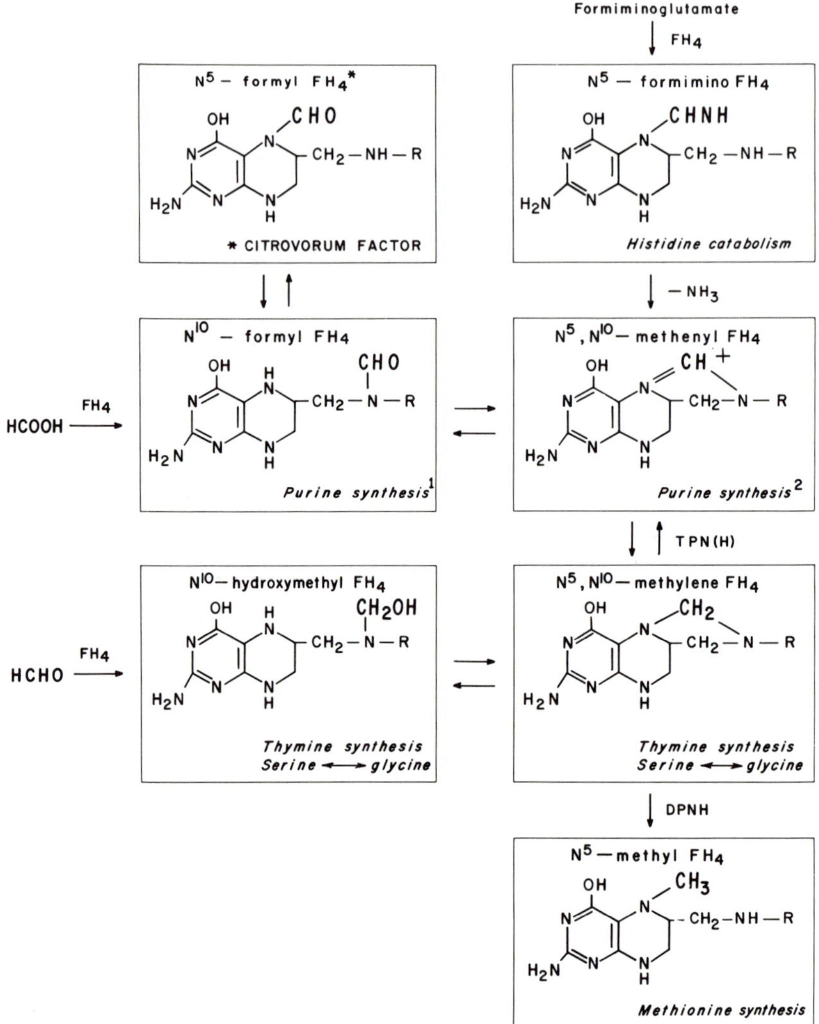

Fig. 6.2
Derivatives of tetrahydrofolic acid (FH_4), their interconversions, and the metabolic pathways in which they participate. One-carbon substituents are shown in boldface. **Purine synthesis**[1] refers to the step in purine synthesis in which 5-amino-4-imidazolecarboxamide ribotide is converted to 5-formamino-4-imidazole carboxamide ribotide; **purine synthesis**[2] refers to the conversion of glycinamide ribotide to formlyglycinamide ribotide. (From W. S. Beck, N. Engl. J. Med. 266[1962]: 765.)

Table 6.1
Activity of Various Folate Derivatives as Bacterial Nutrients

Folic acid derivative	*Pediococcus cerevisiae**	*Streptococcus fecalis*	*Lactobacillus casei*
FH_4 and most derivatives except N^5 methyl FH_4 (form of folate in serum)	+	+	+
F and pteroyl*di*glutamates	−	+	+
N^5-methyl FH_4 (form of folate in serum), N^5-methyl FH_2 and pteroyl*tri*glutamates	−	−	+

* Formerly named *Leuconostoc citrovorum.* Citrovorum factor is the trivial name given to N^5-formyl FH_4, a stable compound essential for the growth of *L. citrovorum.* Note that of the three organisms, only *L. casei* is supported by N^5-methyl FH_4, the folate derivative found in serum.

f. BY MICROBIOLOGIC ACTIVITY

Folate derivatives differ in their ability to serve as nutrients for microorganisms. Table 6.1 summarizes these specificities for three important assay organisms. It is noteworthy that the major form of folate in human serum is N^5-methyl FH_4, which is assayed with *Lactobacillus casei.*

C. Nutritional aspects

1. Sources

The many folate compounds are widely distributed in nature. Green leaves are rich sources and presumably the sites of active synthesis. The richest vegetable sources are asparagus, broccoli, spinach, and lettuce, each of which contains >1 mg of folate per 100 g dry weight. Folates are also found in liver, kidney, yeast, and mushrooms. The vitamin is synthesized by many bacteria. Sulfonamide drugs attack bacteria by interfering competitively with the incorporation of *p*-aminobenzoic into pteroic acid, an intermediate that reacts with glutamate in the presence of ATP to form pteroylglutamate. The major product of the natural synthetic pathway is 7,8-dihydrofolate.

Determination of food folate requires extraction procedures that avoid destruction of labile reduced forms. Since precautions have not always been observed, published values of folate content in foods are often unreliable. Also, results of folate determinations are influenced by the assay method used. As noted in table 6.1, for example, *S. fecalis* is indifferent to N^5-methyl FH_4 or short polyglutamates. Unless pretreated with **conjugase**, higher polyglutamates are unavailable to all assay organisms.

An average daily American diet prepared without special precautions and treated with conjugase contains approximately 200 μg of folate by *S. fecalis* assay and an additional 400–500 μg of folate active only with

L. casei. Values are approximately one-fourth as high without conjugase treatment. The folate in some vegetables (broccoli, lettuce, asparagus) is almost entirely in polyglutamate form. Monoglutamate *L. casei*–active folate activity in cow's milk averages 55 μg/l. Excessive cooking, particulary with large amounts of water, can remove or destroy a high percentage of the folate in foods.

2. *Daily requirements*

The minimum daily adult requirement for folic acid, or its derivatives, is approximately 50 μg. As noted above, the average diet contains several times this amount in the form of various folate compounds, some of which may be unavailable. Body reserves of folic acid are relatively much smaller than those of cobalamin. When a subject receiving a normal intake is switched to a daily intake of 5 μg/day, megaloblastic anemia develops in about 4 months. Folic acid requirements are increased during growth, in pregnancy, and, as will be noted later, in a number of disease states.

D. Role in metabolism

In metabolism, FH_4 is a catalytic self-regenerating acceptor-donor of one-carbon units in reactions involving one-carbon transfers from a carbon-containing donor, X-C, to an acceptor, Y:

$$\begin{array}{llll} \text{X-C} & + FH_4 \rightarrow FH_4\text{-C} + \text{X} & & \\ FH_4\text{-C} & + \text{Y} & \rightarrow \text{Y-C} & + FH_4 \\ \hline \text{Sum: X-C} + \text{Y} & & \rightarrow \text{Y-C} & + \text{X} \end{array}$$

The metabolic systems of animal tissues known to require folic acid coenzymes are summarized in table 6.2. It should be noted that folic acid coenzymes are in the form of polyglutamates (see below).

Table 6.2
Metabolic Systems Requiring Folic Acid Coenzymes in Animal Cells

System	Related transformations of folic acid coenzymes
Serine ⇌ glycine	Serine + $FH_4 \rightleftharpoons N^5, N^{10}$-methylene FH_4 + glycine
Thymidylate synthesis	Deoxyuridylate (dUMP) + N^5, N^{10}-methylene FH_4 → FH_2 + thymidylate (dTMP)
Histidine catabolism	Formiminoglutamate + $FH_4 \rightarrow N^5$-formimino FH_4 + glutamate
Methionine synthesis*	Homocysteine + N^5-methyl $FH_4 \rightarrow FH_4$ + methionine
Purine synthesis[1]	Glycinamide ribotide + N^5, N^{10}-methenyl FH_4 → FH_4 + formylglycinamide ribotide
Purine synthesis[2]	5-amino-4-imidazole carboxamide ribotide + N^{10}-formyl $FH_4 \rightarrow FH_4$ + 5-formamido-4-imidazole carboxamide ribotide

*Pathway also requires a cobalamin derivative (methylcobalamin).

1. Thymidylate synthesis

The reaction, impairment of which in human folate deficiency produces major clinical manifestations, is thymidylate synthesis. Methylation of deoxyuridylate to thymidylate, catalyzed by the enzyme thymidylate synthetase, is an essential preliminary step in the synthesis of DNA (see figure 5.3). The coenzyme of this reaction, N^5, N^{10}-methylene-tetrahydrofolate, is unique among folate coenzymes because it transfers a one-carbon group *and* serves as hydrogen donor in reducing the transferred group to a methyl group. The reaction generates FH_2 (table 6.2), which must be reduced again to FH_4 by dihydrofolate reductase before it can again be utilized as a coenzyme. Thus, the following "thymidylate synthesis cycle" exists, in which the hydroxmethyl carbon of serine is transformed into the methyl carbon of thymine as FH_4 is regenerated from FH_2 at the expense of NADPH:

Serine + $FH_4 \rightarrow N^{10}$-hydroxymethyl FH_4 + glycine

N^{10}-hydroxymethyl $FH_4 \rightarrow N^5$, N^{10}-methylene $FH_4 + H_2O$

dUMP + N^5, N^{10}-methylene $FH_4 \rightarrow FH_2$ + dTMP

FH_2 + NADPH + $H^+ \rightarrow FH_4$ + $NADP^+$

Limitation of thymidylate synthesis in folic acid deficiency impairs DNA synthesis with resulting megaloblastic transformation.

2. Histidine catabolism

Interference with the breakdown of histidine (figure 6.3) and its catabolic product, formiminoglutamic acid (abbreviated FIGlu), in folic acid deficiency has no morbid effects, but it provides the basis for a test that has been used in the diagnosis of folic acid deficiency. When insufficient FH_4 is present to accept the formimino group, FIGlu accumulates, appears in

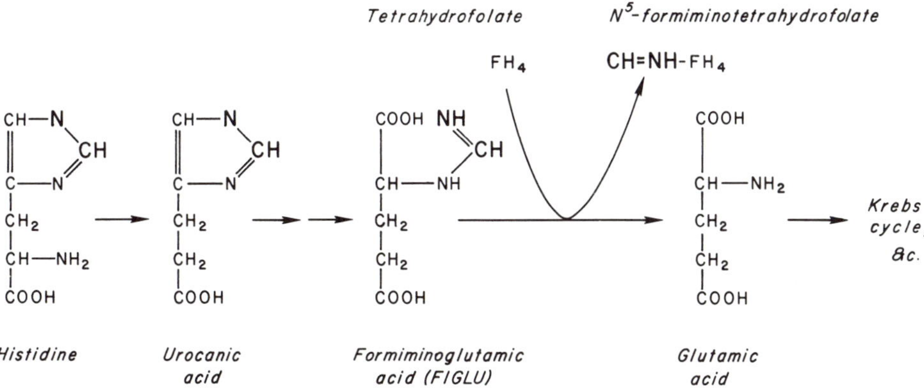

Fig. 6.3
Pathway of histidine catabolism, showing synthesis and FH_4-dependent degradation of FIGlu. (From W. S. Beck. In W. J. Williams et al., *Hematology*, New York: McGraw-Hill, 1972.)

the urine, and is easily detected. Sensitivity is increased with a large oral loading dose (20 g) of histidine. Normal persons excrete little or no FIGlu. The highest levels of FIGlu excretion occur in subjects receiving folic acid antagonists.

3. *Purine synthesis*

Deficiency of folate also diminishes the folate-dependent coversion of 5-amino-4-imidazole carboxamide ribotide (AICAR) to 5-formamido-4-imidazole carboxamide ribotide. AICAR accumulates and is excreted in the urine in excessive amounts in the partially degraded form 5-amino-4-imidazole carboxamide. No clinical manifestations have thus far been related to the block in purine synthesis. FIGlu and AICAR are occasionally excreted in pure cobalamin deficiency, possibly because lack of cobalamin may depress the cobalamin-dependent pathway of methionine synthesis in which N^5-methyl FH_4 is converted to FH_4 (see figure 5.8). For this reason, some workers have decried the specificity of the FIGlu test. When FIGlu excretion is elevated in cobalamin deficiency, however, further study often reveals coexisting folate deficiency.

4. *Role of free pteridine*

In the light of the metabolic functions of folic acid, it is of interest that the free pteridine, **tetrahydrobiopterin**, has been identified as the coenzyme of the enzymatic hydroxylation of phenylalanine to tyrosine, of the oxidation of long-chain alkyl ethers of glycerol to fatty acids, and perhaps of other reactions, for example, the 17-α-hydroxylation of progesterone. FH_4 is weakly active in these systems in vitro but appears to have no such functions in vivo.

E. Physiologic aspects

1. *Significance of folylpolyglutamates*

Recent studies of these naturally occurring peptides have revealed the following points:

- All or most cells contain folate in polyglutamate form and contain a synthetase for converting folylmonoglutamates to polyglutamates.
- Despite this fact, plasma folate consists exclusively and conspicuously of the monoglutamate N^5-methyl FH_4.
- The substrate of synthetase is FH_4, not N^5-methyl FH_4.
- Folylpolyglutamates greatly predominate over folymonoglutamates within cells.
- Folylpolyglutamates exist in reduced and substituted forms just as folylmonoglutamates do.
- Multiple polyglutamate chain lengths exist in all cell types.
- Although most cells contain folylpolyglutamate synthetase and conjugase, the lysosomal locus of the latter serves to separate these enzymes in the cell.

Folylpolyglutamates (and their reduced and substituted forms) are the active coenzymes of folate-dependent enzyme reactions (e.g., thymidylate synthetase and N^5-methyl FH_4-methionine methyltransferase). In cobalamin-deficient humans, the ratio of polyglutamates to monoglutamates is decreased. This pattern evidently signifies a failure of folylpolyglutamate synthesis in cobalamin deficiency. This is probably due to the accumulation or "trapping" of folate as N^5-methyl FH_4, which is a poorer substrate for folylpolyglutamate synthetase. This supports the "methylfolate trap" theory of how cobalamin deficiency impairs DNA synthesis (lecture 5).

2. *Intestinal absorption*

The mechanism of intestinal absorption of folate is imperfectly understood. The proximal jejunum is the principal site of folate absorption. Within minutes of an oral 1-mg dose of folylmonoglutamate, material active with *S. fecalis* and *L. casei* can be detected in plasma. Peak values are reached in 1–2 hr.

Orally administered ^{3}H-folylmonoglutamate and ^{3}H-folylheptaglutamate both increase plasma folate comparably. Since plasma contains only folylmonoglutamate, folylpolyglutamate must be hydrolyzed during intestinal absorption. Although such data may not accurately reflect the disposition of food folate, which is largely in polyglutamate form, it does not appear that much of this folate is nutritionally available. Nonetheless, studies with ingested labeled polyglutamates indicate that fecal losses are greater as the length of the poly-γ-glutamyl side chain increases.

The existence of **conjugases** that convert polyglutamates (once called folate "conjugates") to monoglutamate has long been recognized. Yet the precise role of these exopeptidases in connection with intestinal absorption is still unclear. According to one theory, folylpolyglutamate is hydrolyzed within the lumen of the intestine, and the monoglutamate product is absorbed subsequently. Another holds that hydrolysis occurs on or at the brush border of the intestinal cell, with subsequent transport, reduction, and methylation of the monoglutamate. A third theory is that polyglutamate enters the epithelial cell intact, hydrolysis occurring as an intracellular process followed by transport of the hydrolytic product.

Folate circulates through an enterohepatic cycle. Bile contains 2–10 times the folate concentration of normal serum.

3. *Metabolism*

When a small dose of tritiated folic acid (^{3}H-F) is administered intravenously, 60% is cleared from the plasma in one circulation time and 90–95% is removed in 3 min. The rapidity of clearance suggests either that uptake is active or that it is passive and cells contain binding substances of high affinity—or, perhaps more likely, that folate is both absorbed actively and bound intracellularly. An active transport system for folate is suggested by the slow rate of cellular penetration of 4-amino folate analogues. The nature of intracellular folate binders is discussed below.

Folates are found in all body tissues. The principal form of the vitamin in serum, red cells, and liver is N^5-methyl FH_4; about a third of the serum folate is N^5-methyl FH_2. As noted above, a large portion of the folate in red cells and liver is in the form of polyglutamates. Total body folate has not been measured. That it is at least several miligrams may be surmised from nutritional data.

A portion of folate turned over each day is degraded to *p*-aminobenzoylglutamate and other cleavage products, which along with some intact folate, N^5-methyl FH_4, and citrovorum factor are excreted by the kidney.

4. Folate-binding proteins

Until recently, it was not clear whether a portion of the folate in serum is protein bound. Since serum folate is large dialyzable (and excretable by kidney), it seemed that any binder must be a weak one that leaves most serum folate unbound. Experiments with high specific activity ^{3}H-F and ^{3}H-methyl FH_4 finally produced evidence of some folate binding by a serum protein in about 15% of normal individuals. In these individuals, normal serum binds less than 10% of the serum folate (average, 45 pg/ml) and folate-deficient serum binds greater amounts (average, 333 pg/ml). This elevation appears early in the course of folate deficiency and falls promptly after treatment with folic acid. Elevations of serum folate-binding proteins also occur in pregnancy and a variety of diseases (e.g., uremia, cirrhosis, leukemia). Such changes reportedly are not observed in cobalamin deficiency.

Folate-binding protein from folate-deficient serum appears to consist of two proteins (or classes of proteins) one with a mol. wt. in excess of 200,000, the other with a mol. wt. of 40,000. Similar material is also found in human milk and lymphocyte membranes. A membrane-derived intracellular folate-binding protein may regulate uptake of folate into cell and serve as a storage site for folylpolyglutamates. The binding protein has many properties in common with β-lactoglobulin, the folate-binding protein of cow's milk.

II. FOLIC ACID DEFICIENCY

A. Clinical features

The clinical picture of human folic acid deficiency includes nonspecific manifestations of megaloblastic anemia similar to those observed in cobalamin deficiciency (see lecture 5)—megaloblastic hematopoiesis, glossitis, cytologic abnormalities in various types of epithelium, elevated serum LDH, and so forth—and the following specific features that make the diagnosis of folic acid deficiency, irrespective of the underlying cause:

- Decreased serum folate level.
- Elevated excretion of FIGlu after a loading dose of histidine.

- Full clinical response to therapy with physiologic doses of folic acid.
- Abnormally rapid disappearance from the serum of an intravenously injected standard dose of folic acid.
- Decreased urinary excretion of radioactivity following a standard oral dose of ^{3}H-F.

Features suggestive, but not diagnostic, of folic acid deficiency in a patient with megaloblastic anemia are:

- Lack of neurologic changes of the type seen in cobalamin deficiency.
- Normal serum cobalamin and urine methylmalonic acid levels.
- A history of circumstances almost certain to lead to folic acid deficiency, for example, poor diet, frank malabsorption, or alcoholism.

1. Decreased serum folate level

The serum folate assay, a microbiologic procedure employing *L. casei* (ATCC 7469), is a reliable method for the definitive diagnosis of folic acid deficiency, although satisfactory radioisotope dilution assays are now available. A typical range of normal is 6–20 ng/ml. Serum folate levels are low ($<$3 ng/ml) in folic acid-deficient subjects.

2. Decreased red cell folate

Although assay of red cell folate is said to provide a better assessment of the level of folate coenzymes in tissue than serum folate, the test is not widely used clinically. The normal range is 165–600 ng/ml of packed cells. Folic acid-deficient subjects in one study had levels of 24–135 (mean, 74) ng/ml.

3. Elevated FIGlu excretion

The elevated FIGlu excretion after a histidine-loading dose provides a useful and simple test for folic acid deficiency. However, as noted above, it is less specific diagnostically than the serum folate determination. It becomes abnormal later than serum folate and thus gives a better measure of tissue coenzyme levels. Its greatest usefulness is in subjects taking antifolate drugs, in whom serum folate levels may be normal and tissue coenzyme levels drastically reduced.

4. Response to therapy

The occurrence of a full therapeutic response following administration of a "physiologic" dose of folic acid (i.e., 200–400 μg daily) distinguishes folic acid deficiency from cobalamin deficiency, in which a response to folic acid occurs only after "pharmacologic" doses (i.e., 5 mg daily). Unlike the patient with PA, who cannot assimilate the needed vitamin from food, the folic acid-deficient patient is likely to have a spontaneous response to dietary folic acid unless the hospital diet is restricted in vegetables and liver. Thus, a long control period, which includes the administration of cobalamin in small doses, is necessary for definitive diagnosis by this method.

B. Specific syndromes

Major causes of folic acid deficiency, summarized in table 5.1, are considered here under the headings (1) decreased intake; (2) increased requirements; and (3) blocked activation.

1. Decreased intake

a. POOR DIET

Because the amount of folic acid in the diet is not greatly in excess of the nutritional requirement and because body folate reserves are relatively small, folic acid deficiency develops rapidly in individuals taking an inadequate diet. As mentioned, loss of food folate through excessive cooking may also cause folic acid deficiency, especially among disadvantaged peoples who live on finely divided foods such as rice. Megaloblastic anemia occurring in chronic liver disease is usually due to folic acid deficiency resulting from poor diet and impaired hepatic storage of folic acid. Nutritional folic acid deficiency is often associated with multiple vitamin deficiencies and alcoholism. In such patients, a significant history of gross dietary inadequacy is usually easy to obtain.

b. MALABSORPTION

The importance of intestinal malabsorption as a cause of folic acid deficiency was established by test procedures that assess by microbiologic or isotopic techniques the concentration of folate in the serum, urine, or stool following an oral test dose of the vitamin. These include:

- Comparison of the microbiologically assayed time course of urinary folic acid activity after parenteral and oral administration of 5 mg of folic acid.
- Microbiologic determination of serum folate activity after a standard oral dose of folic acid.
- Determination of urinary radioactivity after an oral dose of ^{3}H-F (40 μg/body weight) accompanied by a parenteral flushing dose of 15 mg of unlabeled folic acid.
- Assay of fecal radioactivity after an oral dose of ^{3}H-F.

Each of these procedures has advantages and disadvantages.

Various forms of malabsorption are common causes of folic acid deficiency. **Nontropical sprue** (adult celiac disease) is now recognized to be a generalized disorder of absorption in children or adults that is related to the ingestion of wheat protein (i.e., gluten) or its glutamine-rich polypeptide components. Patients display many signs of malabsorption, including weight loss, iron deficiency, osteomalacia, decreased prothrombin levels, and so forth. The diagnosis rests on:

- Clinical evidence of folic acid deficiency.
- A jejunal biopsy showing villous atrophy and other changes that are characteristic if not pathognomonic.
- Demonstrable malabsorption of folic acid and steatorrhea.
- Folic acid treatment corrects the deficiency without affecting the absorptive defect.
- A response to therapy with a gluten-free diet.

Tropical sprue, in many ways similar to nontropical sprue, is a malabsorptive disorder of unknown etiology with a wide spectrum of clinical manifestations. It occurs frequently and endemically in the tropics—notably the West Indies, the Indian subcontinent, and southeast Asia—and can be acquired by residents of temperate climates who go to the tropics; sometimes it persists long after return from the tropics. It may be due in part to deficiency of dietary folate, the malabsorption resulting from secondary gastrointestinal changes. Treatment with folic acid alone usually reverses all abnormalities, including defective folate absorption.

Other causes of malabsorption are noted in table 5.1. Low serum folate levels in patients receiving diphenylhydantoin (Dilantin®) have been attributed to a reversible drug-induced malabsorption of pteroylpolyglutamate. Oral contraceptives have recently been shown to block deconjugation of pteroylpolyglutamate in certain women.

2. *Increased requirements*

a. PREGNANCY

Anemia is diagnosed by unique criteria in pregnancy because the physiologic hydremia accompanying gestation decreases hemoglobin concentration by a few grams per deciliter despite a concurrent increase in total hemoglobin mass. Large surveys of pregnant women show that anemia of pregnancy is common and is due (in order of decreasing frequency) to combined deficiency of iron and folic acid; combined deficiency of iron, folic acid, and cobalamin; iron deficiency alone; iron and cobalamin deficiency; and folic acid deficiency alone. Thus, although anemia is commonly due to multiple nutritional deficiencies, two-thirds of anemic women are folic acid deficient during pregnancy, and folic acid deficiency is the major cause of megaloblastic anemia during pregnancy. Its frequency is attributable to low reserves of folic acid and the fact that pregnancy increases daily requirements for folic acid five- to tenfold, especially in the last trimester. The presence of multiple fetuses, poor diet (a frequent result of anorexia or nausea), infection, and lactation may further increase requirements. An unexplained phenomenon is the capacity of the fetus to take up folic acid (and other nutrients) at the expense of the mother, even when the available supply is markedly reduced. Despite controversy, most workers agree that routine folic acid supplementation is desirable during pregnancy because not only are folic acid requirements increased but clinical evidence suggests an association between severe folic acid deficiency and complications of pregnancy other than anemia, for example, abruptio placenta, embryopathology, spontaneous abortion, and bleeding.

b. HYPERACTIVE HEMATOPOIESIS

The requirement for folic acid rises sharply in hemolytic anemias associated with acute or chronic overactivity of the bone marrow (lectures 11–15). Indeed, megaloblastic changes may appear in the bone marrow almost simultaneously with the onset of a severe acute hemolytic process.

c. NEOPLASTIC DISEASE

Moderate to severe folic acid deficiency is frequently observed in patients with neoplastic disease, especially metastatic cancer and the leukemias. The deficiency presumably reflects competitive utilization of the vitamin by tumor cells, a phenomenon that resembles the preemption of maternal nutrients by a fetus. However, other explanations for deficiency in a given patient may be valid, among them poor diet, cachexia, malabsorption, and hepatic insufficiency.

3. Blocked activation

a. FOLIC ACID ANTAGONISTS

The 4-aminopteroylglutamates Aminopterin® and methotrexate are powerful inhibitors of dihydrofolate reductase that can cause deficiency of folate coenzymes in tissues within hours. Other enzymes of folic acid metabolism are inhibited only weakly. Major toxic effects of these drugs are:

- Necrotic mouth lesions
- Ulcerations of the esophagus, small intestine, and colon with abdominal pain, vomiting, and diarrhea
- Megaloblastic anemia and subsequent bone marrow hypoplasia and pancytopenia
- A miscellany of effects including alopecia and increased sensitivity to infection

Citrovorum factor effectively counteracts the actions of methotrexate and is useful in the treatment of toxicity.

b. VITAMIN C DEFICIENCY

Because the metabolic relations of folic acid and vitamin C are unresolved, vitamin C deficiency merits comment in a discussion of folate-responsive megaloblastic anemias resulting from impaired reduction of folic acid. The anemia accompanying scurvy has no characteristic pattern. Usually it is normoblastic, due to hemolysis or tissue bleeding, with resulting iron deficiency. Occasionally it is megaloblastic. The megaloblastic anemia appears in some patients to respond to therapy with ascorbic acid alone and in others to folic acid alone. Despite reports of response to ascorbic acid therapy, it is usual for ascorbic acid therapy to be ineffective until folic acid is given. The following data have suggested that ascorbic acid participates in the reduction of folic acid to FH_4: (1) dietary deficiency of vitamin C may cause an otherwise barely adequate intake of folic acid to become insufficient; (2) in scurvy, oral vitamin C augments the erythropoietic effect of 125 μg of folic acid given daily; and (3) in experimental megaloblastic anemias induced in monkeys by folic acid and vitamin C deficiencies, citrovorum factor is more active erythropoietically than folic acid. Such a double deficiency is the presumed basis for megaloblastic anemia in infants fed exclusively on unsupplemented formulas containing dried milk deprived of vitamin C in the manufacturing process. Despite these findings, a biochemical role for ascorbic acid in the reduction of folic acid remains to be established. It is more likely that ascorbic acid increases the stability of FH_4 and its derivatives.

III. MEGALOBLASTIC ANEMIA UNRESPONSIVE TO COBALAMIN OR FOLIC ACID

Megaloblastic anemia is occasionally unaccompanied by cobalamin or folic acid deficiency and fails to respond to therapy with either vitamin. In some cases, folic acid or cobalamin deficiency coexists with megaloblastic anemia but is not responsible for it. These relatively uncommon occurrences arise in three situations (see table 5.1):

- Therapy with an antimetabolite drug that interferes with DNA synthesis
- Inborn error of metabolism
- Refractory megaloblastic anemia of undetermined etiology

Except for the dysplastic features to be described, megaloblasts in these marrows generally resemble those in vitamin-deficiency megaloblastic anemia. It can be assumed, therefore, that the defect in all is an impaired capacity to duplicate DNA at a normal rate.

A. Antimetabolite drugs

The many antimetabolites employed in the chemotherapy of leukemia, lymphoma, and solid tumors include agents that block the synthesis of DNA, either as a solitary effect or in concert with similar effects on RNA or protein synthesis. Agents that block DNA synthesis inhibit either single or multiple steps in the biosynthetic pathway. We shall consider here only major examples of each class of agents. Notes on their chemotherapeutic applications will be found in lectures 22 and 23. Consideration is also omitted of agents (like methotrexate) that block DNA synthesis by mechanisms that are neutralized by simultaneously administered folic acid or citrovorum factor. These were discussed above.

1. Inhibitors of purine synthesis

The most commonly employed purine analogues are the thiopurines, **6-mercaptopurine** (6-MP), **thioguanine** (6-TG), and **azathioprine** (Imuran®). Although much is known about the multiple sites of action of the thiopurines and their nucleotide derivatives, the mechanism of their chemotherapeutic effects is not precisely known. For example:

- 6-MP competes with hypoxanthine for a binding site in inosinic acid pyrophosphorylase and is itself converted to thioinosinic acid (TIMP), which inhibits the conversions of inosinic acid (IMP) to xanthylic acid (XMP) and adenylic acid (AMP).
- 6-MP is incorporated into RNA and DNA.
- TIMP mimics AMP and GMP as a feedback inhibitor of the first step of purine synthesis, in which phosphoribosylamine is formed from glutamine and phosphoribosylpyrophosphate.

These considerations suggest that the thiopurines can inhibit RNA and DNA synthesis; they can be incorporated into both nucleic acids, thereby causing malfunctions of the several forms of nucleic acid; and they can inhibit coenzyme formation and function, thereby interfering with cell metabolism. The main toxic effects of the thiopurines are bone marrow depression with resulting leukopenia, anemia, and thrombocytopenia. Before hypoplasia occurs, the marrow is megaloblastic. Serum folate and cobalamin levels are normal, and vitamin therapy is unavailing. The megaloblastosis, usually mild, disappears when durgs are withdrawn. If thiopurines interfere equally with the synthesis of RNA and DNA, the appearance of megaloblastosis suggests that effects on DNA synthesis are physiologically more critical than those on RNA synthesis.

2. Inhibitors of pyrimidine synthesis

Two groups of chemotherapeutic agents block the synthesis of pyrimidine nucleotides: (1) those that block methylation of deoxyuridylate (dUMP) to deoxythymidylate (dTMP) and (2) those that block de novo synthesis of the pyrimidine ring. The former includes **5-fluoro-2′-deoxyuridine** (FUdR), the deoxyribonucleoside of 5-fluorouracil (FU). The thymine deficiency produced by the inhibitory FUdR (or its in vivo product, FdUTP) on thymidylate synthetase is in part the basis of its chemotherapeutic action. Interestingly, FdUTP is incorporated into DNA (like dUTP) in place of dTTP. It is also attacked by dUTPase (like dUTP), as discussed in lecture 5. Consequently when dUTPase levels are exceeded, both FU and U (uracil) are misincorporated into DNA, and both are excised by

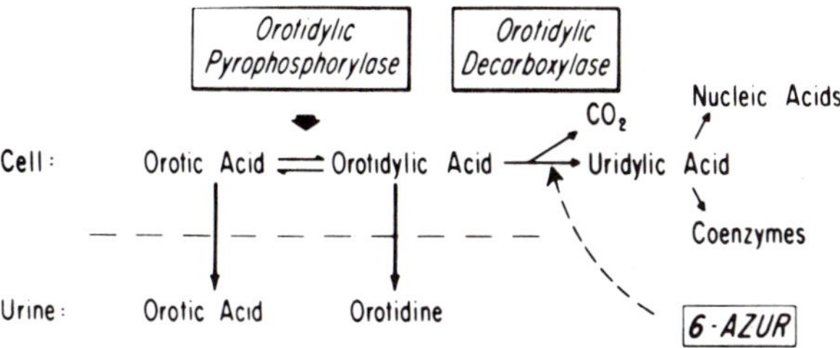

Fig. 6.4
Terminal portion of de novo pathway of pyrimidine synthesis, showing locus of action of 6-azauridine (6-AzUR). Dashed lines indicate inhibition.

uracil-DNA-glycosylase with resulting DNA fragmentation. Administration of FUdR produces a mild megaloblastic anemia along with other toxic effects in rapidly proliferating tissues—glossitis, diarrhea, and so forth. Bone marrow eventually becomes hypoplastic.

The second category of inhibitors of pyrimidine synthesis is exemplified by **6-azauridine** (6-AzUR). It blocks the conversion of orotidylic acid to uridylic acid (figure 6.4) and may occasionally produce megaloblastosis associated with the accumulation of renal excretion of orotic acid and orotidine.

3. *Inhibitors of deoxyribonucleotide synthesis*

Two antitumor agents that appear to act by inhibiting ribonucleotide reductase, the enzyme that catalyzes the reductive conversion of ribonucleotides to deoxyribonucleotides (see figure 5.3), are 1-β-D-**arabinofuranosylcytosine** (ara-C, cytosine arabinoside) and **hydroxyurea**. Ara-C is a nucleoside in which the sugar component is arabinosyl, an analogue of both ribosyl and deoxyribosyl. It is believed to block the conversion of CDP to dCDP and inhibit DNA polymerase. It produces severe megaloblastosis that is indifferent to vitamin therapy. Hydroxyurea also produces marked megaloblastosis. It inhibits the reductive conversion of CDP to dCDP by complexing with the nonheme iron prosthetic group of ribonucleotide reductase.

B. Inborn errors

1. *Hereditary orotic aciduria*

Hereditary orotic aciduria is a rare disorder of pyrimidine metabolism manifested by severe megaloblastic anemia refractory to vitamin therapy, growth impairment, and the renal excretion of orotic acid in large quantities. The disease has been described in several children in whom orally administered preparations of uridylic and cytidylic acids produced clinical improvement with reduction of orotic aciduria. The defect is attributable to a genetically determined block in either the orotidylic pyrosphosphorylase and orotidylic decarboxylase reactions or both (figure 6.4).

2. *Errors of folate metabolism*

Inborn errors have been reported in folate absorption, folate interconversion (e.g., FH_2 reductase deficiency, N^5, N^{10}-methylene FH_4 reductase deficiency), and folate utilization (e.g., N^5-methyl FH_4-homocysteine methyltransferase deficiency, glutamate formiminotransferase deficiency). Although rare, inborn errors should be considered in patients who are not cobalamin deficient and who display:

- Very low serum folate levels and poor response to oral folate
- Mental retardation
- Extreme elevation of serum folate level
- Excessive urinary excretion of homocysteine or FIGlu
- Megaloblastic anemia in infancy

In most cases, the diagnosis is established by enzyme assays in fibroblast cultures of skin biopsy material.

C. Unexplained disorders

There remains a group of disorders associated with megaloblastic transformation, sometimes of severe degree, that does not respond to therapy with cobalamin or folic acid and that has not yet been associated with an enzyme deletion or defect (but which may nevertheless result from such a defect).

1. *Pyridoxine-responsive anemia*

The rare disorder of hemoglobin synthesis known as pyridoxine-responsive anemia is discussed in lecture 7. It is mentioned here because about 20% of such cases are associated with megaloblastosis. The mechanism of megaloblastic transformation in these cases is unknown. Since pyridoxine and folic acid both participate in the serine-glycine interconversion (see table 6.2), it is conceivable that a defect of this enzyme induces a requirement for pharmacologic doses of pyridoxine in the absence of which folic acid metabolism is impaired. In attempting to classify these complex disorders, Vilter pointed out that each type is characterized by variable combinations of ring sideroblasts, excess body iron, and refractory megaloblastic erythropoiesis. All are presumably due to metabolic errors—some hereditary and sex-linked, others apparently acquired. Megaloblastic changes are usually confined to the erythroid series. Thus, unless there is associated folic acid or cobalamin deficiency, hypersegmented neutrophils are not observed in the blood. Megaloblastosis is often atypical with dysplastic features (e.g., binucleate cells, clover-leaf nuclei). Serum lactic dehydrogenase is only moderately elevated. When megaloblastic transformation is severe and extensive, the disorder is indistinguishable from erythremic myelosis.

2. *Erythremic myelosis (Di Guglielmo's syndrome)*

Erythremic myelosis is considered elsewhere (lecture 22). It is mentioned here because it is associated with severe refractory megaloblastic anemia. Its major features are:

- Abnormal proliferation of erythroid and myeloid precursors in marrow
- Dysplastic and megaloblastic PAS-positive erythroid precursors in blood, marrow, and tissues (e.g., large multinucleate cells, clover-leaf nuclei) and bizarre red cell morphology
- Anemia due to ineffective erythropoiesis and variable hemolysis
- Sideroblastic features
- Elevated serum cobalamin levels in many but not all patients
- A tendency to appear as a complication or evolutionary stage of refractory anemia, polycythemia vera, or myelocytic leukemia
- A tendency to evolve into acute myelocytic leukemia.
- A notably poor response to therapy with antimetabolites, cobalamin, or folic acid

The nature and pathogenesis of erythremic myelosis are as unclear as those of the other refractory magaloblastic anemias. The writer suspects that in these disorders the bone marrow has acquired a hardy clone of somatically mutated cells in which the defect is loss of one or another of the enzymes in the pathway of DNA synthesis, for example, ribonucleotide reductase, thymidylate synthetase, DNA polymerase, or deoxyribonucleotide kinase.

SELECTED REFERENCES

Reviews

Beck, W. S. Metabolic aspects of cobalamin and folic acid. In Williams, W. J., Beutler, E., et al., eds. *Hematology*, 3rd ed. New York: McGraw-Hill Book Co. (Blakiston Division), 1983, pp. 311–331.

Beck, W. S. Megaloblastic anemias. In Wyngaarden, J. B., and Smith, L. H., Jr., eds. *Cecil's Textbook of Medicine*, 18th ed. Philadelphia: W. B. Saunders Co., 1988, pp. 900–907.

Hitchings, G. H., Jr. Nobel lecture in physiology or medicine—1988. Selective inhibitors of dihydrofolate reductase. *In Vitro Cell. Dev. Biol.* 25(1989): 303–310.

Kisliuk, R. L. Pteroylpolyglutamates. *Mol. Cell Biochem.* 39(1981): 331–345.

Rosenberg, I. H. Folate absorption: clinical questions and metabolic answers. *Am. J. Clin. Nutr.* 51(1990): 531–534.

Original articles

Beck, W. S. Drugs and the intestinal absorption of folate [editorial]. *J. Lab. Clin. Med.* 108(1986): 263–264.

Bernstein, L. H., Gutstein, S., et al. The absorption and malabsorption of folic acid and its polyglutamates. *Am. J. Med.* 48(1970): 570–579.

Bertino, J. R. Leucovorin rescue revisited. *J. Clin. Oncol.* 8(1990): 193–195.

Bhandari, S. D., Gregory, J. F., III, et al. Properties of pteroylpolyglutamate hydrolase in pancreatic juice of the pig. *J. Nutr.* 120(1990): 467–475.

Erbe, R. W. Inborn errors of folate metabolism. *N. Engl. J. Med.* 293(1975): 753–757.

Fox, R. M., Wood, M. H., et al. Hereditary orotic aciduria: types I and II. *Am. J. Med.* 55(1973): 791–798.

Kane, M. A., and Waxman, S. Biology of disease: role of folate binding proteins in folate metabolism. *Lab. Invest.* 60(1989): 737–743.

Kornberg, A., Segal, R., et al. Folic acid deficiency, megaloblastic anemia and peripheral polyneuropathy due to oral contraceptives. *Isr. J. Med. Sci.* 25(1989): 142–145.

Milunsky, A., Jick, H., et al. Multivitamin/folic acid supplementation in early pregnancy reduces the prevalence of neural tube defects. *JAMA* 262(1989): 2847–2852.

Reisenauer, A. M., Krumdieck, C. L., et al. Folate conjugase: two separate activities in human jejunum. *Science* 198(1977): 196–197.

Rosenberg, I. H. Folate absorption and malabsorption. *N. Engl. J. Med.* 293(1975): 1303–1308.

Schirch, V., and Strong, W. B. Interaction of folylpolyglutamates with enzymes in one-carbon metabolism. *Arch. Biochem. Biophys.* 269(1989): 371–380.

Smith, L. H., Jr. Hereditary orotic aciduria—pyrimidine auxotrophism in man. *Am. J. Med.* 38(1965): 1–6.

Subar, A. F., Block, G., et al. Folate intake and food sources in the US population. *Am. J. Clin. Nutr.* 50(1989): 508–516.

LECTURE 7

Hypochromic Anemias I. Iron Deficiency and Excess

William S. Beck

EDITOR'S COMMENT

Like folate deficiency, iron deficiency is one of the most common of all clinical disorders, in many cases occurring in undeveloped countries as a pandemic that seriously affects the growth, intellectual development, and overall health of children. In addition, many important issues remain to be resolved surrounding the fortification of food with iron and the development of possible methods for surveying populations for iron deficiency. This lecture summarizes our knowledge of iron metabolism, iron deficiency, and the various syndromes of iron excess.

I. INTRODUCTION

A. Major causes of anemia (revisited)

As noted in lecture 1, anemia may be due either to increased loss of red cells (as in hemorrhage or hemolysis) or decreased production of red cells. Increased loss or destruction is associated (at least in early stages) with effective erythropoiesis and marrow hyperproliferation, as manifested by elevation of the reticulocyte count. Anemias due to decreased red cell production are associated with low reticulocyte counts. This category includes anemias assocated with ineffective erythropoiesis (as in hypochromic and megaloblastic anemia) or hypoproliferative defects of the erythroid marrow (as in aplastic aneima or myelophthisis) (see table 4.1)

This lecture concerns the **hypochromic anemias**, a group of disorders in which the primary defect is a quantitative decrease in hemoglobin synthesis. DNA synthesis and the capacity for cell division are not impaired—at least in the early stages.

B. Hypochromia and microcytosis

Whatever the reason for impairment of hemoglobin synthesis, the main result is a decreased mean cell hemoglobin concentration (MCHC). A useful hypothesis holds that in the course of erythroid maturation, cell divisions continue to occur until the MCHC of the developing cell reaches a certain critical value. In hypochromic anemia, one or more extra divisions may occur because the MCHC is depressed. Since each cell division reduces cell size, abnormal extra divisions yield red cells of abnormally small mean corpuscular volume (MCV). This state is termed **microcytosis**. The converse situation, in which fewer divisions occur, results in **macrocytosis**.

C. Major causes of hypochromic anemia

1. *Impaired heme synthesis*

- Unavailability of iron for synthetic process
  Iron deficiency
  "Pyridoxine-responsive" anemia and the several related "sideroblastic" anemias
  Lead poisoning
- Defective iron reutilization

2. *Impaired globin synthesis*

- α-thalassemia (see lecture 11)
- β-thalassemia (see lecture 11)
- Hemoglobin Lepore trait (see lectures 10, 11)

II. IRON METABOLISM

A. Total body iron

Daily iron intake and iron loss are small, and body iron is repeatedly reutilized. Quantitative considerations are therefore uniquely important for an understanding of iron metabolism and its pathophysiology.

1. *Amount*

The average adult body contains a total of about 3.5 g of elemental iron (range, 2–5 g). For convenience, we shall consider that a 70-kg man contains in round numbers 50 mg/kg or about 3500 mg.

2. *Compartments in adult*

	Total (mg)	% of total
• Hemoglobin iron	2300	66
• Tissue iron	1140	33
Available, or storage, iron (ferritin 500, hemosiderin 500)	1000	29
Nonavailable, or essential, iron (myoglobin, 130; cytochromes, catalase 10)	140	4
• Other tissue iron	8	0.2
• Plasma or transport, iron	3	0.1

B. Nutritional requirements

The minuteness of daily iron losses, revealed in classic studies of McCance and Widdowson in 1936 and confirmed by balance studies using ^{59}Fe, implies that daily iron intake is equally minute. If this were not so the body would accumulate iron.

1. Content in diet

The average diet contains considerably more iron than is needed, though exact amounts are in dispute. Food iron consists largely of heme iron. Moreover, heme iron in the diet is relatively unavailable unless enhancers such as ascorbic acid are present. Typical Western diets contain about 6 mg elemental iron per 1000 calories. Hence, an adult consuming a 2500-calorie diet ingests about 15 mg/day. Appreciable amounts of iron can come from iron cooking pots. Despite the seeming excess of dietary iron over need, iron deficiency is common in the world's populations, and many countries have chosen to fortify flour, infant formulas, and other foods with medicinal iron. In Sweden today, 42% of all ingested iron comes from fortification. This and other factors (popularity of self-administered ascorbic acid, use of iron prophylaxis in pregnancy, etc.) have decreased the incidence of iron deficiency but have alarmed those who fear the effects of increased iron intake in individuals with undiagnosed hemochromatosis and other iron-loading disorders (see below).

2. Amount absorbed

A normal individual absorbs 4–10% of the total iron ingested; an average normal figure is 6%. Hence, about 1 mg of iron is absorbed daily. Much work has been done on percentages of iron absorbed from different foodstuffs. Percentages vary notably, being low for eggs, liver, and leafy vegetables and high for muscle, fish, and soybeans.

3. Factors affecting daily requirement

a. MENSTRUATION

Mean blood loss is 44 ml/menstrual period. Since 1 ml of blood contains about 0.5 mg of iron, normal menstrual losses average 22 mg/month or 0.7 mg/day, but in many women losses are as high as 2 mg/day. Menstrual losses tend to rise with increasing age and parity.

b. PREGNANCY

In the second and third trimesters of pregnancy, the daily requirement is 4–6 mg. In an average normal pregnancy iron loss is spared by cessation of menstruation (saving = 280 days × 0.7 = 196 mg). But expansion of the mother's hemoglobin mass requires 480 mg of additional iron, and formation of the placenta, cord, and fetus requires another 390 mg. Actual loss of blood at delivery—about 660 ml of whole blood (560 ml in the placenta and 100 ml in the lochia)—wastes 330 mg. Thus the total iron cost of pregnancy (over and above normal basal requirement of 1.0 mg/day) = 480 + 390 + 330 − 196 = about 1004 mg, or 3.6 mg/day. Since storage iron equals about 1000 mg, a single pregnancy without supplemental iron inevitably exhausts stores. Lactation also increases iron losses.

c. GROWTH

Requirements are proportionately greater in infancy (3–24 months) than at any other age. They are also high in childhood and adolescence, especially in girls at the time of menarche.

C. Intestinal absorption

1. Locus

Iron is mainly absorbed in the duodenum and upper jejunum, though some absorption occurs in the stomach, ileum, and colon.

2. Regulation

Since the diet contains 10–20 times the amount of iron absorbed, body iron levels can be kept constant only through mechanisms that regulate the amount of iron absorbed in the small intestine.

Absorption of iron by intestinal mucosal cells occurs in two phases: **uptake** of iron from lumen into cells and **transfer** of iron across cells into circulation. Ferrous iron (Fe^{2+}) in the intestinal lumen enters readily into the mucosal cells of the duodenum and upper jejunum. Heme taken up by mucosal cells is degraded to free inorganic iron, bilirubin, and carbon monoxide by **heme oxygenase** (see lecture 8). Within mucosal cells, Fe^{2+} is oxidized to ferric iron (Fe^{3+}), some of which complexes with the protein **apoferritin** to yield **ferritin**. The remainder complexes with **apotransferrin** to form **transferrin**, or a transferrin-like protein (see below)—some of it in minutes, the rest in the course of 12 to 24 hours. Transferrin appears to be the carrier in this transfer process. When the cells are sloughed away at the end of their 1- or 2-day life span, their residual iron is lost with them.

The rate of transfer of mucosal cell iron into the bloodstream is somehow governed by the body's iron requirements. Granick proposed a model, the **mucosal block theory**, according to which the ferritin-apoferritin system in mucosal cells controls the amount of iron absorbed. Ferritin depletion in iron deficiency thus increases absorption. However, mucosal cells also contain transferrin and other iron-binding proteins. When iron deficiency is corrected, absorption returns to normal. Some evidence suggests an unidentified pool of tissue iron somehow communicates information on body iron stores.

This system, if it exists, is quite inefficient. For example:

- As iron ingestion increases, iron absorption may become abnormally high, although the percentage absorbed decreases.
- Although iron traffic from mucosal cells into the body increases in iron deficiency, exceptions cloud the picture. Little iron is absorbed in idiopathic steatorrhea (despite iron deficiency), and iron absorption rises despite lack of need in hemochromatosis.

3. Factors affecting iron absorption

a. AMOUNT OF IRON IN DIET

The proportion of iron absorbed decreases as the level of dietary iron increases; however, the absolute amount of iron absorbed increases.

b. FORM OF IRON IN DIET

As noted above, heme iron, derived chiefly from the myoglobin and hemoglobin in meat, is apparently absorbed by a mechanism different from that for inorganic and nonheme iron. Heme is absorbed as such; the iron is freed of the porphyrin ring after it has been taken up by the mucosal cell. Phytates, oxalates, and phosphates in the intestinal lumen precipitate inorganic iron and decrease its absorption but have no effect on heme iron. Substances in various cereals (bran, wheat, and maize) also bind nonheme iron, as do tannins in tea and polyphenols in spinach and other vegetables. Nonheme iron absorption is enhanced by sugars and ascorbic acid (see below).

c. GASTRIC SECRETIONS

An iron-binding substance(s) in gastric juice has been claimed to facilitate iron absorption in the intestine. Another substance, the protein **gastroferrin**, is said to bind a portion of dietary iron, thereby making it unavailable for absorption and preventing excess iron intake. In view of these conflicting reports, the role of gastric factors is unclear.

d. PANCREATIC SECRETIONS

Some evidence suggests that exocrine pancreatic secretions depress iron absorption and their lack increases iron absorption. For example, iron absorption and tissue iron may be increased in pancreatic (and chronic liver) disease. The mechansims of these effects remain unclear.

e. HYDROCHLORIC ACID

Fe^{3+} is less well absorbed than Fe^{2+}, and a greater or lesser portion of luminal inorganic iron is reduced in the gut before being absorbed. Clinical evidence suggests that HCl in the gut enhances absorption of Fe^{3+} but not of Fe^{2+} or heme iron. Since inorganic Fe^{3+} is insoluble at pH > 5 (forming $Fe(OH)_3$), it has been postulated that HCl solubilizes Fe^{3+}, making it available for absorption.

f. CHELATION

An alternative theory of HCl action is based on its role in **chelation**. Covalent bonds from six iron go to corners of an octahedron. Iron is normally coated with a shell of H_2O molecules that are replaceable by other molecules and ions called **ligands**. Ligands also complex with the several stable and unstable oxidation states of iron. Such complexes vary in stability depending on the ligands. Small changes in the ligand may lead to large changes in the character of the iron complex.

Chelation is a process that results in the formation of stable heterocyclic rings as a consequence of ligand attachment. Simple **monodentate** ligands (e.g., acetate, chloride, NH_3) satisfy only one coordination site of a metal cation and form charged soluble complex ions. **Bidentate** ligands (e.g., $H_2N—NH_2$) satisfy two coordination sites but not with one cation because of strain. Therefore, there is bridging (e.g., $Fe—H_2N—NH_2—Fe$) and, in turn, the formation of lattices. Other lattice-building ligands are OH^- and PO_4^{2-}. When **polydentate** ligands combine to form strain-free heterocyclic rings, the resulting structure is a stable structure called a chelate. For example,

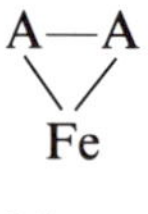

```
A—A
 \/
 Fe
```

Many such examples are found among the derivatives of hydroxamic acid:

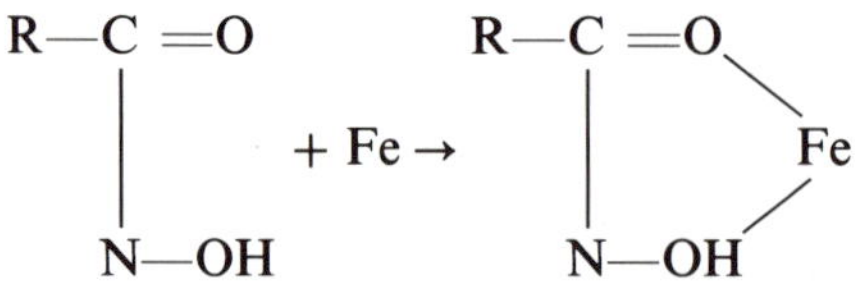

```
R—C =O              R—C =O
  |                   |    \
  |       + Fe →      |     Fe
  |                   |    /
  N—OH                N—OH
```

The bacterial **ferrioxamines** (figure 7.1) are, in effect, three linked hydroxamic acid derivatives. The drug *desferrioxamine* (Desferal®), a potent and specific iron-chelating agent, is essentially an iron-free ferrioxamine. The iron-binding constant is 10^{30}.

Nonheme Fe^{3+} chelates readily with sugars, amino acids, and polyols (e.g., ascorbic acid). Some have proposed that iron is transported across the intestinal mucosal cell membranes as a soluble iron chelate. This may account for the capacity of agents such as sugars, amino acids, and other

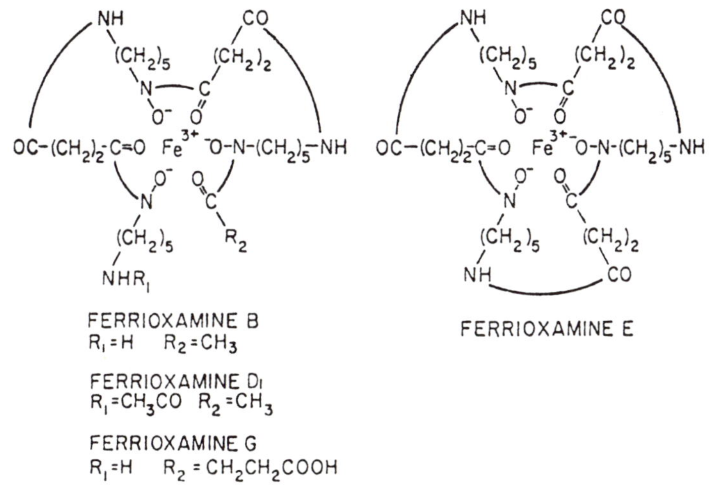

FERRIOXAMINE B
$R_1 = H \quad R_2 = CH_3$

FERRIOXAMINE D_1
$R_1 = CH_3CO \quad R_2 = CH_3$

FERRIOXAMINE G
$R_1 = H \quad R_2 = CH_2CH_2COOH$

FERRIOXAMINE E

Fig. 7.1
Structure of ferrioxamines B, D_1, G, and E. (From V. Prelog, in F. Gross, ed., *Iron Metabolism: An International Symposium*, Berlin: Springer-Verlag, 1964, p. 73.)

organic acids (including ascorbic acid) to promote iron absorption. These are chelating agents; some are also reducing agents. The chelating and reducing functions of these ligands are both important promoters of iron absorption. HCl also promotes chelation of iron. Once chelates have formed at low pH, they remain soluble at an acid or alkaline pH.

D. Transport

1. Transferrin

All body iron is combined (chelated) with one or another protein. Plasma iron is carried in association with the specific iron-binding β_1-globulin **transferrin**.

a. PROPERTIES

Transferrin is a single polypeptide chain of mol. wt. 80,000 on which are arranged two identical branched carbohydrate chains, each anchored to an asparaginyl residue and terminating in sialic acid. The protein is 6.2% carbohydrate by weight. Half-life of transferrin in vivo is 8 days. Asialotransferrin is cleared more rapidly, though early work suggested that asialotransferrin may be an unusual asialoglycoprotein in this respect. Species differences may have been responsible.

Each molecule binds two Fe^{3+} ions with high affinity ($K > 10^{30}$). For each Fe^{3+} bound, a suitable anion must be bound. When available, HCO_3^- is the favored anion. Although there are chemical differences between the two binding sites, iron binding is essentially a random process, and release of iron to erythroid cells is an all-or-none phenomenon. After much controversy, it appears that the two Fe^{3+} are equivalent, the two sites being equivalent as iron donors. However, diferric transferrin is a better iron donor than monoferric transferrin.

The carbohydrate chains may be involved in the binding of transferrin to specific **transferrin receptors** on the erythroid cell surface. When colorless apotransferrin binds iron, the complex undergoes conformational change and becomes salmon-pink. One gram of apotransferrin binds 1.25 mg of iron. Normal plasma concentration of apotransferrin and transferrin (combined) is 1.0–2.5 mg/ml. At least 18 genetic variants of transferrin are known.

Transferrin is required for the growth of many cell lines in culture. It is also a growth factor for fetal cells.

b. TRANSFERRIN RECEPTOR

Transferrin receptors are found on the surfaces of all cells, but in large numbers on erythroid and placental cells, both of which have high iron requirements. The receptor protein is a transmembrane glycoprotein of mol wt. 96,000 with two subunits.

c. PHYSIOLOGIC ROLE

Iron that has crossed the intestinal mucosal cell enters the blood and is there bound to plasma transferrin (figure 7.2). Normal **serum iron** concentration is 100–150 μg/dl. Normal total **iron-binding capacity** (IBC) (i.e., the total amount of iron that can be bound to the sum of apotransferrin and transferrin present) is 300–400 μg/dl. Thus circulating transferrin is normally about one-third saturated. Intravenously injected inorganic iron is rapidly bound to transferrin. Since unsaturated capacity for the total blood volume is about 10 mg (3–4 mg is already bound), injection of more than 10 mg iron can have serious toxic effects.

2. *Plasma-to-cell movement of iron*

In the so-called **plasma-to-cell cycle**, a molecule of diferric transferrin attaches with high affinity to one of more than 250,000 transferrin receptors present on the surface of an early erythroid precursor cell. These receptors decrease in number during red cell maturation. A reticulocyte can still bind 25,000–50,000 iron-laden transferrin molecules. A mature red cell lacks receptors.

Iron is internalized by endocytosis (figure 7.3). In this process the binding of transferrin to surface receptors forms invaginated pits in the cell membrane. A small saclike structure carries the ligand-receptor complex (along with a portion of the external medium) into the cell interior. There a coated vesicle forms, with walls containing clathrin and other proteins. The clathrin coat is soon disassembled and shed. There is then a fusion of several

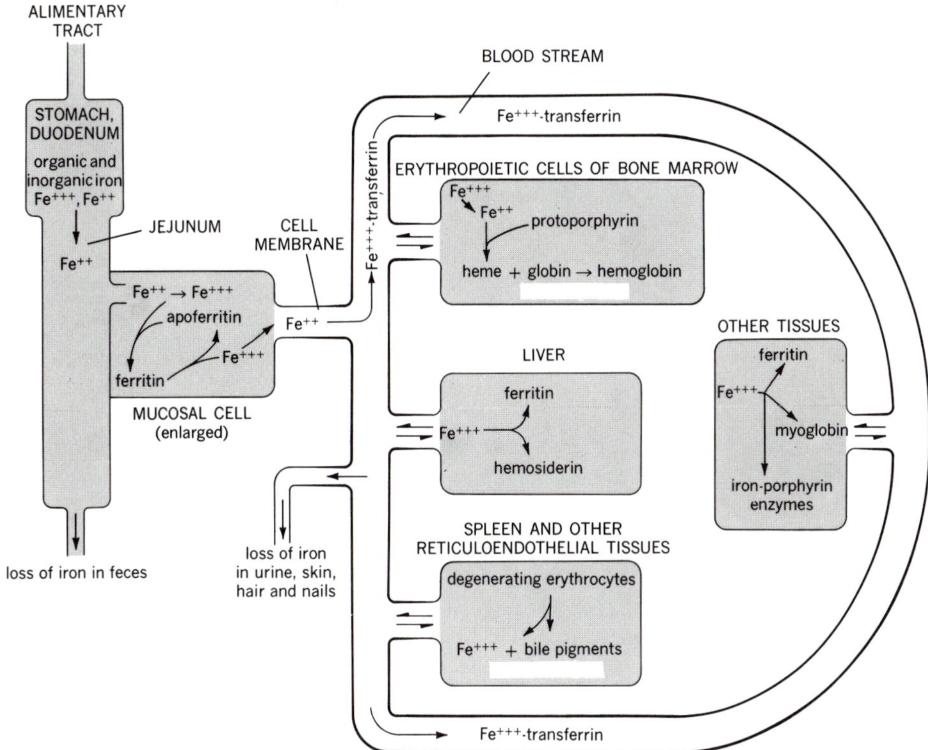

Fig. 7.2
Scheme of iron metabolism. (From W. S. Beck, *Human Design: Molecular, Cellular, and Systematic Physiology*, New York: Harcourt Brace Jovanovich, 1971.)

coated vesicles with an endosome. The pH within the new structure decreases and this dissociates the iron from transferrin. Neither receptor nor transferrin is degraded in the process, both returning to the cell surface.

At neutral pH, free apotransferrin is returned to the plasma, where it can serve again in iron transport. Developing red cells thus have a specific capacity to extract iron from plasma. Although the erythroid marrow receives only 5% of the cardiac output, it extracts 85% of the circulating iron. The remainder goes to parenchymal organs, notably the liver and, if present, the placenta. Interestingly, transferrin and transferrin receptors are found on the surfaces of breast carcinoma cells but not on the cells of normal breast or benign lesions.

The **percentage saturation** of plasma transferrin is an important determinant of the fate of circulating iron. At low saturation, only marrow (and placenta) can extract iron from plasma. At high saturation, the liver takes up more iron. Plasma transferrin levels rise in chronic iron deficiency and drop in hypochromia associated with defective reutilization of iron (see below). Recent work shows that induction of hepatic transferrin synthesis in iron deficiency is regulated directly by an increase in transferrin messenger RNA.

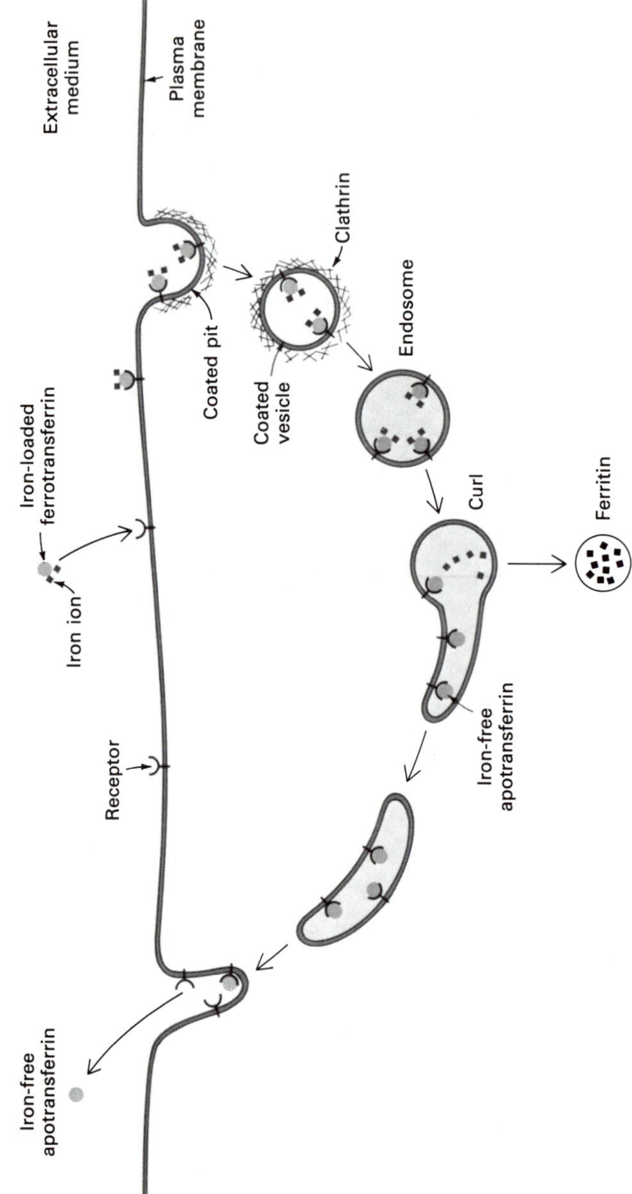

Fig. 7.3
The diagram shows how ferric ions are brought into the cell and eventually enter the cytoplasm, from which the receptors are recycled back to the plasma membrane. (From L. Stryer, *Biochemistry*, 3rd ed. New York: W. H. Freeman, 1988.)

E. Utilization and storage

Injected ^{59}Fe goes to the erythron and to sites of iron storage. However, labeled iron does not mix uniformly with storage iron, and therefore it cannot be used in short-term experiments to measure pool size of storage iron.

1. Storage iron

As noted above, about 30% of body iron is in storage form. The bulk of it is distributed equally between **ferritin** and **hemosiderin**, which are present in RES cells and parenchymal cells of many organs. About one-third is in the marrow; the rest is in spleen, muscle, and so forth.

a. FERRITIN

Ferritin is formed from the combination of iron and apoferritin (figure 7.4). It is a water-soluble complex consisting of an iron core surrounded by 24 apparently identical spherical peptide subunits of mol. wt. about 18,500. Apoferritin has a mol. wt. of about 441,000. The iron content of ferritin is variable; it averages 2,000 atoms per molecule but can reach 4,500 atoms. Thus, the iron can comprise 31% of the weight of ferritin. Usually, ferritin is not maximally saturated and only about 18% iron. Ferritin has a readily identifiable appearance in electron micrographs.

Organ-specific and species-specific (iso)ferritins differing in electrophoretic mobility are now recognized. Ferritn iron is readily mobilized by the

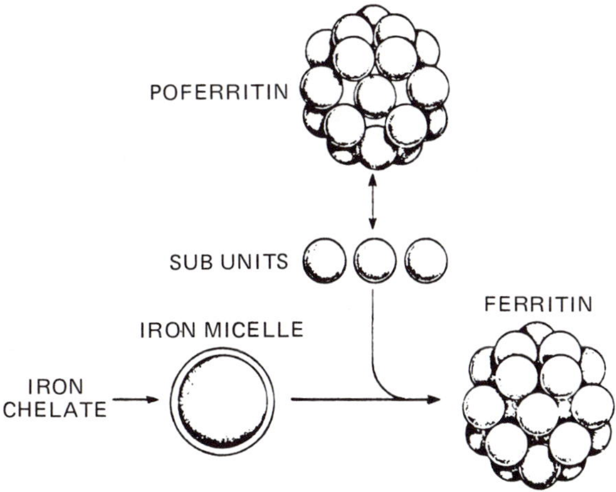

Fig. 7.4
Model showing structure and reconstitution of ferritin. The equilibrium for the dissociation of apoferritin monomers into subunits is assumed to favor the monomer, but removal of subunits by introduction of micellular iron can shift the equilibrium in the direction of ferritin formation. (From R. R. Crichton, *N. Engl. J. Med.* 284[1971]: 1413.)

body when needed, but the mechanism of its mobilization is not clear. Ferritin was once considered an exclusively intracellular protein. It is now known to occur in serum. As noted below, the serum ferritin assay is a valuable index of body iron stores.

b. HEMOSIDERIN

Hemosiderin was first recognized as an amorphous iron-containing granular substance in tissues. The granules are much larger than ferritin molecules and are easily seen by light microscopy, especially when stained with Prussian blue. Hemosiderin is a variable and complex substance formed by aggregation and polymerization of nonferritin micellar iron with natured and denatured protein. Evaluation of the hemosiderin content of liver and RES cells with Prussian blue stain is the best method of assessing body iron stores.

2. *Intracellular events*

Iron in erythroid cells stimulates apoferritin synthesis. Some of it forms ferritin (figure 7.5). By unknown mechanisms, some goes to mitochondria, the loci of heme synthesis. Insertion of iron into protoporphyrin to form

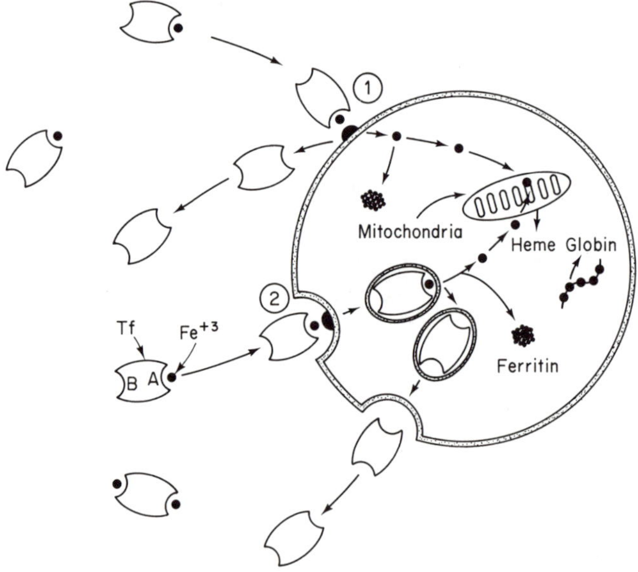

Fig. 7.5
Intracellular events following entry of iron into an immature red cell. (The nucleus is omitted.) As shown, the major mechanism of iron entry is endocytosis of the transferrin-iron complex. When released from transferrin within the cell, iron is transported either to a mitochondrion where it participates in heme synthesis, or to apoferritin, where it forms ferritin, a form of storage iron. (From A. J. Erslev and T. G. Gabuzda, *Pathophysiology of Blood*, 2d ed., Philadelphia: Saunders, 1979.)

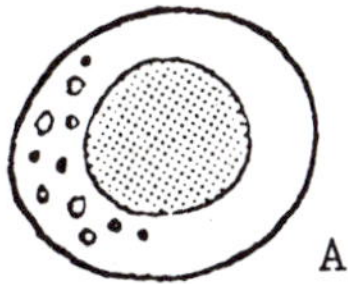

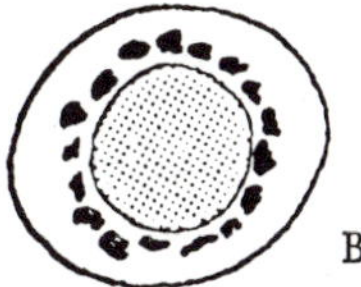

Fig. 7.6
Types of sideroblasts. *A*, Deposits of ferritin. *B*, Mitochondrial loading with ring configuration.

heme is catalyzed in mitochondria by **ferrochelatase (heme synthetase)**, an enzyme system that requires globin and glutathione (-SH). The scheme in figure 7.5 accounts for the appearance of Prussian blue–stained preparations of marrow. In such preparations, approximately 40% of the normoblasts contain small scatered ferritin granules, which appear to be iron storage depots on which the cell can draw as heme synthesis proceeds. At completion of maturation, the iron has gone, leaving apoferritin. Cells containing such deposits are called **sideroblasts** (or, if not nucleated, **siderocytes**). Absence of sideroblasts from marrow is a sign of iron deficiency. Production of heme and globin within the immature cell is precisely balanced, and a decrease in synthesis of either is associated with a parallel decrease in production of the other. However, iron uptake by cells is not regulated, and iron accumulates abnormally if there is a block in porphyrin synthesis (as occurs in "sideroblastic" anemias). Cells in which such iron accumulation has occurred contain large iron clusters of various sizes that are visible with or without special iron stains. These sideroblasts usually contain much more iron than the normal variety. In the sideroblastic anemias, heme synthesis is blocked. Mitochondria become engorged with iron and burst, producing a distinctive **ring sideroblast** (figure 7.6).

3. Cell-to-plasma movement of iron

The **cell-to-plasma cycle** follows the breakdown of red cells at the end of their life span. Since 1% of the total number of circulating red cells breaks down each day, the amount of iron liberated from hemoglobin catabolism is 20–25 mg—the same amount required normally for hemoglobin synthesis each day. (Recall that only 1 mg of iron is ingested and lost each day—only about 0.03% of body iron!) Iron liberated from hemoglobin catabolism remains temporarily in the RES cells. As already noted, assessment of their iron content (by an iron stain) is the best clinical assay of body iron content. As this iron slowly leaves the RES cell, it is again bound by circulating transferrin and returned to the erythroid marrow. Thus, the cycle is as shown in figure 7.7.

F. Ferrokinetics

Kinetic studies, employing ^{59}Fe, are utilized clinically less frequently than the pioneers of the 1950s expected. They are now used mainly for research

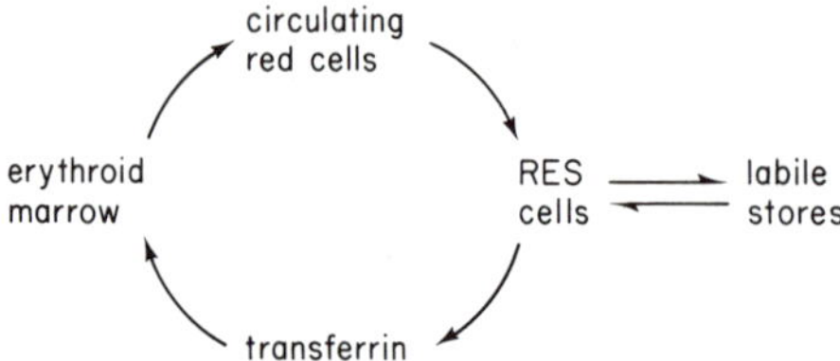

Fig. 7.7
Simplified scheme of iron cycle.

purposes, though occasionally they are of practical value in locating sites of extramedullary erythropoiesis.

1. *Plasma iron clearance*

The clearance from plasma of intravenously injected inorganic ^{59}Fe salts (mixed with serum before injection) is a complex function of time, and several different ways of expressing this complexity have been developed. Over short intervals (1–2 hr), the ^{59}Fe clearance curve is approximately a single exponential function, whose negative slope increases when either serum iron is decreased or when erythroid activity is increased. Conversely, it is reduced when the serum iron is increased or erythroid activity is decreased. The normal half-clearance time is approximately 90 min. It rises when erythropoiesis is hyperactive and decreases when it is depressed.

2. *Plasma iron turnover (PIT)*

The PIT is a measure of the total amount of iron leaving the plasma per unit time. It depends on the size of the circulating iron pool (plasma iron concentration in μg/ml × total plasma volume). It can be expressed in several ways (per hemoglobin mass, blood volume, body weight, etc.) but is most usefully expressed per deciliter of whole blood per day:

$$\text{PIT (mg iron/dl blood/24 hr)} = \frac{\text{plasma iron } (\mu\text{g/dl}) \times (100 - \text{Hct})}{T_{1/2}(\text{min}) \times 100}$$

Normal PIT is 0.6–0.8 mg/dl/day. PIT is a measure of iron taken up by erythroid cells and nonerythroid elements. Appropriate calculations permit correction for nonerythron iron turnover. Thus, total **red cell iron turnover** (RCIT) can be accurately assessed. PIT rises in proportion when erythroid marrow activity increases. PIT correlates well with actual red cell production as long as the serum iron remains between 70 and 200 μg/dl.

3. *Red cell iron utilization rate*

That portion of marrow activity leading to actual production of viable red cells may be estimated from the percentage of injected ^{59}Fe present in the circulating red cell mass 10–14 days after the injection. This is the **red cell iron utilization rate**. Thus, the PIT may be used as an index of **total erythropoiesis**, and the red cell iron utilization (a percentage) times the red cell iron turnover (derived from the PIT) is an index of **effective erythropoiesis**. For convenience, the values of these parameters are usually expressed in relation to the basal level.

4. Organ localization

In addition to the reappearance pattern and time course of incorporation of ^{59}Fe into hemoglobin, the scanning of isotope distribution over various organs (in the intact subject) permits further characterization of abnormal erythropoiesis by demonstrating specific patterns of ineffective or extramedullary erythropoiesis, marrow aplasia, or hemolysis. The graphs in figure 7.8, which depcit the 20-day time courses of marrow, liver, spleen, and blood radioactivity after injection of ^{59}Fe, illustrate these principles in a normal subject and in certain disease states.

5. Serum ferritin

Even though ferritin accounts for only a small fraction of the iron in serum, its concentration is stable and its level proportional to the much larger amount of storage iron in solid tissues. The development of a convenient radioimmunoassay for serum ferritin thus provided a reliable and noninvasive method for evaluating body iron stores. This test along with assays for serum iron and IBC permits a greater degree of diagnostic discrimination. The ferritin in serum arises from the breakdown of iron-containing macrophages of the RES in the liver, spleen, and bone marrow, which derive their iron content largely from senescent red cells.

Serum ferritin levels, in contrast to other measures of iron status such as hemoglobin and serum iron, are usually good indexes of iron stores. The concentration of serum ferritin is about 100 ng/ml in the newborn, rising for about a month to 350 ng/ml, and then declining to 30 at age 6 months, where it remains through puberty. In adults, the concentration reflects the relatively larger iron reserves of males. In one series of men and women from which anemic individuals were excluded, mean levels were 140 and 39 ng/ml, respectively. A normal serum ferritin in most, but not all, instances denotes normal iron stores.

In iron deficiency the concentration is below 12 ng/ml. Concentrations above 200 ng/ml are sometimes (but not always) found in conditions with increased iron stores, such as thalassemia major and hemochromatosis. High serum ferritin levels inappropriate for the level of body iron stores are often seen in malignancy and conditions associated with tissue damage, for example, acute and chronic hepatitis, gastric carcinoma, and other malignant conditions, Hodgkin's disease, and acute myelocytic leukemia.

III. IRON DEFICIENCY

Iron deficiency is a common clinical state in which total body iron is diminished.

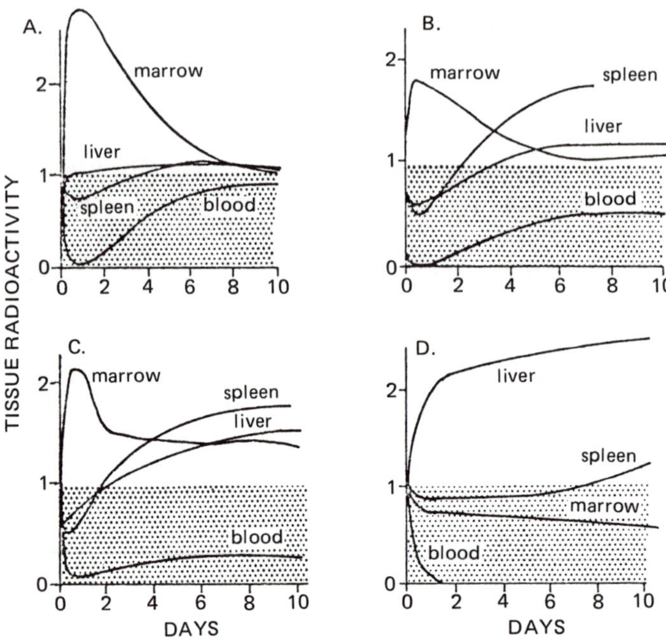

Fig. 7.8
Typical ferrokinetic studies in health and disease. The ordinate value of 1 represents the level of radioactivity immediately after an intravenous ^{59}Fe injection. The blood curve reflects the reappearance of incorporated ^{59}Fe in circulating red cells. If red cell iron utilization were 100%, the curve would reach the 1 level again. *A, normal pattern*: rapid marrow uptake and redelivery of ^{59}Fe as hemoglobin; *B, pattern in hemolytic anemia* (hereditary spherocytosis): rapid marrow uptake and redelivery of ^{59}Fe but less than 60% of injected iron appears in red cells because of splenic destruction of newly formed cells; *C, pattern in ineffective erythropoiesis* (megaloblastic anemia): rapid marrow uptake, but poor redelivery with less than 40% iron utilization because of intramedullary erythroid cell destruction (the other curves suggest splenic uptake of newly produced cells and liver uptake of ^{59}Fe because of high serum iron); *D, pattern in aplastic anemia*: no marrow uptake with 0% iron utilization in hemoglobin synthesis (^{59}Fe is deposited in parenchymal liver cells). (From C. A. Finch et al., *Medicine* 49[1970]: 17.)

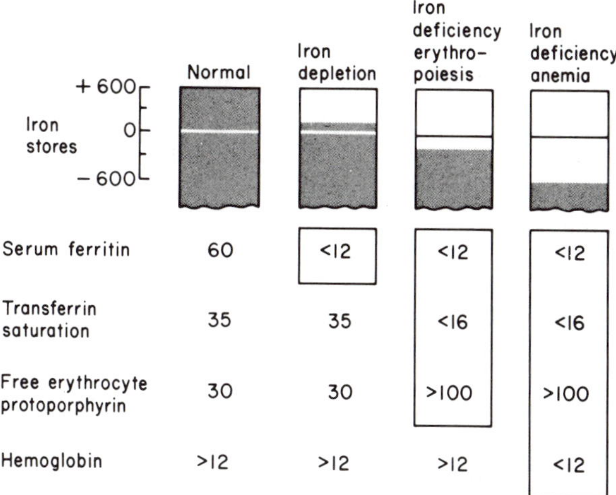

Fig. 7.9
The stages of iron deficiency.

A. Stages

Deficiency occurs in sequential stages (figure 7.9). In **latent iron deficiency**, a stage omitted from some classifications, serum ferritin reveals that body stores are moderately decreased although there is no anemia, no decrease in serum iron, no increase in iron-binding capacity, and no decrease in transferrin saturation. Free erythrocyte protoporphyrin is normal.

In **iron depletion**, stores are exhausted or nearly so, but anemia is still not present. Serum iron may be normal or only slightly decreased and IBC is normal or slightly increased, so that transferrin saturation is normal or nearly so. However, low serum ferritin levels signify sharply decreased iron stores.

Iron-deficient erythropoiesis (also called **iron deficiency without anemia**) is a more advanced stage characterized by decreased or absent strorage iron, low serum iron, elveated IBC, and low transferrin saturation (< 16%), but normal (or nearly normal) hemoglobin or hematocrit levels. If anemia is present, it is mild and normocytic-normochromic. Free erythrocyte protoporphyrin is elevated and serum ferritin minimal.

Iron-deficiency anemia is an advanced stage characterized by decreased or absent iron stores, low serum iron, elevated IBC and low transferrin saturation, elevated free erythrocyte protoporphyrin, low serum ferritin, and low hemoglobin or hematocrit level, with microcytosis-hypochromia.

B. Incidence

Iron deficiency is one of the most common medical disorders, though the precise incidence is hard to judge because differing diagnostic criteria are used in population surveys. Many studies judge iron nutrition by hemoglobin levels, but as noted above, this practice overlooks deficient individuals without anemia. Probably 10–30% of the world population is deficient in iron. In underdeveloped countries, it is a major public health problem, severely limiting work tolerance and productivity. In Western countries, it is the most common nutritional deficiency, affecting mainly women, children, and the poor.

C. Historical notes

Clinical signs of iron deficiency were recognized by the ancients; a good description appeared in an Egyptian papyrus of 1500 B.C. of what was probably a case of ancylostomiasis. **Chlorosis**, or "green sickness," was well known to European physicians after the midsixteenth century. Iron salts were used in France in the midseventeenth century along with other remedies, including phlebotomy.

D. Causes

1. Inadequate intake

a. NEWBORN PERIOD

Deficiency is most often the result of inadequate iron content of unsupplemented milk diets. Prolonged breast or bottle feeding leads to iron deficiency unless supplemental iron is given. During the first year of life, a full-term infant requires 160 mg of iron for erythropoiesis (a premature infant requires 240 mg). About 50 mg of need is met by red cell destruction that occurs physiologically during the first weeks of life. The remainder comes from the diet.

b. CHILDHOOD

During periods of rapid **growth**, diet may provide insufficient iron. Other factors, such as intestinal **parasites**, may also be present.

c. ADULTS

In order to maintain iron balance, the adult male needs to absorb only about 1 mg of iron daily from the diet; hence, iron deficiency in men is only rarely due to dietary deficiency alone. The major cause in men is bleeding (see below). Intestinal malabsorption of iron is an uncommon cause of iron deficiency except in specific malabsorption syndromes (e.g., sprue) or after gastrointestinal surgery. Half of all patients with subtotal gastrectomy develop iron deficiency in later years.

2. Excessive loss

Bleeding is the most common cause of iron deficiency in adult men and postmenopausal women. When bleeding is occult, it is usually from the GI tract (from lesions such as hiatus hernia, neoplasms, esophageal varices). In adult women, iron deficiency is most commonly due to iron losses in **menstruation** and losses in current or previous **pregnancies** that were never repleted. Internal iron loss in kidneys or lungs occurs rarely. In **hemoglobinuria**, iron is retained temporarily in proximal tubular cells but is lost when cells slough off into urine. It is diagnosed by Prussian blue stain of the urinary sediment.

E. Clinical manifestations

1. General symptoms

Clinical manifestations of iron deficiency are in two categories: those related to anemia and impaired oxygen delivery and those unrelated to hemoglobin concentration, which largely reflect decreases in tissue levels of iron-dependent enzymes. Symptoms also include those due to primary disorder (e.g., an anatomic lesion leading to bleeding). A curious and poorly understood manifestation of iron deficiency is the so-called **pica syndrome**, a perversion of the appetite that leads to bizarre practices such as ice-eating (pagophagia), dirt-eating (geophagia), and so forth. Abnormal gnawing behavior occurs in iron-deficient rodents.

2. Epithelial changes

These have been ascribed to deficiency of intracellular iron enzymes. It was once believed that these proteins were never diminished while stores still contain iron. However, recent work shows that even mild iron deficiency depresses cytochrome *c* levels in intestinal mucosa and muscle. The following types of epithelial changes occur.

a. ANGULAR STOMATITIS AND GLOSSITIS

Atrophic changes in epithelium of tongue and corner of mouth are common in iron deficiency. They are more severe in old subjects and in those on a poor diet.

b. POSTCRICOID ESOPHAGEAL WEB

Esophageal webbing is due to atrophic degeneration and keratinization of esophageal epithelium with infiltration by inflammatory cells. Such lesions may become malignant. They occur in certain iron-deficient females. The condition gives rise to dysphagia (Plummer-Vinson syndrome) or may be asymptomatic. Not all patients with webs have iron deficiency, but many did in the past. Webs are not common in iron deficiency. Only 7% in a large British series had dysphagia. They are more uncommon in the United

States and are extremely rare in Africa despite its high incidence of iron deficiency. Such data raise questions whether iron deficiency or other genetic and environmental factors cause webbing.

c. ACHLORHYDRIA AND ATROPHIC GASTRITIS

Histamine-fast achlorhydria is found in many patients with iron deficiency anemia. Many of these have gastric parietal cell antibodies in serum. Proposed explanations are (1) iron deficiency is the initial event that produces atrophic gastritis with achlorhydria; and (2) mucosal atrophy is the initial event and iron deficiency is secondary, being the result of impaired absorption (and intermittent mucosal bleeding).

d. KOILONYCHIA

Flattening or concavity of the nails is seen in severe iron deficiency anemia. Nails return to normal on treatment with iron. Incidence varies in different studies.

3. *Bone marrow*

Marrow shows erythroid hyperplasia with characteristic underhemoglobinized "ragged" normoblasts. Iron is decreased in RES cells. In severe iron deficiency, megaloblastic features are commonly present that respond to iron therapy alone. This is attributable to the fact that ribonucleotide reductase (see figure 5.3) contains an essential nonheme iron atom.

4. *Blood cells*

Red cells are eventually hypochromic and then microcytic. A few are target cells. Poikilocytosis is prominent in severe cases. The reticulocyte count is low. Platelets may be increased or decreased.

Iron-deficient children have decreased percentages of T lymphocytes and impaired incorporation of ^{3}H-thymidine by stimulated lymphocytes in culture. These lymphocyte abnormalities may account for the lower incidence of positive skin tests to various antigens.

Neutrophil function is depressed with decreased capacity to kill *Escherichia coli* or *Staphylococcus aureus* in vitro.

5. *Other metabolic changes*

Serum iron, IBC, transferrin saturation, and serum ferritin are affected as shown in figure 7.9. Other reported changes in iron deficiency are increased catecholamine levels; abnormality in thyroid hormone metabolism (decreased conversion of T4 to T3 in tissues); impaired ability to maintain body temperature; depressed muscle function, probably due to formation of excess lactate, probably as a result of depletion of the iron-containing mitochondrial enzyme α-glycerophosphate oxidase.

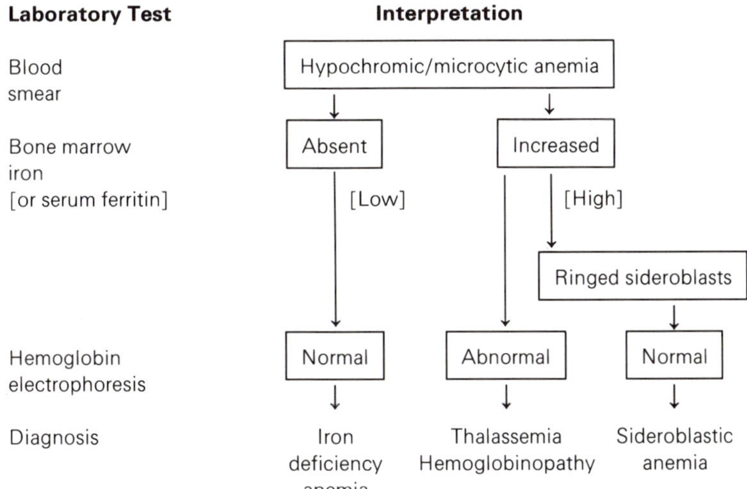

Fig. 7.10
Scheme for investigating patients with hypochromic microcytic anemia.

6. *Therapeutic response*

Significant increase in hemoglobin and reversal of other metabolic abnormalities should follow adequate iron therapy (see below).

F. Diagnosis

As noted below, many hypochromic anemias are not due to iron deficiency. Figure 7.10 summarizes a diagnostic approach to patients with hypochromic anemia.

G. Therapy

Principles of treatment are:

- Correct the underlying disorder.
- Administer the amount of iron needed.
- Observe the response to treatment.

Many preparations of oral iron are available. The usual daily dose is 100–200 mg elemental iron, which is conveniently given as ferrous sulfate, 300 mg, 3 times daily. Parenteral iron is given when the patient is intolerant of all forms of oral iron, rapid response is required, bleeding continues, or when the patient has a gastrointestinal disorder that may be aggravated by iron. In parenteral treatment, calculation should be made of iron deficit and dosage planned accordingly since an overdose cannot be corrected.

Further insight is gained by observing the response to iron therapy. The usual therapeutic dose increases erythrocyte production to about twice normal regardless of the severity of the anemia since production is limited by the 20–40 mg of iron absorbed plus the iron derived from the turnover of circulating cells. Parenteral iron may increase production to about 4 times normal initially, but within a week the response rate is similar to that of oral iron. In following the response to therapy, the increase in hematocrit is a more useful index than the reticulocyte count.

IV. OTHER CAUSES OF HYPOCHROMIC ANEMIA

A. Thalassemias

These is a group of genetically determined disorders in which the synthesis of the α or β chain of globin is impaired. Usually, they are associated with hypochromia and elevated or normal serum iron (see lecture 11). Table 7.1 summarizes major diagnostic differences between iron deficiency and thalassemia minor.

B. Defective iron reutilization

Curiously, this common disorder—one of the most common types of anemia—lacks a suitable name. It is also called "anemia of chronic disease" (even though many associated disorders are not chronic), "anemia of inflammation," "anemia of arthritis," and so forth.

1. Clinical picture

In infection or nonbacterial inflammation (as in rheumatoid arthritis or neoplasm), mild normocytic-normochromic anemia (hematocrit in the 30s) is common (see lecture 4), though MCV and MCHC are depressed in some patients. Such mild anemia often produces few symptoms, but when associated with fever, pulmonary impairment, or cachexia, the anemia can be debilitating.

Typically, the reticulocyte count fails to increase in response to the anemia, and the bone marrow shows no compensatory erythroid hyperpla-

Table 7.1
Points in the Differential Diagnosis of Iron Deficiency and Thalassemia Minor

	Iron Deficiency	Thalassemia Minor
Hemoglobin deficit	Any severity	Rarely <10 g/dl
RBC count	Usually <5 million/μl	Usually >5 million/μl
Serum iron	Reduced	Normal
Serum TIBC	Increased	Normal
Hemoglobin A_2*	<4%	>4%
Basophilic stippling	Usually absent	Present
Family history	No pattern	Mendelian autosomal transmission

*The normal value for hemoglobin A_2 may vary depending on the method of measurement. The upper limit of normal usually is about 4%.

sia. Changes in the white blood count, platelet count, and organ function tests are inconsistent and reflect the underlying disease rather than the anemia.

The serum iron level often falls precipitously, and transferrin synthesis in the liver is evidently depressed. Therefore the serum IBC falls over a period of weeks. Serum iron is low, averaging 30 but ranging from 10 to 70 μg/dl; IBC is moderately depressed, averaging around 200 μg/dl. Thus, saturation is 10–25%. This pattern is diagnostically helpful as it contrasts with the raised IBC of uncomplicated iron deficiency, but often there is difficulty in its interpretation. Ferrokinetic studies show a PIT of 1–2 times normal.

Tissue iron stores can be roughly estimated from a bone marrow aspirate stained for iron. However, serum ferritin is increasingly the preferred method for assessing iron stores. Serum ferritin values above 20 ng/ml usually reflect adequate iron reserves. Since it is an acute phase protein, serum ferritin may rise nonspecifically in acute and chronic disease, and only levels in excess of 60 ng should be taken as evidence of increased iron stores.

In sum, serum ferritin levels are often helpful in distinguishing this disorder from iron deficiency. A normal or elevated ferritin concentration excludes inadequate iron stores and obviates the need for a bone marrow examination. A depressed ferritin concentration signifies depressed iron stores and justifies iron therapy. However, as noted, serum ferritin may be raised in acute or chronic liver disease and in infections and malignant conditions. Where doubt remains, a reliable test of iron deficiency is still a Prussian blue stain of bone marrow aspirate.

2. *Mechanisms*

The characteristic triad—low serum iron, low IBC, and high ferritin—has not been fully explained. Several mechanisms have been proposed: Among these are prostaglandins, interferons, and tumor necrosis factors. These agents are commonly present in chronic disorders.

- A decrease in iron availability for hemoglobin synthesis due to an unexplained block in the release and reutilization of iron from RES macrophages.
- There results an increase in stainable RES iron, depressed plasma iron and transferrin saturation, a decrease in sideroblasts, an increase in red cell protoporphyrin, and mild hypochromia of circulating red cells.
- Moderately increased destruction of circulating red cells, sometimes complicated by such events as intravascular fragmentation associated with vasculitis and/or intravascular clotting. Decrease in the red cell survival increases marrow iron requirements and accentuates consequences of blocked iron release.
- Stem cells in this disorder may be unresponsive to Epo. Also, the many factors and lymphokines released by cells involved in the defense

against infections, inflammations, and tumors may suppress bone marrow function.

3. *Therapy*

The main principle of treatment is: Treat the primary or underlying disorder. Beyond this, treatment is usually unsatisfactory. Oral or parenteral iron has little effect on the anemia (unless there is an additional element of iron deficiency). If anemia becomes symptomatic, transfusion with packed red cells can be used judiciously. Some believe it has not been proved unequivocally that this anemia is detrimental to health. Similarly, a low serum iron, especially when associated with a near-normal iron turnover, may not be harmful either. It is possible that a low serum iron may protect against invasion by iron-dependent bacteria. However, anemia leading to tissue hypoxia does warrant therapy.

Clinical trials with Epo therapy are under way and should soon reveal whether such therapy is feasible.

V. IRON OVERLOAD

Iron overload (iron-loading disorders) is a state in which total body iron is increased.

A. Causes

- Inappropriate increase in intestinal absorption of iron
  - Idiopathic hemochromatosis
  - Various iron-loading anemias (sideroblastic anemias, thalassemia)
- Grossly excessive oral administration of iron over a prolonged period
  - Excessive medicinal iron
  - South African Bantus (who ingest 100–200 mg of iron daily in beer and food cooked in iron pots)
- Excessive blood transfusion (in patients with chronic bone marrow failure)

B. Specific disorders

1. *Hemochromatosis*

Idiopathic hemachromatosis is an inherited iron-loading disease associated with increased intestinal absorption of iron.

a. DESCRIPTION

Clinical features, although not pathognomonic, include lethargy, weight loss, loss of libido, abdominal pain, joint pain, and symptoms related to the onset of diabetes. Prominent physical signs include a darkened skin color, hepatomegaly, testicular atrophy, loss of body hair, arthropathy, and heart failure. An early manifestation in young adults may be cardiac failure. A family history of liver disease, hepatocellular carcinoma, or idiopathic hemochromatosis strongly suggests the diagnosis of idiopathic hemochromatosis in a given patient.

b. DIAGNOSIS

Diagnostic criteria include demonstration of increased total body iron stores in parenchymal locations and evidence of tissue damage. IBC and serum ferritin levels are increased. Parenchymal distribution of iron, as distinguished from RES overload (as occurs in various anemias), is suggested by the presence of >4 mg of iron in a 24-hr urine collection after the intramuscular injection of 0.5 g of desferrioxamine (in subjects with normal renal function). Liver biopsy definitively confirms the increase in parenchymal iron and permits assessment of tissue damage. The major diagnostic problem is in distinguishing idiopathic hemochromatosis and alcoholic liver disease with excess hepatic iron. It was once thought that a minor degree of stainable hepatic iron indicates excess body iron stores. Now it is recognized that stainable iron is common in normal and cirrhotic livers. Those with alcoholic cirrhosis and increased stainable iron include patients with (1) relatively normal iron stores whose liver iron concentration does not exceed twice the upper limit of normal and (2) markedly increased total body iron stores. The majority of such patients probably have idiopathic hemochromatosis as well as alcoholism. Only in these subjects is phlebotomy of benefit. When diagnosis is in doubt, iron stores should be reduced by phlebotomy and family members should be studied.

c. THERAPY

Removal of iron by repeated phlebotomy has modified the prognosis and clinical course of idiopathic hemochromatosis. Aside from cardiac death in the early phase of treatment, mortality is now due chiefly to late hepatoma.

2. *Sideroblastic anemias*

This heterogeneous group of confusingly named chronic disorders is marked by diverse clinical and biochemical manifestations that reflect multiple underlying pathogenetic mechanisms. All are characterized by iron loading and hypochromic anemia.

a. DESCRIPTION

The majority of patients with sideroblastic anemia display the following features:

- Anemia, either hypochromic or dimorphic (i.e., two red cell populations)
- Erythroid hyperplasia of the marrow, often with varying degrees of

megaloblastic change, and clear evidence of sideroblastic features (i.e., significant number of ring sideroblasts)
- Increased iron stores in the RES cells (nearly always present)
- Hyperferremia with an increase in percentage saturation of transferrin
- Increased PIT with subnormal red cell iron utilization
- Decreased levels of various enzymes in mitochondria of erythroid precursors
- Hematologic response to pyridoxine therapy in a few cases

b. CLASSIFICATION

- Refractory sideroblastic anemias (primary, idiopathic)
  - Hereditary (sex-linked hypochromic anemia
  - Acquired
- Reversible sideroblastic anemias (secondary)
  - Toxins, drugs, ethanol, lead, and so forth
  - Other diseases (e.g., lymphoma, myeloma, myeloproliferative disease)
- Pyridoxine-responsive anemia

VI. ACUTE IRON POISONING

Iron poisoning is one of the most common causes of fatal poisoning in young children who find and ingest an excessive quantity of therapeutic iron. The major clinical features are as follows:

- A sequence of stages with abdominal disturbances followed by apparent improvement followed by shock, coma, and death
- Metabolic acidosis and hypovolemia
- Extreme elevation of serum iron

Desferrioxamine therapy may be life saving. Desferrioxamine is also useful in diminishing tissue ferritin and hemosiderin in the various iron-loading disorders, if given in adequate doses and by continuous pump infusion.

SELECTED REFERENCES

Reviews

Beutler, E. Hereditary and secondary acquired sideroblastic anemias. In Williams, W. J., Beutler, E., et al., eds. *Hematology*, 4th ed. New York: McGraw-Hill, 1990, pp. 554–557.

Bothwell, T. H., and Charlton, R. W. Historical overview of hemochromatosis. *Ann. NY Acad. Sci.* 526(1988): 1–10.

Cazzola, M., Bergamaschi, G., et al. Manipulations of cellular iron metabolism for modulating normal and malignant cell proliferation: achievements and prospects. *Blood* 75(1990): 1903–1919.

Crosby, W. H. Unsolved problems in hemochromatosis. *Ann. NY Acad. Sci.* 526(1988): 323–327.

Danford, D. E. Pica and nutrition. *Annu. Rev. Nutr.* 2(1982): 303–322.

Fairbanks, V. F., and Baldus, W. P. Iron overload. In Williams, W. J., Beutler, E., et al., eds. *Hematology*, 4th ed. New York: McGraw-Hill, 1990, pp. 752–758.

Fairbanks, V. F., and Beutler, E. Iron deficiency. In Williams, W. J., Beutler, E., et al., eds. *Hematology*, 4th ed. New York: McGraw-Hill, 1990, pp. 482–505.

Fairbanks, V. F., and Beutler, E. Iron metabolism. In Williams, W. J., Beutler, E., et al., eds. *Hematology*, 4th ed. New York: McGraw-Hill, 1990, pp. 329–339.

Holland, H. K., and Spivak, J. L. Hemochromatosis. *Med. Clin. North Am.* 73(1989): 831–845.

Klausner, R. D. From receptors to genes: insights from molecular iron metabolism. *Clin. Res.* 36(1988): 494–500.

Lee, G. R. The anemia of chronic disease. *Semin. Hematol.* 20(1983): 61–80.

Peters, T. J., Raja, K. B., et al. Mechanisms and regulation of intestinal iron absorption. *Ann. NY Acad. Sci.* 526(1988): 141–147.

Seligman, P. A. Structure and function of the transferrin receptor. *Prog. Hematol.* 13(1983): 131–147.

Theil, E. C. Regulation of ferritin and transferrin receptor mRNAs. *J. Biol. Chem.* 265(1990): 4771–4774.

Yehuda, S., and Youdim, M. B. H. Brain iron: a lesson from animal models. *Am. J. Clin. Nutr.* 50 Suppl. (1989): 618–629.

Original articles

Anderson, G. J., Powell, L. W., et al. Transferrin receptor distribution and regulation in the rat small intestine: effect of iron stores and erythropoiesis. *Gastroenterology* 98(1990): 576–585.

Bacon, B. R., and Britton, R. S. The pathology of hepatic iron overload: a free radical-mediated process. *Hepatology* 11(1990): 127–137.

Bentley, S. A., Ayscue, L. H., et al. The clinical utility of discriminant functions for the differential diagnosis of microcytic anemias. *Blood Cells* 15(1989): 575–582.

Bessman, J. D., McClure, S., et al. Distinction of microcytic disorders: comparison of expert, numerical-discriminant, and microcomputer analysis. *Blood Cells* 15 (1989): 533–540.

Borecki, I. B., Rao, D. C., et al. Percent transferrin saturation in segregating hemochromatosis. *Am. J. Med. Genet.* 36(1990): 301–305.

Burns, E. R., Goldberg, S. N., et al. Clinical utility of serum tests for iron deficiency in hospitalized patients. *Am. J. Clin. Pathol.* 93(1990): 240–245.

Cook, J. D. Adaptation in iron metabolism. *Am. J. Clin. Nutr.* 51(1990): 301–308.

Cook, J. D., Carriaga, M., et al. Gastric delivery system for iron supplementation. *Lancet* 335(1990): 1136–1139.

Crosby, W. H. Pica: a compulsion caused by iron deficiency. *Br. J. Haematol.* 34(1976): 341–342.

Fillet, G., Beguin, Y., et al. Model of reticuloendothelial iron metabolism in humans: abnormal behavior in idiopathic hemochromatosis and in inflammation. *Blood* 74(1989): 844–851.

Grootveld, M., Bell, J. D., et al. Non-transferrin-bound iron in plasma or serum from patients with idiopathic hemochromatosis. Characterization by high performance liquid chromatography and nuclear magnetic resonance spectrosocpy. *J. Biol. Chem.* 264(1989): 4417–4422.

Guyader, D., Gandon, Y., et al. Evaluation of computed tomography in the assessment of liver iron overload. A study of 46 cases of idiopathic hemochromatosis. *Gastroenterology* 97(1989): 737–743.

Hallberg, L., Rossander-Hulthén, L., et al. Iron fortification of flour with a complex ferric orthophosphate. *Am. J. Clin. Nutr.* 50(1989): 129–135.

Houwen, B. The use of inference strategies in the differential diagnosis of microcytic anemia. *Blood Cells* 15(1989): 509–532.

Hunt, J. R., Mullen, L. M., et al. Ascorbic acid: effect on ongoing iron absorption and status in iron-depleted young women. *Am. J. Clin. Nutr.* 51(1990): 649–655.

Johnston, D. L., Rice, L., et al. Assessment of tissue iron overload by nuclear magnetic resonance imaging. *Am. J. Med.* 87(1989): 40–47.

Lombard, M., Bomford, A. B., et al. Differential expression of transferrin receptor in duodenal mucosa in iron overload. Evidence for a site-specific defect in genetic hemochromatosis. *Gastroenterology* 98(1990): 976–984.

Molloy, A. L., and Winterbourn, C. C. Release of iron from phagocytosed *Escherichia coli* and uptake by neutrophil lactoferrin. *Blood* 75(1990): 984–989.

Pagliuca, A., Mufti, G. J., et al. Lead poisoning: clinical, biochemical, and haematological aspects of a recent outbreak. *J. Clin. Pathol.* 43(1990): 277–281.

Powell, L. W., Summers, K. M., et al. Expression of hemochromatosis in homozygous subjects. Implications for early diagnosis and prevention. *Gastroenterology* 98(1990): 1625–1632.

Saven, A., and Beutler, E. Iron overload after prolonged intramuscular iron therapy. *N. Engl. J. Med.* 321(1989): 331–332.

Sharma, R. J., and Grant, D. A. W. The uptake of iron by hepatocytes is not coincident with transferrin endocytosis. *Biochem. Soc. Trans.* 16(1988): 618–620.

Skikne, B. S., Flowers, C. H., et al. Serum transferrin receptor: a quantitative measure of tissue iron deficiency. *Blood* 75(1990): 1870–1876.

Soewondo, S., Husaini, M., et al. Effects of iron deficiency on attention and learning processes in preschool children: Bandung, Indonesia. *Am. J. Clin. Nutr.* 50 Suppl. (1989): 667–674.

Thompson, W. G. Comparison of tests for diagnosis of iron depletion in pregnancy. *Am. J. Obstet. Gynecol.* 159(1988): 1132–1134.

Zanella, A., Gridelli, L., et al. Sensitivity and predictive value of serum ferritin and free erythrocyte protoporphyrin for iron deficiency. *J. Lab. Clin. Med.* 113(1989): 73–78.

LECTURE 8

Hypochromic Anemias II. Heme Metabolism and the Porphyrias

Stephen H. Robinson

EDITOR'S COMMENT

Although the pathways of heme synthesis were established decades ago, that work still stands as a classic early example of the value of radioisotopes in the delineation of metabolic pathways. Current research is aimed chiefly at understanding the factors regulating and coordinating both heme and globin synthesis—and, on the catabolic side, understanding the pathways and abnormalities of hemoglobin breadown. The latter problem puts hematology in close connection with gastroenterology in clinical situations requiring the differential diagnosis of jaundice.

I. HEME BIOSYNTHESIS

Porphyrinogens, **porphyrins**, and **heme** are composed of a ring of four pyrrole nuclei. Degradation of heme, with cleavage of the α-methene bridge, leads to the linear tetrapyrrole structure of the bile pigments (figure 8.1).

A. Normal pathways

1. Site of synthesis

Most heme is synthesized as the prosthetic group of hemoglobin in erythroid precursors in bone marrow. However, some heme formation occurs in virtually all tissues (cytochromes, catalase and other heme enzymes, myoglobin, etc.). Liver is the second most important site of porphyrin and heme synthesis.

2. Sequence of biosynthetic steps

Formation of δ-**aminolevulinic acid** (ALA) from glycine and succinyl CoA is the major rate-limiting step in heme biosynthesis. This is mediated by the mitochondrial enzyme **ALA synthetase**. It is regulated by end-product repression and possibly also direct end-product inhibition by heme. It requires pyridoxal phosphate as a cofactor and is linked to aerobic metabolism via the Krebs cycle intermediate succinyl CoA.

The pyrrole **porphobilinogen** (PBG) is formed by a condensation of two ALAs that is catalyzed by **ALA dehydrase**. PBG yields a red color when tested with Ehrlich's aldehyde reagent (*p*-dimethylaminobenzaldehyde). The color is not extractable into either chloroform or butanol. These

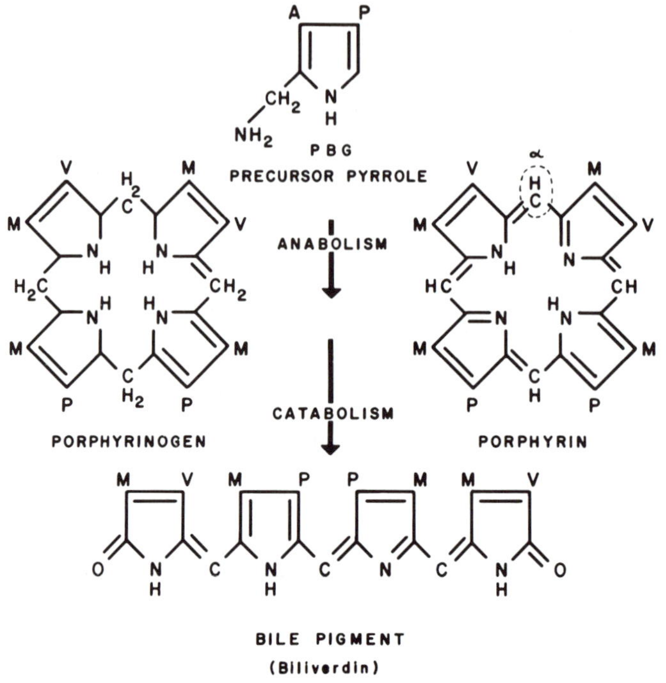

Fig. 8.1
Structure of porphobilinogen, protoporphyrinogen, protoporphyrin, and biliverdin. Bile pigment is formed by cleavage of the α-methene bridge in Fe-protophorphyrin (heme).

procedures make up the modified **Watson-Schwartz test**. A positive test in urine is characteristic of acute intermittent porphyria. **Uroporphyrinogen** (UROgen) is formed by condensation of four PBGs. In the presence of only **UROgen synthetase**, the isomer UROgen I is formed. As shown in figure 8.2, this is a blind alley since heme is derived only from the UROgen III isomer. Normally, when UROgen synthetase and **UROgen cosynthetase** are both present, virtually all UROgen is of the type III isomer. This intermediate is then converted to heme.

Coproporphyrinogen (COPROgen) is formed from UROgen by decarboxylation of the acetic acid side chains to methyl groups on each pyrrole nucleus. **Protoporphyrinogen** (PROTOgen) is formed from COPROgen III by oxidation of the propionic acid side chains on the two topmost pyrroles to vinyl groups. Because PROTOgen has three types of side chain (methyl, propionic acid, and vinyl), there are 15 possible isomers of PROTOgen, as compared to only four for UROgen and COPROgen. PROTOgen 9 is formed from COPROgen III. Porphyrinogens, not porphyrins, are the physiologic intermediates in heme biosynthesis. Porphyrinogens are reduced, unstable, colorless tetrapyrroles that are readily and irreversibly oxidized to porphyrins. Porphyrins are oxidized products of the porphyrinogens. They are resonating molecules (see figure 8.1), with alternating single and double bonds. Largely because of this property, they are colored

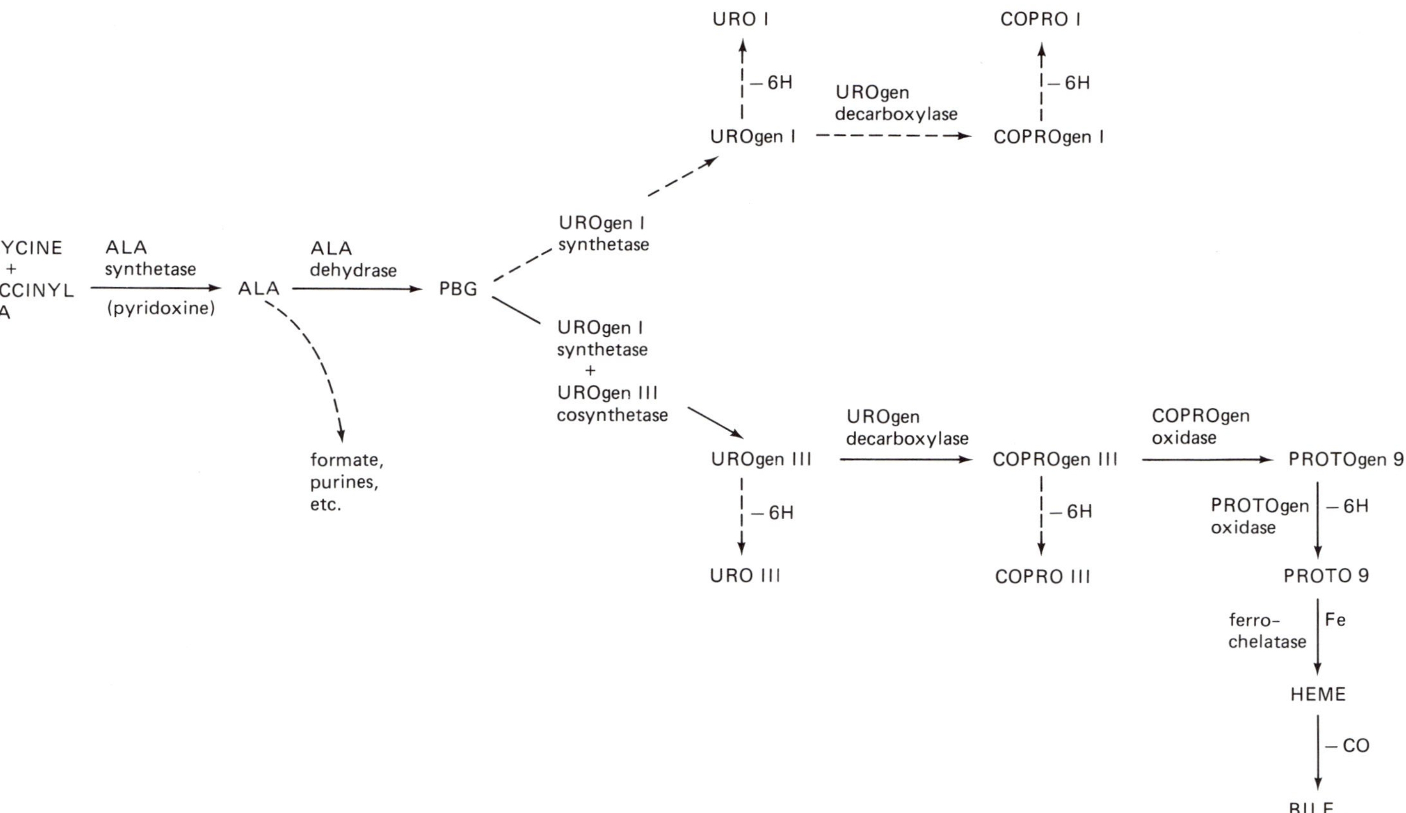

Fig. 8.2
Pathway of heme biosynthesis. Heavy lines refer to the main biosynthetic pathway. Dashed lines refer to potential detours or blind alleys from this route.

(red), fluoresce (red) in UV light, and are highly stable. Normally, little porphyrin is formed. However, porphyrins are formed when excess porphyrinogen production occurs, as in many of the **porphyrias**.

Once formed, porphyrins cannot be rereduced to porphyrinogens. They are lost from the heme biosynthetic pathway and are excreted in bile or urine. The single exception is **protoporphyrin** (PROTO) **9**, which is formed physiologically from PROTOgen 9 in the presence of the enzyme **PROTOgen oxidase**. PROTO 9 is then chelated with iron under the influence of the enzyme **ferrochelatase (heme synthetase)** to yield heme.

When formed in excess, PROTO is excreted via the bile into the feces. **Coproporphyrin** (COPRO) is found mainly in the feces, but some occurs in urine when produced in excess. **Uroporphyrin** (URO) is found primarily in urine.

Like ALA synthetase, ferrochelatase, PROTOgen oxidase, and COPROgen oxidase are mitochondrial enzymes. The physical proximity of these enzymes perhaps facilitates direct end-product inhibition of ALA synthetase by heme. The intermediate biosynthetic reactions occur in the soluble fraction of the cell. In erythroid but not hepatic cells, ferrochelatase, in addition to ALA synthetase, has a major regulatory role in heme biosynthesis. Heme is the prosthetic group of hemoglobin, myoglobin, catalase, the cytochromes, and certain other enzymes.

B. Defects in heme biosynthesis

1. Hypochromic anemias

These anemias, resulting from impaired synthesis of heme or hemoglobin, are discussed in lecture 7. In the light of the foregoing discussion concerning the major locus of heme synthesis, it is of interest that iron-laden mitochondria are the basis of the ring sideroblast of sideroblastic anemia.

2. Porphyrias

a. PATHOPHYSIOLOGY

Porphyrias are characterized not by decreased heme synthesis or hypochromia but by **overproduction of porphyrins** and/or the porphyrin precursors ALA and PGB (table 8.1). These disorders are due to partial blocks at one or another step in the biosynthetic pathway. Heme synthesis remains normal either because these steps are not rate limiting or because of a negative feedback loop that involves heme and ALA synthetase. Excessive production of porphyrin or porphyrin precursor originates in either the **bone marrow** (erythropoietic porphyria) or the **liver** (hepatic porphyria), the two major sites of heme biosynthesis. Many patients with different types of porphyria have the biochemical abnormalities unaccompanied by clinical symptoms. These are considered to have "latent" porphyria.

Increased activity of the rate-controlling enzyme ALA synthetase has been found in many forms of **hepatic porphyria**. In **acute intermittent porphyria** (AIP), this is due to a decrease in UROgen synthetase, which potentially limits heme synthesis. In this disorder and in **coproporphyria** and **variegate porphyria**, the enzyme deficiencies are not truly limiting (table 8.1), and ALA synthetase activity is normal but "sensitized" to induction by drugs, glucose deprivation, or other factors. The resulting increase in ALA synthetase activity accounts for the excessive production of ALA and PBG that is characteristic of acute attacks of hepatic porphyria, which has been termed the "precursor syndrome."

b. RELATION TO DRUGS

Barbiturates, griseofulvin, sulfonamides, stilbestrol, and many other agents may precipitate attacks of AIP in persons with latent AIP, variegate porphyria, or coproporphyria, or they may exacerbate the disorder in symptomatic patients with these disorders. Most of these drugs act by increasing the activity of hepatic ALA synthetase, which is already enhanced or sensitized because of an underlying defect in heme synthesis. Hexachlorobenzene has caused **porphyria cutanea tarda** in normal subjects by inhibiting UROgen decarboxylase activity in the liver.

c. GLUCOSE EFFECT

Glucose blocks the induction of ALA synthetase in the liver. A high carbohydrate diet prevents the chemical induction of hepatic porphyria in experimental animals and is used with partial success in the treatment of patients with acute hepatic porphyrias. Conversely starvation, as with intercurrent illness, may precipitate clinical attacks.

d. CLINICAL FEATURES

There are two general forms of porphyria. In **true porphyrias**, excessive production of porphyrins is associated with photosensitivity and dermatitis. These symptoms result from the fluorescence of porphyrins in skin, which leads to photooxidative and photocatalytic effects. Hemolytic anemia in congential erythropoietic porphyria is presumably related to fluorescence of porphyrins in and around erythrocytes. Urine is red if there is an excess of uroporphyrin.

In **precursor syndromes** (e.g., acute intermittent porphyria) excessive production of the porphyrin precursors ALA and PBG, as the result of increased ALA synthetase activity, is associated with protean neurologic and endocrinologic abnormalities. The pathophysiology is still unclear, although excess ALA may be toxic to nerve tissue. Alternatively, there may be a subliminal but critical deficiency of heme in neuronal cells. There

Table 8.1
Types of Human Porphyria

Type (synonyms)	Clinical manifestations	Chemical findings
I. Erythropoietic		
A. Congenital erythropoietic porphyria; Gunther's disease[t]	Severe photosensitivity and dermatitis; erythrodontia (stained teeth); hemolytic anemia with splenomegaly	Large amounts or URO and COPRO I in bone marrow, red cells, urine; COPRO I in stool; urine red, fluoresces red in UV light
B. Congenital erythropoietic protoporphyria[t]	Mild photosensitivity and dermatitis ("solar urticaria"), hemolytic anemia rarely	Increased PROTO 9 (and some COPRO III) in bone marrow, red cells, plasma, and stool; urine normal (URO not increased)
C. Chronic lead toxicity*	Photodermatitis absent; abdominal colic, neuropathy, encephalopathy; hypochromic anemia with stippled red cells, some hemolysis	Increased urinary ALA (not PBG) and COPRO III; increased red cell COPRO and PROTO
II. Hepatic		
A. Acute intermittent porphyria; porphyria hepatica; "pyrrolia"; Swedish porphyria[p]	Acute attacks of abdominal colic, CNS and peripheral nerve involvement, psychic changes, hypertension, constipation; photosensitivity and dermatitis absent	ALA and PBG (pyrrole) in liver and urine; fresh urine usually has normal color (porphyrins not increased); urine becomes dark on standing
B. Variegate porphyria; mixed hepatic porphyria; South African porphyria[t,p]	Moderate (or absent) photodermatitis; in some cases acute attacks of abdominal pain and neurologic disorder as in AIP, usually precipitated by drugs	Increased COPRO, PROTO, and "X-porphyrin" in liver, stool; increased COPRO in urine; ALA and PBG in urine during acute attacks
C. Coproporphyria[t,p]	Photodermatitis mild or absent; acute attacks may be induced by drugs	Increased COPRO in stool, urine; ALA and PBG in urine during acute attacks
D. Porphyria cutanea tarda; symptomatic porphyria[t]	Photodermatitis	Increased URO in liver, urine; urine may be red
E. Hexachlorobenzene toxicity[t]	Photodermatitis	Increased URO in liver, urine; urine may be red

Note: t = true porphyria (photosensitivity, excretion of true porphyrins);
p = precursor syndrome (neuropsychiatric disorder, excretion of ALA, PBG).
*Lead intoxication is listed because of its resemblances to porphyria.

Table 8.1 (continued)

Inheritance	Biochemical defect
Homozygous for abnormal gene (recessive)	Decreased UROgen cosynthetase in developing red cells, causing abnormal production of type I isomers
Heterozygous for abnormal gene (dominant); latent cases frequent	Decreased ferrochelatase (? unstable enzyme) in developing red cells, causing overproduction of PROTO 9
None (acquired)	Complex defect in developing red cells: decreased ALA dehydrase, ferrochelatase, COPROgen oxidase, and possibly ALA synthetase; decreased intracellular iron transport; depressed globin synthesis; abnormal mitochondria and ribosomes. Relation of symptoms to excess ALA production is unclear
Heterozygous for abnormal gene (dominant); latent cases frequent	Defect in liver: decrease in UROgen synthetase with secondary increase in ALA synthetase in patients with active disease, causing increased ALA and PBG production; basis of abdominal and CNS symptoms unclear (possibly related to excess ALA or PBG)
Heterozygous for abnormal gene (dominant); latent cases frequent	Defect in liver; decrease in PROTOgen oxidase (or possibly ferrochelatase) with secondary "sensitization" of ALA synthetase
Heterozygous for abnormal gene (dominant); latent cases very frequent	Defect in liver: decreased COPROgen oxidase with secondary sensitization of ALA synthetase
In some cases latent genetic defect (dominant) brought out by liver disease or drugs (e.g., estrogens); possibly an entirely acquired defect in other cases	Defect in liver: decrease in UROgen decarboxylase; ALA synthetase probably not increased. Typically associated with iron overload in the liver; may be ameliorated by phlebotomies
None	Hexachlorobenzene inhibits UROgen decarboxylase in liver

is no photosensitivity or red urine in the absence of an excess of true porphyrins.

e. GENETICS

Most porphyrias are inherited abnormalities. However, the following acquired forms occur: (1) Lead intoxication is associated with excessive production of ALA and coproporphyrin, of unknown significance in the genesis of clinical symptoms that may resemble those of AIP (e.g., abdominal colic, neuropathy, encephalopathy). (2) Porphyria cutanea tarda apparently develops as the result of alcoholic liver disease (with iron loading) or in response to certain drugs (e.g., estrogens). However, it now appears that some of these patients have a latent genetic defect (decreased UROgen decarboxylase activity), which is made overt by the liver dysfunction or the drug. (3) Hexachlorobenzene can cause a true acquired form of porphyria cutanea tarda, as demonstrated in a famous outbreak in the 1950s in Turkey, where this drug was being used as a fungicide in grain.

II. HEME DEGRADATION AND BILE PIGMENT PRODUCTION

A. Normal pathways

Bile pigments include biliverdin, bilirubin, urobilinogen, urobilin, and related compounds. Bile pigment is formed by enzymatic cleavage of the α-methene bridge of heme, with release of the linear tetrapyrrole biliverdin and carbon monoxide. Biliverdin is then enzymatically reduced to bilirubin within the same cell. This two-step conversion occurs in mononuclear-phagocytic cells in spleen, liver, and elsewhere (figure 8.3). Bilirubin is rapidly excreted into bile by the liver. Bile pigments are excretory products that cannot be reconverted to porphyrinogens or heme. Urobilinogen is a bile pigment (i.e., it is a product of heme catabolism); uroporphyrin is a cyclic (ring) tetrapyrrole that is a by-product of heme synthesis (i.e., it is related to the anabolic pathway).

1. Sources of bile pigment

Most bile pigment is normally derived from hemoglobin at the end of the red cell life span. In addtion, an "early-labeled" fraction of bile pigment is observed within the first few days after administration of a labeled heme precursor such as ^{14}C-glycine. It normally accounts for about 15% of the total labeled pigment (figure 8.4). This early-labeled fraction originates partly from nonhemoglobin hemes, largely in the liver, but probably also in all tissues in which heme is synthesized. There is also an erythropoietic component that becomes prominent when red cell production in the bone marrow is accelerated or abnormal, especially with ineffective erythropoiesis. This component is presumably derived from the hemoglobin of prematurely destroyed erythroid precursors.

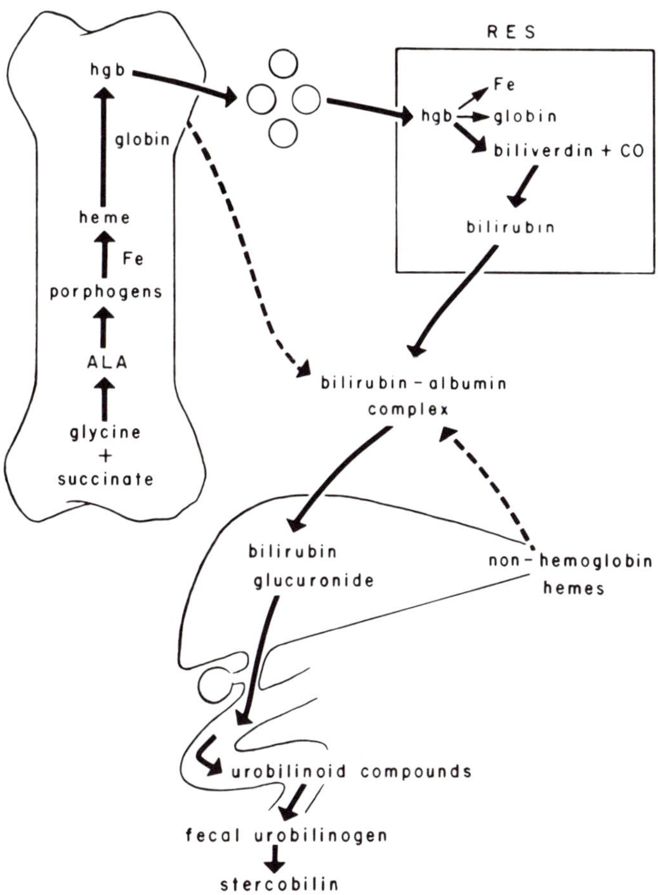

Fig. 8.3
Schematic summary of heme and bilirubin metabolism.

2. *Bilirubin excretion*

Bilirubin is transported in plasma bound to albumin (see figure 8.3). Hepatic excretion occurs in three phases: (1) uptake of unconjugated bilirubin from plasma into liver cell; (2) enzymatic conjugation of bilirubin, primarily with glucuronic acid; and (3) secretion of conjugated bilirubin into the bile canaliculus.

After excretion via bile into the intestine, bilirubin is reduced to a series of urobilinogen compounds by the intestinal bacteria.

B. Overproduction of bile pigment

1. *Mechanisms of jaundice*

In broad terms, hyperbilirubinemia may be due to increased production of bilirubin (less common) or decreased hepatic excretion (more common). In overproduction states, there is unconjugated ("indirect-reacting") hyperbilirubinemia in which the unconjugated bilirubin does not gain

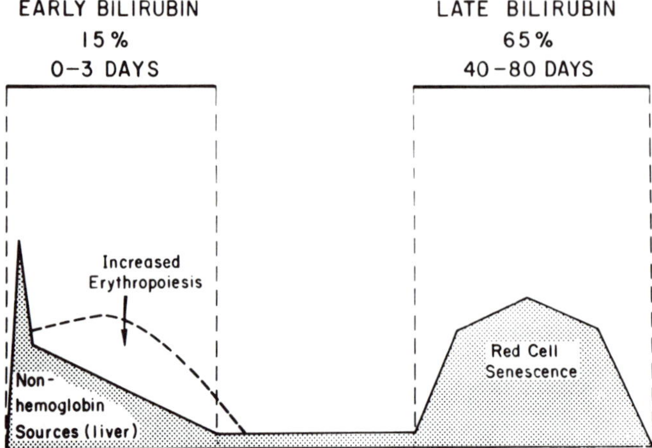

Fig. 8.4
Sources of bile pigments in the rat. This scheme also applies in general to humans, although in them the early-labeled fraction is formed from 0–5 days and the late fraction from 90–150 days. These data were derived from studies employing glycine-2-^{14}C as heme precursor. (From S. H. Robinson, in F. Stohlman, Jr., ed., *Hemopoietic Cellular Proliferation*. New York: Grune & Stratton, 1970.)

access to the urine. Fecal urobilinogen is increased. Unconjugated hyperbilirubinemia also occurs with defects in the uptake or conjugation phases of hepatic excretion. With impaired hepatic secretion, dysfunction of the bile canaliculi, or extrahepatic biliary obstruction, there is some regurgitation of conjugated ("direct-reacting") bilirubin from the liver into the plasma with some spillover into the urine.

2. *Causes of bilirubin overproduction*

- Increased rate of destruction of circulating red cells (hemolytic anemia). This is by far the most common cause of overproduction jaundice (see lecture 12).
- Abnormal hepatic heme metabolism in liver disorders, with an increase in early-labeled bilirubin production. This has been documented thus far only in experimental liver injury.
- Ineffective erythropoiesis (i.e., destruction of defective red cell precursors within the marrow or soon after release into the peripheral blood). This occurs in thalassemia, megaloblastic anemia, sideroblastic anemia, erythroleukemia, and a few other disorders. Some hemolysis of circulating red cells usually also occurs in these states. Ineffective erythropoiesis is associated with an increase in early-labeled bilirubin production.

SELECTED REFERENCES

Reviews

Anderson, K. E. The porphyrias. In Williams, W. J., et al., eds. *Hematology*, 4th ed. New York: McGraw-Hill, 1990, pp. 722–742.

Bloomer, J. R., and Bonkovsky, H. L. The porphyrias. *Dis. Mon.* 35(1989): 1–54.

Bottomley, S. S., and Muller-Eberhard, U. Pathophysiology of heme synthesis. *Semin. Hematol.* 25(1988): 282–302.

Drummond, G. S. Control of heme catabolism by Sn-protoporphyrin. *Semin. Hematol.* 26(1989): 24–26.

Grandchamp, B., and Nordmann, Y. Enzymes of the heme biosynthesis pathway: recent advances in molecular genetics. *Semin. Hematol.* 25(1988): 303–311.

Harrison, P. R., Plumb, M., et al. Regulation of erythroid cell-specific gene expression during erythropoiesis. *Br. J. Cancer Suppl.* 9(1988): 46–51.

Hirsch, R. E. Porphyrins and hemoglobin. *Semin. Hematol.* 26(1989): 47–53.

Kordac, V., Jirsa, M., et al. Agents affecting porphyrin formation and secretion: implications for porphyria cutanea treatment. *Semin. Hematol.* 26(1989): 16–23.

Lim, H. W. Pathophysiology of cutaneous lesions in porphyrias. *Semin. Hematol.* 26(1989): 114–119.

Mustajoki, P., Tenhunen, R., et al. Heme in the treatment of porphyrias and hematological disorders. *Semin. Hematol.* 26(1989): 1–9.

Perutz, M. F. Mechanisms regulating the reactions of human hemoglobin with oxygen and carbon monoxide. *Annu. Rev. Physiol.* 52(1990): 1–25.

Robinson, S. H. Degradation of hemoglobin. In Williams, W. J., et al., eds. *Hematology*, 4th ed. New York: McGraw-Hill, 1990, pp. 407–414.

Straka, J. G., Rank, J. M., et al. Porphyria and porphyrin metabolism. *Annu. Rev. Med.* 41(1990): 457–469.

Traugh, J. A. Heme regulation of hemoglobin synthesis. *Semin. Hematol.* 26(1989): 54–62.

Woods, J. S. Regulation of porphyrin and heme metabolism in the kidney. *Semin. Hematol.* 25(1988): 336–348.

Original articles

Anderson, K. E. LHRH analogues for hormonal manipulation in acute intermittent prophyria. *Semin. Hematol.* 26(1989): 10–15.

Clark, M., Royal, J., et al. Interaction of iron deficiency and lead and the hematologic findings in children with severe lead poisoning. *Pediatrics* 81(1988): 247–254.

Horiguchi, Y., Horio, T., et al. Late onset erythropoietic porphyria. *Br. J. Dermatol.* 121(1989): 255–262.

Needleman, H. L. The persistent threat of lead: a singular opportunity. *Am. J. Public Health.* 79(1989): 643–645.

Nunn, A. V., Norris, P., et al. Zinc chelatase in human lymphocytes: detection of the enzymatic defect in erythropoietic protoporphyria. *Anal. Biochem.* 174(1988): 146–150.

LECTURE 9

Hemoglobin I. Structure and Function

H. Franklin Bunn

EDITOR'S COMMENT

Studies of the structure and function of hemoglobin, one of the most abundant mammalian proteins and one that was long ago isolated in pure form, represents one of the great chapters in the history of hematology, biochemistry, and molecular biology. Not only is this remarkable protein abundant, it has several sharply delineated physiologic functions (i.e., oxygen transport, Bohr effect, cooperativity, among others) that uniquely suit it to studies of the functional consequences of small changes in the primary amino acid sequence. Moreover, the long delayed discovery of the regulatory effects of 2,3-DPG (now called 2,3-BPG in most texts) added an extraordinary dimension to the biology of hemoglobin, and, at the same time, resolved some long-standing puzzles. For example, why does bank blood too long on the shelf do a poorer job of restoring oxygen transport than freshly drawn blood? In these brief notes, Dr. Bunn brings this subject to life.

I. HEMOGLOBIN SYNTHESIS

A. Structural genes

Multiple structural genes govern the biosynthesis of globin in maturing human erythroid cells. Each gene results in the formation of a structurally unique polypeptide chain. The resulting gene products have been named α, β, γ, δ, ε, and ζ chains. The α and ζ genes are located on chromosome 16; the others are located on chromosome 11. Each newly synthesized globin chain links covalently with heme (ferroprotoporphyrin 9), as described in lectures 7 and 8. The globin genes are discussed in more detail lecture 11.

B. Combination of chains

Globin chains (or subunits) combine to form tetramers of mol. wt. 64,500. The physiologic function of hemoglobin depends on the presence of two α chains and two non-α chains. For example, normal adult hemoglobin, or **hemoglobin A**, is $\alpha_2\beta_2$. Normal fetal hemoglobin, or **hemoglobin F**, is $\alpha_2\gamma_2$.

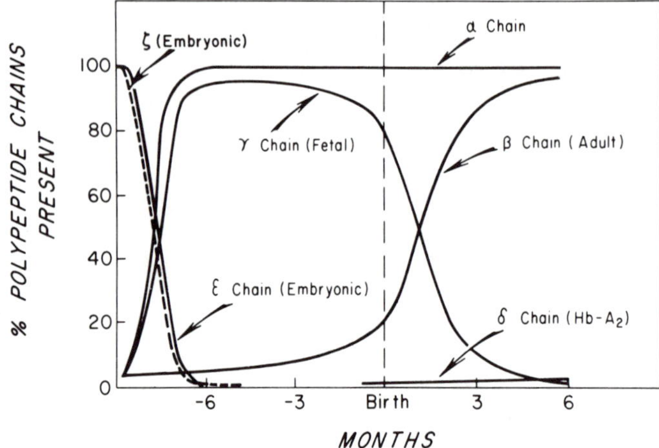

Fig. 9.1
Relative rates of synthesis of different globin chains during embryonic and neonatal life.

C. Synthetic rates of globin chains

Globin chain synthesis is discussed in detail in lecture 11. The synthetic rates of the five globin chains vary during the transition from embryonic and fetal life to neonatal life, as shown in figure 9.1.

D. Chains in normal hemoglobin

Table 9.1 summarizes the nomenclature and chain composition of the several hemoglobins found in normal subjects at various stages of life. The most abundant minor hemoglobin component in adult red cells is hemoglobin A_{1c}, which is a post-translational modification of glucose with the N-terminal amino of the β chain according to the reaction scheme in figure 9.2. This minor component is elevated two- to threefold in red cells of diabetics and provides a useful measurement of the adequacy of diabetic control. Furthermore, this chemical modification occurs in other tissues and may contribute to the long-term complications of diabetes.

II. HEMOGLOBIN STRUCTURE

A. Primary and secondary

The primary amino acid sequences of the normal human hemoglobins, and more than 400 genetic variants, have been established by chemical methods (primarily "fingerprinting" and peptide analyses). The normal α chain contains 141 amino acid residues in linear sequence; the β chain has 146 residues. The δ and γ chains differ from the β chain by 10 and 39 amino acids, respectively. Analysis of hemoglobin F shows it can contain two

Table 9.1
Structure of Normal Hemoglobins

Hemoglobin	Structure	Comments
A	$\alpha_2\beta_2$	Comprises ~92% of adult hemoglobin
A_{1c}	α_2(β-NH-glucose)$_2$	Comprises ~3% of adult hemoglobin. Increased in patients with diabetes
A_2	$\alpha_2\delta_2$	Comprises about ~2% of adult hemoglobin. Elevated in β thalassemia
F	$\alpha_2\gamma_2$	Predominant hemoglobin in fetus from the 3d through 9th month of gestation. Facilitates transfer of oxygen across placenta. Increased in β-thalassemia and other disorders
Gower 1	$\zeta_2\varepsilon_2$	Present in early embryo. Facilitates transfer of oxygen to embryo.
Gower 2	$\alpha_2\varepsilon_2$	
Portland	$\zeta_2\gamma_2$	
H	β_4	Found in α thalassemia (--/-α)*. Low solubility. Nonfunctional
Bart's	γ_4	Trace present in newborns. May comprise 100% of hemoglobin in homozygous α-thalassemia (--/--).* Nonfunctional

*See table 11.1.

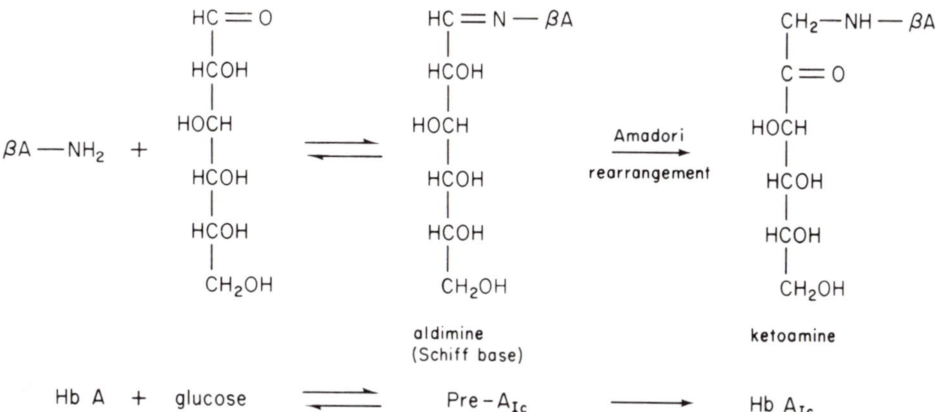

Fig. 9.2
Mechanism of hemoglobin glycosylation.

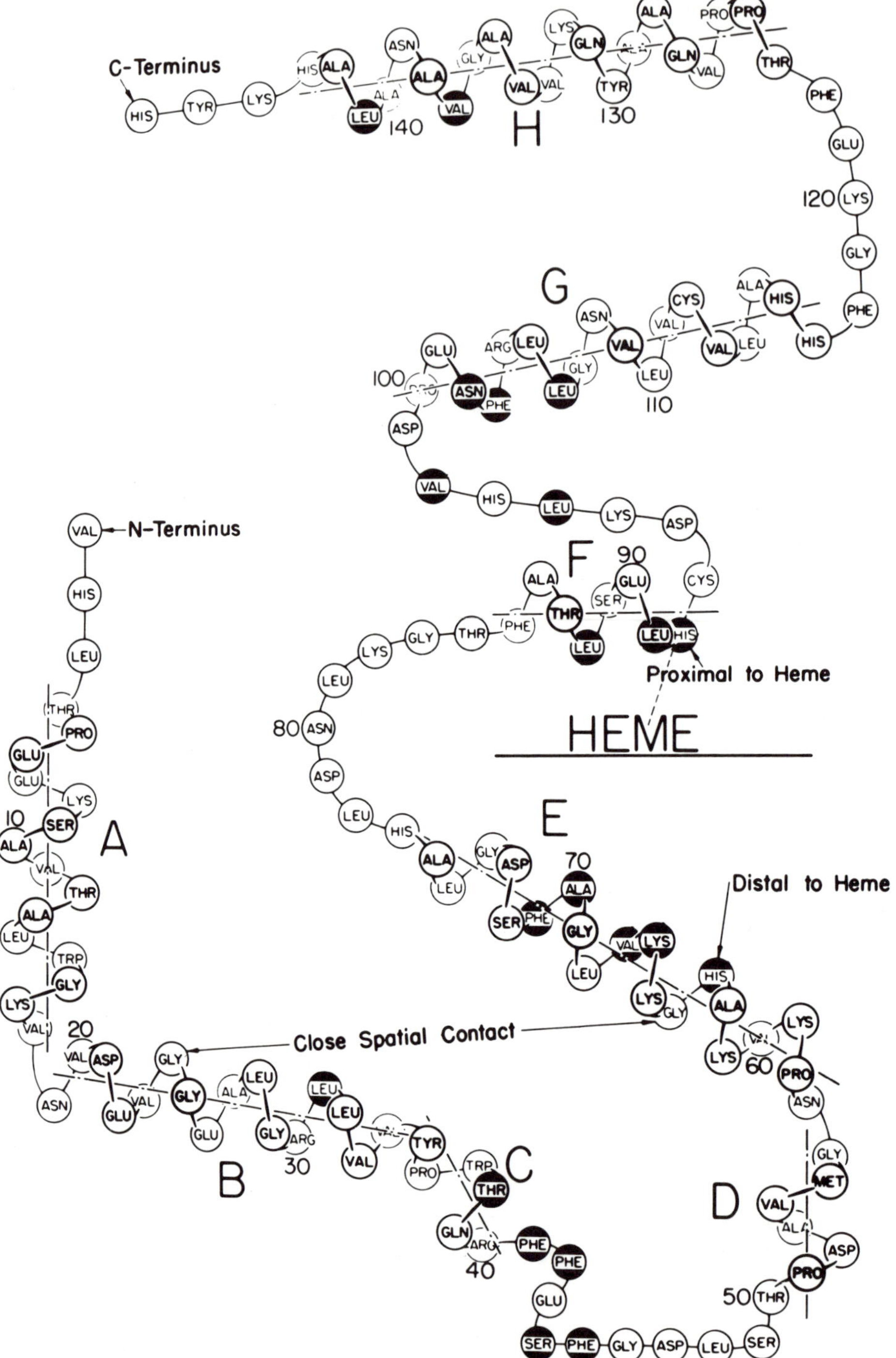

Fig. 9.3
Normal human β chain. Diagrammatic scheme shows the sequence of 146 amino acids from the N-terminal end above to the C-terminal end below. Helical regions are designated by single letters (A, B, E, etc.). Amino acid residues within helical regions are shown. The half-black circles indicate residues that are in contact with the heme group. (From T. H. J. Huisman and W. A. Schroeder, *New Aspects of the Structure, Function and Synthesis of Hemoglobins*. Boca Raton, FL: CRC Press, 1971.)

structurally distinct chains that differ by a single amino acid at position 136. In some chains (termed $^{G}\gamma$), glycine occupies this position; in others ($^{A}\gamma$), alanine does. As described in lecture 10, different structural genes specify $^{G}\gamma$ and $^{A}\gamma$.

About 80% of native hemoglobin is in the α helical form. Many amino acid residues are homologous in comparable helices of the α and β chains of human and animal hemoglobins. These are termed *invariant residues.* An example is the histidine at F8 (β92, α87), the imidazole moiety of which is bonded covalently to heme iron. The primary structure of the normal human β chain is shown diagrammatically in figure 9.3.

B. Tertiary and quarternary

From x-ray analyses of hemoglobin crystals, Perutz and associates have worked out the three-dimensional structure of human hemoglobin. This remarkable achievement has facilitated progress in relating structure to function. The tetramer was shown to be a spheroid with a diameter of about 55 Å and a single axis of symmetry. The four hemes lie in clefts situated equidistantly on the suface of the molecule. Upon deoxygenation all four chains undergo conformational changes (figure 9.4), the distance between β chain hemes increasing by 7 Å. X-ray data indicate that the deoxy conformation is stabilized by intra- and interchain salt bonds, including some dependent on proton binding and others on the presence of 2,3-diphosphoglycerate (2,3-DPG; see below). These are sequentially broken upon addition of oxygen. The primary physiologic properties of the molecule, namely, heme-heme interaction and the Bohr effect, can be

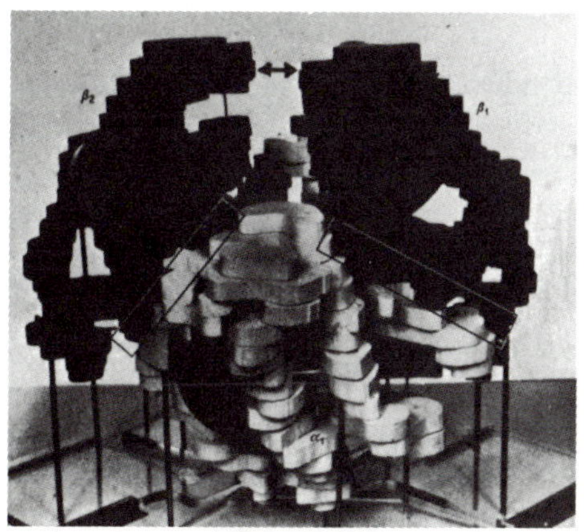

OXY

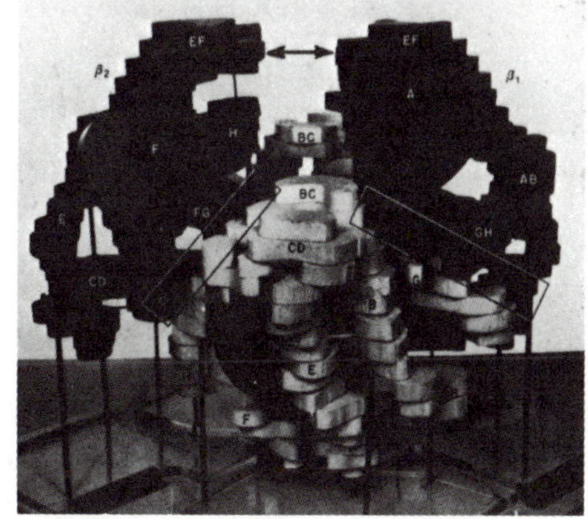

DEOXY

Fig. 9.4
Three-dimensional model of hemoglobin. The β chains are shown in black, the α chains in white. (One α chain is largely hidden from view.) Note the change in the distance between β chains on oxygenation. (From M. F. Perutz, *Nature* 228[1970]: 726.)

explained in terms of such stereochemical transitions. Some of these oxygen-linked salt bonds are shown diagrammatically in figure 9.5. At specific sites, protons are bound preferentially to deoxyhemoglobin. This is the structural basis of the Bohr effect, which is discussed below. The binding of 2,3-DPG to deoxyhemoglobin is shown in figure 9.5A.

III. HEMOGLOBIN FUNCTION

A. Heme-heme interaction

The familiar sigmoid shape of the oxyhemoglobin dissociation curve (figure 9.6) is of great physiologic importance for it permits a considerable transfer of oxygen from hemoglobin to tissues with only a small drop in oxygen tension. In contrast, myoglobin and single α and β chains lack heme-heme interaction and therefore have hyperbolic (nonsigmoid) oxygen dissociation curves. Thus, heme-heme interaction, a critical function of hemoglobin (i.e., $\alpha_2\beta_2$), depends on the interaction of pairs of unlike chains.

B. Bohr effect

The oxygen affinity of hemoglobin is directly related to pH over the pH range 6.0–8.5. A corollary to that statement is that oxyhemoglobin is a stronger acid than deoxyhemoglobin. The conversion from deoxy to oxy conformation decreases the pKs of acid groups of certain specific (and invariant) amino acid residues. Under physiologic conditions, oxygenation releases about 2.8 protons:

$$HbH + 4O_2 \rightleftharpoons Hb(O_2)_4 + 2.8H^+$$

The Bohr effect is physiologically advantageous (1) in **tissues**, where the decrease in pH due to carbon dioxide uptake lowers oxygen affinity and thereby enhances oxygen release; and (2) in **lungs**, where expulsion of carbon dioxide raises pH and thereby increases oxygen affinity and uptake.

C. Role of 2,3-DPG

1. Binding to hemoglobin

Unlike other tissues, red cells contain a high concentration of the organic phosphate ester **2,3-diphosphoglycerate** (2,3-DPG), which is a glycolytic intermediate. Its concentration in normal red cells equals that of hemoglobin tetramer (about 5 mM). It is a highly charged anion, which is partially protonated at physiologic pH:

$$\begin{array}{c} COO^- \\ | \\ HCOPO^{3-}H \\ | \\ H_2COPO^{3-}H \end{array}$$

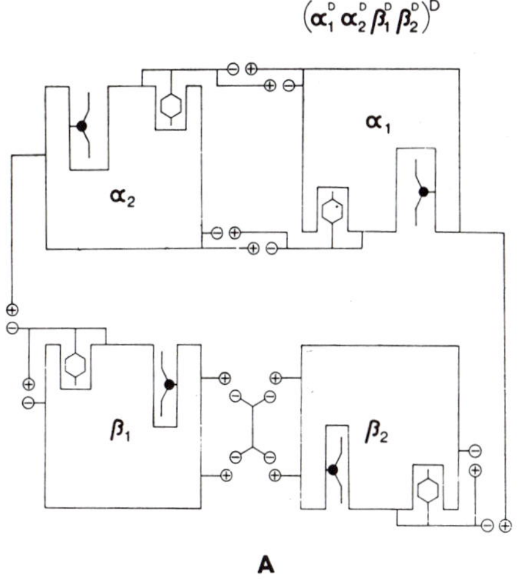

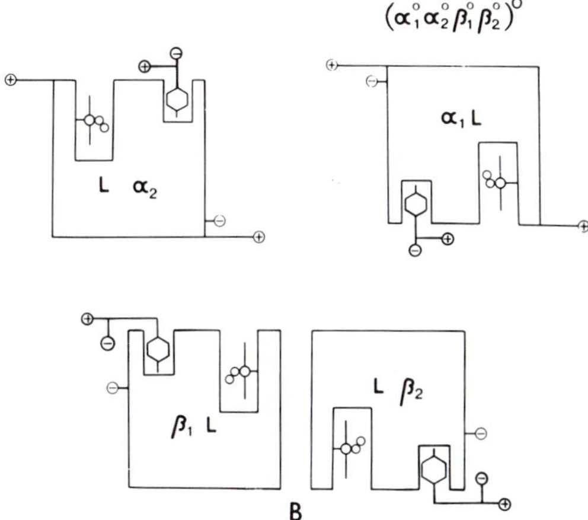

Fig. 9.5
Diagrammatic representation of the quaternary configurations of deoxyhemoglobin (*A*) and oxyhemoglobin (*B*). The salt bonds that stabilize the deoxy conformation are broken when the molecule is oxygenated. The binding of the negatively charged 2,3-DPG to the β chains of deoxyhemoglobin is shown (above *A*). (From M. F. Perutz, *Nature* 228[1970]: 726.)

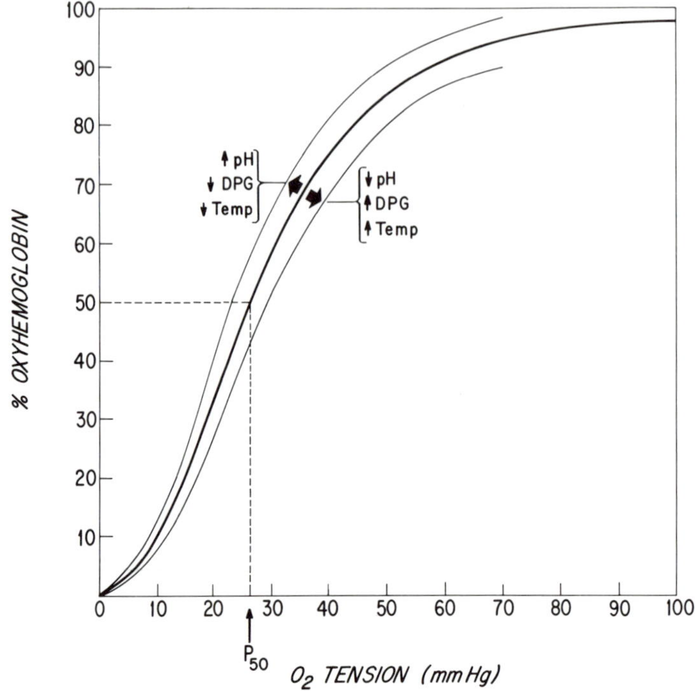

Fig. 9.6
Normal oxyhemoglobin dissociation curve and the effects on oxygen affinity of changes in pH, temperature, and red cell 2,3-DPG level.

When it is added to hemoglobin, 2,3-DPG sharply lowers oxygen affinity without disturbing heme-heme interaction or the Bohr effect. 2,3-DPG has been shown to bind at a specific site to deoxyhemoglobin (much more avidly than to oxyhemoglobin) in a 1 : 1 molar ratio. Thus, the reaction can be written as follows:

$$HbDPG + 4O_2 \rightleftharpoons Hb(O_2)_4 + DPG.$$

This equation should be compared to that given above for the Bohr effect.

2. *Adaptation to hypoxia*

An increased concentration of 2,3-DPG within the red cell favors the lowering of the oxygen affinity of blood in two way: **direct** binding to deoxyhemoglobin as described above; and **indirectly** by lowering the pH within the red cell relative to plasma pH.

The position on the oxyhemoglobin dissociation curve is an important determinant of oxygen delivery to tissues. As diagrammed in figure 9.7, oxygen delivery to an organ or tissue is directly proportional to blood flow, hemoglobin concentration, and the difference in oxygen saturation of arterial and venous blood. Patients with various types of hypoxia may compensate in the following ways:

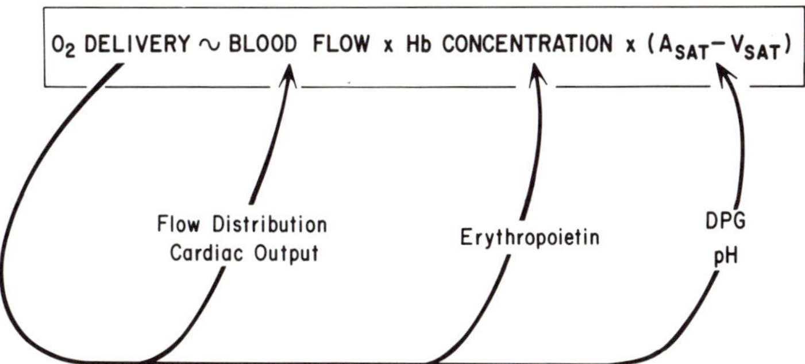

Fig. 9.7
Diagram of factors regulating oxygen delivery to tissues.

- Total cardiac output increases when hypoxia is severe and the distribution of blood flow may be altered so as to maintain the oxygenation of vital organs.
- Erythropoiesis increases as a result of increased erythropoietin production.
- Oxygen unloading ($A_{SAT}-V_{SAT}$) is enhanced by a shift to the right in the oxygen-hemoglobin dissociation curve (with resulting decrease in oxygen affinity) that is mediated by increasing 2,3-DPG in the red cell.

The extent to which oxygen unloading can be enhanced is illustrated in figure 9.8.

The mechanism by which red cell 2,3-DPG is elevated in hypoxic states is not fully understood. Red cell pH is probably the most important determinant of 2,3-DPG levels. Alkalosis causes an increase in 2,3-DPG, and acidosis causes a decrease. The direct effect of pH on red cell affinity (Bohr effect) is opposite to the indirect effect of pH on the 2,3-DPG level.

A "shift to the right" occurs in the various clinical types of hypoxia, among them:

- High-altitude effects
- Pulmonary insufficiency
- Cardiac right-to-left shunt
- Congestive heart failure
- Severe anemia of any type

3. *Shifts to the left*

A "shift to the left" of the oxygen-hemoglobin dissociation curve impairs oxygen release to the tissues. The following conditions can cause such a shift:

- Multiple transfusions with blood that has been stored in liquid preservative and has been depleted of 2,3-DPG
- Rapid correction of metabolic acidosis
- The presence of hemoglobin F (as in fetal blood), which contains γ

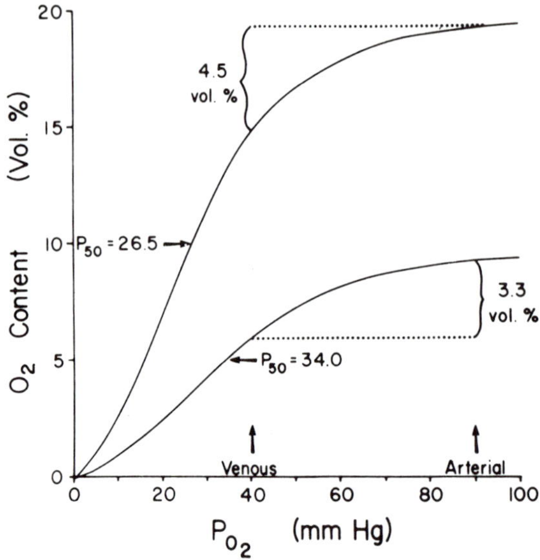

Fig. 9.8
Enhancement of oxygen unloading by decreased red cell oxygen affinity in a patient with anemia. Anemic patient with a 50% reduction in hemoglobin concentration has only a 27% reduction to oxygen unloading. (From R. A. Klocke, *Chest* *69*[1972]: 795.)

chains instead of β chains and thus interacts only weakly with 2,3-DPG, thereby facilitating the transport of oxygen from mother to fetus

- The presence of a chemically altered hemoglobin such as methemoglobin, carboxyhemoglobin (to be discussed below), or certain of the hemoglobin variants to be discussed in lecture 10

IV. ACQUIRED ABNORMALITIES

A. Carbon monoxide poisoning

Carbon monoxide (CO) arises from combustion of organic material, particularly hydrocarbons such as petroleum and tobacco tar. It is an important toxic component of tobacco smoke. It is produced endogenously in the catabolism of heme, which results in formation of 1 mole each of CO and bilirubin per mole of heme (see lecture 8).

1. Toxicology

The hazards of CO intoxication are evident in its frequent use in suicide attempts and its seriousness as an industrial toxin. The mechanism of toxicity depends on the fact that CO and oxygen compete for the same binding site in heme, but CO is bound 210 times more firmly than oxygen. Thus, carbonmonoxyhemoglobin (also called carboxyhemoglobin, abbreviated HbCO), unlike oxyhemoglobin, dissociates with difficulty. This

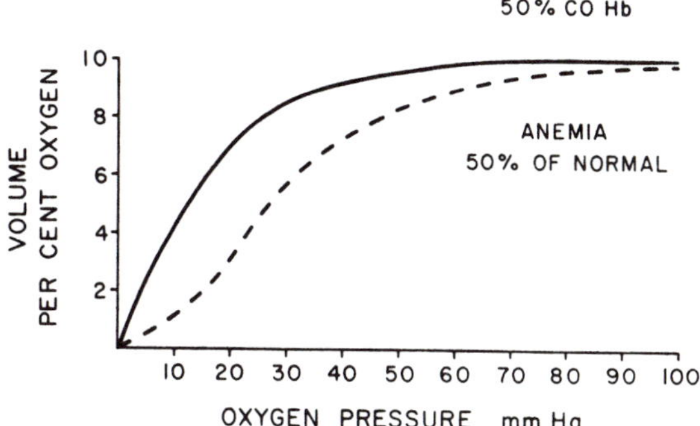

Fig. 9.9
Demonstration that oxygen release to tissues, as determined by shape and position of the oxyhemoglobin dissociation curve, is less abnormal in anemia than in CO poisoning.

relationship may be expressed as follows:

$$\frac{[\text{HbCO}]}{[\text{HbO}_2]} = 210\frac{\text{PCO}}{\text{PO}_2}.$$

The binding of CO to hemoglobin prevents the molecule from assuming the deoxy conformation. As a result, remaining heme groups that have not bound CO have an increased affinity for oxygen. Thus, increasing concentrations of HbCO in blood cause a progressive "shift to the left" and loss of sigmoidicity of the oxygen dissociation curve. This results in decreased release of oxygen to tissues. Figure 9.9 compares oxygen dissociation curves in an anemic patient in whom half of the hemoglobin is missing, with a patient having a normal total hemoglobin level but in whom half the hemoglobin is in the form of HbCO. Because of the increase in oxygen affinity, 50% HbCO results in much less delivery of oxygen to tissues than a 50% decrease in hemoglobin concentration.

2. *Clinical features*

In normal subjects, the maximum level of HbCO is 2% of total hemoglobin. Symptoms of acute poisoning vary with the level of HbCO. At 6–10%, vision and time discrimination are impaired. Unconsciousness followed by death occurs at 40–60%. There are no proven effects of chronic intoxication. Some workers have postulated a relation between chronic CO poisoning and coronary artery disease.

HbCO is a cherry-red pigment. When CO poisoning is suspected because of known exposure or symptoms of anoxia in the absence of cyanosis, the presence of HbCO can be established by studies of the visible absorption spectrum. The intoxicated victim should be immediately removed from exposure to carbon monoxide. Oxygen should be administered, and when necessary ventilation should be supported.

B. Methemoglobinemia

1. Pathophysiology

Methemoglobin is the form of hemoglobin in which the heme iron has been oxidized and is no longer able to bind to oxygen. It is sometimes called ferr*i*hemoglobin or hem*i*globin in contrast to reduced hemoglobin, which has been termed ferr*o*hemoglobin or hem*o*globin. Methemoglobin is continually being formed in normal red cells (in the absence of exogenous oxidant drugs or toxins) and is continually being reduced to hemoglobin. In normal red cells under steady-state conditions, the methemoglobin level does not exceed 1% of the total hemoglobin.

Two enzymatic reduction mechanisms are found in red cells. An enzyme called **cytochrome b_5 reductase** catalyzes the reduction of methemoglobin in a reaction that is coupled with the oxidation of NADH to NAD.

Methemoglobinemia may develop when (1) normal red cells are exposed to excess oxidant drugs or toxins or (2) red cells are congenitally deficient in cytochrome b_5 reductase.

Red cells also contain an **NADPH-dependent methemoglobin reductase** system that requires the presence of an exogenous electron carrier such as methylene blue (MB) and thus does not function physiologically. MB accepts electrons from NADPH (with formation of NADP and MBH) and transfer them to Fe^{3+}-heme to form Fe^{2+}-heme. When MB is present, NADPH-dependent reductase is more active than NADH-cytochrome b_5 reductase (figure 9.10). The significance of methemoglobin lies in the fact that Fe^{3+}-heme cannot bind oxygen. As in the presence of HbCO, an

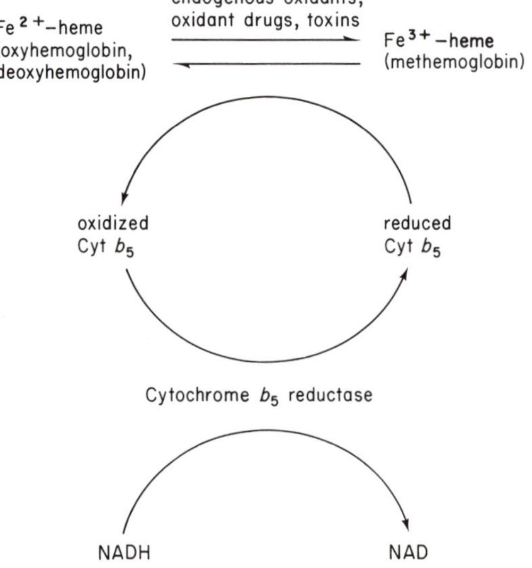

Fig. 9.10
Pathway of oxidation-reduction reactions in NADH-cytochrome b_5 methemoglobin reductase system.

increasing concentration of methemoglobin causes a progressive increase in oxygen affinity of the remaining functioning hemes on the hemoglobin tetramer (see figure 9.9). The result is decreased oxygen release to tissues.

2. *Etiology*

a. CONGENITAL

Causes of congenital methemoglobinemia include (1) deficiency of cytochrome b_5 reductase (2) presence of a hemoglobin M (see lecture 10).

b. ACQUIRED

Causes of acquired methemoglobin include (1) exposure to oxidant drugs or toxins that act directly such as nitrates from well water (that are reduced to nitrites by intestinal flora), chlorates, and quinones, and (2) agents that act indirectly such as aniline, acetanilid, and sulfonamides. Persons heterozygous for cytochrome b_5 reductase deficiency are more susceptible to oxidant agents than normal subjects.

3. *Clinical features*

A methemoglobin level in excess of 1.5 g/dl (10% of total hemoglobin) leads to visible cyanosis. (In contrast, cyanosis does not become visible until the level of reduced (deoxygenated) hemoglobin reaches 5.0 g/dl.) If methemoglobin exceeds 35% of total hemoglobin, headache and dyspnea may result. Levels over 70% are lethal. In some patients with congenital methemoglobinemia, mild polycythemia may result from chronic anoxia (see lecture 26).

4. *Treatment*

In mild cases, intravenous methylene blue administration activates NADPH-dependent methemoglobin reductase and readily corrects methemoglobinemia. In severe cases involving oxidant toxins, renal dialysis and exchange transfusion with fresh blood may be necessary. Orally administered methylene blue or ascorbic acid is a useful maintenance therapy in congenital methemoglobinemia.

C. Sulfhemoglobinemia

Sulfhemoglobinemia is associated with the presence in blood of a poorly characterized hemoglobin derivative with a characteristic absorption spectrum that distinguishes it from methemoglobin. It can be produced in vivo by various oxidant drugs including sulfonamides, phenacetin, and acetanilid. Unlike methemoglobin, sulfhemoglobin cannot be converted back to hemoglobin. When sulfhemoglobinemia occurs, it persists until the red cells containing the abnormal pigment are destroyed.

SELECTED REFERENCES

Reviews

Adams, J. G., and Honig, G. R. *Human Hemoglobin Genetics*. New York: Springer-Verlag, 1986.

Baldwin, J. Structure and cooperativity of haemoglobin. *TIBS* 5(1980): 224.

Bunn, H. F., and Forget, B. F. *Hemoglobin: Molecular, Genetic and Clinical Aspects*. Philadelphia: W. B. Saunders, 1986.

Friedman, J. M. Structure, dynamics, and reactivity in hemoglobin. *Science* 228 (1985): 1273–1280.

Gibson, Q. H. Hemoproteins, ligands, and quanta. *J. Biol. Chem.* 264(1989): 20155–20158.

Gill, S. J., Di Cera, E., et al. New twists on an old story: hemoglobin. *TIBS* 13(1988): 465–467.

Hirsch, R. E. Porphyrins and hemoglobin. *Semin. Hematol.* 26(1989): 47–53.

Perutz, M. F. Hemoglobin structure and respiratory transport. *Sci. Am.* 239(1978): 92–125.

Perutz, M. F. Molecular anatomy, physiology and pathology of hemoglobin. In Stamatoyannopoulos, G., et al., eds. *The Molecular Basis of Blood Diseases*. Philadelphia: W. B. Saunders, 1987.

Perutz, M. F. Myoglobin and haemoglobin: role of distal residues in reactions with haem ligands. *TIBS* 14(1989): 42–44.

Weatherall, D. J., Wood, W. G., et al. The developmental genetics of human hemoglobin. *Prog. Clin. Biol. Res.* 191(1985): 3–25.

Original articles

Bunn, H. F., et al. The glycosylation of hemoglobin: relevance to diabetes mellitus. *Science* 200(1978): 21–27.

Klein, R., Klein, B. E. K., et al. Glycosylated hemoglobin predicts the incidence and progression of diabetic retinopathy. *JAMA* 260(1988): 2864–2871.

LECTURE 10

Hemoglobin II. Sickle Cell Anemia and Other Hemoglobinopathies

H. Franklin Bunn

EDITOR'S COMMENT

The study of sickle cell hemoglobin is a splendid chapter in the history of hematology and molecular biology. This was the first mutant protein to be recognized. It was the first mutation to be attributed to a single amino acid switch. Its prevalence in the population led to important insights on natural selection and polymorphism in evolution. Its clinical importance and severity has led to massive searches for innovative therapies. Since the discovery of hemoglobin S, the many hundreds of hemoglobin mutants that have been (and are still being) recognized have greatly enhanced our understanding of the structure-function connection in the hemoglobin molecule. Significantly, most of these mutations have few clinical consequences because they occur in parts of the molecule that are not critical to hemoglobin functions. In my opinion, we tend to overlook the rarer abnormal hemoglobins in studying our patients. There is truth in the rule, "If you seek, you will find."

I. HEMOGLOBIN VARIANTS

More than 400 human hemogoblin **variants** of known structure have been reported to date. The majority were discovered incidentally in the course of population surveys and are not associated with clinical manifestations.

A. Genetic basis

Over 90% of the human hemoglobin variants are single amino acid substitutions in the α, β, γ, or δ subunits. These can all be explained by single base substitutions in the corresponding triplet codon. As shown in table 10.1, other molecular mechanisms must be invoked to explain the structure of a minority of the known hemoglobin variants.

A hemoglobin variant is inherited as an autosomal codominant trait. A pedigree of a family having genes for hemoglobin S and hemoglobin C is shown in figure 10.1 (right). Statistically, one-quarter of the offspring will be normal (AA), one-quarter will be SA heterozygotes, one-quarter will be CA heterozygotes, and one-quarter will be SC double heterozygotes.

Table 10.1
Molecular Bases of Human Hemoglobin Variants

Basic mechanism	Chain	Example
A. Amino acid substitution(s) (with nucleotide base substitution(s) in codon)		
1. One substitution	α	I Memphis, M Boston [146]
	β	S, C, D, E Seattle [268]
	γ	F Texas, I, F, Hull, etc. [50]
	δ	A_2 Sphakia, A_2 Flatbush, etc. [17]
2. Two substitutions	α	J Singapore
	β	C Harlem, Arlington Park, C Ziguinchor, S Travis, S Antilles, Poissy
B. Amino acid deletions	β	Gun Hill (5)
(nonhomologous crossing-over)	β	Tochigi (4)
	β	Niteroi (3)
	β	St. Antoine (2)
	β	Lyon (2)
	β	Tours (1)
	β	Leiden (1)
	β	Freiburg (1)
	β	Leslie (Deaconness) (1)
	β	Coventry (1)
C. Fusion hemoglobins	$\delta\beta$	The Lepores
(nonhomologous crossing-over	$\beta\delta$	Miyada, P Congo, P Nilotic
between genes encoding for two different subunits)	$\gamma\beta$	Kenya
D. Elongated subunits		
1. Base substitutions in termination codon	α	Constant Spring, Icaria, Koya Dora, Seal Rock
2. Frame shift	α	Wayne
	β	Tak, Cranston, Saverne
3. Retention of initiator methionine	β	Long Island/Marseille, South Florida, Doha

Note: Number of known variants appears in brackets; number of amino acid residues deleted appears in parentheses.

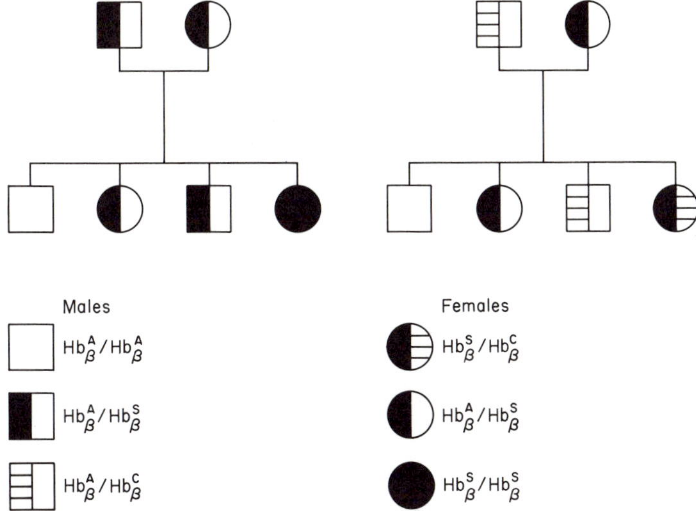

Fig. 10.1
Pedigrees of families with genes for hemoglobin S and A (*left*) and hemoglobin S, C, and A (*right*).

Table 10.2
Effect of Substitution at β6 on Isoelectric Point

Hemoglobin	β chain sequence	Isoelectric point
A	H_2N-Val-His-Leu-Thr-Pro-**Glu**-Glu ...	7.0
S	H_2N-Val-His-Leu-Thr-Pro-**Val**-Glu ...	7.2
C	H_2N-Val-His-Leu-Thr-Pro-**Lys**-Glu ...	7.4

B. Detection

Abnormal hemoglobins are usually detected by electrophoresis of red cell hemolysate. If the substituted amino acid alters the net charge, the isoelectric point and electrophoretic mobility of the variant hemoglobin will differ from those of hemoglobin A. The effects of amino acid substitutions at β6 on the isoelectric point are illustrated in table 10.2 and figure 10.2.

C. Clinical classification

The common clinically significant human hemoglobin variants can be classified as follows:

- Sickle syndromes
  - Sickle cell trait (AS)
  - Sickle cell anemia (SS)
  - Double-heterozygous states (sickle–β-thalassemia; SC disease; SD disease)

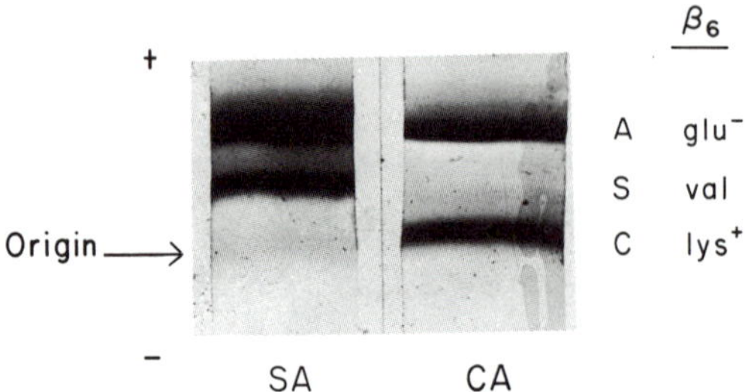

Fig. 10.2
Electrophoresis of hemolysates of individuals with sickle trait (SA) and hemoglobin C trait (CA).

- Unstable hemoglobin variants (congenital Heinz body hemolytic anemias)
- Variants with high oxygen affinity (familial erythrocytosis)
- The M hemoglobins (familial cyanosis)

The sickle syndromes to be described below are clinical problems only in homozygotes or double heterozygotes. In contrast, unstable variants, high-oxygen-affinity variants, and M hemoglobins are encountered only in heterozygotes. In these states, homozygosity would be lethal.

II. SICKLE SYNDROMES

In 1910, Herrick described a black student with a hemolytic anemia and peculiar elongated or "sickled" red cell on the blood smear. The subsequent elaboration of the molecular and genetic basis of sickle cell disease is one of the most absorbing chapters in the history of molecular biology. The various states associated with the presence of hemoglobin S ($\alpha_2\beta_2{}^{6Glu\rightarrow Val}$) are listed in table 10.3, in order of clinical severity.

A. Sickle cell trait

About 8% of black Americans are heterozygous for hemoglobin S. Thus their red cells contain hemoglobin S and A. In parts of central Africa where malaria is endemic, nearly 25% of the population has the sickle trait. The gene has persisted because of balanced polymorphism, whereby heterozygotes are slightly protected against falciparum malaria.

1. Clinical features

Life expectancy and morbidity of individuals with sickle trait resemble those of a comparable group with hemoglobin A. SA red cells sickle far less readily than SS red cells (table 10.4). Accordingly, SA heterozygotes develop sickling crises rarely and only when severely hypoxic. Splenic infarction occurs only occasionally. Since the renal medulla is unusually susceptible to sickling, these patients often display an impaired ability to

Table 10.3
Varying Clinical Severity of the Different Sickle Syndromes

Genotype	% of hemoglobin S	% of non-S hemoglobin	Clinical severity
SS	80–90	5–15 (F)	++/++++
SO, SD	30–40	60–70 (O, D)	++/++++
S-β-thalassemia	80	20 (A + F)	+/+++
SC	50	50 (C)	+/+++
S-HPFH*	70	30 (F)	0
SA	30–40	55–65 (A)	0

* Double heterozygous state for hemoglobin S and hereditary persistence of fetal hemoglobin (see lecture 11).

Table 10.4
Comparison of Intracellular Sickling and Solubility in the Sickling Disorders

Genotype	PO_2-50% sickled cells (mm Hg)	Solubility (g/dl)
SS	30–50	19
S-β-thalassemia	22–32	variable
SC	10–20	26
S-HPFH	~10	24
SA	2–7	28

concentrate urine and rarely have recurrent episodes of painless hematuria due to medullary infarction. Individuals with the sickle cell trait should not be placed in high-risk categories by employers or insurers.

2. *Diagnosis*

The diagnosis rests on the following laboratory tests:

- Sickling preparation. A blood sample mixed with an oxygen-consuming reagent such as metabisulfite is examined under the microscope for sickled cells.
- Solubility tests (e.g., dithionite tube test). These tests depend on the fact that deoxyhemoglobin S has low solubility at high ionic strength.
- Mechanical precipitation tests. Hemoglobin S has an increased rate of surface denaturation and forms a precipitate when a dilute solution is shaken vigorously.
- Hemoglobin electrophoresis (figure 10.2). Individuals with the sickle cell trait have 30–40% hemoglobin S and 55–65% hemoglobin A.

B. Sickle cell anemia

The clinical manifestations of sickle cell anemia are all attributable to a specific molecular lesion: the substitution of valine for glutamic acid at the sixth residue of the β chain.

1. Molecular basis of sickling

Upon deoxygenation, a red cell containing hemoglobin S acquires an elongated crescent shape or sickle shape. Electron micrographs reveal bundles of fibers each with a diameter of 180 Å, running parallel to the long axis of sickling (figure 10.3). Each fiber consists of a 14-strand helical polymer having an inner core of 4 strands and an outer layer of 10 strands (see figure 10.3). Both hydrophobic and electrostatic bonds contribute to the stabilization of the helical polymers. In addition, there are interactions between neighboring fibers. The mechanism of sickling can be studied in vitro by determination of the hemoglobin concentration at which polymerization occurs (i.e., the solubility). As shown in table 10.4, this concentration is relatively low for deoxyhemoglobin S.

Sickling, both within the red cell and in a hemoglobin solution, is greatly affected by the presence of non-S hemoglobin. This can be confirmed by solubility measurements (table 10.4). Hemoglobin F inhibits gelation. These experimental results agree with well-known differences in clinical severity of the various sickle syndromes: SS, SF, and SA. Other less common hemoglobin variants also interact with hemoglobin S. Hemoglobins O Arab and D Los Angeles readily copolymerize with Hb S. Accordingly, double heterozygotes (SO and SD) have clinical severity equivalent to that of SS homozygotes.

Such information has been valuable in localizing the sites on the hemoglobin molecule responsible for the interaction of neighboring tetramers in the polymer. In order for hemoglobin S to form a sickle polymer (or fiber), it must be in the deoxy form.

Kinetic considerations are of importance in determining to what extent sickling occurs in solution or in the red cell. The initial and rate-limiting step is nucleation, that is, aggregation of individual hemoglobin tetramers into helical fibers (figure 10.4). This process is markedly concentration dependent. Once formed, the fibers undergo a phase transition from a random orientation to parallel alignment. This alignment of fibers is responsible for the distortion of the red cell into an elongated sickled form. Upon oxygenation or cooling, the polymers dissolve and the gel readily liquefies or melts (figure 10.4).

2. Events at the cellular level

As sickle polymer forms, red cells become rigid and may further obstruct capillary blood flow. Obstruction of flow leads to local tissue hypoxia, further deoxygenation of hemoglobin, and therefore further intracellular polymerization. This vicious cycle may amplify microscopic obstruction into macroscopic infarction.

Ordinarily, the sickled cell resumes a normal shape upon reoxygenation. However, the membrane of SS red cells may become damaged with resulting formation of **irreversibly sickled cells** (ISC; figure 10.5). Continuous formation and destruction of ISCs probably contributes to the severe

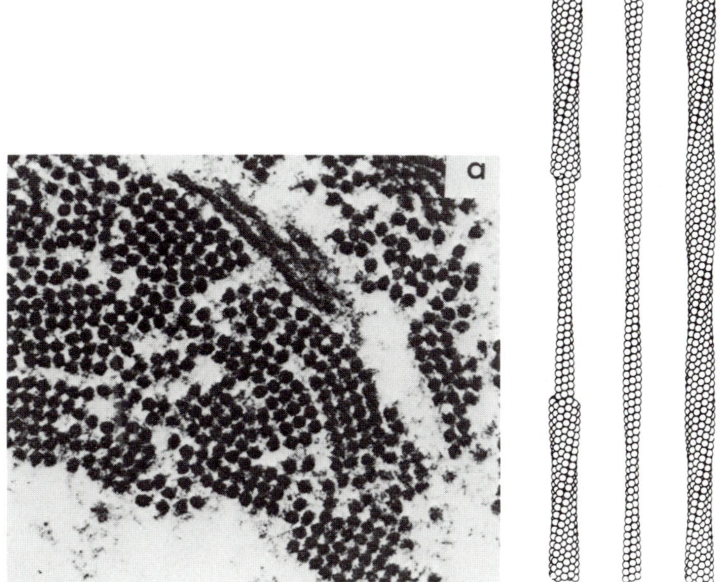

Fig. 10.3A
Electron micrographs of concentrated solution of deoxygenated hemoglobin S (× 57,500). *Left*, Transverse section. *Right*, Longitudinal section showing parallel fibers.

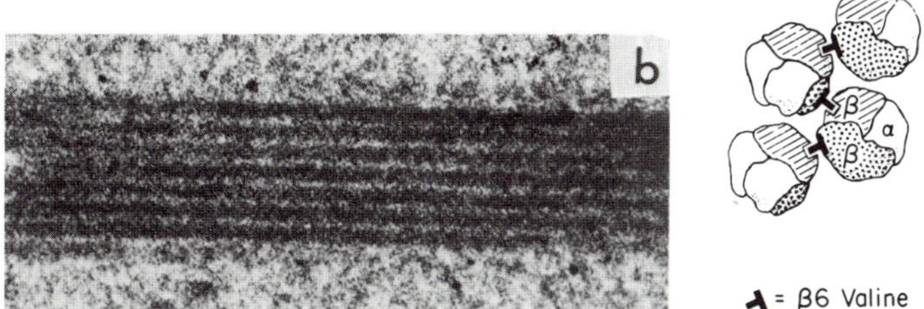

Fig. 10.3B
Left, Model of sickle fiber showing an inner core and outer layer. Each deoxyhemoglobin S tetramer is represented as a sphere. (From Dykes et al., *J. Mol. Biol.* 130[1978]: 451.) *Right*, Interaction of hemoglobin S molecules within the sickle fiber. The β6 valine in hydrophobically bonded to a complementary site on the β chain of an adjacent hemoglobin molecule.

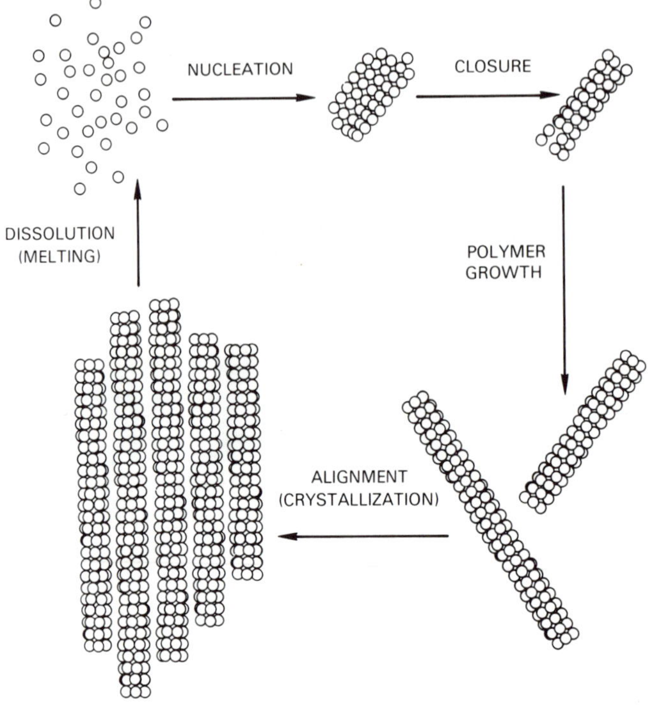

Fig. 10.4
Model of the polymerization of deoxyhemoglobin S. Monomeric hemoglobin aggregates in supersaturated solutions to form the compact nucleus for a single fiber. The fibers grow and then align into an ordered structure (tactoid or nematic crystal). (Courtesy of Dr. J. Hofrichter and Dr. W. Eaton.)

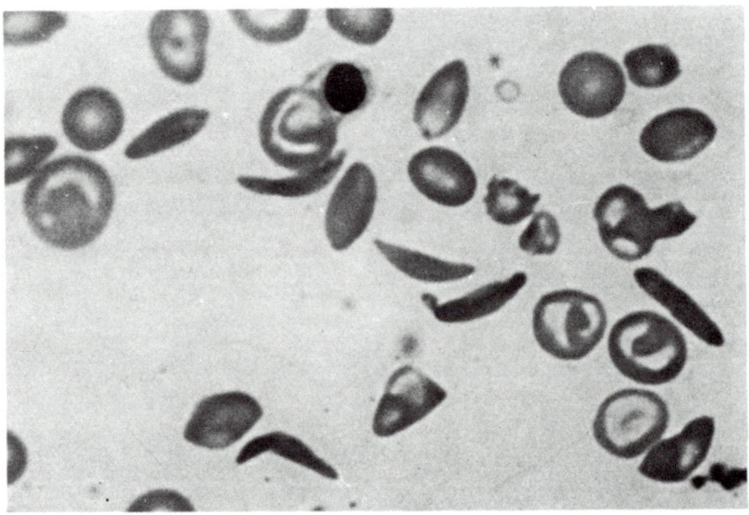

Fig. 10.5
Blood smear of patient with sickle cell anemia showing irreversibly sickled cells. (Photomicrograph by C. von Kapff.)

hemolytic anemia occurring in sickle cell anemia. Furthermore, these rigid cells may initiate small vessel occlusion.

Several independent factors promote intracellular polymerization of Hb S. Increased corpuscular hemoglobin concentration is the most important since the rate of polymerization is so concentration dependent. The rate and extent of deoxygenation is another critical factor. Finally, both acidosis and increased red cell 2,3-DPG promote polymerization of sickle hemoglobin by lowering oxygen affinity (see lecture 9) and therefore increasing levels of deoxyhemoglobin S.

3. *Clinical features*

a. CONSTITUTIONAL SIGNS

Children with SS disease have impaired growth and development; general failure to thrive; and increased tendency to develop serious infections (especially with pneumococcus). These patients have marked impairment of splenic function (see lecture 3) with inadequate clearance of blood-borne bacteria. The spleen develops recurrent infarcts and in time becomes a nubbin of fibrous tissue. Infection is a common complication owing in part to the absence of splenic function. Infection frequently triggers the development of painful crises.

b. ANEMIA

SS homozygotes have a severe hemolytic anemia, hematocrit values ranging between 18 and 30%. Those red cells with relatively low hemoglobin F levels are likely to become ISCs and therefore have the shortest life spans. Anemia becomes increasingly severe if erythropoiesis is also suppressed. The two main causes of such suppression are aplastic crises due to infection and megaloblastosis due to folic acid deficiency. A decrease in red cell production, however transient, can rapidly depress the hematocrit.

c. VASOOCCLUSIVE PHENOMENA

As noted, the morbidity and mortality of sickle cell disease is due primarily to recurrent vasoocclusive phenomena. These can be divided into two groups: painful crises and chronic organ damage. Painful crises may appear suddenly in any part of the body. The common sites are abdomen, chest, and joints. About a third of painful crises are preceded by a viral or bacterial infection. The frequency and severity of painful crises are highly variable. It may be difficult to distinguish between painful sickle crisis and another acute process. Abdominal crisis may mimic biliary colic, appendicitis, or perforated viscus. A sickle crisis in the extremities may mimic osteomyelitis or an acute arthritis such as gout or rheumatoid arthritis.

The incidence, severity, and duration of pain crises vary markedly among patients and even in a given patient.

- **Chronic organ damage** consisting of anatomic or functional damage to various tissues is due to the cumulative effect of recurrent vasoocclusive episodes. Any organ or system may be involved, but the following are most commonly encountered:
- **Cardiopulmonary system**. Impairment of pulmonary function is common. Patients have hypoxemia due in part to intrapulmonary arteriovenous shunting. Congestive heart failure develops frequently owing to the burdens of chronic severe anemia and hypoxemia. Although more oxygen is extracted by the myocardium than any other tissue, myocardial infarction is rare.
- **Hepatobiliary system**. Icterus and increased tendency to form gallstones commonly results from chronic hemolysis and impaired liver function. Hepatic infarction may occur. Splenic infarction is inevitable.
- **Genitourinary system**. The hypertonic and acidic environment in the renal medulla promotes sickling with resulting microinfarcts. Virtually all patients have isosthenuria. Like those with sickle trait or SC disease, SS homozygotes may develop significant and prolonged painless hematuria as a result of papillary infarcts. Male patients with sickle cell disease occasionally develop priapism (spontaneous, painful, and continued engorgement of the penis).
- **Skeletal system**. The development of bone infarcts produces characteristic x-ray abnormalities. Biconcave "fish-mouth" vertebrae are pathognomonic of sickle cell disease (figure 10.6). Aseptic necrosis of the femoral head is common and can lead to disability.

Like infarcts in other organs, bony infarctions often become infected. Osteomyelities is frequently due to salmonella.

- **Eye**. Ocular complications include retinal infarcts, peripheral vascular disease, arteriovenous anomalies, vitreous hemorrhage, retinitis proliferans, and retinal detachment. Major ocular complications are more common in SC disease than in SS homozygotes.
- **Skin**. Chronic skin ulcers often occur in the distal lower extremities, particularly in severely anemic patients and in tropical areas.
- **Nervous system**. A quarter of all patients with SS disease eventually develop some type of neurological manifestation. Hemiplegia is the most fequent. Coma, convulsions, or visual disturbances also occur. Patients generally recover from these episodes.

4. Diagnosis

The diagnosis is usually suspected from the clinical appearance of the patient and the appearance of the blood smear (see figure 10.5). Hemoglobin electrophoresis shows 80–95% hemoglobin S, 0–20% hemoglobin F, and a normal amount of hemoglobin A_2. The diagnostic tests for sickling described about are positive.

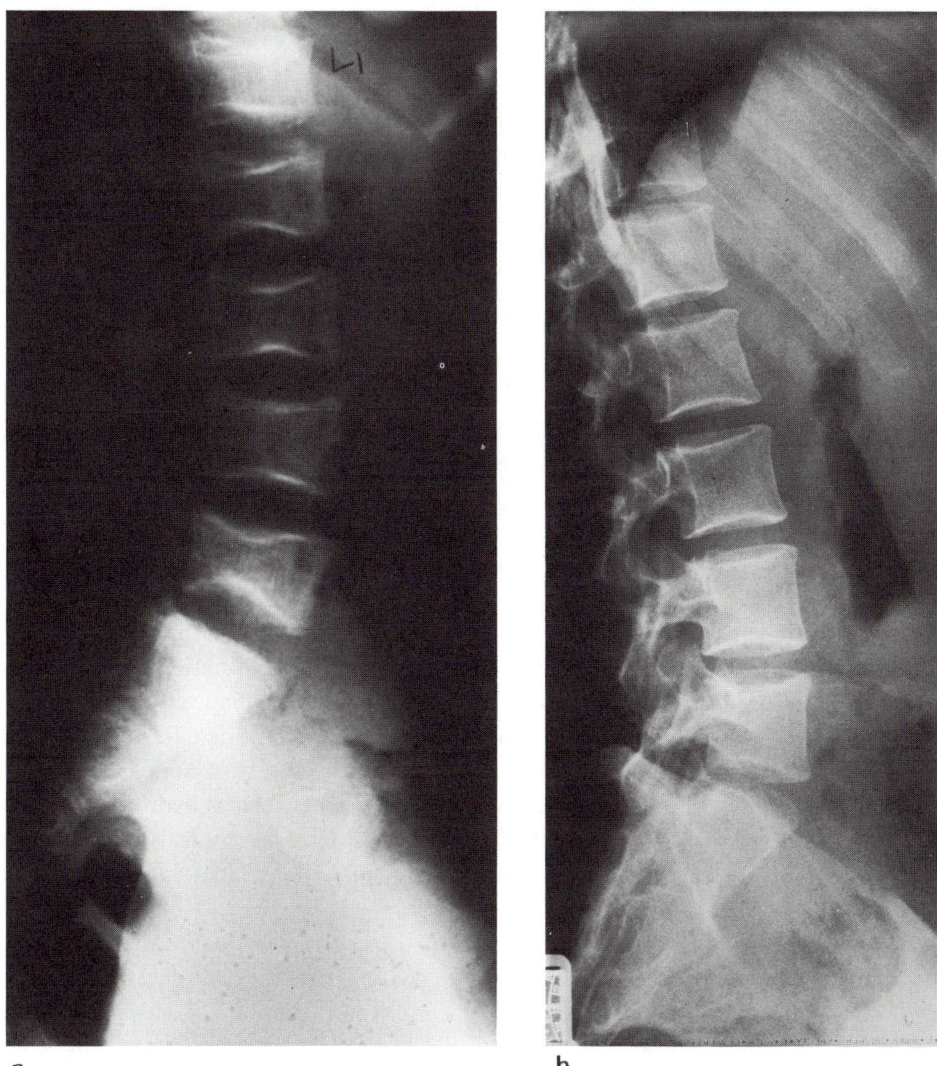

Fig. 10.6
A, Lateral view of lumbar spine of patient with sickle cell anemia. Note biconcave fish-mouth vertebrae. *B*, Comparable view of a normal lumbar spine.

5. *Therapy*

Many antisickling regimens have been proposed to date, but none has stood the test of time. Currently accepted management of sickle cell anemia is primarily supportive and conservative. Since these patients risk developing infections, which may trigger painful and aplastic crises, it is important to detect infection early and treat promptly with antibiotics. Pneumococcal vaccination and prophylactic penicillin are effective in preventing the development of meningitis. Anemia increases markedly if the patient becomes folic acid deficient. Since these patients have an increased folic acid requirement, they should be given a daily supplement.

Painful crises should be treated promptly with analgesia and hydration. Since crises may be aborted if treated early, it is advisable to give patients a supply of analgesics (e.g., codeine) that can be self-administered.

Blood transfusions have a limited role in the management of sickle cell anemia. Between crises, patients usually tolerate anemia well and do not derive much subjective benefit from transfusions. Replacement of 70% of the patient's SS red cells with normal AA red cells (hypertransfusion) reduces the recurrence rate of strokes in children. Furthermore, hypertransfusion may be a useful way of getting a patient through a limited period of risk such as surgery. However, the risks of isoimmunization, iron overload, and hepatitis are sufficient reasons to minimize transfusion.

Currently a number of investigators are attempting to treat sickle cell disease by inducing an increase in Hb F. This can be accomplished by the administration of certain antineoplastic agents such as hydroxyurea. The mechanism underlying the increase in the Hb F synthesis is unclear. Unfortunately, high doses of recombinant erythropoietin are ineffectual.

6. *Prevention*

Genetic counseling may be useful in the prevention of sickle cell anemia. If both marital partners are SA heterozygotes, they may decide not to have children, knowing that there is a 25% chance that an offspring will be an SS homozygote.

The antenatal diagnosis of sickle cell anemia can now be made early in the 18th to 20th week of pregnancy by the testing of a small sample of amniotic fluid. There are endonucleases that can distinguish between the normal β globin gene and the β^S gene at the site of base substitution. If it is established that a fetus is an SS homozygote, the parents may elect to interrupt a pregnancy.

7. *Prognosis*

The clinical course of homozygous SS disease is highly variable. Most published assessments of prognosis have been unduly pessimistic. In the United States, an increasing number of patients are surviving into adulthood and bearing offspring. Although patients who have relatively high hemoglobin F levels tend to have milder clinical manifestations, this relation is of little prognostic value in a given patient.

C. Other sickle syndromes

1. Sickle–β-thalassemia

β-thalassemia, a disorder characterized by absent or diminished β chain synthesis, is fully discussed in lecture 11. In sickle–β-thalassemia, both β-globin genes are defective, one producing an abnormal β chain and the other affecting the rate of β chain synthesis. The disease is variable in its clinical manifestations. It occurs primarily in Mediterranean people. Like homozygous β-thalassemia, sickle–β-thalassemia is milder in blacks than in Mediterranean people. Patients have moderately severe hemolytic anemia (hematocrit 25–35%). Splenomegaly occurs in 70% of the cases. Patients who are unable to make any Hb A (S-β^0 thal) have disease as severe as that of SS patients. Those with S-β^+ thal have milder hemolysis and vasoocclusive phenomena.

2. Diagnosis

The blood smear reveals hypochromic microcytic red cells with polychromatophilia, target cells, stippling, and rare ISCs (figure 10.7).

Hemoglobin electrophoresis reveals that 60–90% of the hemoglobin is S and 10–30% is F. Hemoglobin A is about 10–30% if the patient is capable of producing some β^A chains (see β^+ thalassemia in lecture 11). Hemoglobin A_2 is moderately elevated in sickle–β-thalassemia.

3. Prognosis and therapy

Therapy is the same as that for SS disease. If the spleen is sequestering red cells in significant amounts, splenectomy may be beneficial.

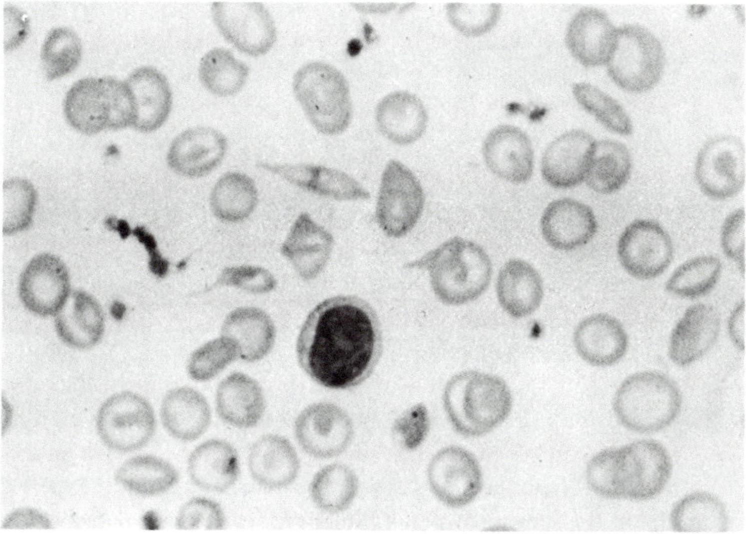

Fig. 10.7
Blood smear of patient with sickle–β-thalassemia. (Photomicrograph by C. von Kapff.)

D. Sickle-C disease

The gene frequency for hemoglobin C ($\alpha_2\beta_2^{6Glu \rightarrow Lys}$) is a quarter of that for hemoglobin S. Nevertheless, SC disease is almost as common among adults as SS disease since life expectancy in SC disease is nearly normal. There are two reasons why SC is a disease whereas SA is benign. First, intracellular hemoglobin concentration is significantly higher in SC red cells owing to the presence of Hb C (see below). Second, SC red cells have at least 10% higher level of hemoglobin S than have SA red cells. Patients have a mild to moderate hemolytic anemia and usually have splenomegaly. The blood smear shows target cells and occasional plump sickled forms (figure 10.8). Painful crises or organ infarcts occur occasionally. Ocular complications are common, as are hematuria from renal medullary infarcts, aseptic necrosis of the femoral head, and various complications during pregnancy.

E. Homozygous C disease

Homozygous hemoglobin C disease produces a mild congenital hemolytic anemia with splenomegaly. Hemoglobin C is less soluble than hemoglobin A, and it tends to form intracellular crystals, particularly if red cells are suspended in a hypertonic medium or CC red cells are dehydrated. The blood smear reveals striking target cells (figure 10.9). Red cell osmotic fragility is decreased. Significant complications are rare, and no specific therapy is required.

III. UNSTABLE HEMOGLOBINS

More than 60 unstable hemoglobin variants are known. These hemoglobins cause hemolysis in heterozygous subjects. In some instances, the homozygous state would be lethal. The molecular abnormality is often an amino acid substitution in the heme pocket of the β chain (figure 10.10). In comparison to hemoglobin A, such hemoglobins readily autooxidize to methemoglobin, whereupon the heme becomes detached and residual relatively insoluble globin forms an intracellular precipitate, or **Heinz body**. Some unstable hemoglobins result from an amino acid subtitution that distorts or interrupts the helical structure of the involved chain. The abnormal subunits of a few unstable variants have deletions of 1–5 amino acid residues (see table 10.1). The precipitated inclusions impair red cell deformability, and the cell becomes trapped in the RES. The inclusions may be "pitted" from the red cell (see lecture 3) or the entire cell may be destroyed (see lecture 12). The heme may be catabolized aberrantly to form **dipyrroles**, which cause the excretion of dark-colored urine. Unstable hemoglobin should be suspected in any patient with congenital hemolytic anemia. Its presence is confirmed by supravital Heinz body stains, hemoglobin electrophoresis, and stability tests in which hemolysate is heated to

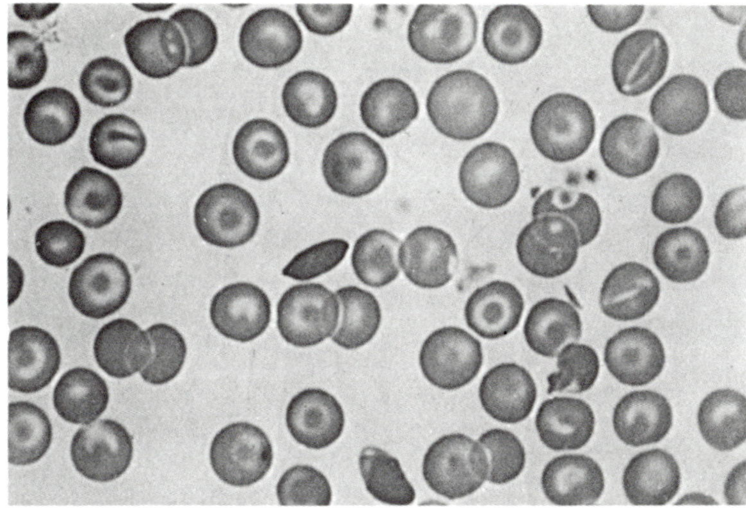

Fig. 10.8
Blood smear of patient with sickle-C disease. (Photomicrograph by C. von Kapff.)

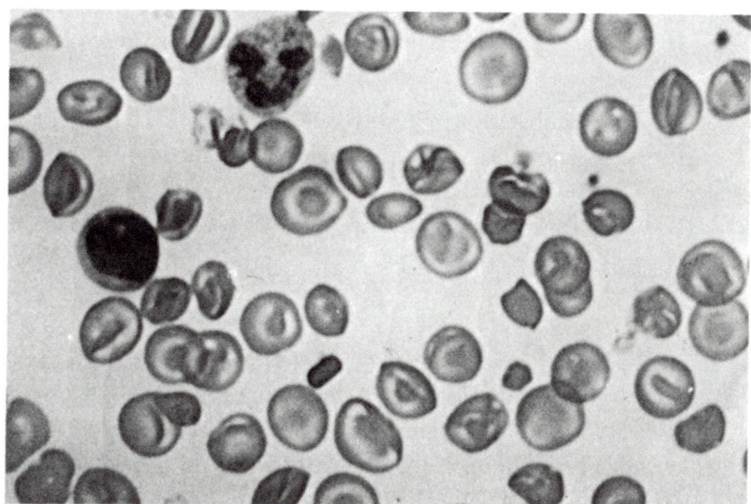

Fig. 10.9
Blood smear of patient with homozygous hemoglobin C disease. (Photomicrograph by C. von Kapff.)

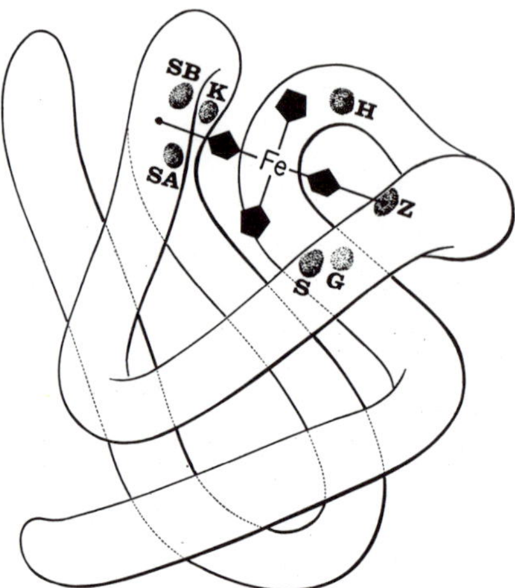

Fig. 10.10
Unstable hemoglobins. The diagram depicts a three-dimensional representation of a β chain. Sites of amino acid substitutions of some of the unstable hemoglobin variants are designated with letters. Note their proximity to the heme group: K = Köln, β98 Val → Met; H = Hammersmith, β42 Phe → Ser; Z = Zurich, β63 His → Arg; G = Genova, β28 Val → Ala; SA = Santa Ana, β88 Leu → Pro. (From H. Jacob and K. Winterhalter, *Proc. Nat. Acad. Sci. USA* 65[1970]: 697.)

50°C or incubated at 37° with 17% isopropanol. Unstable hemoglobins form a precipitate; normal hemoglobins do not.

IV. HEMOGLOBINS WITH ABNORMAL OXYGEN AFFINITY

A. High-oxygen-affinity variants

Familial erythrocytosis may be due to the inheritance of a stable hemoglobin variant having increased oxygen affinity. More than 20 different **high-oxygen-affinity hemoglobin variants** have been discovered to date. Like unstable hemoglobins, they are found only in heterozygotes. The amino acid substitution is likely to be in the $\alpha_1\beta_2$ contact area, or at the C-terminus of the β chain. Interference in the normal conformational isomerization between deoxyhemoglobin and oxyhemoglobin leads to altered oxygen affinity and decreased heme-heme interaction.

The major pathophysiologic consequences of the presence of a high-oxygen-affinity hemoglobin are the following:

- Decreased unloading of oxygen in tissues
- Increased erythorpoietin production
- Familial erythrocytosis

Table 10.5
The M Hemoglobins

Amino acid substitution	Name of hemoglobin (location of propositus)
$\alpha_2^{58\mathrm{His}\to\mathrm{Tyr}}\beta_2$	Boston, Osaka, Gothenburg
$\alpha_2^{87\mathrm{His}\to\mathrm{Tyr}}\beta_2$	Iwate, Kankakee, Oldenburg
$\alpha_2\beta_2^{63\mathrm{His}\to\mathrm{Tyr}}$	Saskatoon, Chicago, Emory, Kurme, Radom
$\alpha_2\beta_2^{92\mathrm{His}\to\mathrm{Tyr}}$	Hyde Park
$\alpha_2\beta_2^{67\mathrm{Val}\to\mathrm{Glu}}$	Milwaukee

B. Low-oxygen-affinity variants

A number of variants have slightly decreased oxygen affinity but no clinical consequences. A few such as hemoglobins Kansas, Beth Israel, and St. Mandé have such low oxygen affinity that arterial blood is partially unsaturated, with resulting cyanosis. These variants have substitutions that destabilize the "oxy" quaternary structure.

V. THE M HEMOGLOBINS

As noted in lecture 9, familial cyanosis may be due to inheritance of one of the M hemoglobins. This group includes five variants. In four, tyrosine is substituted for the invariant distal(E7) or proximal (F8) heme-linked histidine of the α or β chain (see figure 9.2). The fifth variant (M Milwaukee) involves substitution of glutamic acid for valine at the β^{67} locus. These changes stabilize the hemes of the abnormal globin chains in the ferric form. This alters the absorption spectrum and gives the hemoglobin a brown color. It also alters the oxygenation of the normal (nonmutant) chains.

Families with the same hemoglobin M have been discovered in many widely separated areas (table 10.5). Variants have been designated by the place of origin, sometimes with competing names. Heterozygotes are usually asymptomatic except for cyanosis, though hemoglobins M Saskatoon and M Hyde Park are also unstable and may cause mild hemolysis.

SELECTED REFERENCES

Reviews

Adams, J. G., and Honig, G. R. *Human Hemoglobin Genetics*. New York: Springer-Verlag, 1986.

Briehl, R. W. The rheology of sickle cell hemoglobin. *Ann. NY Acad. Sci.* 565 (1989): 279–283.

Briehl, R. W., and Mann, E. S. Hemoglobin S polymerization: fiber lengths, rheology, and pathogenesis. *Ann. NY Acad. Sci.* 565(1989): 295–307.

Bunn, H. F., and Forget, B. F. *Hemoglobin: Molecular, Genetic and Clinical Aspects*. Philadelphia: W. B. Saunders, 1986.

Charache, S. Treatment of sickle cell anemia. *Annu. Rev. Med.* 32(1981): 195.

Embury, S. The clinical pathopysiology of sickle cell disease. *Annu. Rev. Med.* 37(1986): 361–376.

Luzzatto, L., and Goodfellow, P. Sickle cell anaemia: a simple disease with no cure. *Nature* 337(1989): 17–18.

Powars, D. R., Chan, L., et al. The influence of fetal hemoglobin on the clinical expression of sickle cell anemia. *Annu. NY Acad. Sci.* 565(1989): 262–278.

San Biagio, P. L., Hofrichter, J., et al. Current perspectives on the kinetics of hemoglobin S gelation. *Ann. NY Acad. Sci.* 565(1989): 53–62.

Sergeant, G. R. *Sickle Cell Disease*. New York: Oxford University Press, 1985.

Ueno, H., Bai, Y., et al. Covalent chemical modifiers of sickle cell hemoglobin. *Ann. NY. Acad. Sci.* 565(1989): 239–246.

Zinkham, W. H., and Winslow, R. M. Unstable hemoglobins: influence of environment on phenotypic expression of a genetic disorder. *Medicine* (*Baltimore*) 68 (1989): 309–309.

Original articles

Bunn, H. F., Bradley, T. B., et al. Structural and functional studies on hemoglobin Bethesda ($\alpha_2\beta_2{}^{145His}$), a variant associated with compensatory erythrocytosis. *J. Clin. Invest.* 51(1972): 2299–2309.

Castle, W. B. From man to molecule and back to mankind. *Semin. Hematol.* 13(1976): 159.

Dover, G. J., and Charache, S. Chemotherapy and hemoglobin F synthesis in sickle cell disease. *Ann. NY Acad. Sci.* 565(1989): 222–227.

Eaton, W. A., and Hofrichter, J. Hemoglobin S gelation and sickle cell disease. *Blood* 70(1987): 1245.

McDade, W. A., Carragher, B., et al. On the assembly of sickle hemoglobin fascicles. *J. Mol. Biol.* 206(1989): 637–649.

Messmann, R., Gannon, S., et al. Mechanical properties of sickle cell membranes. *Blood* 75(1990): 1711–1717.

Platt, O. S. Is there treatment for sickle cell anemia? *N. Engl. J. Med.* 319(1988): 1479–1480.

Rodgers, G. P., Dover, G. J., et al. Hematologic responses of patients with sickle cell disease to treatment with hydroxyurea. *N. Engl. J. Med.* 322(1990): 1037–1045.

Samuel, R. E., Salmon, E. D., et al. Nucleation and growth of fibres and gel formation in sickle cell haemoglobin. *Nature* 345(1990): 833–835.

Watowich, S. J., Gross, L. J., et al. Intermolecular contacts within sickle hemoglobin fibers. *J. Mol. Biol.* 209(1989): 821–828.

LECTURE 11

The Thalassemias

David G. Nathan

EDITOR'S COMMENT

Although often described as a hemoglobinopathy, the thalassemias are not as a rule associated with an abnormal hemoglobin molecule. The problem rather relates to depressed rates of synthesis of normal hemoglobin chains. As a result of unbalanced chain synthesis, there is a web of clinical consequences that varies with the severity of the biosynthetic block and the chain that is blocked. A long list of mutations affecting virtually every step in protein synthesis is now known to account for thalassemias in various regions of the world. It is fair to assume that these mechanisms, which have clinically visible consequences when they affect the synthesis of hemoglobin, are more or less relevant to the biosynthesis of all proteins. Those other proteins, however, are present only in micro quantities and are correspondingly harder to study. Once again, we may assume that what is true of blood, an accessible tissue, applies to disorders of less accessible tissues.

I. INTRODUCTION

A. Definitions

The thalassemias (named from the Greek word for sea) are a heterogeneous group of inherited disorders of hemoglobin synthesis characterized by absent or diminished synthesis of one or the other of the globin chains of hemoglobin A. In the **α-thalassemias**, α chain synthesis is absent or diminished; in the **β-thalassemias**, β chain synthesis is absent or diminished. Diverse molecular mechanisms account for the various thalassemias. Clinical manifestations vary with the nature and severity of the defect.

The terms **Mediterranean anemia** and **Cooley's anemia** were used in the older literature to denote β thalassemia. The term **thalassemia major** has also been used to refer to the homozygous state and **thalassemia minor** and **thalassemia intermedia** to heterozygous states of various degrees of severity.

B. Geographic distribution

Although the thalassemias are found all over the world, specific forms occur with high frequency in certain populations—notably in Mediterranean populations (i.e., from southern Italy and Greece) and Oriental populations (i.e., from Thailand, China, and the Philippines). β-thalassemia is

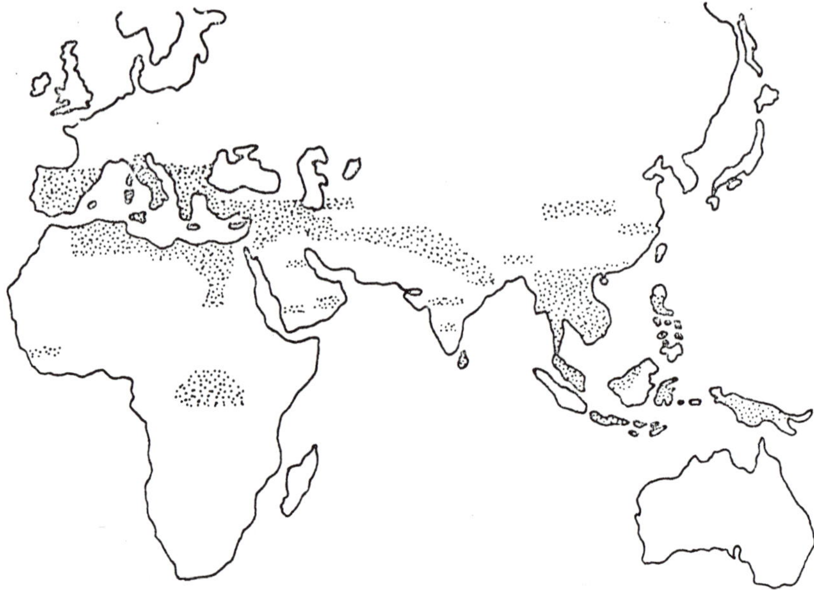

Fig. 11.1
Geographical distribution of the thalassemias, indicated by speckled regions.

more common in Mediterranean populations: α-thalassemia is prevalent in Oriental populations. In Italy and Greece, 5–10% of the population are heterozygous for β-thalassemia. In Thailand, the gene frequency for the various forms of heterozygous α-thalassemia reaches 25%. Sporadic cases of thalassemia are common among Africans and American blacks. Generally, the distribution of thalassemia follows the malaria belt (figure 11.1). The high frequency of thalassemia in these areas may be attributable to the fact that the heterozygous thalassemias enhance resistance to malaria.

C. Pathophysiology

1. Basic mechanisms

A unifying concept underlies our understanding of the pathophysiology of all the thalassemias: Deficient or absent synthesis of a specific globin chain leads to unbalanced chain synthesis. This has two effects: (1) inadequate hemoglobinization of developing erythroid cells with resulting hypochromia; and (2) more important, various specific sequelae of unbalanced globin chain synthesis. For example, chains present in relative excess, particularly when of the α type, precipitate in the developing erythroid cell. This damages surface membranes in both developing and mature cells. Cells thus handicapped either die in the bone marrow (thus causing ineffective erythropoiesis) or, if released from the marrow, are promptly removed by the RES (thus causing hemolysis). Both phenomena compound the anemia and lead to compensatory erythropoietin-induced marrow hyperplasia. This in turn leads to a hypermetabolic state, skeletal changes, and

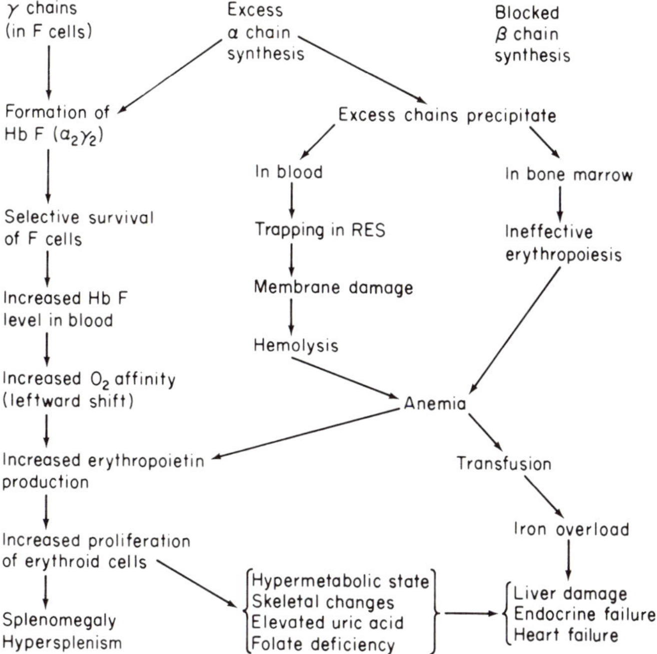

Fig. 11.2
Pathophysiology of homozygous β-thalassemia.

increased intestinal absorption of iron and iron overload. This web of causes and effects in homozygous β-thalassemia is diagrammed in figure 11.2. The blood also contains many target cells.

2. *Clinical implications*

Clinical severity varies broadly, ranging from benign to lethal. The severity of a particular thalassemia is related to

- Patterns of inheritance, that is, heterozygosity or homozygosity
- Severity of the particular thalassemia defect
- Degree of compensation, especially with respect to γ globin chain production (see below and figure 11.2)
- Presence of interacting thalassemia defects (e.g., simultaneous inheritance of α- and β-thalassemia defects, presence of β^S, β^E)
- Presence of interacting factors of unknown character.

D. Molecular biology of globin genes

1. *Hemoglobin structure*

Molecular structure of various normal hemoglobins (summarized in table 9.1) should be reviewed because it is essential to an understanding of the basis of thalassemia. It also permits a classification of these disorders on the basis of primary defect rather than by overlapping and somewhat confusing clinical descriptions. It will be recalled that all normal hemoglobins are formed as tetramers of two α (or α-like) chains and two non-α globin chains. Hemoglobin A is $\alpha_2\beta_2$. Hemoglobin A_2, $\alpha_2\delta_2$, comprises about 2% of adult hemoglobin, and hemoglobin F, $\alpha_2\gamma_2$, is predominant in fetal life and is only 1–2% in normal adults.

2. *Reactivation of hemoglobin F*

The time sequence of hemoglobins present in fetal and adult life is shown in figure 9.1. This evidence of hemoglobin "switching" reflects a changing pattern of erythroid progenitors, each expressing different programs of gene expression in the differentiated erythroid cells to which they give rise. The substantial disappearance of hemoglobin F in the first 6 months of neonatal life reflects the cessation of γ chain synthesis. Reactivation of hemoglobin F synthesis often occurs in normal pregnancy and in severe disorders of erythropoiesis, including hemolytic anemias such as thalassemia and sickle cell anemia and leukemia. This occurs in a restricted subset of red cells (F cells), which increase in number in anemia. They produce an amount of hemoglobin F that rarely exceeds 20% of the total. In contrast, all of the red cells in a fetus produce hemoglobin F, so that the amount of hemoglobin F is a substantial percentage of the total.

3. *Organization of globin genes*

The α chain genes are on a different chromosome from the non-α chain genes (figure 11.3). Ordinarily, the α chain gene is duplicated—that is, there are two α genes per haploid set of chromosomes. Recent work employing restriction endonuclease techniques of gene mapping and gene cloning has revealed many details of globin gene arrangements in DNA.

The **α genes** are on chromosome 16:

	5′	α_2		α_1	3′
nucleotide distance		|	3700	|	

The **β genes** (and the γ and δ genes which are linked to the β genes) are on the short arm of chromosome 11:

	$^G\gamma$		$^A\gamma$		δ		β
nucleotide distances	|	3500	|	14,000	|	5500	|

The difference between $^G\gamma$ and $^A\gamma$ is explained in lecture 9.

In sum, there are per diploid cell

α genes	4
β genes	2
δ genes	2
γ genes	4

The extensive homology of duplicated α and γ genes can lead to a high potential rate of deletion due to unequal crossing over. The $\delta\beta$ area is at lower risk because homology is less and intergenic distance greater. Like other eukaryotic genes, globin genes are discontinuous or split—that is,

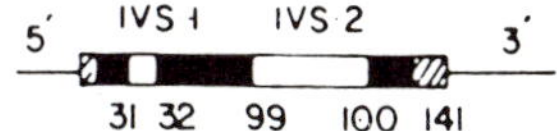

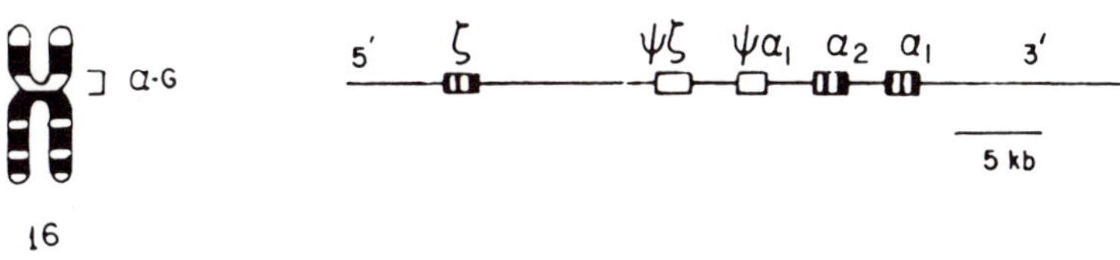

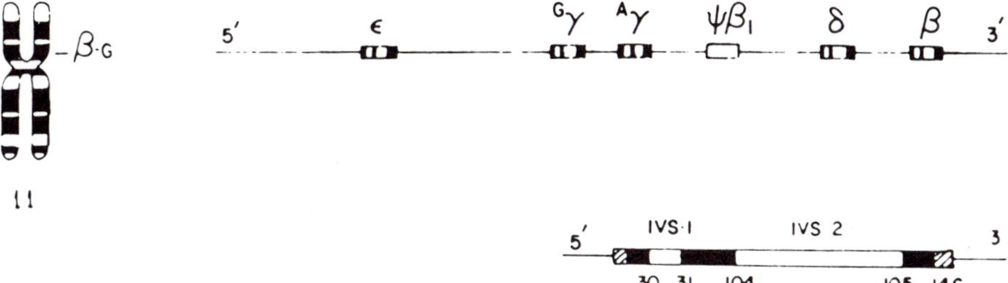

Fig. 11.3
The chromosomal localization and genomic organization of the human globin genes. To the left, the α- and β-globin gene complexes are positioned on chromosomes 16 and 11, respectively. In the center, the arrangement of genes in the two complexes is depicted. The general structures of the genes are shown at the top and bottom with the location of the IVS shown by the codon numbers below the schematics. Coding regions are shown by closed boxes and IVS by open boxes.

coding sequences (exons) are interrupted by sequences of DNA that do not encode globin chains (introns or intervening sequences). The intervening sequences, larger in δ, γ, and β genes than in α genes, are transcribed into a primary transcript RNA or pre-mRNA in erythroid cell nuclei. Then in a maturation process these sequences are removed in precise splicing reactions to yield mature mRNA.

The molecular basis of thalassemia is discussed below.

II. CLINICAL ASPECTS

As noted the thalassemias are named for the affected chain(s). Due to hemoglobin switching, β-thalassemias are usually not clinically apparent until the age of about 6 months.

A. Classification

Figure 11.4 shows a simple, broad classification.

α-thalassemias
α+-thalassemia:
some α chains present,
benign to moderate
α0-thalassemia:
α chains absent,
lethal, homozygous

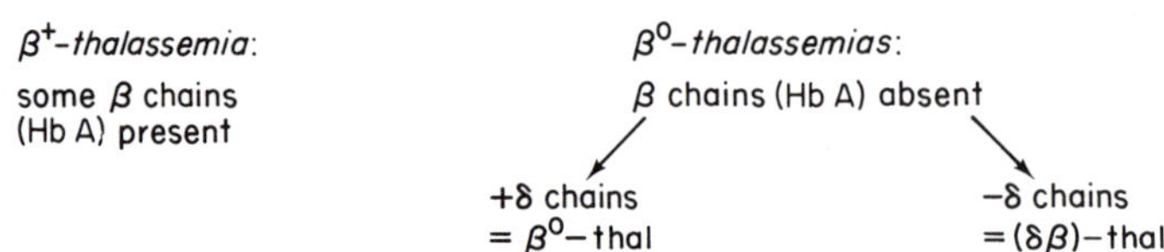

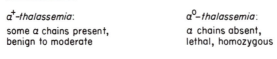

Fig. 11.4
Classification of the thalassemias.

Table 11.1
The α-Thalassemias

Diagnosis	Common name	α globin output (%)	Number of functional α genes	Gene configuration
Normal	Normal	100	4	αα/αα
1 α-thal	Silent carrier	75	2	-α/αα
2 α-thal	Trait	50	2	-α/-α or --/αα
3 α-thal	Hb H disease	25	1	--/-α
4 α-thal	Hydrops fetalis	0	0	--/--

B. The α-thalassemias

1. *Clinical states*

The α-thalassemias have been studied extensively in Asian populations. Four principal clinical states are encountered that differ in clinical severity. Each is associated with a different number of deletions of functional α genes. These are summarized in table 11.1. Clinical and genetic features of these syndromes are given in table 11.2. Note that hemoglobin H is β_4. Hemoglobin Bart's is γ_4.

2. *Patterns of inheritance*

The following matings produce the indicated progeny:

silent carrier × normal → normal (50%) and silent carrier (50%);

silent carrier × trait → trait (25%), normal (25%), Hb H (25%), silent carrier (25%);

trait × trait → hydrops fetalis (25%), normal (25%), trait (50%).

Table 11.2
Clinical Aspects of α-Thalassemias

Condition	Parental genotypes	Risk	Hemoglobin pattern	Severity	α mRNA	Genes
Silent carrier (1 α-thal)	Silent carrier, normal	$\frac{1}{2}$	Approximately 1–2% Hb Bart's in cord blood	0	Presumed slight deficiency	1 of 4 α genes deleted
Heterozygous α-thalassemia (α-thal trait) (2 α-thal)	α-thalassemia trait, normal	$\frac{1}{2}$	Approximately 5% Hb Bart's in cord blood	Mild; very mild in blacks	Presumed deficiency	2 of 4 α genes deleted; ? 1 of 3 deleted in blacks
Hb H disease (3 α-thal)	(i) α-thalassemia trait, silent carrier (ii) α-thalassemia trait, Hb CS heterozygote	$\frac{1}{4}$ $\frac{1}{4}$	4–30% Hb H in adults: approximately 25% Hb Bart's in cord blood; when Hb CS gene present, 2–3% Hb CS	Variable, usually thalassemia intermedia	Marked deficiency	(i) 3 of 4 α genes deleted (ii) 2 of 4 deleted; 1 normal; 1 Hb CS gene
Homozygous α-thalassemia (hydrops fetalis with Hb Bart's) (4 α-thal)	Both α-thalassemia trait	$\frac{1}{4}$	80% Hb Bart's; remainder, Hb H and Hb Portland*	Lethal	Absent	All α genes deleted
Heterozygous Hb Constant Spring (CS)	Hb CS heterozygote, normal	$\frac{1}{2}$	Approximately 1% Hb CS	0	Presumed deficiency	3 of 4 α genes present; 1 Hb CS gene

* Hb Portland ($\zeta_2\gamma_2$) is derived from the product of the embryonic α-like gene called zeta (ζ) and the product of the gamma genes.

3. Distribution of α genes

Deletion of α genes, often a result of unequal crossing over between two chromosomes, can cause different gene distributions and different risks. For example, blacks with so-called 2 α-thal (see above) usually have a single α gene deleted on each chromosome 16 rather than deletions of both α genes on a single chromosome 16. Therefore blacks with the phenotype 2 α-thal have two deletions in *trans* (i.e., on different chromosomes) rather than two deletions in *cis* (i.e., on the same chromosome). This explains the absence in blacks of homozygous α-thalassemia with hydrops fetalis due to total α gene deletion. The frequency in blacks of chromosomes with two α genes deleted is so low and of chromosomes with single α genes so high that homozygosity for no α genes is very rare. In contrast, it is common among the Chinese. In some individuals unequal crossing over can lead to three α genes on one chromosome. This leads to genetic interchange among three types of chromosomes. Duplication of α genes and their flanking regions increases the likelihood of genetic recombination and heterogeneity.

C. The β-thalassemias

The β-thalassemias are characterized by deficient synthesis of β chains and persistent synthesis of γ chains. This results in variable elevations of Hb F. However, γ chain production is usually inadequate to compensate fully for the β chain deficiency. The combination of hemoglobins present in the blood reflects the genotype. It also reflects the selection of the hardiest cells (i.e., usually those with Hb F). Nevertheless, a rough categorization of "homozygous" β-thalassemias may be based on hemoglobin patterns, as following:

	β^+-thal	β^0-thal	δβ-thal	Normal
Hb A	Present (↓)	Absent	Absent	Normal
Hb A_2	Increased	Increased	Absent	Normal
Hb F	Increased (but < 100%)	Increased (nearly 100%)	Increased (100%)	Low

Patients with "homozygous" β- or β^0-thalassemia usually have lower **total** hemoglobin levels than those with "homozygous" δβ-thalassemia.

1. Clinical states

As noted, β-thalassemia can be divided into two general types, β^+-thal and β^0-thal. As shown in table 11.3, the clinically severe thalassemias may not in fact be homozygous. In addition, there is considerable mechanistic heterogeneity at the molecular level. This may also lead to clinical heterogeneity. Clinical features of the β-thalassemias are summarized in table 11.4.

Table 11.3
Characteristics of the "Homozygous" β-Thalassemias

	Hemoglobin patterns			
Genotype	Hb A ($\alpha_2\beta_2$)	Hb A_2 ($\alpha_2\delta_2$)	Hb F ($\alpha_2\gamma_2$)	Clinical severity
β^+/β^+	Variable	Variable	↑	Depends upon severity of β gene impairment and extent of γ gene compensation
β^+/β^0	Usually low	Variable	↑	Usually more severe than β^+/β^+
β^0/β^0	Absent	Variable	↑	Very severe unless γ gene compensation is unusually high
$\beta\delta/\beta^+$	Low	Low	↑↑	Relatively mild due to increased γ chain production
$\beta\delta/\beta^0$	Absent	Low	↑↑	Somewhat more severe than $\beta\delta/\beta^+$ due to absent β chain production
$\beta\delta/\beta\delta$	Absent	Low	↑↑↑	Mild due to increased γ chain production

Note: The term **homozygous** is misleading when applied to patients who have inherited two different kinds of thalassemia genes.

D. Therapy

Definitive treatment is not yet available. Therapy is entirely supportive. Carrier states do not require treatment. The following remarks concern management of the β-thalassemias.

1. Transfusion

When untreated, patients with homozygous β-thalassemia may die by the age of 2 or 3 years with hematocrits as low as 5–6%. Blood transfusions prevent this outcome. Patients maintained by frequent transfusions from an early age avoid many complications. If hemoglobin levels are kept between 10 and 12 g/dl by repeated transfusions, marrow hyperplasia is repressed. Bones do not become demineralized and weakened, and facial changes do not develop. There is less cardiomegaly and hepatosplenomegaly, better growth and development, and better quality of life. Frequent transfusions, however, inevitably lead to iron overload and its serious complications, including intractable congestive heart failure. Transfusion with young red cells ("neocytes") increases the interval between transfusions. These patients, incidentally, have increased folic acid requirements and require regular supplements.

2. Splenectomy

Splenectomy is often needed to reduce blood volume and red cell pooling. Splenomegaly often causes a gradual increase in the transfusion requirement. Splenectomy reverses this trend. If possible, splenectomy should be

Table 11.4
Clinical Aspects of β-Thalassemias

Condition	Parental genotypes	Risk	Hemoglobin pattern	Severity	β mRNA	Genes
Homozygous states						
β^+-thalassemia	Both β^+/β	$\frac{1}{4}$	↓ Hb A, ↑ Hb F, variable Hb A_2	Variable; usually Cooley's anemia	Marked deficiency of β mRNA	β genes present
β^0-thalassemia	Both β^0/β	$\frac{1}{4}$	0 Hb A, variable Hb A_2, residual Hb F	Cooley's anemia	(i) absent β mRNA (ii) mutant, nonfunctional β mRNA present in rare Oriental cases	β genes present
$\delta\beta^0$-thalassemia	Both $\delta\beta^0/\delta\beta$	$\frac{1}{4}$	0 Hb A, Hb A_2; 100% Hb F	Thalassemia intermedia	δ and β mRNAs absent	β genes deleted; probable δ gene deletion
Hb Lepore	Both Hb Lepore/β	$\frac{1}{4}$	0 Hb A, Hb A_2; 75% Hb F, 25% Hb Lepore	Cooley's anemia	β-like mRNA present in reduced amount	β-δ fusion genes present; no normal β and δ genes
Heterozygous states						
β^+-thalassemia	β^+/β, normal	$\frac{1}{2}$	↑ Hb A_2, slight ↑ Hb F	Thalassemia minor	Deficient β mRNA	β genes present
β^0-thalassemia	β^0/β, normal	$\frac{1}{2}$	↑Hb A_2, slight ↑ Hb F	Thalassemia minor	Deficient β mRNA, or rarely nonfunctional β mRNA present	β genes present
$\delta\beta^0$-thalassemia	$\delta\beta^0/\delta\beta$, normal	$\frac{1}{2}$	5–20% Hb F	Thalassemia minor	Presumed deficiency of β and δ mRNAs	β and probable δ gene deletion on 1 homologous chromosome
Hb Lepore	Hb Lepore/β, normal	$\frac{1}{2}$	↑ Hb F, ↓ Hb A_2, 5–15% Hb Lepore	Thalassemia minor	β-like mRNA present	Hb Lepore gene replaces normal β and δ genes on 1 chromosome

deferred until age 5–6 years, after which there is a lessened risk of overwhelming infection (usually pneumococcal septicemia).

3. Iron-chelating agents

As discussed in lecture 7, the iron-chelating agent desferrioxamine is used successfully in the treatment of acute iron poisoning. However, until recently the effectiveness of such therapy in removing iron accumulations from heart, liver, and endocrine organs has been disappointing. The drug must be given parenterally. Recent work shows that continuous subcutaneous infusion (under the control of a portable infusion pump) for 12 hr each day leads to significant negative iron balance. It is not yet known whether chronic desferrioxamine therapy will prolong survival in patients on frequent transfusion regimens.

4. Modulating Hb F synthesis

A variety of drugs, including 5-azacytidine, cytosine arabinoside, and hyroxyurea, have been given in an attempt to increase Hb F synthesis. Only 5-azacytidine has given encouraging results. This drug inhibits the postsynthetic methylation of DNA and may in this way increase expression of the γ-globin gene. Repeated courses are needed and in time the drug may suppress erythropoiesis. It also may be leukemogenic.

E. Prevention

The severity of the thalassemias has prompted serious efforts at prevention. Current methods involve genetic counseling and prenatal diagnosis.

1. Genetic counseling

In principle, genetic counseling of patients with various heterozygous β-thalassemia syndromes should reduce the number of pregnancies for which homozygous β-thalassemia is a risk. Once the type of thalassemia is established, advice concerning the probability of its occurrence among offspring can usually be offered. In practice, it has not yet been established that extensive population surveys and genetic counseling can actually achieve this goal.

2. Prenatal diagnosis

Prenatal diagnosis of the α-thalassemias is of little importance since infants with Hb Bart's and hydrops fetalis usually die in utero and Hb H is compatible with a normal life expectancy. However, a method for the prenatal diagnosis of β-thalassemia would be of great value. Two approaches have been used.

a. PHENOTYPIC METHOD

In the first trimester of normal fetal development, β chain synthesis is at a low level. The actual level can be accurately quantified by appropriate biosynthetic studies on fetal blood cells. Thus, even if the β chain gene is only minimally expressed in fetal development, it is possible to diagnose qualitative and quantitative abnormalities of β chain synthesis in the first 18–20 weeks. By various techniques (e.g., chorionic villous sampling, placental aspiration , or fetoscopy, which permits needle aspiration under direct visualization of blood vessels on the placental surface), it is usually possible without harming the fetus to obtain relatively pure samples of fetal blood, which can then be subjected to isotopic analysis of the rates of α, γ, and β chain synthesis. This procedure is capable of diagnosing all forms of thalassemia and hemoglobinopathy. Risk to the fetus is about 5%.

b. GENETIC METHOD

This procedure analyzes the DNA of amniotic cells or chorionic villi for primary defects or associated polymorphisms. The techniques involve (1) direct restriction enzyme analysis of deletions or single mutations that produce restriction enzyme pattern shifts, or (2) application of oligonucleotide hybridization to detect single base alterations. This technique permits diagnosis of all deletion syndromes, all cases of sickle cell anemia, and most cases of thalassemia. The risk relates to the need to obtain sufficient numbers of amniotic or chorionic cells.

III. MECHANISMS IN THALASSEMIA

A. Genetic defects

The central problem is, Why in thalassemia are specific hemoglobin chains not synthesized effectively? It will be recalled that normal synthesis of a protein involves (1) the presence of a normal structural gene in the DNA; (2) transcription of the DNA into a primary RNA product; (3) processing of the initial RNA product to a mature mRNA; (4) transport of mature globin mRNA to cytoplasm, where it associates with ribosomes; (5) translation of mRNA on ribosomes into the amino acid sequence of protein; and (6) structural changes that enhance the stability of the protein products. The first three steps occur in the nucleus of developing erythroid cells.

B. Specific defects

Defects have been demonstrated in the thalassemias at almost every level of this process. Genetically, all lesions act in *cis* as regards their linkage to the globin gene. Defects can always be ultimately traced to the mRNA

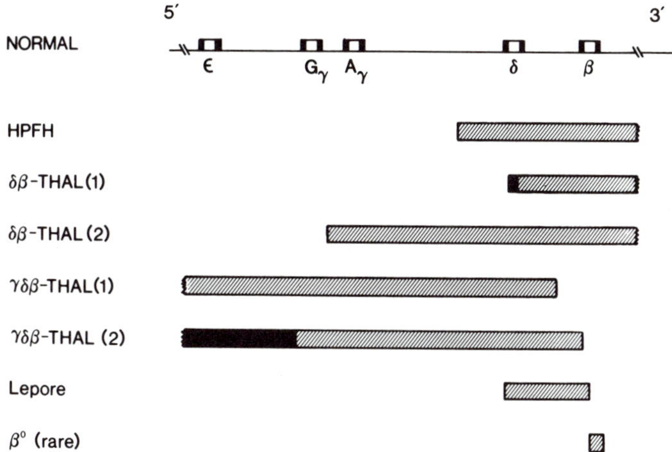

Fig. 11.5
Gene map of the various forms of hereditary persistence of fetal hemoglobin. Bars denote deleted portions. Black areas denote uncertainty.

for a specific globin chain that is quantitatively or qualitatively abnormal. The following are examples of specific defects.

1. *Deletion of globin structural genes*

An **entire gene** may be missing. This is the case in most α-thalassemia mutations. The β gene may be deleted in rare types of δβ thalassemia and HPFH (see below). There may also be deletions of both β and δ genes (figure 11.5).

2. *Partial gene deletion*

Partial gene deletions account for rare types of β^0-thal and α-thal. Varying degrees of deletion appear to be associated with different clinical syndromes in which Hb F expression is markedly increased. This leads to the syndrome termed **hereditary persistence of fetal hemoglobin**, or HPFH (figure 11.5).

3. *Fused globin chains*

Nonhomologous crossing over may lead to fused or "hybrid" hemoglobin chains in which a non-α chain contains amino acid sequences corresponding in two different non-α chains. In the Lepore hemoglobins (figure 11.6), a portion of the δ chain and a portion of the β chain have been lost in the process of crossing over. The resulting non-α chain has the character of a δ chain at its N-terminal end and of a β chain at its C-terminal end. The point of fusion is variable. At least three different Lepore hemoglobins are known that differ in the locus of this point. Hemoglobin Lepores have an electrophoretic mobility similar to that of hemoglobin S. Hemoglobin Kenya contains a fused γβ chain.

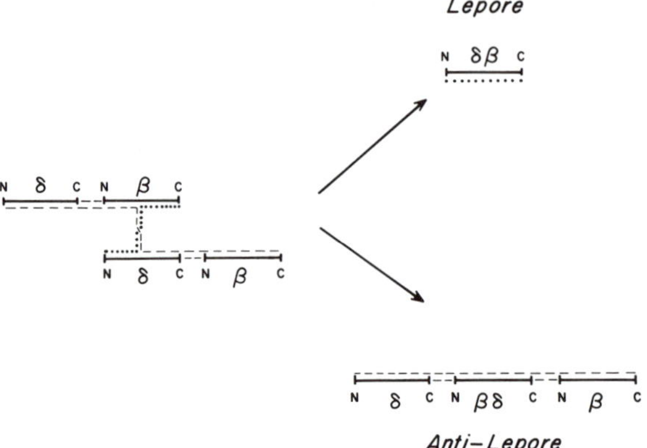

Fig. 11.6
Diagram of nonhomologous crossing-over between δ and β globin genes with resulting formation of Lepore and anti-Lepore globin genes. (From D. G. Nathan and F. A. Oski, eds., *Hematology of Infancy and Childhood*. Philadelphia: Saunders, 1974.)

4. Production of nonfunctional mRNA

Point mutations within the β gene may lead to production of defective mRNAs. The mRNA is present, but it cannot be translated into globin. This is the case in about 50% of β^0-thalassemias in which there is a nonsense point mutation that halts translation of β globin early in its synthesis.

5. Abnormal gene transcription

Other point mutations occur that affect the processing of globin pre-mRNA. Aberrant processing with the resulting unstable mRNA product probably explains the majority of β^+-thalassemias and perhaps some α-thalassemias. An example of a common processing defect is shown in figure 11.7.

6. Production of elongated chain

Globin chains (when present) are usually structurally normal in the thalassemias. An exception occurs in five known α chain variants characterized by the presence of additional amino acid residues at the C-terminal end of the α chain. The prototype example is hemoglobin Constant Spring, in which the α chain is elongated due to a mutation in the codon that normally terminates translation. For unknown reasons, the abnormal α chain is synthesized at a low rate. Therefore, the clinical picture (phenotype) mimics α-thalassemia (see table 11.1).

7. Production of unstable globin

In the rare case in which a mutaton leads to the production of an unusually unstable hemoglobin, degradation may occur almost immediately after synthesis. This leads to the clinical picture of thalassemia. Hb Indianapolis,

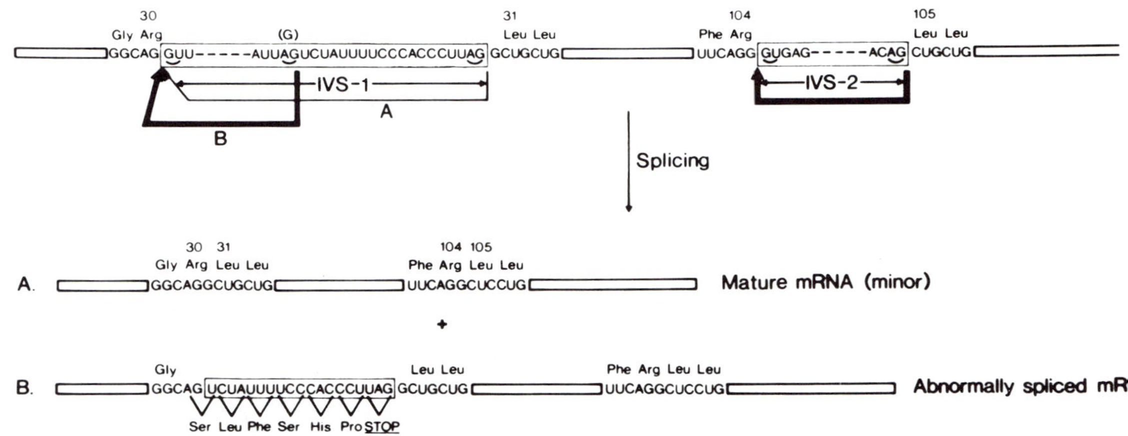

Fig. 11.7
Abnormal processing of β-mRNA precursor in one type of β-thalassemia. A section of transcribed mRNA precursor in the most common type of β^+-thalassemia is shown above. Note that the first intron contains a substitution of an A for G that creates a new 3′ splice acceptor (AG) that resembles the normal splice acceptor just 5′ to the codon for amino acid 31. This new 3′ splice acceptor combines with the splice donor GU (just 3′ to the codon for amino acid 30) at a rate 10 faster than the normal splice acceptor (indicated by the heavy arrow). Therefore two mature mRNAs are formed. One, a minor component, is normal. The other, 90% of the total, retains a segment of intron 1 that contains a stop codon. It cannot produce globin chains. Hence severe thalassemia with some hemoglobin A is produced.

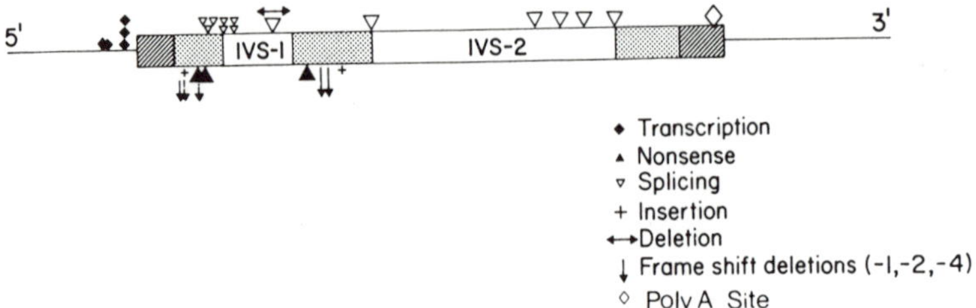

Fig. 11.8
A summary of β-thalassemia point mutations.

a β chain mutant, is an example of such a hemoglobin. The clinical picture resembles β-thalassemia.

8. *Molecular polymorphisms*

Abnormalities of the gene map (as determined by restriction enzyme techniques) are found in certain populations. These consist of DNA sequence differences (polymorphisms) in regions flanking the structural genes. Demonstration of these polymorphic DNA sequences permits detection of abnormal globin genes that are closely linked to them. This approach is currently in clinical use in the prenatal diagnosis of both sickle cell anemia (see lecture 10) and thalassemia.

9. *Summary of point mutations*

As a result of molecular cloning and sequencing studies, over 30 point mutations causing β-thalassemia have been detected. Some affect transcription and clearly demonstrate the importance of 5′ promoter sequences. Other cause nonsense mutations or splicing defects. A summary of some defects and their locations is set out in figure 11.8.

C. Future possibilities

Recombinant DNA technology now permits isolation of abnormal genes and the characterization of their structure and function. Thalassemia research is currently at the forefront of molecular biology, and it is reasonable to expect in the near future

- Elucidation of specific defects in various thalassemias including those affecting gene transcription or RNA processing.
- In vitro gene replacement in bone marrow cells.
- Improved understanding of gene function and application of this knowledge to other human disorders.
- Possible reversal by molecular or cellular approaches of the fetal hemoglobin switching mechanism. This would ameliorate the severity of all forms of β-thalassemia.

SELECTED REFERENCES

Reviews

Boyer, S. H. The emerging complexity of genetic control of persistent fetal hemoglobin biosynthesis in adults. *Ann. NY Acad. Sci.* 565(1989): 23–36.

Cohen, A. Current status of iron chelation therapy with deferoxamine. *Semin. Hematol.* 27(1990): 86–90.

Higgs, D. R., Vickers, M. A., et al. A review of the molecular genetics of the human α-globin gene cluster. *Blood* 73(1989): 1081–1104.

Kazazian, H. H., Jr., and Boehm, C. D. Molecular basis and prenatal diagnosis of β-thalassemia. *Blood* 72(1988): 1107–1116.

Shinar, E., and Rachmilewitz, E. A. Oxidative denaturation of red blood cells in thalassemia. *Semin. Hematol.* 27(1990): 70–82.

Talacki, C. A., Larner, J., et al. The effect of alpha thalassemia on the clinical course of hemoglobin SC disease. *Ann. NY Acad. Sci.* 565(1989): 365–366.

Weatherall, D. J. The thalassemias. In Williams, W. J., et al., eds. *Hematology*, 4th ed. New York: McGraw-Hill, 1990, pp. 510–539.

Original articles

Cai, S.-P., Chang, C. A., et al. Rapid prenatal diagnosis of β thalassemia using DNA amplification and nonradioactive probes. *Blood* 73(1989): 372–374.

Cai, S.-P., and Kan, Y. W. Identification of the multiple β-thalassemia mutations by denaturing gradient gel electrophoresis. *J. Clin. Invest.* 85(1990): 550–553.

Feingold, E. A., and Forget, B. G. The breakpoint of a large deletion causing hereditary persistence of fetal hemoglobin occurs within an erythroid DNA domain remote from the β-globin gene cluster. *Blood* 74(1989): 2178–2186.

Gonzalez-Redondo, J. M., Stoming, T. A., et al. Severe Hb S-β^0-thalassaemia with a T → C substitution in the donor splice site of the first intron of the β-globin gene. *Br. J. Haematol.* 71(1989): 113–117.

Green, R., and King, R. A new red cell discriminant incorporating volume dispersion for differentiating iron deficiency anemia from thalassemia minor. *Blood Cells* 15(1989): 481–495.

Hershko, C., Link, G., et al. Principles of iron chelating therapy. *Semin. Hematol.* 27(1990): 91–94.

Houwen, B. The clinical utility of discriminant functions for the differential diagnosis of microcytic anemias. *Blood Cells* 15(1989): 583–584.

Jankovic, L., Efremov, G. D., et al. Two novel polyadenylation mutations leading to β^+-thalassaemia. *Br. J. Haematol.* 75(1990): 122–126.

Lindeman, R., Volpato, F., et al. Detection and characterization of the Hb Lepore (Boston) defect by the polymerase chain reaction. *Br. J. Hzematol.* 73(1989): 566–568.

Lucarelli, G., Galimberti, M., et al. Bone marrow transplantation in patients with thalassemia. *N. Engl. J. Med.* 322(1990): 417–421.

Martin, D. I. K., Tsai, S.-F., et al. Increased gamma-globin expression in a non-deletion HPFH mediated by an erythroid-specific DNA-binding factor. *Nature* 338(1989): 435–438.

McDonagh, K. T., Dover, G. J., et al. Manipulation of HbF production with hematopoietic growth factors. *Progr. Clin. Biol. Res.* 316B(1990): 307–315.

Rouyer-Fessard, P., Garel, M.-C., et al. A study of membrane protein defects and α hemoglobin chains of red blood cells in human β thalassemia. *J. Biol. Chem.* 264(1989): 19092–19098.

Schrier, S. L., Rachmilewitz, E., et al. Cellular and membrane properties of alpha and beta thalassemic erythrocytes are different: implication for differences in clinical manifestations. *Blood* 74(1989): 2194–2202.

Shinar, E., Rachmilewitz, E. A., et al. Differing erythrocyte membrane skeletal protein defects in alpha and beta thalassemia. *J. Clin. Invest.* 83(1989): 404–410.

Thein, S. L., Hesketh, C., et al. Molecular characterization of a high A_2 β thalassemia by direct sequencing of single strand enriched amplified genomic DNA. *Blood* 73(1989): 924–930.

Thein, S. L., and Weatherall, D. J. A non-deletion hereditary persistance of fetal hemoglobin (HPFH) determinant not linked to the β-globin gene complex. *Progr. Clin. Biol. Res.* 316B(1990): 97–111.

Van der Weyden, M. B., Fong, H., et al. Red cell ferritin and iron overload in heterozygous beta-thalassemia. *Am. J. Hematol.* 30(1989): 201–205.

Zurlo, M. G., De Stefano, P., et al. Survival and causes of death in thalassaemia major. *Lancet* 2(1989): 27–30.

LECTURE 12

Hemolytic Anemias I. Introduction

W. Hallowell Churchill, Jr., and James H. Jandl

EDITOR'S COMMENT

Hemolysis is the premature destruction of red cells. This and the next three lectures show that it can occur because of an extracorpuscular defect, such as an anti-red cell antibody, or because of some defect in the membrane or metabolism of the red cell itself. The list of circumstances in which hemolysis, mild or severe, can occur is very long and physicians must remain alert to its possible presence. In many cases, it is a significant clue to some underlying condition. This lecture discusses hemolysis in general terms, summarizing the clinical signs that should arouse suspicion of hemolysis. Significantly, when hemolysis becomes chronic, supervening events such as folate deficiency secondary to marrow hyperplasia can blunt such signs as elevation of the reticulocyte count.

I. RED CELL LIFE SPAN AND SURVIVAL

A. Determining factors

Red cells have a life span of about 120 days. As the cells age, glycolysis slows, enzyme activity diminishes, and the content of ATP, potassium, and membrane lipids declines. How these and other age-dependent changes lead to removal of senescent red cells from the circulation is uncertain. The **life span** of the red cells—their potential longevity—must be distinguished from their actual **survival**, which encompasses all factors, including premature aging, that may cause their untimely destruction.

B. Measurement

Measurement of red cell survival requires use of a label. Labeled cells may be of **mixed ages** or they may constitute a **cohort**—a group of cells of identical age.

1. Mixed-age labeling

a. DIFFERENTIAL AGGLUTINATION (ASHBY TECHNIQUE)

The normal red cell life span was first determined by the Ashby technique, which now is used only in a research setting. The technique utilizes antigenic differences between the red cells of a donor and the cells of the recipient. Usually type O donor red cells lacking the M antigen are given to a recipient whose cells possess the antigen. Thereafter, the recipient's blood is sampled periodically, and antibodies that agglutinate type M cells are added. Survival of donor cells is calculated from the declining number of inagglutinable cells.

The technique has two disadvantages: (1) it does not measure survival of an individual's own red cells; and (2) transfusion of another individual's cells incurs risk of sensitization to minor blood group antigens and premature destruction of donor cells.

b. DIISOPROPYL FLUOROPHOSPHATE (DFP) METHOD

An alternative technique employs diisopropyl fluorophosphate (DFP) labeled with ^3H. DFP binds covalently to a serine residue in the cholinesterase of cell membranes. This permits study of the life span of autologous cells. A disadvantage is the loss during the first several days of cells injured by the labeling process. Consequently this technique is not useful in patients with brisk hemolysis.

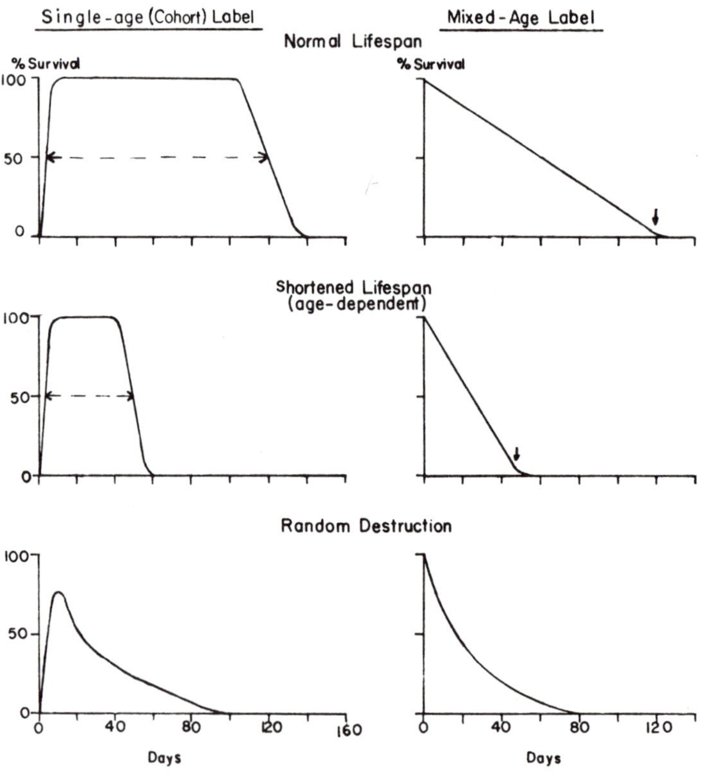

Fig. 12.1
Patterns of red cell survival and life span as revealed by cohort and mixed-age labeling of red cell population. *Left*, A single-age cohort of red cells was labeled with the biosynthetic precursor, [2-^{14}C]glycine. *Right*, A population of cells, evenly distributed as to age, was labeled with [^{3}H]DFP.

c. PATHOPHYSIOLOGY

Normally both the Ashby and DFP techniques measure the fate of red cells that are evenly distributed as to age from 1 to 120 days. Thus labeled cells diminish at a rate of approximately 1/120 of the infused cells daily (figure 12.1, top right). In **premature destruction**, the red cell survival curve has a similar straight-line pattern, but the descent is steeper (figure 12.1, middle right).

In most hemolytic anemias, the labeled red cells are destroyed by a process that is indifferent to cell age. In **random destruction**, a constant fraction of labeled cells is destroyed daily. The rate of this destruction is governed by chance exposure to injury, as by passage through a particular vascualr region. When hemolysis is severe, the red cell survival curve usually conforms to a first-order pattern, for the cells do not survive to die a "natural death" (figure 12.1, bottom right). In such patients, most red cells are only a few days old, and those surviving 50–60 days may be too few to measure.

As the Ashby and DFP methods are unsatisfactory for measuring red cell destruction in hemolytic anemias, where a measurement is most needed, other techniques are employed. The most widely used label is radioactive chromium (^{51}Cr).

2. *Cohort labeling*

a. METHODS

In cohort labeling, a red cell population similar in age is labeled biosynthetically by injecting a radioactive precursor that is incorporated by immature erythroid cells of the bone marrow. Cells so labeled enter the circulation for up to 6 or 7 days, even as some are being destroyed. Some label appears in circulating reticulocytes shortly after injection.

Cohort labeling is unsuitable for studying rapid hemolytic processes and is used primarily in determining red cell life span. During hemoglobin catabolism, the amino acids released are not reutilized; thus [2-^{14}C]glycine provides a good cohort label. On the other hand, ^{59}Fe is not suitable because it is extensively retuilized after lysis of labeled cells (see lecture 7).

b. PATHOPHYSIOLOGY

Normally, the percentage of cohort-labeled red cells in the circulation remains constant for about 100 days (figure 12.1, top left). By 120 days radioactivity has declined 50%, and within 140 days it is inappreciable. When red cell life span is shortened, the survival curve has a similar but abbreviated plateau pattern. Cohort labeling is most useful in mild or moderate hemolytic processes. However, the more severe hemolytic anemias associated with random red cell destruction are not accurately characterized by cohort labeling (figure 12.1, bottom left).

3. Measurement of survival in hemolytic anemia: ^{51}Cr method

a. METHODS

The only practicable method for studying red cell survival in hemolytic anemias involves labeling a sample of the patient's red cells with ^{51}Cr in its stable form as a chromate anion ($^{51}CrO_4^{2-}$). Chromate rapidly permeates red cells, wherein it is trapped by reduction to the nearly impermeant $^{51}Cr^{3+}$ ion. In small amounts, chromate is harmless to red cells. After reinfusion of ^{51}Cr-labeled red cells, total red cell mass can be determined, for red cells remain confined to the vascular compartment. By periodically assaying blood samples for radioactivity, one can ascertain the red cell survival pattern. However, correction must be made for the fact that about 1% of intracellular ^{51}Cr is eluted daily and excreted in the urine.

The ^{51}Cr method also permits determinations of (1) the **site** at which red cells are destroyed (figure 12.2); (2) **vascular pooling** of red cells within organs; (3) **kinetics of mixing** of ^{51}Cr-labeled red cells in the spleen; and (4) extent of **gastrointestinal blood loss**. Neither Cr^{3+} nor CrO_4^{2-} is excreted via the normal GI tract.

b. PATTERNS

^{51}Cr elution has a marked effect on the shape of the survival curve of normal red cells, transforming it from a rectilinear to a curvilinear pattern. The Ashby and DFP techniques yield a normal half-survival of about 60 days. The half-survival time for ^{51}Cr-labeled normal red cells, however, is about 30 days owing to ^{51}Cr elution. The error introduced by ^{51}Cr elution is minimal in severe hemolytic anemias, in which red cell survival studies are most needed. Figure 12.2 depicts the effects of elution and tissue excretion of ^{51}Cr upon measurements of red cell survival and of splenic sequestration.

II. HEMOLYSIS

A. Types

As a clinical term, **hemolysis** means premature red cell destruction, whether due to reduction in red cell life span or to random cell destruction.

1. Extravascular and intravascular sites

In most cases, hemolysis involves the trapping of red cells in spleen or liver sinuses; the cells are then lysed and most of the hemoglobin is catabolized within the sequestering organ. This process is termed **extravascular hemoly-**

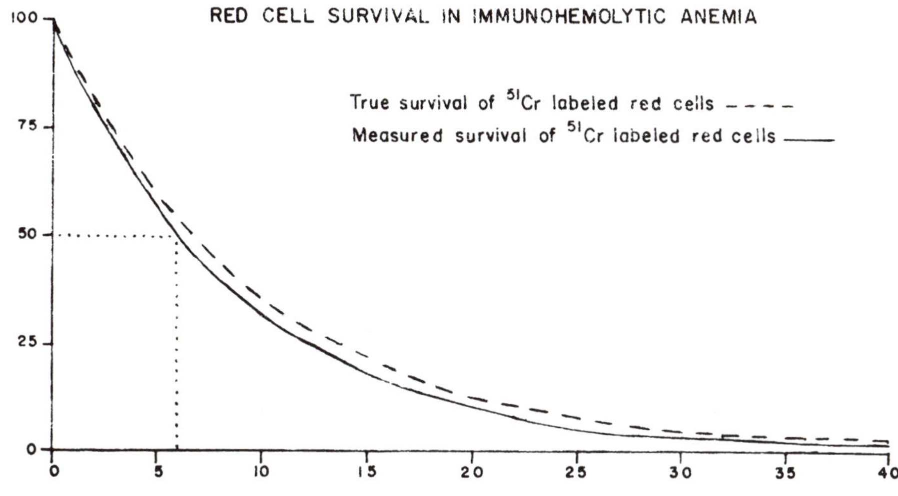

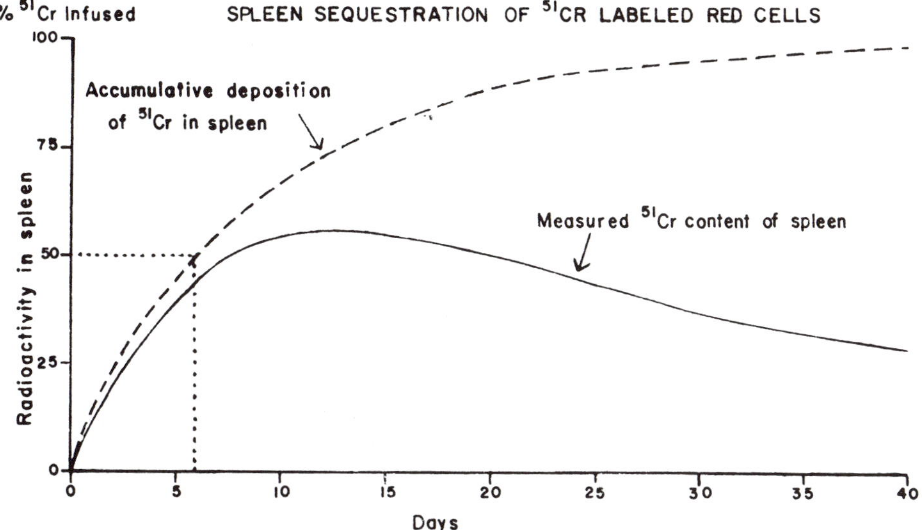

Fig. 12.2
Use of ^{51}Cr method in a patient with immunohemolytic anemia associated with random destruction of 10% of the red cells daily. *Top*, Red cell survival studies show that the "true" half-survival time is 6.9 days and the measured half-survival time, diminished by ^{51}Cr elution, is 6.0 days, a difference having no practical significance. *Bottom*, Spleen sequestration studies show the effect of tissue excretion of ^{51}Cr on the measured ^{51}Cr deposition in the spleen. The accumulated radioactivity would be as shown by the dashed line if all ^{51}Cr deposited in the spleen remained there. Spleen excretes 2.5–3% of its ^{51}Cr daily, and accumulation is diminished accordingly (*solid line*). Half of injected ^{51}Cr was deposited in the spleen by day 6 (*dashed line*), but half of the radioactivity was not measurable in the spleen until day 7.5. ^{51}Cr localization is best determined during period in which about 3/4 of labeled cells are hemolyzed.

sis. Less often, red cells are destroyed within the systemic circulation, and hemoglobin is released into plasma and catabolized only when it is taken up by the liver or lost through the kidneys. This is termed **intravascular hemolysis**.

2. *Extracorpuscular and intracorpuscular defects*

Hemolytic anemias can also be classified according to whether the initiating event is extrinsic (an **extracorpuscular defect**) or intrinsic (an **intracorpuscular defect**) to the red cell.

3. *Hereditary and acquired disorders*

A third basis for cataloging hemolytic disorders differentiates those that are **hereditary** from those that are **acquired**.

B. Clinical features

Hemolytic disorders are marked by signs of increased hemoglobin catabolism combined with signs of increased erythropoiesis.

1. *Accelerated hemoglobin catabolism*

The principal indicators of accelerated catabolism of hemoglobin are:

- Jaundice
- Hemoglobinemia and decreased plasma haptoglobin
- Hemoglobinuria and hemosiderinuria
- Methemalbuminemia

a. JAUNDICE

In extravascular hemolysis, macrophages (RES cells) convert most of the hemoglobin from destroyed red cells to bilirubin. As described in lecture 8, this process liberates 1 mole each of iron, carbon monoxide, and bilirubin per mole of heme catabolized. The indirect-reacting (or unconjugated) serum bilirubin is elevated. In brisk hemolysis, direct-reacting (or conjugated) serum bilirubin may also rise.

b. HEMOGLOBINEMIA AND DECREASED PLASMA HAPTOGLOBIN

Severe hemolysis of any sort elevates the plasma hemoglobin concentration (normal level, <1 mg/dl). During intravascular hemolysis, the plasma hemoglobin is high enough to be visible. Levels of 10–20 mg/dl give plasma an amber coloration; at 50–100 mg/dl, it is reddish.

Plasma **haptoglobin** is an α_2 globulin that binds free hemoglobin and so prevents leakage of hemoglobin from the vascular compartment and excretion into the urine. Haptoglobin and hemoglobin form a complex that is rapidly cleared by the liver. Thus hemoglobinemia diminishes the level of haptoglobin. Plasma normally possesses sufficient haptoglobin to bind 100–150 mg/dl of hemoglobin. During hemoglobinemia, haptoglobin is depleted and the level of unbound or free hemoglobin increases. Free hemoglobin is oxidized rapidly to methemoglobin, which lends a mahogany red-brown color to the plasma. A significant portion (40–50%) of circulating free hemoglobin (or methemoglobin) is cleared by the kidneys.

c. HEMOGLOBINURIA AND HEMOSIDERINURIA

The rapidity with which hemoglobin, despite its molecular weight of 64,500, is filtered by glomeruli is attributable to its dissociation in dilute solution into half-molecules, pairs of peptide chains, termed **dimers** or **αβ dimers**, having molecular weight of about 32,000 (figure 12.3). Proximal tubule cells reabsorb and catabolize most of the filtered hemoglobin, preventing it from appearing in urine. At normal perfusion pressures, plasma hemoglobin concentrations must exceed 30 mg/dl before hemoglobinuria ensues. The renal threshold of about 150 mg/dl for plasma hemoglobin therefore reflects two conserving mechanisms: (1) binding of hemoglobin by haptoglobin and (2) absorption of hemoglobin by proximal tubule cells.

After filtration by the glomerulus, hemoglobin tetramers and dimers reequilibrate within the renal tubule (figure 12.3). Organic components of hemoglobin are catabolized rapidly in the proximal tubule cells. Although half the globin and porphyrin are degraded in <30 min, iron atoms are handled differently. Iron released from hemoglobin stimulates synthesis of apoferritin, and ferritin iron soon appears within the tubule cells (see lecture 7). The iron of ferritin and hemosiderin leaves the kidney slowly ($T_{1/2}$ > 30–40 days) both by excretion into the urine and by absorption

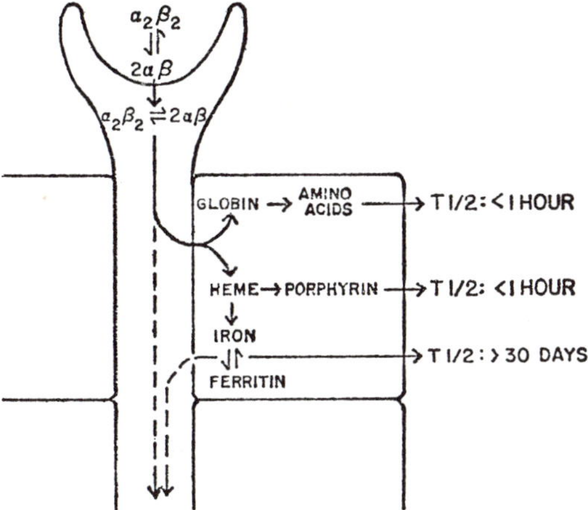

Fig. 12.3
Renal catabolism and excretion of hemoglobin. (From H. F. Bunn and J. H. Jandl, *J. Exp. Med.* 129(1969): 925.)

Table 12.1
Differential Diagnosis of Hemoglobinuria and Myoglobinuria

Observation	Hemoglobinuria	Myoglobinuria
Appearance of plasma	Amber to red-brown	Normal[a]
Bilirubin level	Slightly to moderately elevated	Normal
Effect of 80% saturation with ammonium sulfate	Precipitates hemoglobin	Does not precipitate myoglobin (in fresh specimen containing undenatured myoglobin)
Agarose electrophoresis of plasma at pH 8.6	Free plasma hemoglobin migrates near transferrin in β_1-globulin region; addition of haptoglobin[b] moves it into α_2 region. Albumin band may appear yellow or brown due to methemalbumin	Myoglobin migrates near C3. Addition of haptoglobin[b] has no effect

a. Except when associated with renal failure.
b. By addition of normal serum to sample prior to electrophoresis.

from tubules into the blood. When hemoglobin uptake and iron accumulation by proximal tubule cells is extenstive, the cells exfoliate into the urine, where they can be detected by the Prussian blue reaction. Hemoglobinuria imparts a red-brown color to urine, reflecting the admixture of hemoglobin and methemoglobin. Hemoglobin may be distinguished from myoglobin in the urine spectroscopically or spectrophotometrically, but only with some difficulty. Table 12.1 lists several simpler means for differentiating hemoglobinuria and myoglobinuria.

d. METHEMALBUMINEMIA

When hemoglobinemia persists for an hour or more and the free hemoglobin undergoes oxidation to methemoglobin, **methemalbumin** accumulates. This brown pigment, a hallmark of intravascular hemolysis, forms because of the affinity of albumin for oxidized heme (ferriheme) groups. Plasma albumin possesses two sites that selectively bind ferriheme but not methemoglobin (ferrihemoglobin). The ferriheme is in an exchange equilibrium with the heme of other molecules of free methemoglobin and with heme bound to plasma albumin. Although the affinity of globin for ferriheme far exceeds that of free hemoglobin. Consequently, most of the ferriheme of methemoglobin is shifted onto the albumin, and the level of plasma methemalbumin (ferriheme-albumin) rises disproportionately due to its longer retention in circulation. (Unlike hemoglobin, methemalbumin is not filtered by the normal glomerulus.) Thus, the plasma becomes brown rather than red, while fresh voided urine shows the reddish color of hemoglobin or red-brown of methemoglobin.

Hemopexin, a plasma glycoprotein having the electrophoretic mobility of β_{1B} globulin, also binds ferriheme, and does so with a greater affinity than albumin. Like albumin, it does not bind intact hemoglobin. The hemopexin concentration in normal plasma is 50–100 mg/dl. The heme-hemopexin complex is removed from the circulation during hemolysis; thus its level declines.

2. Increased erythropoiesis

The acceleration of erythropoiesis that occurs in hemolytic anemia in response to diminished oxygen transport (see lecture 2) induces intramedullary erythroid hyperplasia. When severe and extended over a long period the following may be observed:

- Intramedullary erythroid hyperplasia
- Extramedullary erythropoiesis
- Skeletal deformities
- Bile pigment gallstones
- Nucleated red cells in the blood

a. INTRAMEDULLARY ERYTHROID HYPERPLASIA

In acute hemolytic anemia, a sharp increase in iron utilization by the bone marrow occurs within 12–24 hr. Within 2 days, the bone marrow manifests erythroid hyperplasia; and on the third day, barring factors that inhibit the marrow's proliferative response, the reticulocyte count increases (see lecture 2). Erythroid hyperplasia at first occurs only in regions of bone marrow that are normally hematopoietic, the rate of erythropoiesis rising about threefold. If hemolytic anemia persists, erythroid hyperplasia spreads througout the marrow cavity. Should anemia contiune, the entire marrow cavity becomes occupied by hematopoietic cells, the rate of erythropoiesis increasing as much as tenfold.

b. EXTRAMEDULLARY ERYTHROPOIESIS

In some patients, particularly those with congenital hemolytic anemias (e.g., hereditary spherocytosis and thalassemia), tumorlike erythropoietic masses may appear outside the marrow cavity, often adjacent to the spine. The masses are smoothly rounded or lobulated, often multiple, and when seen in chest films may resemble large encapsulated neoplasms. At autopsy, it s usually possible to demonstrate connections, often by narrow stalks, to the marrow of the vertebral bodies, for they are extrusions from the marrow cavity. Small, and from an erythropoietic standpoint, insignificant, colonies, of erythropoietic cells may be found in the spleen, liver, lymph nodes, and perinephric tissues.

c. SKELETAL DEFORMITIES

Severe chronic hemolytic anemia beginning in infancy or early childhood may expand the marrow space sufficiently to deform the patient's appearance. Children with thalassemia or other severe forms of chronic hemolytic anemia often develop **hemolytic facies** with broad cheekbones and protruding maxillae resulting from expansion of marrow space in these bones. This may create severe dental malocclusion and a chipmunk appearance. X-rays show broadening of the medullary cavity throughout most of the skeleton. In the skull, this leads to wide separation of the two tables of the calvarium and eventual demineralization of the outer table. The thin trabecular extensions radiating from the inner table create a "hair-on-end" appearance. During growth, vertebrae become broadened, demineralized, and coarsely trabecular with small radiolucent lakes resembling osteolytic lesions of malignancy. Intervertebral disks are commonly pressed into the thinned-out centers of softened adjacent vertebrae, and intervertebral spaces develop a fish-mouth appearance.

d. BILE PIGMENT GALLSTONES

Gallstones containing bile pigments are common in patients with congenital hemolytic disorders, whether or not there is frank anemia, but are uncommon in patients with acquired hemolytic disorders. They are usually small, numerous, and multifaceted.

e. NUCLEATED RED CELLS AND OTHER ABNORMALITIES IN BLOOD

Nucleated red cells commonly enter the circulation within several days of the onset of severe, acute hemolytic anemia. In sustained and severe hemolytic anemia, nucleated red cells may be a persistent feature of the blood. The majority are late normoblasts. Many show the nuclear deformities of normal karyorrhexis, such as lobulation, cloverlike deformities, and nuclear fragmentation. Nuclear fragments that are 1 or 2 μm in diameter are known as **Howell-Jolly bodies**. Blood often contains spherocytes.

C. Classification according to mechanisms

Types of hemolytic anemias were categorized above from three broad viewpoints: site of hemolysis, locus of defect, and genetic mechanism. In reality, no simplified classification is fully adequate because categories often overlap. In almost all instances, hemolytic anemias cuused by extrinsic or extracorpuscular factors are acquired. In some cases, an intrinsic defect may render the red cell abnormally susceptible to environmental factors that cause little damage to normal red cells. Excepting paroxysmal nocturnal hemoglobinuria, virtually all intrinsic red cell defects are hereditary. The following list is a working classification of the major hemolytic anemias based on the fundamental underlying abnormality.

1. Extracorpuscular defects

- Immunohemolytic anemias (see lecture 13)
- Microangiopathic and other hemolytic anemias caused by physical or thermal injury to red cells (see lecture 14)
- Oxidative hemolysis (Heinz body anemias) caused by exposure to exogenous chemicals or drugs that promote oxidation of red cell constituents (see lecture 15)
- Hemolysis caused by splenic enlargement: the splenomegaly syndrome or "hypersplenism" (see lecture 3)
- Hemolysis caused by alteration of red cell membrane lipids, spur cell anemia; hemolysis caused by bacterial phospholipases; others. (see lecture 14)

2. Intracorpuscular defects

- Defects of the red cell membrane: hereditary spherocytosis; hereditary elliptocytosis (see lecture 14)
- Metabolic defects due to hereditary deficiencies of red cell enzymes: glucose-6-phosphate dehydrogenase deficiency; pyruvate kinase deficiency; deficiencies of other enzymes of the Embden-Meyerhof glycolytic pathway and hexose monophosphate shunt (see lecture 15)
- Hemoglobinopathic defects associated with hereditary abnormalities in hemoglobin structure: sickle cell anemia; hemoglobin C disease; hemoglobins unstable to oxidation; others (see lecture 10)
- Hereditary impairment in rate of synthesis of a hemoglobin polypeptide chain: the thalassemias (see lecture 11)

3. Combined defects

- Megaloblastic anemia (see lectures 5 and 6)
- Hypochromic anemias (see lecture 7)
- Most disorders of the erythron if severe

SELECTED REFERENCES

Reviews

Berlin, N. I. The biological life of the red cell. In Surgenor, D. M., ed., *The Red Blood Cell*, 2nd ed. Orlando, FL: Academic Press, 1975, pp. 957–1019.

Berlin, N. I., and Berk, P. D. Quantitative aspects of bilirubin metabolism for hematologists. *Blood* 57(1981): 983–999.

Danon, D., and Marikovsky, Y. The aging of the red blood cell. A multifactor process. *Blood Cells*. 14(1988): 7–18.

Erslev, A. J. Erythrokinetics. In Williams, W. J., et al., eds. *Hematology*, 4th ed. New York: McGraw-Hill, 1990, pp. 414–422.

LaCelle, P. L. Destruction of erythrocytes. In Williams, W. J., et al., eds. *Hematology*, 4th ed. New York: McGraw-Hill, 1990, pp. 398–407.

Mayer, K., and Freeman, J. E. Techniques for measuring red cell, platelet, and WBC survival. *CRC. Crit. Rev. Clin. Lab. Sci.* 23(1986): 201–217.

Mohandas, N., and Groner, W. Cell membrane and volume changes during red cell development and aging. *Ann. NY Acad. Sci.* 554(1989): 217–224.

Original articles

Alam, J., and Smith, A. Receptor-mediated transport of heme by hemopexin regulates gene expression in mammalian cells. *J. Biol. Chem.* 264(1989): 17637–17640.

Brus, I., and Lewis, S. M. The haptoglobin content of serum in haemolytic anaemia. *Br. J. Haematol.* 5(1959): 348–355.

Hillman, R. S., and Finch, C. A. Annotation: the misused reticulocyte. *Br. J. Haematol.* 17(1969): 313–315.

Singcharoen, T. Unusual long bone changes in thalassaemia: findings on plain radiography and computed tomography. *Br. J. Radiol.* 62(1989): 168–171.

LECTURE 13

Hemolytic Anemias II. Immunohemolytic Anemias

W. Hallowell Churchill, Jr., and James H. Jandl

EDITOR'S COMMENT

The discovery by R. A. Coombs of the antiglobulin test, also called the Coombs test, was a great and many-faceted achievement. Although a mainstay of hematologic practice today, the Coombs test was discovered as recently as 1945. Its first application to the analysis of hemolytic anemia took place in 1946. The discovery of "globulin-coated" red cells in certain hemolytic anemias proved that hemolysis can have an immunologic basis, but often has some other basis. Soon thereafter, antibodies against red cells were divided into warm- and cold-active types and there arose the major new branch of hematology now called immunohematology. Its clinical and biologic implications have been broad and deep, extending into such diverse fields as blood group testing procedures, basic immunology, and other branches of clinical medicine.

I. INTRODUCTION

Immunohemolytic anemias (also termed **autoimmune hemolytic anemias**) are acquired disorders in which premature red cell destruction is mediated by an immunologic process. Diagnosis is based on evidence that autologous antibodies (usually IgG) and or one or more components of **serum complement** (primarily C′3d and some C4) are attached to the patient's red cells.

B. Detection

1. Direct antiglobulin test

Red cells coated with small amounts of antibody and/or complement may not agglutinate in vitro without an additional antibody acting as a bridge between red cells that are separated by their net negative charge (see lecture 16).

In the **direct antiglobulin test**, commonly called the **direct Coombs test**, cells are exhaustively washed to remove serum proteins and proteins that are nonspecifically adsorbed to red cells. The red cells are then tested for residual immunoglobulin and/or complement components by addition of a polyspecific antibody with specificity for the Fc portion of immunoglobulin and for complement components (C′3, C′4 and their degradation products). Cells coated with immunoglobulin or complement will form agglutinates because the "antibody," also called **Coombs reagent**, reacts with immunoglobulin or complement on different cells and thus causes clumping.

If agglutination is produced by addition of a polyspecific Coombs reagent, various monospecific Coombs reagents—directed against either IgG or complement—can be used to identify the proteins present on the red cell surface.

2. *Indirect antiglobulin test*

Unlike the direct antiglobulin test, which detects red cells coated by antibodies in vivo, the **indirect antiglobulin test** identifies antibodies present in serum, which under test conditions coated red cells in vitro.

This is accomplished by incubation of indicator type O red cells with serum from the patient being tested. The red cells are then washed and tested for the presence of cell surface antibody and/or complement by addition of a Coombs reagent. In this way, indirect test detects antibody in serum while the direct test identifies antibody or complement already on the cell surface.

Antibody in serum in the absence of cell-bound antibody usually indicates allogeneic immunization. The indirect Coombs test is the main procedure used in detection of allogeneic red cell antibodies and in pretransfusion compatibility testing (see lecture 16).

Routine antiglobulin tests can detect between 100 and 500 molecules of IgG and about 100 molecules of C′3d per red cell. If a lower number is present, routine antiglobulin tests may be negative, but immunohemolysis may still occur.

C. Classification

Classification of the immunoholytic anemias is based on three considerations:

- Whether antibody attaches to cells at body temperature (**warm-active antibody**) or is active primarily at cooler temperatures (**cold-active antibody**)
- Whether the antibody is IgG or IgM, and whether it activates complement
- Whether the hemolytic antibody reacts with an antigenic constituent of the cell

As less than half these cases are associated with defined causative agents or disorders, the best initial approach is to determine the kind of protein present in a given Coombs-positive patient. The immunologic process responsible for hemolytic anemia in most patients is unknown.

Drug-induced hemolytic anemias are usually classified separately from other immunohemolytic anemias because the etiologic agent is known and the process is usually reversible.

II. MECHANISMS OF RED CELL INJURY

The following discussion considers mechanisms of immune hemolysis that are mediated by IgG warm-active antibodies and IgM or IgG cold-active antibodies.

A. Warm-active antibodies

1. Properties

Characteristics of warm-active antibodies are summarized in table 13.1. Although the thermal range may vary, maximum antibody activity is almost always about 37°C. Most severely affected patients have a strongly positive test when Coombs antiserum is directed against IgG. In some patients, appropriate Coombs antisera reveal that the red cell is also coated with a fragment of inactivated C3.

In IgG-mediated, warm-active antibody, immunohemolytic anemias, antibody specificity is usually directed at some component of the Rh system.

- In two-thirds of cases, Rh specificity can be demonstrated by the failure of autoantibodies from these patients to react with Rh null cells, which are devoid of Rh antigens.
- In the remaining third, the autoantibodies react with all red cells, including Rh null cells. The specificity of these antoantibodies is not known (see lecture 16).

2. Factors determining locus of hemolysis

Warm-active 7S IgG antibodies that are profoundly hemolytic in vivo cause no injury to red cells in vitro, irrespective of the amount of antibody or the presence or absence of complement; there is no change in appearance, metabolism, viscosity, rigidity, or ability to pass through capillary-sized filters.

Infused plasma containing 7S IgG autoantibodies induces spherocytosis, increases osmotic fragility of the patient's red cells, and causes hemolysis in vivo.

The change in activity of autoantibodies in vivo is the result of the interaction of coated red cells with fixed or circulating phagocytic cells. The mechanisms of these interactions have been elucidated by studies of the ingestion of red cells by fixed or circulating phagocytes.

a. STUDIES OF ERYTHROPHAGOCYTOSIS

An antibody that activates "hemolytic complement" while reacting with red cell antigens typically causes abrupt and extensive erythrophagocytosis, provided that fresh serum complement (at physiologic pH) and phagocytic cells are present. In the blood, most erythrophagocytosis involves

Table 13.1
Antibodies Associated with Immunohemolytic Anemia

Properties	Warm-active antibodies	Cold-active antibodies
Immunoglobulin class[a]	Usually IgG	Usually IgM
Heavy chain subclass[a]	IgG1 and IgG3	
Sedimentation coefficient	7S	19S
Mol. wt.	160,000	~1,000,000
Temperature optimum	37°C	4°C (0–10°C)
Activation of complement	None or little	Yes, but sequence seldom completed
Agglutination of normal red cells	None or little	Yes (titer > 1:300)
Direct Coombs test with		
Antihuman serum	+++/++++	+/++
Anti-IgG	+++/++++	0/++
Anti-IgM	0	0
Anti-C3	0/++	++/+++
Anti-C4	0/+	+/++
Indirect Coombs test with		
Antihuman serum	0/+++	0/++[b]
Anti-IgM	0/+++	0
Anti-IgM	0	0
Anti-C3	0	0/+++[b]
Effective affinity	++/++++	tr/+ (at >30°C)
Antigenic specificity	Nonspecific (but often requires Rh locus)[c]	I, i (also H, M, N)
Number of antibody molecules per red cell	10^3–10^5	10^5 or more
Frequency of etiologies		
Idiopathic	55–60%	30–40%
Drug-induced	25–30%	1–5%
Lymphoproliferative disorder	10–15%	15–20%
Mycoplasma infection	0%	25–35%
Other	5–10%	5–10%

a. See lecture 25.
b. Test negative unless fresh, complement-replete serum incubated with cells at cold temperatures.
c. See lecture 16.

granulocytes. Virtually all granulocytes can engage in erythrophagocytosis, many gorging themselves to the point of rupture. Aggregation of numerous red cells with two or more granulocytes leads to characteristic ragged mixed agglutinates (figure 13.1A). Monocytes also engage in complement-mediated erythrophagocytosis, although a smaller percentage of them actually ingests red cells and does so more slowly than granulocytes.

The extent of erythrophagocytosis is influenced by the presence or absence of both IgG and C3b on the red cell because the interaction of C3b with its receptor, called CR1, on the macrophage causes close apposition with the red cell—and phagocytosis is stimulatd by the additional presence of IgG interacting with the macrophage Fc receptor. These receptors react specifically with certain regions of the Fc fragments of the heavy chain subclasses IgG1 and IgG3. (Immunoglobulin structure is fully discussed in lecture 25.)

IgG antibodies frequently coat red cells without fixing complement. In these cases, the physical attributes of red cells coated with IgG antibody are not altered, but the cells are trapped in the proximal (and later the entire) splenic red pulp because of the Fc interactions with macrophage receptors (figure 13.2).

b. MECHANISM OF SPHEROCYTOSIS

Variable numbers of red cells may become bound to activated lining cells, undergo membrane contraction (and thus become spherocytic), and still escape back into the circulation for a time (figure 13.3). Immunohemolytic anemia secondary to IgG warm antibodies is uncommonly associated with erythrophagocytosis because IgG autoantibodies usually are so widely dispersed on the cell surface that doublet formation required for activation of C1 of the classic pathway does not occur. Without the additional signal provided by the C3b-macrophage interaction, the rate of phagocytosis is insignificant. The injury to IgG-coated red cells trapped, thus, occurs on the external surface of the macrophages and is mostly likely due to the random loss of small fragments of red cell membrane (see figure 14.7).

3. Factors determining hemolytic potency

Immune hemolysis by warm-active IgG antibodies in humans is influenced by the four major factors:

- Number and distribution of antigens on red cell surface
- Heavy chain subclass
- Amount of IgG in fluid phase
- Functional capacity of the RES

a. NUMBER AND DISTRIBUTION OF ANTIGENS

This factor determines the spacing of the antibodies. The D antigen and other antigens of the Rh locus—typical of antigens interacting with warm-

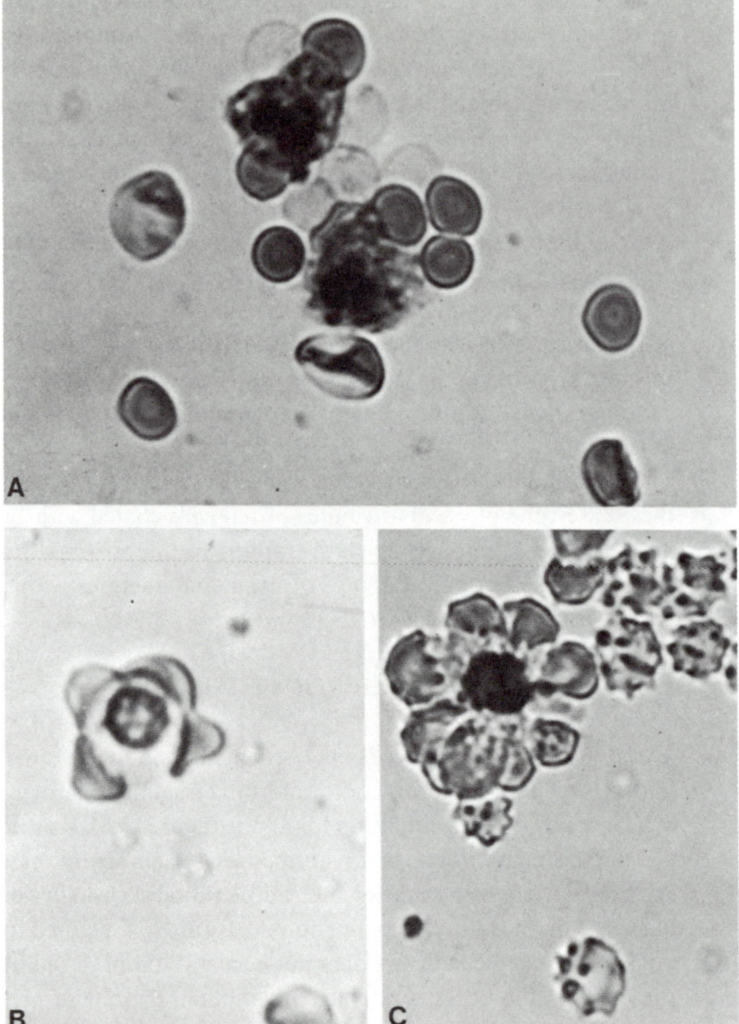

Fig. 13.1
Photomicrographs comparing interactions of red cells with granulocytes (mediated by complement-activating antibodies) and with lymphocytes and monocytes (mediated by Rh antibodies) ($\times 425$). *A*, Mixed agglutination, showing red cell-granulocyte aggregation, involving several cell types, induced by complement-activating antibodies. *B*, Attachment of several anti-D coated red cells to a lymphocyte, showing characteristic red cell deformation induced by stubby lymphocytic processes. *C*, Rosette, in which monocyte is surrounded by numerous adherent anti-D coated red cells, showing severe red cell deformation by long, grasping monocytic processes. (In *A*, cells are suspended in fresh, complement-replete serum; in *B* and *C*, cells are suspended in saline.)

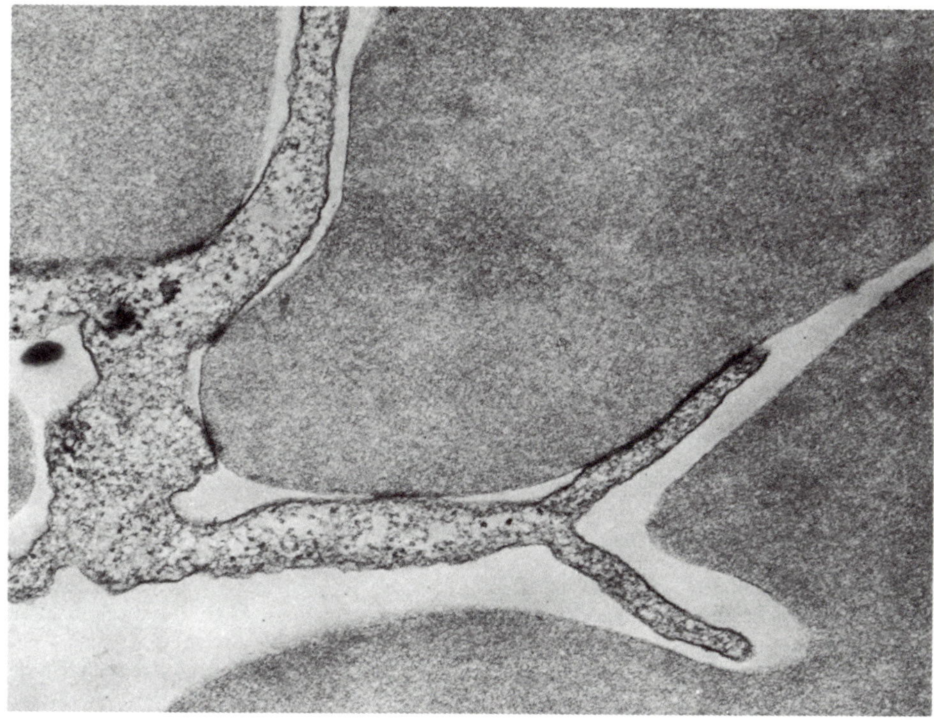

A

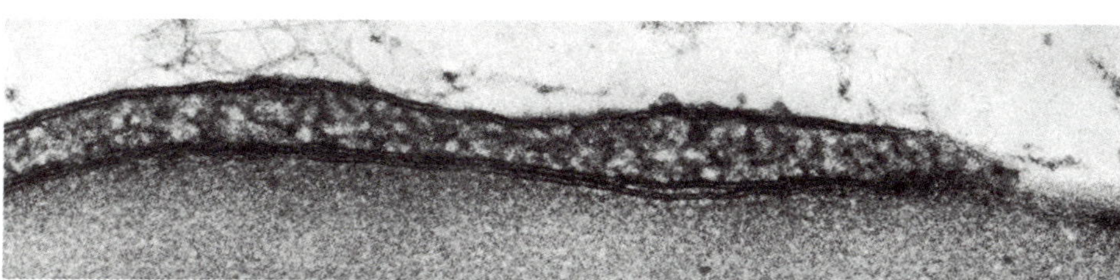

B

Fig. 13.2

Binding of red cells to monocytes. *A*, Electron micrograph demonstrating complex, long, branching processes extending around and enmeshing red cells coated with IgG (× 21,300). Processes at right (particularly thin end-processes with a diameter of 0.1 μm) adhere to red cells and form the trilaminar pattern characteristic of cell-cell fusion. *B*, Detail of fusion pattern (× 42,600). Complex arborizing and adherent processes of monocytes (and macrophages) are capable of extending around two or even three "orbitals" of attached red cells. Those few lymphocytes that form incomplete rosettes with IgG-coated red cells appear incapable of extending cytoplasmic processes beyond about 1.5 μm. (From N. Abramson, R. Cotran, and J. H. Jandl, *J. Exp. Med.* 132[1970]: 1191.)

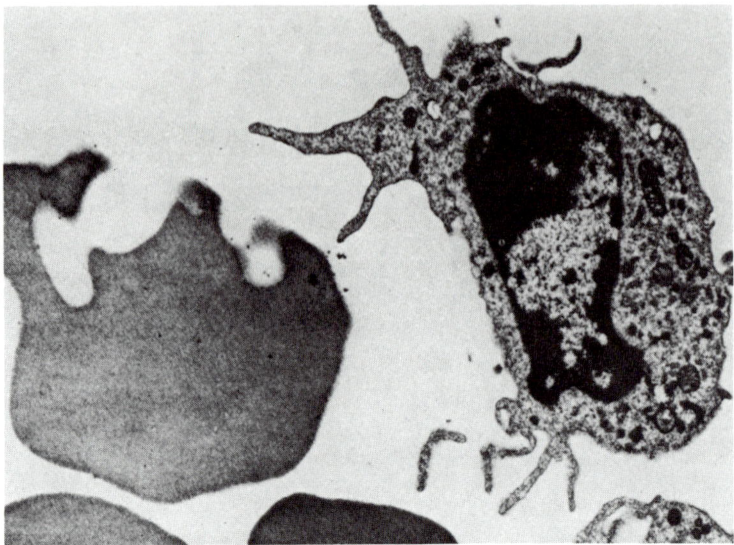

Fig. 13.3
Mechanism of spherocytosis. Electron micrograph (×4400) of red cell (left) and monocyte (right) 15 min after addition of papain (and cysteine) to a suspension of IgG-mediated rosettes (such as those in figure 13.1C). The released red cell is intact. It is osmotically fragile and would appear as a spherocyte by light microscopy. However, electron microscopy reveals the persisting deformities induced by the monocyte. (From N. Abramson, R. Cotran, and J. H. Jandl, *J. Exp. Med.* 132[1970]: 1191.)

water antibodies—are widely spaced on the red cell surface (about 1.5 μm apart, a distance over 10 times the span of an IgG molecule). This explains why antibody, even when in excess, fails to induce agglutination. A sparsity of antigenic sites also may render IgM antibodies weak inducers of agglutination. By reacting with single antigens on each of two cells, several IgM molecules may induce weak agglutination that is easily disrupted, particularly at body temperature.

b. HEAVY CHAIN SUBCLASS

IgG3 is more efficient that IgG1. IgG3 requires as few as 230 molecules/cell for phagocytosis whereas IgG1 requires about 2000. IgG2 and IgG4 are inactive.

c. IgG IN FLUID PHASE

Fluid-phase IgG inhibits the interaction of red cell–bound IgG with macrophage Fc receptors. Because of plasma skimming, the relative amount of IgG in the high hematocrit environment of the spleen is much reduced. The probability of red cell–bound IgG interacting with macrophage Fc receptors is, therefore, increased in this environment. Furthermore, lightly coated red cells are more likely to be retained in the spleen where the inhibitory effect of the fluid-phase IgG is minimized. With more heavily coated cells, the inhibitory effect of fluid-phase IgG is relatively less important, so red cells are sequestered at sites of larger phagocytic cell mass such as the liver.

d. FUNCTIONAL CAPACITY OF RES

As discussed in lecture 3, the capacity of RES cells (macrophages, monocytes, activated endothelial lining cells, and so on) for destroying antibody-coated red cells depends on (1) the number of cells that are phagocytic or are capable of binding the Fc portion of IgG molecules; (2) the number of antibody-coated cells circulating through these organs; and (3) the regional blood flow to major organs of the RES.

These factors influence the sites of red cell clearance. Small quantities of IgG-coated red cells are cleared almost exclusively by the spleen. Splenic blood flow per minute is normally 3–5% of cardiac output. The rate of clearance of anti-D-coated red cells infused into the circulation is approximately 3%/min with a half-life of clearance of about 20 min. Thus, when the number of antibody-coated red cells is small relative to the mass of available RES cells, all or most of the splenic arterial blood is cleared of the antibody-coated cells. In contrast, when an immunohemolytic anemia is associated with intravascular agglutination, agglutinated red cells are cleared from the blood at a rate approximating the rate of blood flow through the entire RES, the bulk of which is in the liver. In this instance, th rate of clearance would approximate hepatic blood flow—about 37% of cardiac output.

The rate of red cell destruction in warm antibody immunohemolytic anemia is determined by saturation kinetics. At a given level of antibody per red cell, half-life for red cell clearance may be several days. However, as splenic proliferation occurs in response to the trapped red cell debris, all splenic components increase in number by five- or tenfold. Consequently, splenic blood flow and clearance capability increase proportionately.

B. Cold-active antibodies

1. Properties

Most cold-active antibodies are 19S IgM immunoglobulins (see Table 13.1). The temperature optimum for these antibodies is 2–4°C. Above 10°C, effective affinity of antibody for red cell antigen diminishes; above 30°C, attached antibodies dissociate rapidly from the cells. On electron microscopy, cell–bound IgM appears as a strand positioned so as to bridge the 200- to 300-Å gap that normally separates blood cells. By bridging cells and forming a lattice structure, IgM antibodies cause agglutination. As most IgM antibodies bind red cell antigens primarily at low temperatures, agglutination in vivo is restricted to blood perfusing superficial vessels subject to environmental cooling. However, as cool blood is returned to the warm central circulation, antibody is released quickly and agglutinates disperse.

2. *Cold agglutinin titer*

In order to quantify antibodies that agglutinate red cells in the cold, serial dilutions of patient's serum are mixed with a 1% suspension of normal type O red cells. The highest dilution (often expressed as its reciprocal) at which visible agglutination occurs denotes the **cold agglutinin titer**. Patients may have cold agglutinin titers in excess of $1:10^6$.

3. *Antigen specificity: the I-i system*

The **I-i system** of red cell antigens is related to the ABO(H) system, which will be discussed in lecture 16. The I antigen is present in the red cells of most adults, and a low concentration of cold-active IgM with anti-I specificity is present in healthy individuals. In early infancy, i antigen, which is found on fetal and cord red blood cells, becomes more branched and, thus, acquires I specificity. (see lecture 16).

Consequently, a cold-active antibody may be identified as anti-I if it strongly agglutinates normal adult red cells and fails to agglutinate cord blood cells in comparable fashion. Some anomalous cold-active antibodies possess **anti-i** specificity.

4. *Factors determining hemolytic potency*

These include:

- Effects of mechanical trauma on circulating agglutinates
- Participation of the complement system
- Thermal range of the antibodies
- The presence of anti-I IgG
- Structure of the C3b receptor

a. MECHANICAL FACTORS

Mechanical trauma to circulating agglutinates is probably not an important cause of hemolysis unless severe cold exposure is accompanied by muscular exertion.

b. SERUM COMPLEMENT

If IgM antibody binds to red cells long enough to activate the complement sequence (several seconds at most), "hemolytic complement" is generated and hemolysis occurs. When activation is sustained, severe intravascular hemolysis ensues.

Activation of the classic complement pathway generates several hundred C3b sites for every fully lytic site. C3b is further inactivated so that only a small fragment, called C3d, remains on the cells that return to circulation. The C3d, clustered around sites of antibody attachment, inhibits further attachment of C3b and thus has the effect of decreasing the sequestration of complement-coated red cells in the reticuloendothelial system. An anti-C3 Coombs reagent recognizes both C3b and C3d. Therefore, because of the blocking effect of C3d, a strongly positive anti-C3 Coombs reaction in patients with cold antibodies does not always signify extensive hemolysis.

c. TEMPERATURE

The striking thermal dependence of cold-active antibodies is determined mainly by effects of temperature on the distribution and reactivity of antigen on the red cell membrane.

d. ANTIGEN DENSITY

There are roughly 1 million I antigens per red cell—a density comparable to that of blood group antigens A_1 and B. The close proximity of I-combining sites permits some anti-I IgG to bind to red cells in the steric arrangement required for activation of complement. Red cells of patients with high titers of cold-active antibodies often are agglutinated by both anit-C3 and anti-IgG Coombs sera.

e. REARRANGEMENT OF THE C3b RECEPTOR

Using two-dimensional gel analysis, studies of red cell membranes from patients with chronic cold agglutinin disease have shown the appearance of a polymeric glycophorin that is not present in normal membranes. This polymeric glycophorin appears after normal red cells are treated with purified cold agglutinin antibody (anti-I specificity) and results in increased efficiency of C3b binding.

C. Activation of complement

When antibodies reacting with red cell antigens cause all complement components to be sequentially converted to their active forms, "hemolytic complement" is generated and the red cell undergoes hemolysis.

1. Mechanism of complement-mediated hemolysis

Lysis of red cells by "hemolytic complement" is due to profound alteration in membrane permeability. The terminal components, C5bC789, form a cylindrical structure with a hydrophobic outer structure that associates with membrane lipid and a hydrophilic inner core through which leakage of small ions eventually leads to cell lysis. This structure appears as a large (80–100 Å) circular depression on electron microscopy. In cross-section, these structures are imperforate craters in which the bilaminar membrane structure is thinned out to a single layer.

2. *Pathways of complement activation*

In reacting with red cell antigens, IgM activates the first complement (C1) and launches the "classic pathway" of the complement cascade. The C1q subunit of C1 bears a combining site for the exposed Fc portion of IgM. Its addition to the antibody-antigen complex activates C1r, which then converts C1s to an esterase reactive with C4. This step leads to the generation of large amounts of the complex C4b2a (the C3 convertase), which activates hundreds of C3 molecules. This key amplification step liberates split products of C3, including a major fragment, C3b, that adheres to nearby cells surfaces and facilitates their phagocytosis by neutrophils and macrophages which have C3b receptors (CR1 receptors).

In the alternate pathway, activation is achieved without involvement of antibody. A convertase is generated from a hydrolytic fragment of C3 and a cleavage product of factor B. This alternate pathway convertase can also generate C3b from native C3.

3. *Noncompletion of complement sequence*

In addition to the regulatory effect already described for residual C3d, several other regulatory proteins have been identified. These include:

- Decay-accelerating factor, which inhibits synthesis and accelerates destruction of C3 convertase
- C8 binding protein, which binds to C8 and thus inhibits lysis

These proteins play a role in IgM-mediated hemolysis. Absence or decrease of these proteins is probably responsible for the abnormal hemolysis of paroxysmal nocturnal hemoglobulinuria.

III. CLINICAL DISORDERS

A. With warm-active antibodies

Immunohemolytic anemias associated with warm-active antibodies are idiopathic in almost 60% of the patients (see tabel 13.1). They are drug induced in 25–30%, associated with lymphoproliferative disorders in 10–15%, and with other disorders in 5–10%.

1. *Idiopathic type*

a. CLINICAL FEATURES

Idiopathic immunohemolytic anemia occurs in both sexes at all ages. Hemolysis may be acute and occasionally explosive in onset, severe anemia occurring within several days, In most patients, the disorder is self-limited, duration varying from 2–3 weeks to several years. One or more relapses may occur over a period of years. In some, hemolysis is chronic and unremitting. The early symptoms are those of acute anemia (see lecture 1) —dyspnea, weakness, dizziness upon rising, pounding in the ears, pallor, and so on. Mild icterus is common. Symptoms of the initial severe phase often disappear as the patient establishes a compensatory erythropoietic response. Splenomegaly, with some tenderness, initially occurs within a few days of the onset. If the hemolytic process continues and reaches a steady state, the spleen may enlarge to 10–12 times its normal weight, extending 2–6 cm below the left costal margin. Massive splenomeglay is not encountered unless the spleen is affected by an associated disease (e.g., chronic lymphocytic leukemia). Hepatomegaly may result from congestive heart failure induced by anemia. Reduction in red cell mass is usually not offset by an increase in plasma volume, and blood volume may be diminished by 1–2 liters.

b. LABORATORY FINDINGS

The direct anti-IgG Coombs test is typically positive, but occasionally it is initially negative or doubtful. When this occurs, antisera from several sources should be tried, and the test should be performed at several dilutions; a prozone may be caused by an excess of antiglobulin relative to its antigen (IgG). Hemolysis may precede the appearance of detectable antibody. Other early findings in severe cases may include hemoglobinemia, methemalbuminemia, hemosiderinuria, and hemoglobinuria.

When anemia enters a steady state 2–3 weeks after onset, hematologic examination may reveal a hematocrit of about 20%; a reticulocyte count of 10–30% (with large reticulocytes); nucleated red cells; spherocytosis affecting 10–60% of the red cells; normal or slightly elevated white count; and a normal platelet count. In a few patients, platelet levels decline sharply, inducing thrombocytopenic purpura (Evans' syndrome). In most cases, a patient's ^{51}Cr-labeled red cells are sequestered entirely, or primarily, in the spleen (see figure 12.2). When confined to the spleen, the rate of red cell destruction gradually becomes equilibrated by increased red cell formation as the marrow response is established. When hepatic red cell destruction in appreciable, the hemolytic rate may exceed the proliferative capacity of the marrow. Factors that commonly interfere with the compensatory response of marrow include folic acid deficiency and infection. In chronic hemolysis, the nutritional requirement for folic acid, which is needed in DNA synthesis (see lecture 6), may increase two- to threefold. Administration of folic acid is advisable in such cases. Infection, by viruses such as parvovirus, may dangerously suppress cell proliferation in the bone marrow. Less frequent causes of relative marrow failure include exposure to myelosuppressive drugs (e.g., chloramphenicol, various cytotoxic drugs) and uremia.

2. ***Drug-induced immunohemolytic anemias***

Many drugs and chemicals have been found to induce Coombs-positive hemolytic anemia. A summarized listing of offending compounds, grouped according to the three different mechanisms of action, is presented in table 13.2.

a. HAPTEN-TYPE MECHANISM (STIBOPHEN MODEL)

Stibophen is the archetypical drug of this class. Other drugs that may act similarly include quinine, quinidine, sulfonamide and sulfanilylurea derivatives, five or six congeners of phenacetin, and PAS. These drugs induce Coombs-positive hemolytic anemia by binding to a plasma protein. The **drug-protein complex** is antigenic, the drug serving as a hapten. Antibodies form to the drug-protein complex, and antigen-antibody complexes formed in the plasma are deposited on red cell surfaces. Cell-bound **immune complexes** tend to activate the complement system; additionally, the complexes may activate complement in the serum, in which case complement fragments are deposited on circulating red cells (which are "innocent bystanders"). The cells become agglutinable by anti-C3 Coombs antiserum. When the elicited antibody is IgM, it is seldom demonstrable on washed red cells because most IgM antibodies dissociate readily at ambient temperatures. As with cold antibodies, evidence for an immune reaction is inferred from finding complement components (primarily C3d) on the red cells. In some patients, the antibody elicited by the drug-protein complex is IgG; complement components and IgG are both detected on the red cell in such cases.

b. HAPTEN-TYPE MECHANISM (PENICILLIN MODEL)

An analogous but sequentially different mechanism for drug-induced Coombs-positive hemolytic anemia occurs in patients receiving large doses of penicillin intravenously. Penicillin also acts as a hapten, but in a different manner. When added to red cells suspended in saline, or in greater amounts to whole blood, penicillin binds covalently to proteins in the red cell membrane. The **cell-drug complex** is antigenic, eliciting IgG antibodies directed against "penicillinized" red cells. The IgG Coombs tests is positive; the C3 Coombs test is usually negative. In some cases, IgM may also participate, although this antibody to penicillin is ordinarily harmless.

Immune hemolysis induced by hapten-type mechanisms occurs only when all three reactants—drug, protein (or red cells), and antibody—are present. In both hapten-type mechanisms, the hematologic picture resembles idiopathic immunohemolytic anemia. The term **autoimmunity** is inappropriate since antibody is specific for an exogenous compound. Cases now considered idiopathic may later be attributable to exogenous compounds in the environment. Therapy consists of withdrawing the causative

Table 13.2
Drug-Induced Immunohemolysis: Proposed Mechanisms

	Hapten type		
Features	Binding of drug to protein	Binding of durg to red cell	Unknown
Representative drug	Stibophen	Penicillin	Aldomet®
Positive Coombs test	Rare	Uncommon (only at high doses)	Common (varies with dose)
Hemolysis in those with positive Coombs test (and severity)	Usual (occ. severe)	Frequent (mild to moderate)	Uncommon (occ. severe)
Effect of drug withdrawal			
On Coombs test	Negative in few weeks	Negative in 2–3 months	Negative in 3–18 months
On hemolysis	Rapid, complete improvement	Rapid, complete improvement	Improvement in several weeks; recovery in several months
Direct Coombs test	C3 (occ. IgG)	IgG (occ. C3)	IgG
Antibody causing positive Coombs test and hemolysis	IgM (occ. IgG)	IgG (occ. IgM)	IgG
Antibody (from red cell eluate or serum)*			
Binds to red cells only if drug present	Yes	Yes	No
Causes red cell to adhere to mononuclear cells			
Drug present	No	Yes	Yes
Drug absent	No	No	Yes

* The diagnosis may be missed if the assay for antibody is not carried out with addition of drug to the reaction mixture or, in the case of a drug bound to red cell membranes, if drug-coated cells are not used as indicator cells in the indirect Coombs test.

agent. Hemolysis ceases when drug elutes from the cells or drug-coated red cells are removed.

Recent studies indicate some overlap of mechanisms, especially for drugs that work by hapten-related mechanisms. For example:

- Some cephalosporins cause a positive direct antiglobulin test by a hapten mechanism and severe hemolysis by immune complex formation.
- Antibodies associated with Nomifensine® (a nonsteroidal anti-inflammatory drug) in some cases require the presence of the drug or its metabolite for activity. In other cases, the antibodies appear to be autoantibodies.
- In hydrochlorthiazide-induced hemolytic anemia, the immune complexes are absorbed by all red cells except -D- cells and Rh null cells (see lecture 16).

c. UNKNOWN MECHANISM (ALDOMET® MODEL)

Doubt as to whether exogenous drugs or chemicals commonly cause Coombs-positive hemolytic anemia was dispelled when it was recognized that the antihypertensive drug α-methyl dopa or Aldomet® (α-methyl-3,4-dihydroxy-L-phenylalanine) often causes a typical positive IgG Coombs test. Complement is not activated. The frequency of this reaction in patients receiving Aldomet® for >3 months is dose related, ranging from about 10% at a daily dose of 0.75 g to almost 40% at 2.0 g. The IgG Aldomet® antibody is similar in different patients. It appears to react with the Rh locus, showing little or no reaction with Rh null red cells or with red cells of species lacking the Rh locus. Affinity of the Aldomet® antibody for red cells is less that that of warm isoantibodies of the anti-D type (see lecture 17). Consequently, fewer than 1% of those who develop a positive Coombs test during Aldomet® therapy have significant hemolytic anemia. In Coombs-positive but nonanemic patients, the Coombs test is usually 1–2+; on withdrawal of drug, it becomes negative in 3–4 months. In patients with hemolytic anemia, the Coombs test is 3–4+; on withdrawal it becomes negative in 6–24 months.

Aldomet®, its congeners, and degradation products cannot be shown to affect or participate in the interaction between eluted antibody and normal red cells. Proof that the antibody is drug induced is entirely epidemiologic—that is, a positive Coombs test is rare in normal individuals and in hypertensive patients not receiving Aldomet®. Another medication known to cause Aldomet®-like Coombs-positive hemolytic anemia is the anti-inflammatory drug mefenamic acid. L-dopa, which is administered to patients with Parkinson's disease, causes a positive Coombs test in 5% to 8% of patients. Unlike α-methyl dopa (a synthetic analogue), L-dopa (a physiologic compound) does not cause hemolytic anemia. Presumably, other medications or chemical agents may cause immunohemolytic anemia of the Aldomet® type.

Procainamide is associated with an immunohemolytic anemia, in which the autoantibody resembles that found in Aldomet® immunohemolysis. Interestingly, procainamide initiates hemolysis but is not required to sustain a hemolytic process in which the antibodies come to resemble those of idiopathic IgG-mediated immunohemolytic anemia. The mechanisms may relate to changes in suppressor cells and/or the clearance capacity of the RES.

3. Therapy

Therapy of immunohemolytic anemia induced by warm-active antibodies, whether the antibodies are idiopathic or drug induced, varies with the clinical situation.

a. TRANSFUSION

Catastrophic hemolysis with severe anemia requires prompt infusion of fluids and red cells. Normal ABO-compatible red cells will survive at least as long as the patient's red cell, and usually longer. Cross-matching (discussed in lecture 17) may be difficult in some patients but should not deter administration of life-saving transfusion of ABO-compatible blood or packed cells.

b. CORTICOSTEROIDS

Most patients (80%) respond initially to treatment with large doses of steroids which act by suppressing antibody synthesis, by decreasing binding of autoantibody to red cells, and by down-modulating macrophage Fc receptors. The reticulocyte count begins to rise in 48 hr. The indirect Coombs test, if positive, soon becomes negative, and in a few weeks the direct Coombs test usually weakens and may disappear. About one-third of patients relapse unless large doses of corticosteroids are continued. Continuation of steroid therapy beyond 2–3 months poses serious risks.

c. SPLENECTOMY

Patients who do not respond to corticosteroids within several weeks of therapy are candidates for splenectomy. Those nonresponders with moderate or severe hemolysis who neither develop splenomegaly nor accumulate ^{51}Cr-labeled red cells in their spleens rarely benefit from splenectomy. Those with splenomegaly (which is invariably present when splenic sequestration is extensive) and striking ^{51}Cr uptake should undergo splenectomy, provided the patient is an acceptable candidate for surgery. Splenectomy removes the filter of antibody-coated red cells but does not alter antibody levels. The Coombs test may remain positive or become even more strongly positive despite a good remission after splenectomy.

d. IMMUNOSUPPRESSIVE DRUGS

Occasional patients partially benefit from therapy with immunosuppressive cytotoxic drugs; these agents depress the entire immune system, but in some cases disproportionately affect the vigorous immunohemolytic process.

e. OTHER THERAPY

Danazol is a modified androgen that appears to be useful in the management of IgG-mediated immunohemolytic anemia. The mechanism of action is not understood but may be related to reduction of cell surface antibody and possibly modulation of macrophage Fc receptors. Intravenous γ-globulin in large doses may be effective and is worth trying when there are reasons to avoid immunosuppressive therapy.

f. TREATMENT OF ASSOCIATED DISEASES

As indicated in table 13.1, Coombs-positive hemolytic anemia is common in patients with lymphoproliferative disorders, particularly chronic lymphocytic leukemia and certain lymphomas. It may also be associated with teratomas, dermoid cysts, carcinoma, systemic lupur erythematosus, and ulcerative colitis. Successful treatment of the underlying disorders usually improves the hemolytic process.

B. With cold-active antibodies

1. Classification

Most normal serum contains low concentrations of IgM anti-I that causes red cells to agglutinate in the cold.

Elevated titers of cold-active antibodies occur in three clinical circumstances (table 13.3):

- During recovery phase of *Mycoplasma pneumoniae* and, less often, of infectious mononucleosis (the former has anti-I specificity, the latter anti-i).
- In association with lymphoproliferative disease.
- In idiopathic cold agglutinin disease.

2. Clinical features

Symptoms are due to vasoocculsion in regions of the circulation exposed to cooling and may include painful stiff fingers and toes; blanching or stagnant cyanosis of the skin overlying affected joints; urticaria, generalized or restricted to exposed areas; mottled cyanosis and painful blanching of skin; and local dry gangrene in acrocyanotic regions.

Table 13.3
Characteristics of Various Cold Agglutinins

Clinical setting	Antigenic specificity	Usual titer*	Clonal characteristics	Associated hemolysis
Normal	Anti-I Anti-i Anti-H	<50	Polyclonal	None
Postinfection	Anti-I Anti-i	10^2–10^4	Polyclonal	None to severe
Lymphoproliferative disorders	Anti-I	10^2–10^6	Often monoclonal	Mild to severe
Idiopathic cold agglutinin disease	Anti-I	10^2–10^6	Often monoclonal	Mild to severe

* Expressed as reciprocal of titer.

Affected patients are generally older than those with warm-active antibodies. Overt hemolytic anemia develops in a minority of patients. Hemolysis, when it occurs, is usually mild, but it may be severe. In patients with cold-active antibody hemolysis, ^{51}Cr-labeled red cells are usually sequestered in the liver. Splenomegaly is uncommon.

3. *Therapy*

Antibody titers may be brought down by therapy with an alkylating agent such as chlorambucil. Except for the unusual case in which IgG cold agglutinin is present, splenectomy and/or corticosteroid therapy is usually of little benefit. As IgM is largely intravascular, plasmapheresis has been used to reduce antibody levels in some acute cases. The best therapy is preventive; avoidance of cold exposure and use of measures such as mittens and long underwear. When the cold agglutinin syndrome is associated with lymphoproliferative disorder, improvement may follow antileukemic or antilymphoma therapy (see lectures 22–24).

4. *Paroxysmal cold hemoglobinuria*

Paroxysmal cold hemoglobinuria (PCH) is a rare, potentially life-threatening, episodic disorder caused by acquisition of the **Donath-Landsteiner (D-L) antibody**, a cold-active complement-fixing antibody. More common at the turn of the century, PCH is usually associated with syphilis, particularly congenital syphilis, or various viral infections.

A paroxysm of hemolysis begins with the binding of D-L antibody to red cells at or below 20–25°C. When blood temperature rises several degress, complement is rapidly are fully activated. The resulting lysis of circulating red cells is accompanied by pronounced erythrophagocytosis and abrupt granulocytopenia. A weakly positive anti-C3 or anti-IgG Coombs test may appear and persist for a day or two. D-L antibody is invariably an autoantibody directed at the P antigen (see lecture 16). If antibody persists, recurrence is prevented simply by avoidance of cold.

SELECTED REFERENCES

Reviews

Ahn, Y. S., Harrington, W. J., et al. Danazol therapy for autoimmune hemolytic anemia. *Ann. Intern. Med.* 102(1985): 298–301.

Churchill, W. H. Transfusion problems in immunohemolytic anemias. In Churchill, W. H. and Kurtz, S. R., eds. *Transfusion Medicine.* Boston: Blackwell Scientific Publications, 1988, pp. 265–274.

Frank, M. M. Complement in the pathophysiology of human disease. *N. Engl. J. Med.* 316(1987): 1525–1530.

Frank, M. M., Chreiber, A. D., et al. Pathophysiology of immune hemolytic anemia. *Ann. Intern. Med.* 87(1977): 210–222.

Freedman, J. The significance of complement on the red cell surface. *Trans. Med. Rev.* 1(1987): 58–70.

Garraty, G. The significance of IgG on the red cell surface. *Trans. Med. Rev.* 1(1987): 45–57.

Multiple authors, NIH conference. Pathophysiology of immune hemolytic anemia. *Ann. Intern. Med.* 87(1977): 210–222.

Salama, A., and Mueller-Eckhardt, C. On the mechanisms of sensitization and attachment of antibodies to RBC in drug-induced immune hemolytic anemia. *Blood* 69(1987): 1006–1010.

Sinha, A. A., Lopez, M. T., and McDevitt, H. O. Autoimmune diseases: the failure of self-tolerance. *Science* 248(1990): 1380–1388.

Original articles

Fries, L. F., Brickman, C. M., and Frank, M. M. Monocyte receptors for the Fc portion of IgG increase in number of autoimmune hemolytic anemia and other hemolytic states and are decreased by glucocorticoid therapy. *J. Immunol.* 131(1983): 1240–1245.

Jaffe, C. J., Atkinson, J. P., and Frank, M. M. The role of complement in the clearance of cold agglutinin sensitized erythrocytes in man. *J. Clin. Invest.* 58(1976): 942–949.

Kelton, J. G. Impaired reticuloendothelial function in patients treated with Methyldopa. *N. Engl. J. Med.* 313(1985): 596–600.

Kirtland, H. H., Mohler, D. N., and Horwitz, D. A. Methyldopa inhibition of suppressor-lymphocyte function. *N. Engl. J. Med.* 302(1980): 825.

Kleinman, S., Nelson, R., et al. Positive direct antiglobulin tests and immune hemolytic anemia in patients receiving procainamide. *N. Engl. J. Med.* 311(1984): 809–812.

Parker, C. J., Frame, R. N., and Elstad, M. R. Vitronectin (S protein) augments the functional activity of monocyte receptors for IgG and complement C3b. *Blood* 71(1988): 86–93.

Parker, C. J., Soldato, C. M., and Jelen, M. J. Increased efficiency of binding of nascent C3b to the erythrocytes. *J. Clin. Invest.* 74(1984): 1050–1062.

Rosse, W. F. The control of complement activation by the blood cells in paroxysmal nocturnal hemoglobinuria. *Blood* 67(1986): 268–269.

Salama, A., Gottsche, B., et al. "Immune complex" mediated intravascular hemolysis due to IgM cephalosporin-dependent antibody. *Transfusion* 27(1987): 460–463.

Shirey, R. S., Bartholomew, J., et al. Characterization of antibody and selection of alternative drug therapy in hydrochlorothiazide-induced immune hemolytic anemia. *Transfusion* 27(1987): 70–72.

Silberstein, L. E., Berkman, E. M., and Schreiber, A. D. Cold hemagglutinin disease associated with IgG cold-reactive antibody. *Ann. Intern. Med.* 106(1987): 238–242.

Symposium on innovative use of IV gammaglobulin. *Am. J. Med.* (1987): Suppl. 4A.

Victoria, E. J., Pierce, S. W., et al. IgG red blood cell autoantibodies in autoimmune hemolytic anemia bind to epitopes on red blood cell membrane band 3 glycoprotein. *J. Lab. Clin. Med.* 115(1990): 74–88.

Zupanska, B., Brojer, E., et al. Monocyte-erythrocyte interaction in autoimmune haemolytic anaemia in relation to the number of erythrocyte-bound IgG molecules and subclass specificity of autoantibodies. *Vox Sang* 52(1987): 212–218.

LECTURE 14

Hemolytic Anemias III. Membrane Disorders

William S. Beck and Robert I. Tepper

EDITOR'S COMMENT

This lecture deals with a group of common disorders that are both hereditary and acquired. It also discusses a number of rare entities whose importance lies in the remarkable contributions their study has made to our understanding of the structure of cell membranes and cytoskeletons. In many ways, these advances resemble those that took place in the clotting field—when rare patients were encountered whose clotting defects could not be explained by then current understanding of the clotting reaction. Thus were new clotting factors discovered. In the same way, patients are constantly turning up with hemolysis and some sort of membrane disorder, in whom subsequent investigation reveals a lacking or defective cytoskeletal component that had previously gone unrecognized. Indeed, we are still discovering new components and properties of these structures by finding them missing or defective. Needless to say, much that has been learned in the study of red cell structure is relevant for the membranes of all eukaryotic cells.

I. RED CELL MEMBRANE

Hemolysis of red cells in hypotonic solution leaves a membranous residue known as red cell **ghosts** or **stroma**. Ghosts are remnants of red cell membranes, which surround red cells and perform various essential functions.

Much is now known about this readily available membrane. Because it is structurally and functionally similar to the outer membrane of diverse cell types (e.g., brain, kidney, and other blood cells), the red cell membrane serves as a useful model.

A. Structure and composition

The primary membrane structure is a bilayer that by weight is half lipid and half protein.

1. Membrane lipids

The outer and inner layers of the red cell membrane include many different lipid components, but despite their diversity, they occur in a limited number of categories:

- A matrix of **cholesterol** and **phospholipid** molecules. A single red cell contains about 1.9×10^8 cholesterol molecules and 2.4×10^8 phospholipid molecules.
- **Glycosphingolipids**, which have an outer end that is a branching structure of simple sugars and a tail end that anchors them to the membrane surface. The root *-sphingo* identifies them as a special class of glycolipids that includes a structural component, sphingosine.
- Other **glycolipids**, less well understood, which are confined to the outer monolayer. A red cell contains about 1.2×10^7 glycolipid molecules.

a. MAJOR COMPONENTS

Phospholipids and nonesterified cholesterol account for more than 95% of the total lipids present. On a molar basis, phospholipids and cholesterol are equal in amount. Phospholipids (other than sphingomyelin) are named for the base attached to the third glycerol carbon. Fatty acids are attached to the other two carbons, except in **lysophosphatides**, which contain only one fatty acid. The parent compound of sphingomyelin is sphingosin, a more complex alcohol.

One milliliter of red cells contains about 3 mg of phospholipids. The major ones and their relative abundance are:

- Phosphatidylcholine, 30%
- Phosphatidylethanolamine, 29%
- Phosphatidylserine, 10%
- Sphingomyelin, 25%
- Lysolecithin, 2%

b. PHYSICAL ORGANIZATION

The lipids are asymmetrically organized in the membrane.

- Choline phosphatides (phosphatidylcholine and sphingomyelin) are primarily on the outer leaf of the bilayer, which faces the plasma.
- Amino phosphatides (phosphatidylethanolamine and phosphatidylserine) are on the inner leaf, which faces the cytoplasm.
- Cholesterol is approximately equally distributed.
- Lysophosphatides, being equally lipophilic and hydrophilic, collect at phase inferfaces. Under certain circumstances, these molecules are potent detergents that can lyse red cell membranes—hence, their name.

Two lipid-related properties of bilayers critically influence membrane functions:

- Hydrophobic conditions within the membrane makes it impermeable to most polar biomolecules (amino acids, sugars, macromolecules), ions, and other compounds that are water-soluble and lipid-insoluble.
- The lipids have many properties of a fluid. The hydrophobic tails of phospholipid molecules can wiggle about in a relatively nonresistant

medium. In addition, each lipid monolayer is itself a two-dimensional fluid in which individual lipid molecules—and many (but not all) proteins—are free to "creep" sideways as though diffusing in a thin film—and they do so millions of times a second at a measurable rate of speed (120 μm/min). Only rarely do phospholipids flip from one monolayer to the other. Cholesterol enhances membrane fluidity.

Although mature red cells do not synthesize lipids, membrane lipids are in dynamic equilibrium with the lipids of plasma lipoproteins and the red cell constantly remodels its lipids.

- Membrane cholesterol exchanges rapidly with plasma unesterified cholesterol but not with esterified cholesterol. The cholesterol content of red cells may decrease 40% without detectable change in membrane function.
- Some membrane phospholipids exchange with plasma phospholipids. Others do not. Phospholipid exchange is slow relative to cholesterol exchange. No appreciable loss of phospholipid can take place without membrane damage.
- Lysophosphatides exchange rapidly with plasma lysophosphatides, which are albumin-bound.

2. *Membrane proteins*

The membrane contains 10 major and perhaps as many as 200 minor proteins (figure 14.1). These are also asymmetrically organized. Membrane lipids form a permeability barrier, but specific membrane proteins mediate most other membrane functions.

a. CLASSIFICATIONS

Membrane proteins are roughly classified into two categories according to their structure:

- Chunky globular proteins that are embedded in the lipid bilayer
- Single polypeptide chains in the form of an α-helix that extend through the membrane, sometimes weaving back and forth across the membrane with the intramembrane portion consisting of as many as seven α-helical regions

Ends of both types of proteins exposed to the extracellular environment may bear attached carbohydrate chains and thus are glycoproteins. Glycoproteins on the outer surface include proteins carrying red cell antigens (see lecture 16) and/or receptors (e.g., glycophorins A and B) or transport proteins (e.g., band 3, the anion exchange channel). Note that protein "band names" relate to their sequential position after electrophoresis in SDS-polycrylamide gel.

Another classification of membrane proteins is based on their position in the membrane.

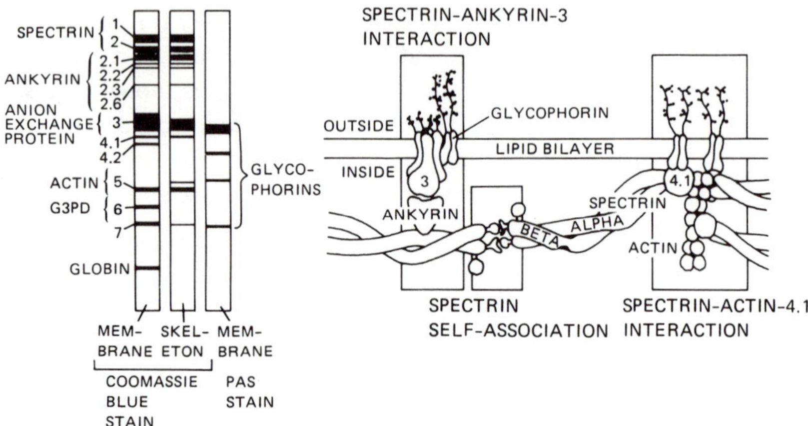

Fig. 14.1
Composition and arrangement of red cell membrane proteins. *Left*, SDS-polyacrylamide gel patterns of the major proteins (stained with Coomassie blue) and sialoglycoproteins (stained with periodic acid Schiff, PAS) of the red cell membrane and membrane skeleton. *Right*, Schematic illustration of the organization of the major proteins and sialoglycoproteins. The major integral proteins, band 3 and the glycophorins, traverse the lipid bilayer. The major peripheral membrane proteins, spectrin, actin, ankyrin, and band 4.1 form a protein meshwork (the membrane skeleton) that is attached to the inner membrane surface. Like ankyrin, bands 4.2 and 6 (not shown) bind to the cytoplasmic portion of band 3. The location of band 7 is unknown.

- **Integral** (or **intrinsic**) **proteins** are deeply embedded in the lipid bilayer and only a small part of the molecule reaches the inner or outer surface, or both surfaces. In penetrating the lipid bilayer, these proteins interact with the hydrophobic lipid core and are tightly bound to the membrane.
- **Peripheral** (or **extrinsic**) **proteins** are not embedded in the bilayer but rest upon one surface or the other. They often bind to each other or to integral proteins. Peripheral proteins include certain enzymes (e.g., glyceraldehyde-3-phosphate dehydrogenase), structural proteins such as spectrin and actin, and hemoglobin.

b. MEMBRANE SKELETON

Studies employing freeze-fracture, differential extraction with nonionic detergents, and protein cross-linking techniques reveal a remarkable membrane skeleton that serves to modulate cell shape and deformability. A dense, two-dimensional network of interconnected peripheral membrane proteins, the skeleton lies along the inner membrane surface (figure 14.2).

When the skeleton is isolated by extracting intact red cells or ghosts with nonionic detergents, its principal components are shown to be the following:

- Spectrin, α and β (bands 1 and 2)
- Actin (band 5)

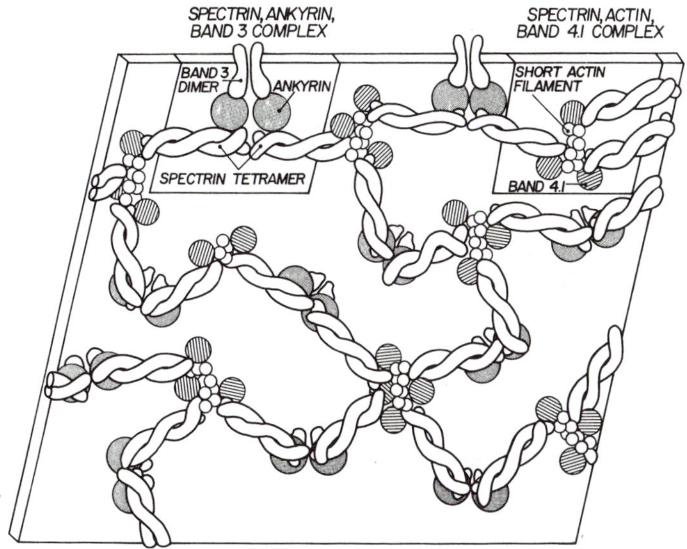

Fig. 14.2
Red blood cell membrane and its protein skeleton. The diagram shows scaffolding of membrane skeleton to underside (cytoplasmic side) of red cell membrane. Transmembrane proteins are anchored on the cytoplasmic side by fibrous proteins that help to maintain the characteristic biconcave shape of the cell. Note that spectrin binds directly to ankyrin, which is anchored to the membrane by a linkage to band 3. Actin is also present. It binds to spectrin and the actin-spectrin complex binds to a membrane glycoprotein called glycophorin. (From S. E. Lux, in W. S. Beck, ed., *Hematology*, 4th ed. Cambridge, MA: MIT Press, 1985.)

- Band 4.1
- Ankyrin (bands 2.1, 2.2, 2.3, and 2.6)

Spectrin, the major skeletal protein, is a heterodimer composed of two long chains (α and β subunits) that are aligned in parallel and variably twisted around each other. Bands 1 and 2 are dimeric and monomeric forms of spectrin. Spectrin dimers self-associate at their head ends to form tetramers or higher oligomeric forms.

At their tail-end, spectrin dimers interact with short filaments of actin and band 4.1. The latter bind to spectrin near the actin binding site. Because multiple spectrins can bind to each actin filament, this interaction serves as a molecular junction, which allows the spectrin to branch and form a two-dimensional network.

The whole skeleton is anchored to the overhead lipid bilayer by ankyrin, which tightly binds to β-spectrin near its head end and links it to the inner pole of the integral membrane protein band 3.

A second membrane binding site for the skeleton connects band 4.1 with the integral membrane protein **glycophorin C.** Still another is the interaction of band 4.1 with band 3.

The net effect of this complex series of spectrin-spectrin interactions and skeleton-membrane interactions is to produce a supporting structure of great strength and integrity. The skeleton stabilizes the asymmetric organization of membrane phospholipids. It also interacts with and immobilizes most of the membrane spanning (integral) proteins and thus determines, at least in part, their arrangement on the external membrane surface. Because membrane fusion, endocytosis, and certain cell-to-cell interactions require rearrangement of integral membrane proteins, these processes are also influenced by the organization state of the membrane skeleton.

c. GLYCOPHORINS

The glycophorins are a family of transmembrane integral protein that forms a hydrophilic, anionic, carbohydrate coat around red cells. The major component, **glycophorin A** (75% of the total) is a single polypeptide chain with 16 attached oligosaccharide units comprising 60% of the molecular mass (figure 14.3). It was the first integral membrane protein to be sequenced.

Glycophorin consists of three parts:

- An N-terminal region containing all of the carbohydrate units, which is located on the extracellular face of the membrane.
- A hydrophobic middle region that is buried within the hydrocarbon core of the membrane.
- A C-terminal region rich in polar and ionized side chains, which is exposed on the cytosolic face of the red cell membrane.

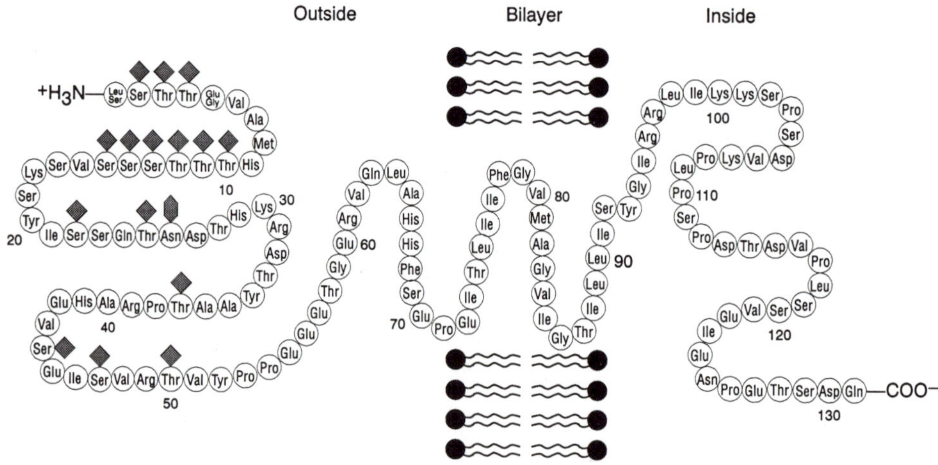

Fig. 14.3
Amino acid sequence and transmembrane disposition of glycophorin A from the red-cell membrane. The diagram shows 15 *O*-linked carbohydrate units and one *N*-linked unit. The hydrophobic residues buried in the bilayer form a transmembrane α helix. The carboxyl-terminal part of the molecule, located on the cytosolic side of the membrane, is rich in negatively charged and positively charged residues. (From L. Stryer, *Biochemistry*, 3rd ed. New York: W. H. Freeman, 1988.)

Some glycophorin molecules are phosphorylated. Surprisingly, individuals lacking glycophorin A appear otherwise normal.

B. Major functions

1. Membrane skeletal functions

As noted above, the membrane skeleton is a major determinant of red cell shape, flexibility (deformability), and integrity. Thus it permits red cells to resist strong shearing forces. Red cell morphologic abnormalities and hemolytic disorders are associated with qualitative and quantitative abnormalities of membrane skeleton proteins. For example:

- Selective extraction of spectrin and actin, or heat denaturation of spectrin produces membrane vesiculation.
- Mice with genetic spectrin deficiency have fragile red cells that spontaneously lose membrane fragments in the circulation, leading to marked spherocytosis and severe hemolysis.
- Deficiency of band 4.1 occurs in hereditary elliptocytosis.

Other such abnormalities are discussed below.

2. Maintenance of cell volume

The red cell controls its volume and water content by controlling its Na^+ and K^+ content. Increase in red cell volume as a result of excessive water is prevented by two mechanisms:

- The relative impermeability of the cell membrane to cations.
- Active extrusion of cations (primarily Na^+) by a process that is linked to K^+ influx, three molecules of Na^+ being "pumped" out for every two molecules of K^+ "pumped" in. These active linked processes require ATP and depend upon a **Na-K–ATPase** in the membrane.

Clearly, preservation of the membrane's selective permeability properties is vital to cell survival. If the rate of Na^+ influx is increased to 3–4 times normal, the limited capacity of membrane cation pumps is exceeded, and red cell volume increases. Red cells swell when Na^+ leaking in exceeds K^+ leaking out. They shrink when K^+ leaking out exceeds Na^+ leaking in.

Since glycolysis, the metabolic source of ATP, cannot increase to more than twice the normal rate, ATP levels decline in such circumstances. Cell swelling occurs and osmotic hemolysis ensues (see lecture 15).

3. Ca^{2+} homeostasis

The membrane contains an efficient calcium pump protein, which is an ATP-dependent calcium pump (**Ca^{2+}–ATPase**) that actively extrudes potentially deleterious Ca^{2+} from the cell interior. Intracellular Ca^{2+} is normally almost undetectable. If ATP levels fall (to 20% of normal) or if Ca^{2+} leakage exceeds the capacity of the calcium pump, rising intracellular Ca^{2+} may disassemble the skeletal lattice with resulting change in cell shape from a biconcave disk to an **echinocyte**, a spiculated sphere with short, regular projections.

Elevated intracellular Ca^{2+} also causes a selective loss of K^+ and H_2O (**Gardos effect**). The result is a crenated, dehydrated, almost indeformable cell that is highly susceptible to splenic sequestration and destruction. The calcium pump is regulated by a cytoplasmic Ca^{2+}-binding protein called **calmodulin**. When intracellular Ca^{2+} rises, Ca^{2+}-calmodulin activates Ca^{2+}–ATPase, accelerating Ca^{2+} egress.

4. *Anion exchange*

The red cell is a critical participant in CO_2 transport. They carry HCO_3^- ions to the lungs, where they are exchanged for Cl^-. The massive exchange process (7×10^{10} anions per red cell per second) requires about 5×10^5 exchange channels. The channel is formed by band 3, a major red cell membrane component.

II. INTERACTIONS BETWEEN RED CELLS AND SPLEEN

A. Flow patterns

Although the spleen comprises only 0.2% of body weight, it receives 6% of the cardiac output. Thus about 300 ml of blood per minute courses through the unique blood vessel network shown in figure 3.6, which has alternative open (90% traffic) and closed (10% traffic) channels.

Red cells in the rapid-transit open circuit must repeatedly squeeze their 7-μm-diameter bodies through the narrow 3-μm, elliptical fenestrations that separate the splenic cords and sinuses (figure 14.4). A normal red cell traverses the spleen 120 times per day and completes the journey in approximately 30 sec, but abnormal red cells—those with abnormal shapes, attached antibodies, inclusion bodies, parasites etc.—may be detained for minutes to hours in the stagnant, acidic, hypoxic, hypoglycemic environment of the splenic cords. We saw in lecture 10 the disastrous consequences of this sequence in sickle cell anemia. This is an exacting test for abnormal red cells. Often old and defective red cells fail to meet it and are destroyed. Sometimes bits of membrane are removed and the cell becomes a spherocyte (see below). Sometimes inclusion body may be removed and leave a "pitted out," misshapen red cell remnant.

B. Red cell deformability

Red cells are detained in the splenic cords if they are poorly deformable or if they bear proteins (e.g., IgG1, IgG3, or C3b) that can bind to receptors on splenic phagocytes (see lecture 13). Other, still undefined alterations in the membrane surface may also attract the attention of phagocytes and lead to red cell destruction. Decreased red cell deformability may result from:

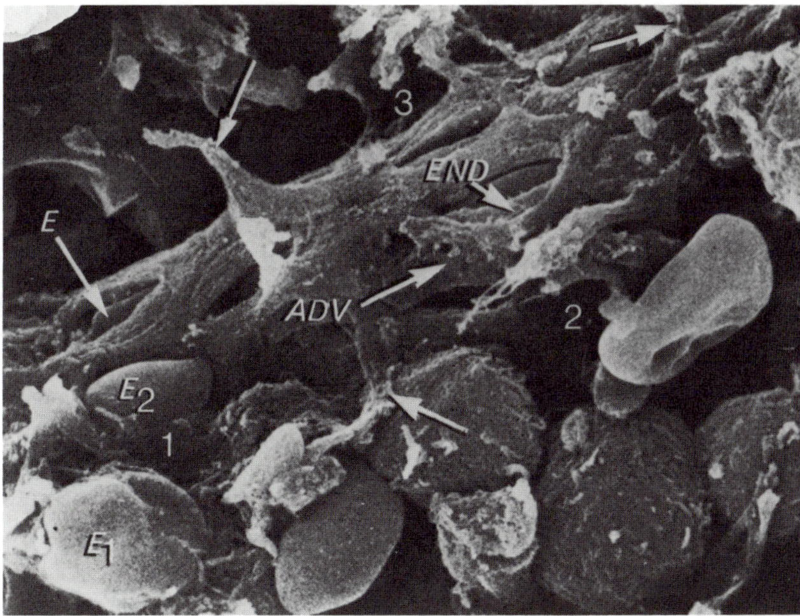

Fig. 14.4
Scanning electron micrograph of a splenic sinus wall viewed from a splenic cord. A portion of the overlying cordal structure has been removed. The narrow transmural slits between the endothelial (END) cells of the sinus wall are easily seen. It is likely that these cells are normally opposed and that the slits are potential structures rather than fixed pores. They are evident here because of a drying artifact. Note that the adjacent erythrocytes (E) are considerably larger than the slits and hence must be flexible to pass into the splenic sinuses. (ADV, adventitial cell.)

- An increase in cytoplasmic viscosity (e.g., sickled cells, dehydrated red cells)
- Intracellular debris (e.g., Heinz bodies)
- Membrane rigidity (e.g., due to oxidant-induced cross-linking of the membrane skeleton)
- A decrease in red cell surface-to-volume ratio

C. Surface-to-volume ratio

1. Spherocytosis

Spherocytosis occurs when the surface-to-volume ratio decreases. The term **microspherocytosis** is used when a decreased ratio is due to diminution of surface area. **Macrospherocytosis** results from increase in cell volume within a normal cell membrane. Both changes (membrane loss and transient swelling) accompany most hemolytic processes involving spherocytosis.

Because the red cell membrane is flexible but not stretchable, the red cell becomes progressively less deformable as its spheroidicity increases. A useful analogy is the progressive filling of a plastic bag with water. When half-filled, the bag (like a spherocyte) is almost indeformable.

2. *Target cells*

When the surface-to-volume ratio increases, the resulting flattened cells appear in blood smears as **target cells**. This results from redundancy of membrane and from disorders causing cell volume to decrease but intracellular hemoglobin to decrease even more proportionately (e.g., iron deficiency, thalassemia.) The targeted appearance results from the puddling of hemoglobin during drying. Poorly soluble hemoglobins (e.g., hemoglobins C and S) precipitate more rapidly than normal during air-drying of blood smears. Consequently, target cells, usually smaller than those of high surface area disorders (see below), are seen in these hemoglobinopathies.

3. *Osmotic fragility*

The **osmotic fragility test** is a useful indirect measure of the surface-to-volume ratio. As shown in figure 14.5, the test measures the ability of red cells to swell in hypotonic media.

Spherocytes, with a decreased surface-to-volume ratio, are highly fragile; that is, they can tolerate less osmotic swelling than normal red cells before they burst. Target cells, in contrast, are relatively osmotically resistant, given their excess surface-to-volume ratio.

III. DISORDERS OF RED CELL SHAPE

Certain membrane disorders are classified by the shape changes they produce. Red cell shape may be viewed in terms of associated changes in membrane surface area and cellular volume (figure 14.6). A more detailed presentation of this concept appears in figure 14.7.

A. Hereditary spherocytosis (HS)

Hereditary spherocytosis is a common hemolytic anemia of varying severity that affects 1 in every 5000 individuals in the United States and probably more in view of recent data on the carrier state. It is usually inherited as an autosomal dominant.

1. *Pathogenesis*

Two major factors operate in HS:

- An underlying defect in the red cells, which is reflected in shortened survivals of HS red cells transfused into normal subjects and normal survivals of normal red cells transfused into HS patients
- An intact spleen that selectively retains and destroys HS red cells

a. MEMBRANE INSTABILITY

The primary defect is membrane instability due to dysfunction or deficiency of a skeletal protein. As a result, cell membranes fragment easily

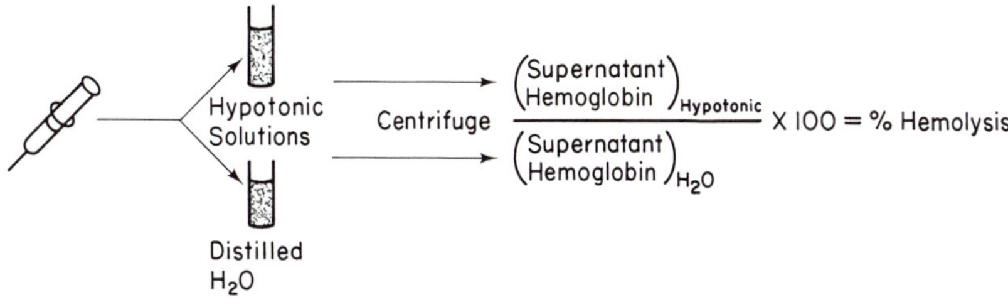

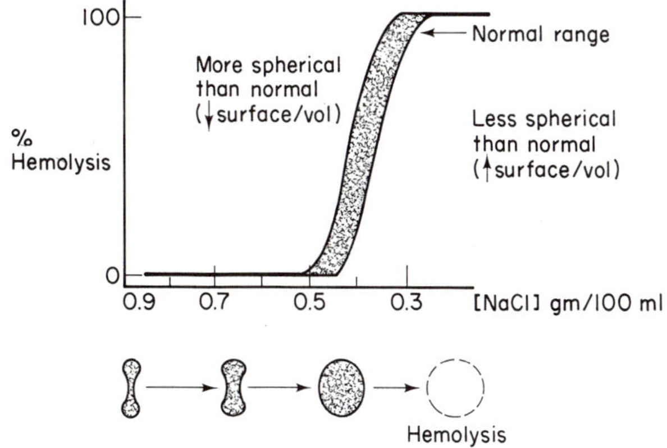

Fig. 14.5
Schematic illustration of the osmotic fragility test. Equal aliquots of blood are placed in equal volumes of buffered salt solutions of varying osmolarity or in distilled water. After a brief incubation, the unhemolyzed red cells are removed by centrifugation and the supernatant hemoglobin released at each salt concentration is compared to the distilled water sample (100% lysis) to determine the percentage hemolysis. The osmotic fragility (OF) curve is a plot of the percentage hemolysis vs. the sodium chloride concentration (conventionally plotted as decreasing from left to right on the *x*-axis). (From S. E. Lux, in W. S. Beck, *Hematology*, 4th ed. Cambridge, MA: MIT Press, 1985.)

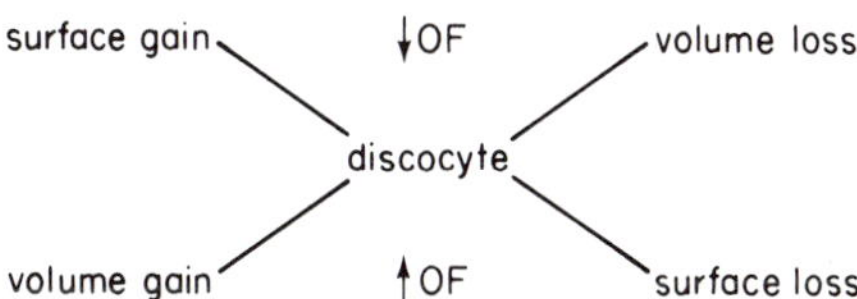

Fig. 14.6
Changes in surface area and volume associated with disorders of red cell shapes. (From S. E. Lux, in W. S. Beck, *Hematology*, 4th ed. Cambridge, MA: MIT Press, 1985.)

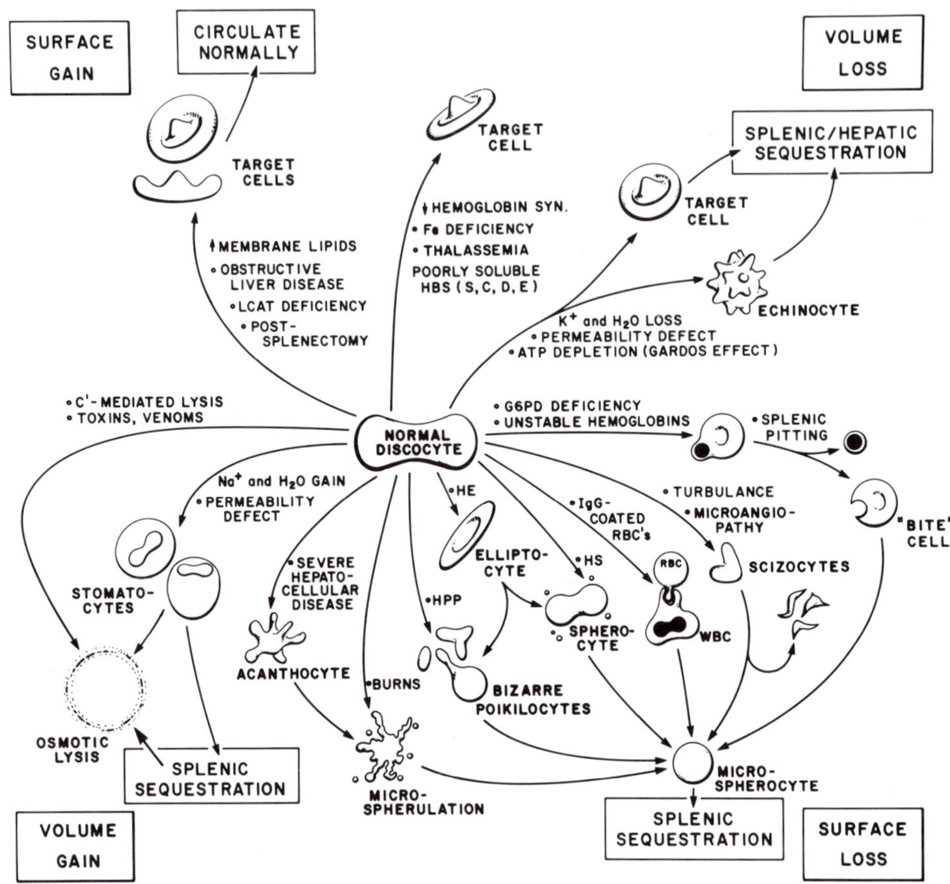

Fig. 14.7

Summary of the major abnormalities of red cell surface area, volume, and shape. (From S. E. Lux, in W. S. Beck, *Hematology*, 4th ed. Cambridge, MA: MIT Press, 1985.)

under mechanical stress and are leaky to Na^+. Recent studies have revealed a variety of membrane skeleton defects in different HS families:

- **Spectrin deficiency**. In these patients, the degree of spectrin deficiency correlates with the degree of spherocytosis and with clinical severity. Most HS patients have mild deficiencies—spectrin content is 75–90% of normal—but in rare, apparently homozygous patients, spectrin content may be 30–50% of normal. These patients have severe hemolysis and are transfusion-dependent. It is not yet certain whether spectrin deficiency is the primary molecular defect.

- **β-Spectrin dysfunction**. In 10% of HS patients, half of the spectrin molecules lack the ability to bind band 4.1. As a result, spectrins bind poorly to actin, weakening the skeleton. This defect can be corrected in vitro with reducing agents. The availability of cDNA probes for α- and β-spectrin and band 4.1 should soon clarify these abnormalities.

- **Ankyrin deficiency**. An abnormal ankyrin molecule is unstable and rapidly degraded.
- **Band 4.2 deficiency**. Occurs in a few families.

b. SPLENIC CONDITIONING

As shown in figure 14.8, membrane weakness leads to repeated loss of membrane fragments as the HS red cell circulates and a gradual decrease in surface-to-volume ratio and increased spheroidicity. This causes HS red cells to be detained in splenic cords, where for unknown reasons membrane surface loss is augmented by the cordal environment. In vivo, splenic conditioning involves multiple episodes of splenic stasis. In vitro, it can be partially stimulated by incubating red cells in the absence of glucose for 24 hours. In this setting, as in the spleen, HS red cells rapidly lose membrane fragments. This is the basis of the **incubated osmotic fragility test**.

Conditioned red cells escaping from the splenic pulp into the blood account for the "tail" on osmotic fragility curves. In blood smears, they appear as dense, hyperchromic microspherocytes characteristic of HS. Many HS red cells never escape the spleen and are destroyed. Those that do escape are vulnerable to recapture by the spleen where their nondeformability leads to eventual destruction.

2. *Clinical features*

Neonatal jaundice is common and may require exchange transfusion (see lecture 7). After the neonatal period, most patients develop a partially compensated hemolytic state with the following consequences:

- Mild to moderate anemia.
- Mild or intermittent jaundice—especially during virus infections.
- Splenomegaly.
- Bilirubin gallstones secondary to hemolysis.
- Occasional leg ulcers.
- In a quarter of HS patients, the picture is mild owing to marrow compensation. There is an elevated reticulocyte count, but no anemia and little jaundice or splenomegaly.
- In contrast, a few patients are severely anemic and transfusion-dependent.
- In some cases the diagnosis is first made in old age.

3. *Laboratory features*

The following findings are characteristic:

- **Blood smear**: spherocytosis and an increase in reticulocytes.
- **Bone marrow**: normoblastic erythroid hyperplasia.
- Mild elevation of indirect-reacting serum bilirubin and increased urobilinogen, but no bilirubin in the urine.
- Negative Coombs test.

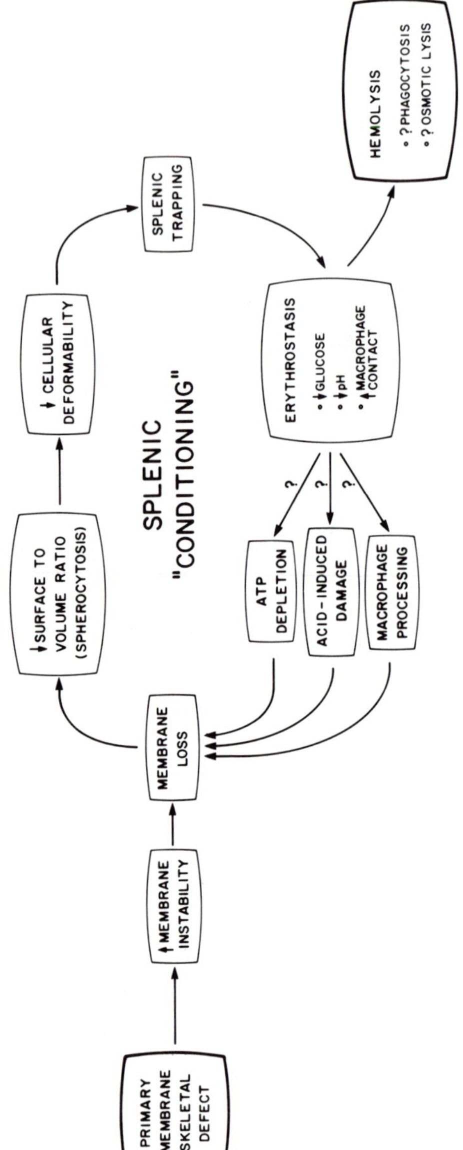

Fig. 14.8
Currently model for the pathophysiology of HS.

Table 14.1
Types of Crises Seen in Patients with Hemolysis

Type of crisis	Anemia	Reticulocytes	Jaundice	Cause	Comment
Hemolytic	↑	↑	↑	Infection	Frequent, mild
Aplastic	↑	↓	↓	Infection	Infrequent, severe
Megaloblastic	↑	↓	↑	Relative folate deficiency	Infrequent

Spherocytosis, the hallmark of the disease, is always present, but in 20–25% of patients, typical microspherocytes are sparse. In these patients, the unincubated osmotic fragility test may be normal or only slightly abnormal since it simply quantifies what is seen in the smear. However, the *incubated* osmotic fragility test is almost always abnormal and is the most reliable simple diagnostic test available.

4. Crises

The course in most patients is punctuated by "crises" characterized by worsening anemia. Three types occur (table 14.1):

- **Hemolytic** crises are the most common. These are often mild. They are probably due to the reticuloendothelial hyperplasia accompanying many infections.
- **Aplastic** crises, due to viral suppression of erythropoiesis, are less frequent, but are often severe enough to require transfusion. Many are caused by a human parvovirus. They are common in the flu season. Major diagnostic clues are: depressed reticulocyte count and decreased erythroid precursors in the marrow.
- **Megaloblastic** crises occur when dietary intake of folic acid is inadequate to the increased folate requirement of hyperactive erythropoiesis, especially in pregnant patients (see lecture 6). These may be prevented by administration of folic acid.

5. Therapy

Splenectomy dependably halts both red cell conditioning and hemolysis in most HS patients although the basic red cell defect (which produces spherocytosis, increased Na^+ flux, and so forth) remains. Thus, spherocytosis persists, but conditioned microspherocytes disappear. The blood smear also acquires the changes typical of the postsplenectomy state (Howell-Jolly bodies, target cells, siderocytes, and acanthocytes).

Since splenectomy increases susceptibility to infection from pneumococci and other encapsulated bacteria, especially in infancy and childhood (lecture 3), it is usually delayed until age 5 or 6 years.

B. Hereditary elliptocytosis (HE) and related disorders

Hereditary elliptocytosis is inherited as an autosomal dominant and is common (1:2500), particularly the mild form. It is due to defects in the membrane skeleton, since ghosts and isolated skeletons retain the elliptical shape. The many observed molecular abnormalities in HE and a variety of related disorders include the following:

- Dysfunctional spectrins of various kinds
- Spectrin deficiency
- Band 4.1 defects
- Glycophorin C deficiency

It is unclear how the various molecular defects of the membrane skeleton relate to the abnormal red cell shapes and the presence or absence of hemolysis in the HE syndromes. The elliptocytic shape change is acquired in the circulation. HE red cells are disk-shaped. Since normal red cells are caused to undergo elliptical deformation by shear stress in capillaries, it may be that HE red cells, with their weakened skeletons, simply are rearranged to this configuration by repeated passages through the microcirculation. When the skeletal defect is severe, the red cells cannot withstand circulatory shear stresses and fragment in the circulation. In these disorders the compliant skeletons are grossly deformed, and bizarre pokilocytosis results.

The following syndromes are well recognized.

1. Mild HE

This is the common form of HE (90% of cases). It is often, though not always, caused by structural defects in the head end of spectrin, which interfere with spectrin self-association, causing impaired conversion of dimers to tetramers. Most patients have no anemia or splenomegaly, only mild hemolysis, and reticulocyte counts of 1–4%. The blood smear shows prominent elliptocytosis. Note that a few elliptocytes are seen in normal blood.

In some patients, the low number of elliptocytes is confusing. In them, the diagnosis rests on evidence that one of the parents has typical mild HE. A minority (10–20%) displays moderate hemolysis. Although classified in some texts as "sporadic hemolytic variant," this pattern may be due to such other factors as infection, splenomegaly due to other diseases, and so on. Patients with mild HE require to therapy.

2. HE with neonatal poikilocytosis

Neonates in some HE families (often black families) may have moderately severe hemolysis with red cell budding, fragmentation, and poikilocytosis. This is attributed to a curious chain of events, in which the spectrin-band 4.1 interaction is destabilized by increased levels of 2,3-DPG resulting from its low affinity for fetal hemoglobin. In a year or two, the picture evolves into mild HE.

3. Hereditary pyropoikilocytosis (HPP)

This rare autosomal recessive disorder is characterized by severe hemolytic anemia, marked red cell fragmentation, and microspherocytosis, bizarre poikilocytosis, and often (because of red cell shape abnormalities) an MCV as low as 50. It is most common in blacks. The red cells demonstrate striking thermal instability. HPP red cells fragment (and their isolated spectrin denatures) at 45–46°C instead of the normal 49°C. This is the primary test for the disease.

Hemolysis decreases after splenectomy, but bizarre red cell morphology and heat sensitivity remains. HPP is probably a subset of mild HE because (1) HPP patients often have relatives with mild HE, and (2) the defect in spectrin self-association is qualitatively similar to that in mild HE but more severe.

A current notion is that HPP patients are either homozygous for mild HE, homozygous for a related "silent" mutation, or doubly heterozygous for mild HE and the putative silent gene defect. Factors determining red cell shape and clinical severity in the HE and HPP syndromes are probably the fraction of unassembled, dimeric spectrin and the total spectrin content of the cells.

4. Spherocytic HE

This variant (10% of cases), also called **hereditary ovalocytosis**, resembles HS in that patients have moderate hemolysis, mild anemia, and splenomegaly. Elliptocytes are less prominent and more spheroidal than in typical mild HE. Spherocytes are often present and may predominate. However, a family member will have clear-cut elliptocytosis.

Patients with this form of HE, like those with HS, have osmotically fragile cells and respond well to splenectomy. A deficiency of band 4.1 occurs in some but not all families with this disorder.

IV. OTHER CAUSES OF MEMBRANE LOSS

A. Mechanical injury

An important hemolytic anemia results from the **mechanical damage** to red cells in the high-pressure arterial or arteriolar circulation by pathologic blood vessels. These circumstances cause red cell fragmentation (helmet cells, triangular fragments, and other schistocytes) and intravascular hemolysis (see lecture 12). Such cells in a blood smear suggests several possible underlying disorders:

- **Microangiopathic** hemolytic anemia may result from damage to arteriolar endothelium or from fibrin deposition within these vessels. This picture arises in the many disorders listed in table 14.2.

Table 14.2
Major Causes of Microangiopathic Hemolytic Anemia

Disseminated intravascular coagulation (see lecture 29)
Abruptio placenta
Purpura fulminans
Septicemia
Localized intravascular coagulation (see lecture 29)
Cavernous hemangioma
Collagen-vascular disease
Polyarteritis nodosa
Scleroderma
Systemic lupus erythematosus
Wegener's granulomatosis
Renal vascular disorders
Malignant hypertension
Preeclampsia
Renal transplant rejection
Disseminated carcinomatosis
Thrombotic thrombocytopenic purpura and hemolytic-uremic syndrome (see lecture 28)

- Excessive turbulence around an **artificial heart valve** (especially the aortic valve) or other intraventricular prosthesis. The shear stress produced literally tears the red cells apart. Hence, it has been called the **Waring blendor syndrome**. It is also called **macroangiopathic** hemolytic anemia.

B. Immunohemolytic anemia

As discussed in lecture 13, phagocytes bearing receptors for IgG1, IgG3, and C3b bind and detain red cells coated with these substances, remove portions of their membranes, or, in some cases, phagocytize them completely. Escaped red cells that return to the blood as spherocytes are destined for splenic detention and recapture by phagocytes.

C. Heinz body hemolytic anemias

Intracellular precipitation of hemoglobin to form Heinz bodies occurs in unstable hemoglobinopathies (see lecture 10) and oxidant hemolysis, e.g., G-6-PD deficiency (see lecture 15). Splenic "pitting" of Heinz bodies may lead to the appearance of "bite cells" (see lecture 3), and occasionally to spherocytes.

D. Thermal injury

Spherocytes appear when blood is heated to temperatures above 49°C, due to damage to spectrin, which becomes denatured. The spherocytes result from marked membrane fragmentation (microspherulation). Spherocytic hemolytic anemia may result from third-degree burns covering more than 20% of the body surface.

E. Toxins and infections agents

Red cell life span may be moderately or severely shortened in infectious or inflammatory diseases, especially if the patient has G-6-PD deficiency (see lecture 15) or splenomegaly. In infections with the following organisms hemolysis is a prominent part of the clinical picture:

- The major malarial organisms
- *Bartonella bacilliformis*
- *Clostridium perfringens*
- *Babesia microtic* and *Babesia divergent*

In addition, various chemicals and venoms (e.g., of snakes and brown spiders) can cause membrane injury and spherocytosis.

F. Spiculated red cells

1. Acanthocytes (spur cells)

Acanthocytes are rounded red cells with **irregular**, thorny projections. They occur in some patients with severe hepatocellular disease (where they are often called **spur cells**) and in a variety of other rare conditions.

a. LIVER DISEASE

In severe liver disease (especially that due to alcoholism), acanthocytosis occurs in two stages: **cholesterol loading** and **splenic remodeling** (figure 14.9). In the first stage, abnormal cholesterol-laden lipoproteins, produced by the diseased liver, transfer their excess cholesterol to circulating red cells and increase membrane cholesterol, the cholesterol-phospholipid ratio, and the membrane surface area. This is an acquired process and can be mimicked in vitro by incubating normal red cells in plasma containing spur cells or in artificial media containing cholesterol-rich lipid dispersions. Microoscopically, these cholesterol-laden red cells are flattened (leptocytes) with a scalloped periphery. In vivo these cells are converted into spur cells by splenic conditioning. Over several days, membrane lipids and surface area are lost, cellular rigidity increases, and the cells assume a typical acanthocytic form (figure 14.9). Splenectomy prevents formation of spur cells and their premature destruction, but it is a high-risk procedure in these patients and is seldom indicated.

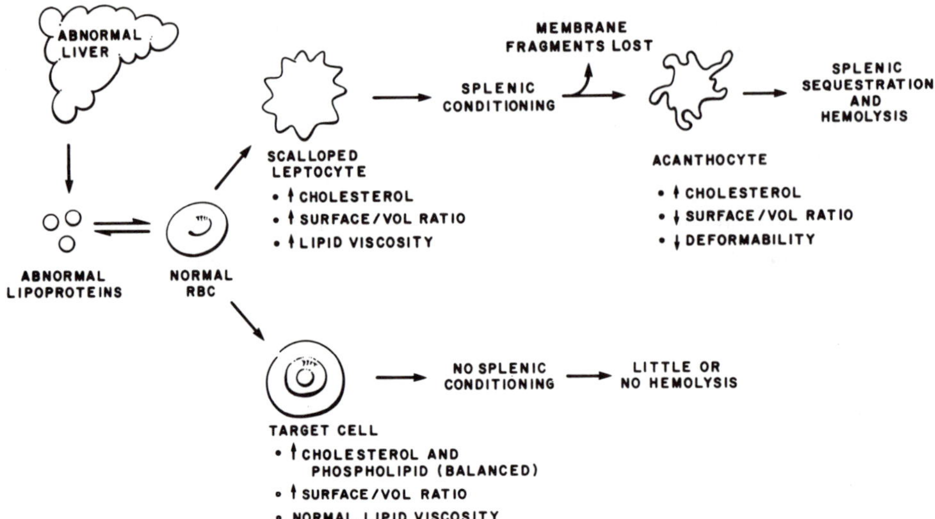

Fig. 14.9
Schematic illustration of the pathophysiology of acanthocyte (spur cell) and target cell formation in liver disease.

b. OTHER CAUSES

Acanthocytes are prominent in:

- Patients with a rare anomaly of the Kell blood group antigens (McLeod phenotype) (see lecture 16)
- The rare disease **abetalipoproteinemia**, in which there is an increase in membrane sphingomyelin, and thus decreased membrane fluidity
- Severe malnutrition, including that due to anorexia nervosa and cystic fibrosis
- Postsplenectomy state
- Hypothyroidism in some patients

2. *Echinocytes (burr cells)*

Unlike irregularly spiculated acanthocytes, echinocytes (crenated cells, burr cells) are covered with short, uniform spicules arranged in a **regular** array. This difference is easily appreciated in scanning electron micrographs, but may be difficult to discern in blood smears.

Echinocytes are common in severe **uremia** and occur in small numbers in normal newborns, in splenectomized patients, and in various hemolytic anemias. They have a nearly normal survival. Less viable echinocytes occur in conditions associated with **cell dehydration** and decreased intracellular volume (to be discussed) and rarely in patients with disseminated carcinomatosis or microangiopathic hemolytic anemia.

V. INCREASED MEMBRANE SURFACE AREA

A. Biliary obstruction

As noted earlier, **target cells** form when the red cell surface-to-volume ratio rises. Patients with liver disease associated with **biliary obstruction** often develop target cells. The pathogenesis of the shape change parallels that of spur cells (i.e., the red cells acquire excess lipids from abnormal lipoproteins), except that the lipid transfer involves both *cholesterol* and *phospholipids* in a ratio similar to that normally existing in red cell membranes (see figure 14.9). As a result, membrane surface area expands, but the cholesterol-phospholipid ratio remains normal. Because cellular deformability is unimpaired, these cells survive well, and the abnormality produces no clinical consequences.

B. Other causes

Other causes of excess membrane and targeting include the following:

- **Splenectomy**. The spleen normally removes some membrane lipid and protein components from reticulocytes soon after their release into the circulation. In splenectomized patients, this excess membrane material expands surface area, and small numbers of target cells appear on the blood smear.
- **Deficiency of the plasma enzyme lecithin–cholesterol acyltransferase (LCAT)**. This rare autosomal recessive disorder is also associated with corneal opacities, proteinuria, and premature atherosclerosis.

VI. VOLUME LOSS

A. Hemoglobin abnormalities

Target cells are also seen in pateints with abnormal hemoglobin synthesis, e.g., iron deficiency (see lecture 7) and thalassemia (see lecture 11) and in patients with certain abnormal hemoglobins, e.g., hemoglobins S, C, D, and E (see lecture 10).

B. Cation abnormalities

Loss of intracellular water leads to red cell dehydration or **xerocytosis**. As noted, cell water is regulated by intracellular monovalent cation content. If red cell membrane permeability is altered so that loss of K^+ (the predominant intracellular cation) exceeds gain of Na^+ (the predominant extracellular cation), total cation content and cell water decline.

This occurs as a primary disorder in the rare disease **hereditary xerocytosis** and as a secondary event in disorders associated with intracellular

Ca^{2+} accumulation (e.g., sickle cell anemia) (see lecture 10) or **ATP depletion** (e.g., pyruvate kinase deficiency) (see lecture 15).

Morphologically, dehydrated red cells are typically either targeted or contracted and spiculated. Because dehydration elevates intracellular viscosity, these cells are relatively rigid and risk splenic sequestration and hemolysis.

VII. VOLUME GAIN

A. Water volume

The analogous but opposite disorder to hereditary xerocytosis is **hereditary hydrocytosis**. In this rare condition, an inherited defect in Na^+ permeability causes **massive Na^{2+} influx**, which overwhelms the Na-K pump and leads to an increase in intracellular cations and water. Severe hemolysis results. The partially swollen blood cell appear on blood smears as **stomatocytes** (i.e., red cells with a mouthlike band of pallor across the center of the stained cell).

B. Other causes

Stomatocytes are also seen as an acquired defect, not associated with cation changes—particularly in patients with acute **alcoholism** and in various types of liver disease. Little hemolysis is present.

C. Complement-mediated intravascular hemolysis

Complement-mediated hemolysis may be considered a form of volume gain since red cell destruction occurs by rapid osmotic swelling (colloid osmotic hemolysis). Practically, however, complement lysis is so rapid that swollen macrospherocytes, which must occur as intermediates in this process, are not seen. Clinically, complement-mediated hemolysis occurs in some immunohemolytic anemias (e.g., PCH), in some transfusion reactions (e.g., ABO blood group incompatibility), and in **paroxysmal nocturnal hemoglobinuria** (PNH).

1. Paroxysmal nocturnal hemoglobinuria (PNH)

A notable feature of this fascinating disorder is its frequent misclassification in older texts. Commonly considered a type of hemolytic anemia, PNH is in fact a clonal, honmalignant, hematopoietic stem cell disorder that results in the formation of defective red cells, white cells, and platelets (figure 14.10).

- The **red cell** abnormality predisposes them to intravascular complement-mediated lysis, which waxes and wanes in severity. Hence, the cyclic variation in hemoglobinuria that is a feature of this disease.

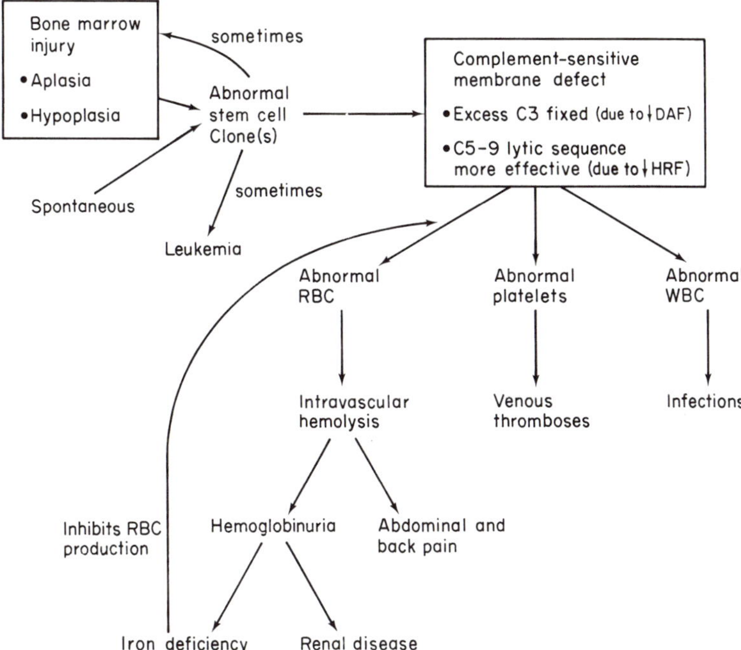

Fig. 14.10
Pathophysiology of PNH.

- The **white cell** abnormality is manifested by a decrease in leukocyte alkaline phosphates (LAP). This is one of the few diseases other than chronic myelocytic leukemia in which LAP is low (see lecture 22).
- The **platelet** abnormality is believed responsible for frequent venous thrombosis or bleeding.

a. PATHOPHYSIOLOGY

PNH is an **acquired** membrane disorder. Most abnormal PNH clones arise from a mutagenic event occurring in the course of aplastic anemia or **marrow hypoplasia**, but sometimes they occur without hypoplasia.

The pathophysiologic sequence is summarized in figure 14.10. The red cell defect, which leads to the most prominent clinical findings, is intracorpuscular, not extracorpuscular. Normal red cells survive normally in patients with PNH. PNH red cell membranes are deficient in two glycoproteins: **decay-accelerating factor** (DAF) and **homologous restriction factor** (HRF), which normally function to impede complement activation. The functional consequence is an **increased sensitivity to activated complement** due to an increased ability of PNH membranes to fix C3 and to more efficient penetration of the PNH membrane by the terminal lytic sequence of complement. All three cell lines are affected in this way.

Activation of complement is caused in various ways: lowering of pH, as in **acid hemolysis test**; reducing ionic strength, as in the **sucrose hemolysis**

test; treatment with cobra venom; increasing the Mg^{2+} concentration; or exposure to antibodies such as anti-A. Wide variations in the degree of complement sensitivity (and symptoms) is due, in part, to variability in the proportion of stem cells in the abnormal clones and, in part, to the degree of complement sensitivity of each of the clones.

In addition to complement sensitivity, there is diminished acetylcholinesterase activity in PNH red cells and increased susceptibility to hemolysis by hydrogen peroxide.

b. CLINICAL FEATURES

PNH patients present with the following clinical picture:

- **Hemoglobinuria** is present that, for unknown reasons, is worse at night and remits during the day. However, it is often irregular and not nocturnal. Some patients have chronic hemolysis without hemoglobinuria.
- Most patients have chronic **hemosiderinuria** and many eventually develop iron deficiency and/or renal injury owing to iron deposition. Iron therapy may be necessary, but is hazardous when iron-induced reticulocytosis produces new complement-sensitive cells that exacerbate hemolysis.
- During hemolytic episodes, patients may experience severe abdominal or back **pain** that may mimic a surgical emergency. There is often severe anemia, mild to moderate reticulocytosis, and erythroid hyperplasia in the marrow.
- There is often severe anemia, mild to moderate reticulocytosis, and erythroid hyperplasia in the marrow.
- There is typically a low white count (with low LAP) and a low or normal platelet count.
- Infection occurs due to leukopenia and/or abnormal function of PNH phagocytes.
- Some develop (or revert) to aplastic anemia.
- Others suffer from recurrent venous thromboses, especially of the portal venous system. These may be due to activation of the complement-sensitive platelets by C3.
- The PNH clone occasionally evolves into acute myelocytic leukemia (see lecture 22).

c. DIAGNOSTIC LABORATORY FEATURES

PNH can be present in many guises and is frequently considered in differential diagnoses. The diagnosis depends on:

- Detection of complement-sensitive red cells. In humans complement fixes to red cells at a slightly acid pH. PNH red cells lyse under these conditions even in the absence of antibody. The **acid-hemolysis test**, or **Ham test**, is a measure of this property.

- In the **sucrose hemolysis test** (or **sugar water test**), a medium of low ionic strength (i.e., isotonic sucrose) is used to aggregate serum globulins onto the red cell surface. This activates complement and promotes hemolysis of PNH red cells. Diagnostically this test is slightly more sensitive and the Ham tset is slightly more specific.

d. THERAPY

There is no specific therapy. Symptomatic treatment is given for anemia (red cell transfusions), iron deficiency (iron therapy), thrombocytopenia (platelet transfusions), and thromboses (anticoagulants). As in all diseases characterized by intravascular hemolysis, splenectomy produces little benefit. In patients with severe PNH-induced marrow aplasia, bone marrow transplantation may be life saving.

SELECTED REFERENCES

Reviews

Beutler, E. Paroxysmal nocturnal hemoglobinuria. In Williams, W. J., Beutler, E., et al., eds. *Hematology*, 4th ed. New York: McGraw-Hill, 1990, pp. 188–192.

Davies, K. A., and Lux, S. E. Hereditary disorders of the red cell membrane skeleton. *TIG* 5(1989): 222–227.

Larzarides, E., and Woods, C. Biogenesis of the red blood cell membrane-skeleton and the control of erythroid morphogenesis. *Annu. Rev. Cell Biol.* 5(1989): 427–452.

Palek, J. Acanthocytosis, stomatocytosis, and related disorders. In William, W. J., Beutler, E., et al., eds. *Hematology*, 4th ed. New York: McGraw-Hill, 1990, pp. 582–590.

Palek, J. Hereditary elliptocytosis and related disorders. In Williams, W. J., Beutler, E., et al., eds. *Hematology*, 4th ed. New York: McGraw-Hill, 1990, pp. 569–581.

Palek, J. Hereditary spherocytosis. In Williams, W. J., Beutler, E., et al., eds. *Hematology*, 4th ed. New York: McGraw-Hill, 1990, pp. 558–569.

Rosse, W. F. Paroxysmal nocturnal hemoglobinuria and decay-accelerating factor. *Annu. Rev. Med.* 41(1990): 431–436.

Rotoli, B., and Luzzatto, L. Paroxysmal nocturnal hemoglobinuria. *Semin. Hematol.* 26(1989): 201–207.

Shohet, S. B., and Beutler, E. The red cell membrane. In Williams, W, J., Beutler, E., et al., eds. *Hematology*, 4th ed. New York: McGraw-Hill, 1990, pp. 368–377.

Original articles

Brecher, M. E., and Taswell, H. F. Paroxysmal nocturnal hemoglobinuria and the transfusion of washed red cells: a myth revisited. *Transfusion* 29(1989): 681–685.

Chasis, J. A., Prenant, M., et al. Membrane assembly and remodeling during reticulocyte maturation. *Blood* 74(1989): 1112–1120.

Eber, S. W., Lande, W. M., et al. Hereditary stomatocytosis: consistent association with an integral membrane protein deficiency. *Br. J. Haematol.* 72(1989): 452–455.

Evans, E. A. Structure and deformation properties of red blood cells: concepts and quantitative methods. *Methods Enzymol.* 173(1989): 3–34.

Holguin, M. H., Fredrick, L. R., et al. Isolation and characterization of a membrane protein from normal human erythrocytes that inhibits reactive lysis of the erythrocytes of paroxysmal nocturnal hemoglobinuria. *J. Clin. Invest.* 84(1989): 7–17.

Horne, W. C., Leto, T. L., et al. Preparation of red cell membrane skeleton proteins. *Methods Enzymol.* 173(1989): 380–391.

Lux, S. E., John, K. M., et al. Analysis of cDNA for human erythrocyte ankyrin indicates a repeated structure with homology to tissue-differentiation and cell-cycle control proteins. *Nature* 344(1990): 36–42.

Lux, S. E., John, K. M., et al. Cloning and characterization of band 3, the human erythrocyte anion-exchange protein (AE1). *Proc. Natl. Acad. Sci. USA* 86(1989): 9089–9093.

Lux, S. E., Tse, W. T., et al. Hereditary spherocytosis associated with deletion of human erythrocyte ankyrin gene on chromosome 8. *Nature* 345(1990): 736–739.

Okuda, K., Kanamaru, A., et al. Membrane expression of decay-accelerating factor on neutrophils from normal individuals and patients with paroxysmal nocturnal hemoglobinuria. *Blood* 75(1990): 1186–1191.

Reid, M. E., Takakuwa, Y., et al. Glycophorin C content of human erythrocyte membrane is regulated by protein 4.1. *Blood* 75(1990): 2229–2234.

Sachs, J. R. Cation fluxes in the red blood cell: Na^+-K^+ pump. *Methods Enzymol.* 173(1989): 80–93.

Taguchi, R., Funahashi, Y., et al. Analysis of PI (phosphatidylinositol)-anchoring antigens in a patient of paroxysmal nocturnal hemoglobinuria (PNH) reveals deficiency of 1F5 antigen (CD59), a new complement-regulatory factor. *FEBS Lett.* 261(1990): 142–146.

LECTURE 15

Hemolytic Anemias IV. Metabolic Disorders

William S. Beck and Robert I. Tepper

EDITOR'S COMMENT

All who are old enough to have lived (medically) through World War II will recall the urgency of this nation's search for antimalarial drugs that could substitute for quinine, whose source had been lost. In the testing of primaquine, discovery of its occasional toxicity led in the years just after the war to the discovery of glucose-6-phosphate deficiency in individuals who responded to primaquine with severe hemolysis. This field continues to expand to this day, as other red cell enzyme deficiencies are uncovered and large numbers of genetic variants of G-6-PD are revealed. Presumably, the pattern of genetic abnormalities displayed by these enzymes of the HMP shunt in red cells is occurring in other cells and in other enzymatic pathways. Study of red cells—and indeed of this particular pathway—is greatly facilitated by the accessibility of these cells and the clinical consequences of some of these mutations.

I. RED CELL METABOLISM

A. Major features

Red cell metabolism has a number of distinctive features:

- Glucose enters red cells by a carrier process that is independent of insulin.
- Glucose, the main substrate of red cells, is metabolized via two major pathways: (1) the **Embden-Meyerhof**, or **glycolytic**, **pathway**; and (2) the **hexose monophosphate (HMP) shunt pathway** (figure 15.1). Compared to other cells, these pathways in red cells generate a meager yield of ATP and reducing power.
- Mitochondria and microsomes are lost as reticulocytes mature into adult red cells. Hence, adult cells utilize little oxygen and synthesize no protein.

1. Embden-Meyerhof pathway

The metabolic needs of the red cell are met almost exclusively by the conversion of glucose to lactic acid. About 95% of the glucose metabolized to lactate traverses the Embden-Meyerhof pathway.

The major metabolic events of glycolysis are the following:

- Each glucose molecule (a hexose) is converted to two pyruvate molecules (a triose).

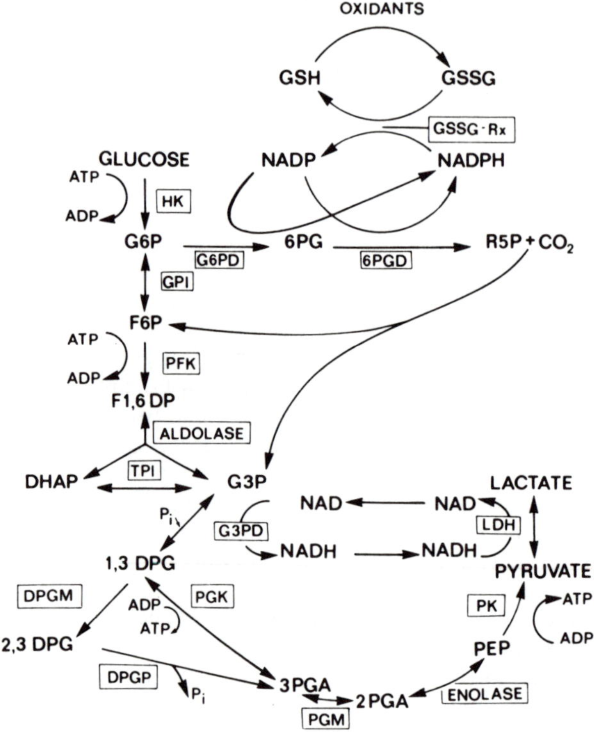

Fig. 15.1

Erythrocyte glucose metabolism. *Abbreviations of enzymes (boxed)*: HK, hexokinase; GPI, glucose-phosphate isomerase; PFK, phosphofructokinase; TPI, triosephosphate isomerase; G3PD, glyceraldehyde-3-phosphate dehydrogenase; PGK, phosphoglycerate kinase; DPGM, diphosphoglyceromutase; DPGP, diphosphoglycerophosphatase; PGM, phosphoglyceromutase; PK; pyruvate kinase; LDH, lactic dehydrogenase; G6PD, glucose-6-phosphate dehydrogenase; 6GPD, 6-phosphogluconate dehydrogenase; GSSG-Rx, glutathione reductase. *Abbreviations of substrates*: G6P, glucose 6-phosphate; F6P, fructose 6-phosphate; F1,6DP, fructose-1,6-diphosphate; DHAP, dihydroxyacetone phosphate; G3P, glyceraldehyde-3-phosphate; 1,3DPG, 1,3-diphosphoglyceric acid; 2,3DPG, 2,3-diphosphoglyceric acid; 3PGA, 3-phosphoglyceric acid; 2PGA, 2-phosphoglyceric acid; PEP, phosphoenolpyruvate; 6PG, 6-phosphogluconate; R5P, ribulose-5-phosphate; GSH, reduced glutathione; GSSG, oxidized glutathione. Cofactors are given standard abbreviations: NAD, NADP, NADH, NADPH, and Pi (inorganic phosphate). (From S. E. Lux, in W. S. Beck, ed., *Hematology*, 4th ed. Cambridge, MA: MIT Press, 1985.)

- For every glucose molecule, two molecules of an intermediary triose (glyceraldehyde 3-phosphate) are oxidized. This oxidation liberates two pairs of hydride ions, which then reduce two molecules of NAD^+ to NADH and H^+. These in turn reduce pyruvate to lactate.
- Two molecules of ATP are utilized in the early phosphorylations that launch the glycolytic sequence.
- Four molecules of ATP are synthesized from four molecules each of inorganic phosphate and ADP. This compensates for the two ATPs utilized earlier and yields a net profit of two ATP molecules.

2. *ATP*

In mature red cells, only the Embden-Meyerhof pathway is capable of synthesizing ATP. Compared to cells with mitochondria and an active Krebs cycle (which in theory generates 36–38 ATP molecules per glucose unit), the ATP yield from glycolysis is small. Nonetheless, it is more than sufficient to permit renewal of total red cell ATP, generating 1.0–1.5 mmole/liter red cells per hour.

The major ATP-dependent systems in red cells are the following:

- Initiation of glycolysis.
- Active transport of Na^+ and K^+ across the cell membrane.
- Maintenance of low intracellular Ca^{2+} levels.
- Phosphorylation of membrane proteins.

3. *NADH*

Glycolysis is the source of NADH, the cofactor of several oxidation-reduction reactions. One such reaction, catalyzed by **NADH-cytochrome b_5 reductase**, maintains heme iron in the reduced state (Fe^{2+}). Oxidation of heme iron to Fe^{3+} produces methemoglobin, which is incapable of oxygen transport (see lecture 9).

4. *2,3-DPG*

Red cells have a uniquely high concentration of 2,3-DPG—about 4–5 mmoles/liter of red cells compared to the traces present in other cells (see lecture 9). This compound is formed in the **Rapaport-Luebering shunt**, a two-step detour from the glycolytic pathway that branches off at 1,3-DPG (see figure 15.1). Both steps are nearly irreversible.

Because this shunt pathway is energetically unprofitable, it was widely ignored and the role of 2,3-DPG as an allosteric effector of hemoglobin was overlooked until 1967.

B. Hexose monophosphate (HMP) shunt

Approximately 5–10% of utilized glucose is normally metabolized through the HMP shunt, which is concerned chiefly with the generation of reducing power. The HMP shunt is the major source of NADPH in red cells, two molecules of NADPH being produced for each molecule of glucose metabolized. Traffic through the shunt pathway increases whenever NADPH oxidation is accelerated. The major reactions associated with NADPH oxidation are related to glutathione metabolism.

C. Glutathione metabolism

Red cells contain a high concentration (2 mM) of reduced glutathione (GSH), a tripeptide (γ-glutamyl-cysteinyl-glycine), that is synthetized de novo by mature red cells and serves as a sulfhydryl buffer, cycling between its reduced form (GSH) and an oxidized form (GSSG), which links two tripeptides by a disulfide bond.

GSH acts intracellularly to protect red cells against injury by exogenous and endogenous oxidants, such as superoxide anion (O_2^-) and hydrogen peroxide (H_2O_2), which are produced by macrophages in infection and by red cells in the presence of certain drugs (see lecture 19). Accumulation of these agents leads to injury of cell proteins and lipids. This is normally prevented by GSH, which inactivates such oxidants. This detoxification can occur spontaneously, but it is accelerated by **glutathione peroxidase**, a remarkable selenium-containing enzyme. As hydrogen peroxide is reduced in the peroxidase reaction, GSH is oxidized to GSSG and mixed disulfides with protein-thiols (GS-S-protein). (Catalase also degrades peroxides, but under physiologic conditions it is less important.)

Regeneration of GSH is catalyzed by **glutathione reductase**, a flavoprotein. In this NADPH-mediated reaction, both GSSG and mixed disulfides are reduced to GSH as NADPH is simultaneously oxidized. This in turn stimulates HMP shunt activity, which regenerates NADPH. The tight coupling of HMP shunt and glutathione metabolism efficiently protects red cells from oxidant injury.

II. DEFECTS IN HMP SHUNT OR GLUTATHIONE METABOLISM

A. Introduction

HMP shunt defects are common; glycolytic pathway defects are relatively rare. The majority of shunt defects are associated with diminished **glucose-6-phosphate dehydrogenase** (G-6-PD) activity. This is the most common enzyme abnormality associated with hemolytic anemia—and one of the most common of all human disorders, affecting millions of people throughout the world. In contrast, **pyruvate kinase** (PK) deficiency, the most common glycolytic abnormality, affects only hundreds or thousands of individuals.

B. G-6-PD deficiency

Severe hemolysis was first noted in certain individuals treated with the antimalarial drug pamaquine in 1926 and primaquine during World War

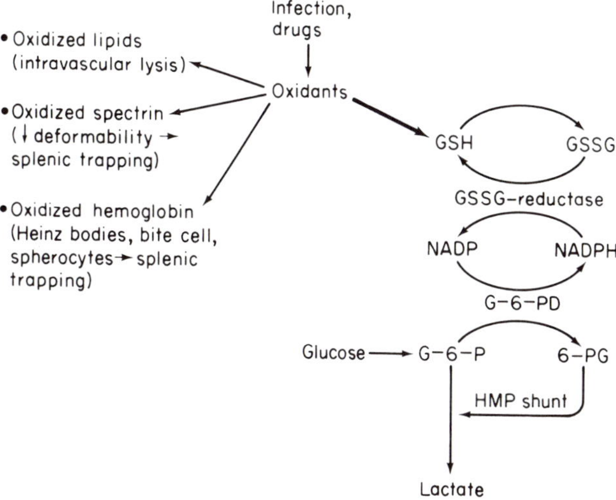

Fig. 15.2
Pathophysiology of hemolysis associated with G-6-PD deficiency.

II. A genetic abnormality was suspected because hemolysis occurred only in black soldiers. Later it was found that 10% of American black males have red cells that are vulnerable to these drugs. In 1956, this sensitivity was attributed to the presence in these red cells of an unstable variant of the polymorphic enzyme G-6-PD. We now recognize multiple genetic abnormalities that diminish G-6-PD activity in red cells.

1. Pathophysiology

Since red cells lack mitochondria, enzymatic defects in the HMP shunt and associated pathways of glutathione metabolism can sharply diminish NADPH synthesis, and thus impair resistance to oxidative stress. The relevant sequence is shown in figure 15.2. Oxidants of various kinds are normally reduced by GSH. But in G-6-PD deficiency and other disorders, GSH levels fall because NADPH syntehsis is diminished. Oxidants are thus free to damage cell constituents. Oxidation of hemoglobin produces methemoglobin (in which Fe^{3+} cannot bind oxygen) and denatured hemoglobin (in which globin has been oxidized). The latter precipitates as intracellular **Heinz bodies**.

Heinz bodies are not visible in ordinary Wright's stained blood smears but are demonstrable with supravital stains such as **methyl violet**. Heinz bodies attach to the red cell membrane by unknown mechanisms.

In vitro, this causes:

- Increased membrane leakiness to cations
- Increased osmotic fragility
- Decreased deformability

In vivo, Heinz bodies are "pitted" from circulating red cells by the spleen (see lecture 3)—and thus are plentiful in splenectomized patients. "Bite cells," that is, hyperchromic red cells with a localized invagination (presumably at the site of Heinz body removal), appear in the circulation during acute hemolytic episodes. Red cells with a submembranous hemoglobin-free area (blister cells) may also be seen.

Small numbers of spherocytes are also observed. They arise from repetitive loss of small amounts of membrane surface during the pitting of Heinz bodies. Membrane damage occurs due to oxidative cross-linking of spectrin and lipid peroxidation. The damage inflicted on hemoglobin and the membrane skeleton leads to diminished red cell deformability and splenic trapping. Lipid damage probably produces direct intravascular hemolysis. Oxidation of intracellular enzymes (e.g., Ca^{2+}-ATPase) may also contribute to red cell damage in G-6-PD deficiency.

2. G-6-PD variants

Surprisingly, more than 350 G-6-PD variants have been described, though few have been sequenced. Table 15.1 lists those in which the mutation has been precisely defined. Note that several conventions are used to name variants in the literature. Thus, the normal enzyme is designated **Gd^B**, or **G-6-PD^B**, or **G6PD B**. We will use the short term.

Of the known variants, the following are the most important clinically:

- **Gd^B**, the phenotype considered normal, is present in 70% of Caucasians.
- **Gd^A** is a normal variant present in 20% of American blacks. Replacement of asparagine with aspartic acid makes it electrophoretically faster than Gd^B.
- **Gd^{A-}**, the most common variant associated with hemolysis, is found in 11% of American blacks and in higher percentages in many African populations. Its electrophoretic mobility is identical to that of Gd^A, but its catalytic activity is impaired. Because it has two nucleotide substitutions (table 15.1), it may be that the A$^-$ mutation occurred when A was the predominant genotype.
- **Gd^{Med}**, the second most common abnormal variant (and the most common among Caucasians) is found in many ethnic groups in the Mediterranean area basin (Italians, Greeks, Sardinians, Sephardic Jews, Arabs, etc.), and in India and southeastern Asia. Its electrophoretic mobility is normal, but its catalytic activity is markedly reduced. It may include several discrete variants.
- **Gd^{Canton}** is a common variant in Oriental populations that produces a clinical syndrome like that associated with Gd^{A-}.

3. Genetics

The G-6-PD gene is on the X chromosome and its inheritance is sex-linked.

- Males have only one type of G-6-PD and any genetic defect is fully expressed.
- Females have two types of G-6-PD—i.e., Gd^B and Gd^A, or Gd^B and Gd^{A-}.

Table 15.1
Several of the Mutations That Have Been Associated With G-6-PD Variants

	Base Position											
G-6-PD Variant	172	202	376	466	563	844	968	1003	1156	1311	1339	Proposed Designation
A			A → G									G6PD A^{376G}
A–		G → A	A → G									G6PD A–$^{202A/376G}$
A–			A → G				T → C					G6PD A–$^{376G/968C}$
Matera		G → A	A → G									G6PD Matera$^{202A/376G}$
Betica		G → A	A → G									G6PD Betica$^{202A/376G}$
Betica			A → G				T → C					G6PD Betica$^{376G/968C}$
Metaponto	G → A											G6PD Metaponto^{172A}
Ilesha				G → A								G6PD Ilesha^{466A}
Mediterranean					C → T							G6PD Mediterranean^{563T}
Sassari					C → T					C → T		G6PD Sassari$^{563T/1311T}$
Cagliari					C → T					C → T		G6PD Cagliari$^{563T/1311T}$
Santiago de Cuba											G → A	G6PD Santiago de Cuba^{1339A}
Iowa									A → G			G6PD Iowa^{1156G}
Original amino acid	Asp	Val	Asn	Glu	Ser	Asp	Leu	Ala	Lys	Tyr	Gly	
Substitution	Asn	Met	Asp	Lys	Phe	His	Pro	Thr	Glu	Tyr	Arg	

Adapted from E. Beutler (1989) *Blood* 73:1397–1401.

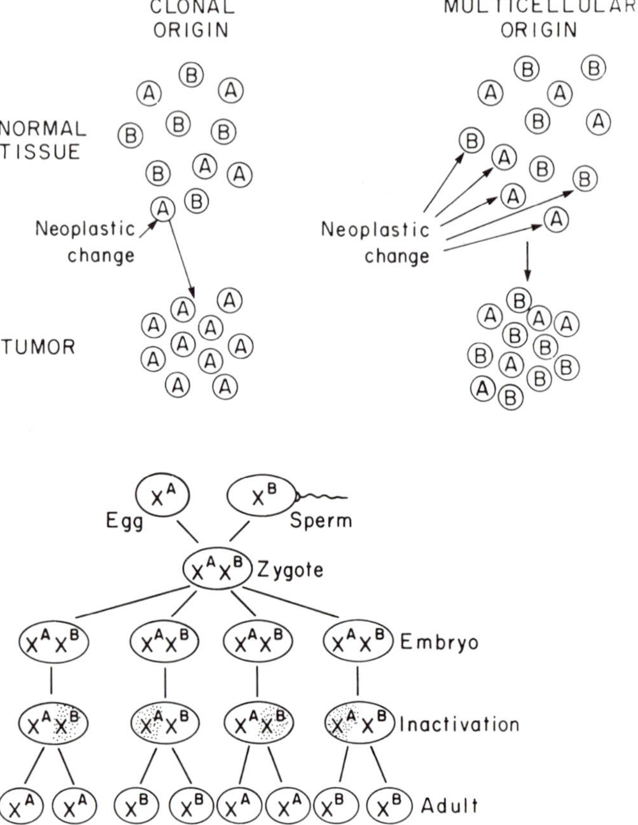

Fig. 15.3

Top, The concept of cellular mosaicism. A normal tissue consisting of cell types A and B can give rise to tumors of clonal origin (containing either type A or type B cells) or tumors of multicellular origin (containing both A and B cell types). *Bottom*, The Lyon hypothesis and the origin of tumors. The G-6-PD gene is X-linked and can be used as a marker to determine tumor origins. A female exhibiting two forms of the gene X^A and X^B) will be expressing either one form or the other in any given cell. This can be used to determine the clonal or multicellular origin of tumors. (Note that the inactivated X is not shown.) (From W. S. Beck et al., *Life: An Introduction to Biology*, 3rd ed. New York: HarperCollins, 1991.)

According to the **Lyon hypothesis** (the validity of which is strongly supported by G-6-PD genetics), only one X chromosome is active in any somatic cell. Thus, individuals red cells of females contain only one G-6-PD type—and a given red cell in heterozygous-deficient females is either normal or deficient. The presence of two cell populations is confirmed by red cell stains. Mean enzyme activity in deficient females may be normal or moderately reduced (the usual pattern), or grossly decreased, depending on the degree of "lyonization." Deficient cells in females are as susceptible to oxidant injury as deficient cells in males. The severity of hemolysis is less, however, because fewer vulnerable cells are present.

The phenomenon of random X-inactivation permits useful studies of the cellular origin of tumors (figure 15.3). Isolation of enzyme from tumor cells in women heterozygous for Gd^B and Gd^A shows that tumors may be of either unicentric or multicentric origin.

Despite the adverse effects of G-6-PD gene mutations, it is a common gene in many areas. Its prevalence has been attributed to a selective advantage it may provide in making individuals resistant to *Plasmodium falciparum* malaria. This thesis is supported by epidemiologic studies and by demonstrations in infected Gd^B/Gd^{A-} females that parasites are rarely found in Gd^{A-} red cells. Indeed, G-6-PD deficiency impairs parasite growth. However, the prevalence of Gd^A in blacks is unexplained in terms of genetic polymorphism.

4. *Relation between enzyme defect and hemolysis*

As normal red cells age in vivo, the activity of intracellular Gd^B slowly decays with a half-life of about 60 days (figure 15.4). Nonetheless, older red cells are still able to produce enough NADPH to maintain adequate levels.

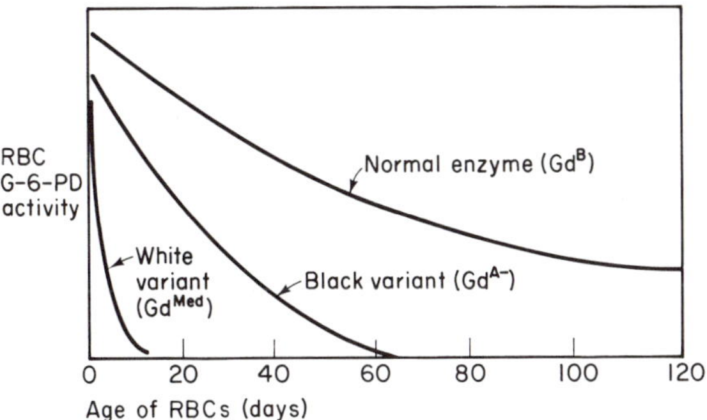

Fig. 15.4
Intracellular decay of red cell G-6-PD as a function of cell age. G-6-PD normally decays as red cells age. The top curve shows the decay rate for Gd^B, the normal enzyme. The middle and lower curves show the greater than normal decay rates for Gd^{A-} and Gd^{Med} variants. (From S. E. Lux, in W. S Beck, ed., *Hematology*, 4th ed. Cambridge, MA: MIT Press, 1985.)

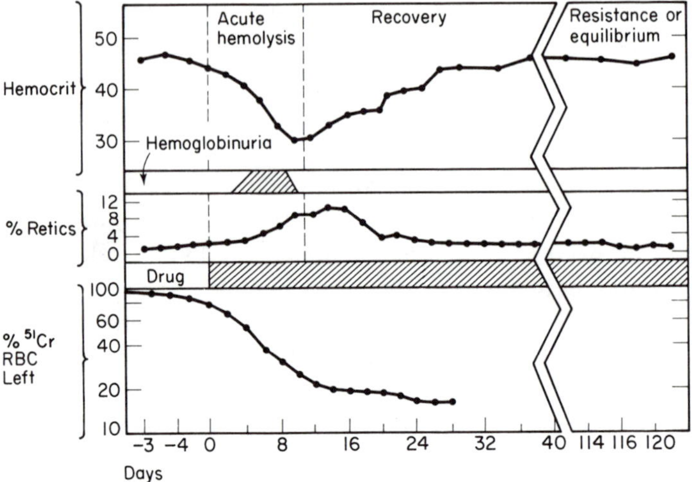

Fig. 15.5
Course of drug-induced hemolysis in an individual with Gd^{A-}. Note that hemolysis abates, and apparent resistance to the drug develops after the initial hemolytic episode due to repopulation with young red cells. (From A. S. Alving et. al. *Bull. World Health Organ.* 22[1960]: 621.)

Gd^{A-} is a labile enzyme that decays with a half-life of about 13 days. Young red cells have normal enzyme activity; older red cells are severely deficient. As a result, hemolysis is self-limited in individuals with Gd^{A-}. Figure 15.5 shows the course of primaquine-induced hemolysis in individuals with Gd^{A-}. When the drug is first administered, there is hemolysis with hemoglobinuria and decreased red cell survival. But this is followed by abatement of the anemia, reticulocytosis, and improved red cell survival despite continued administration of the drug. The reason is clear: Once the oxidant-sensitive older red cells have been destroyed, remaining young cells are relatively oxidant-resistant. Since only half the cells are oxidant-sensitive (in Gd^{A-}), the bone marrow can compensate by simply doubling its output. This apparent drug resistance persists as long as the drug is continuously administered. If the drug is stopped for 2–3 months, older red cells again accumulate and the patient can again become drug-sensitive.

Gd^{Med} is much more unstable than Gd^{A-} (figure 15.3) Very little activity is present in mature red cells. Nonetheless, chronic hemolysis does not occur, presumably because endogenous oxidant stress is normally low. Exposed to oxidant drugs or infections, however, these patients are at profound risk because their entire red cell population can be destroyed.

5. *Clinical features*

The clinical features of the Gd^{A-} and Gd^{Med} syndromes are compared in table 15.2. The following findings are commonly seen:

- Acute intravascular hemolysis is the most dramatic presentation.

Table 15.2
Clinical Comparison of the Two Common Forms of G-6-PD Deficiency

	Gd^{A-}	Gd^{Med}
Frequency	Common in black populations	Common in Mediterranean populations
Degree of hemolysis	Moderate	Severe
G-6-PD defect	Old red cells	All red cells
Hemolysis with:		
Drugs	Unusual	Common
Infection	Common	Common
Need for transfusions	No	Sometimes
Chronic hemolysis	No	No

- Usually, there is hemoglobinemia (pink to brown plasma), hemoglobinuria (dark or even black urine), and jaundice—acutely with an infection or within 1–3 days of exposure to the offending drug.
- More often, hemolysis is less dramatic, and a modest decline of hemoglobin (3 or 4 g/dl) occurs without hemoglobinuria or prominent symptoms. These episodes are easily overlooked unless the physician is alert.
- In severe cases, there is abdominal or back pain.
- Symptoms of acute anemia (e.g., dizziness, palpitations, dyspnea) are common (see lecture 2).
- Heinz bodies appear in red cells, and some bite cells, blister cells, and/or spherocytes appear on the blood smear. However, red cell morphology may be relatively normal.

a. OXIDANT DRUGS

The discovery of G-6-PD deficiency followed observations on soldiers receiving primaquine. Many other oxidant drugs were later implicated as causative agents (table 15.3).

b. INFECTION

The most common cause of hemolysis is infection. Virtually every type of infection has been implicated. The initiation of free radical chain reactions by superoxide (O_2^-) and hydrogen peroxide and the generation of longer-lived oxidants (e.g., monochloroamines) in activated phagocytes likely play a role in damaging nearby red cells.

c. FAVISM

Sudden severe hemolytic episodes occasionally follow exposure to **fava beans** or their pollen. Fava beans contain high concentrations of certain β-glucosides (e.g., vicine, convicine) which, following enzymatic action in

Table 15.3
Drugs Commonly Leading to Hemolysis in G-6-PD Deficiency

Antimalarials	**Analgesics**
Primaquine	Acetanilid
Quinacrine (Atabrine®)	Acetylsalicylic acid*
	Acetophenetidin (Phenacetin®)*
Sulfonamides	**Sulfones**
Sulfanilamide	Diaminodiphenyl sulfone (Dapsone®)
Salicylazosulfapyridine (Azulfidine®)	
Sulfisoxazole (Gantrisin®)*	
Other Antibacterials	**Miscellaneous**
Nitrofurantoin (Furadantin®)	Dimercaprol (BAL)
Nitrofurazone (Furacin®)	Naphthalene (moth balls)
Chloramphenicol*	Methylene blue*
Para-aminosalicylic acid	Vitamin K (water-soluble analogues)*
Nalidixic acid	Ascorbic acid*

Note: A more comprehensive list of drugs that have been implicated in oxidant-induced hemolysis appears in E. Beutler, *Pharmacol. Rev.* 21(1969): 73.
*Hemolysis is infrequent and generally requires high concentrations of the drug. Probably a risk in Gd^{Med} but not in Gd^{A-} or Gd^{Canton}.

the presence of oxygen, generates hydrogen peroxide and free radicals. This rare phenomenon occurs mainly in individuals with Gd^{Med}. It is not seen with Gd^{A-}. Interestingly, not all patients with Gd^{Med} are susceptible.

d. HEREDITARY NONSPHEROCYTIC HEMOLYTIC ANEMIA (HNHA)

In some patients with rare variants of G-6-PD, chronic hemolysis occurs in the absence of obvious oxidants. These individuals have an enzyme that is unable to sustain adequate NADPH production. Such variants generally have either a high K_m for NADP or a low K_i for NADPH. Consequently, enzyme activity measured under ideal conditions in vitro (high [NADP], low [NADPH]) may be nearly normal, while enzyme activity in vivo under physiologic conditions (low [NADP], high [NADPH]) may be depressed.

6. Diagnosis

Several tests for the diagnosis of G-6-PD deficiency available. All are indirect or direct assays of G-6-PD activity in red cells. The tests differ in sensitivity and their usefulness depends on the clinical situation (sex of patient, ethnic background, and proximity to hemolytic episode). Commercial kits are available for many of these procedures.

- Commonly used **screening tests** are based on (1) fluorescence of NADPH, (2) NADPH-mediated dye decolorization, or (3) the reduction of methemoglobin in the presence of methylene blue. These procedures should always include normal red cell controls. They are of limited sensitivity since 30–40% of the cells must be abnormal if deficiency is to be detected.

- **Quantitative G-6-PD assay** relies on direct spectrophotometric measurement of NADPH production. This is more sensitive than screening tests, but still does not show depressed activity unless 20–30% of red cells are deficient. A useful control is the simultaneous assay of other age-dependent enzymes. When these are compared with G-6-PD, G-6-PD deficiency can be detected even after a hemolytic episode.
- The **cyanide-ascorbate test** assays the ability of red cells to prevent ascorbate-induced oxidation of hemoglobin. Unlike the others, this test uses intact red cells instead of hemolysates. Thus, as few as 10–15% enzyme-deficient cells can be detected. This sensitivity is useful in the diagnosis of G-6-PD deficiency in female heterozygotes and in males following a hemolytic episode. This test can also detect other abnormalities of the HMP shunt or glutathione metabolism (see below).
- **Cytochemical estimation** of G-6-PD activity in individual red cells is possible with tetrazolium dyes. This test can detect the presence of less than 5% G-6-PD deficient cells and is useful in identifying female heterozygotes.
- **Identification of G-6-PD variants** requires electrophoresis, kinetic studies, and other biochemical techniques.

C. Other defects of glutathione metabolism

Abnormalities of GSH metabolism, the first line of defense against oxidants, are also associated with hemolysis.

1. Glutathione synthetase deficiency

Defects in the enzymes responsible for GSH synthesis occur rarely. Red cells lacking these enzymes have very low GSH levels. Clinically, the disorders resemble G-6-PD deficiency, that is, mild-to-moderate hemolytic anemia following oxidant stress.

2. Glutathione reductase deficiency

In early reports, GSSG reductase deficiency was associated with a variety of other hematologic abnormalities. It was then discovered that flavin adenine dinucleotide (FAD) is a cofactor of GSSG reductase, and many apparent enzyme deficiencies were later attributed to abnormalities of riboflavin metabolism. Actual genetic deficiency of GSSG reductase does exist but is rare.

3. Other defects

Deficiency of **GSH peroxidase**, found in newborn infants and others, produces little hemolysis. Deficiency of **glutathione S-transferase** causes mild hemolysis.

III. DEFECTS OF GLYCOLYSIS

A. General features

Abnormalities in virtually every glycolytic enzyme have been described, in both clinically normal individuals and in patients with hereditary nonspherocytic hemolytic anemia (HNHA) but pyruvate kinase (PK) deficiency accounts for about 90% of all cases associated with hemolysis.

1. Genetics

Glycolytic enzymopathies display an autosomal recessive pattern of inheritance. Hemolysis occurs in homozygotes. Heterozygotes are clinically normal, but their red cells display enzyme deficiencies. Phosphoglycerate kinase (PGK) deficiency is an exception since this disorder may be sex-linked.

2. Relation between enzyme defect and hemolysis

Hemolysis of red cells deficient in glycolytic enzymes presumably reflects impairment of the ATP-dependent reactions that control membrane function. However, red cell ATP content is not invariably decreased because:

- The mean cell age is very young (and reticulocytes have high ATP levels).
- Defective cells with low ATP content are promptly removed from the circulation.
- ATP may be compartmentalized within red cells, in which case one critical locus may be sufficient to cause cell injury.

3. Clinical features

Most patients with HNHA manifest only the signs and symptoms of chronic hemolysis.

- Unlike the vast majority of cases of G-6-PD deficiency, hemolysis due to glycolytic enzyme defects is typically chronic and not affected by drugs.
- Splenomegaly is usually present owing to the stagnation of cells in this organ. The acidic, hypoxic, and nutrient-poor environment of the spleen is an added insult to the metabolically abnormal red cells. Thus, the hemolytic rate frequently decreases following splenectomy.
- The blood smear often contains some dense spiculated red cells (echinocytes), particularly after splenectomy, but this is not invariable or unique to these disorders.
- In most cases, red cell morphology is unremarkable in unsplenectomized patients.
- Varying degrees of anemia and reticulocytosis are present. Heinz bodies are absent.

4. *Diagnosis*

A major problem in the diagnosis of glycolytic enzyme abnormalities is the fact that the most seriously affected cells are removed in vivo and thus are unavailable for analysis in vitro. Definitive diagnosis requires spectrophotometric enzyme assays performed under a variety of conditions (e.g., with varying substrate and cofactor concentrations) in order to detect enzymes with abnormal kinetics. Measurement of glycolytic intermediates may reveal subtle enzyme abnormalities since the concentration of intermediates is usually increased proximal to a defect and decreased distal to it.

B. Pyruvate kinase (PK) deficiency

Since PK catalyzes one of the major reactions responsible for ATP production in glycolysis, it is not surprising that deficiency of this enzyme causes hemolytic anemia. Hemolysis can be mild and compensated or severe enough to require frequent transfusions. The improvement of severe hemolysis following splenectomy is related to the fact that **PK-deficient reticulocytes** depend on mitochondrial oxidative phosphorylation as an ATP source. In vitro incubation of PK-deficient reticulocytes under hypoxic conditions or with inhibitors of oxidative phosphorylation causes ATP levels to fall; cells subsequently gain Ca^{++}, lose K^+ and water, and become rigid. PK-deficient reticulocytes sequestered in the hypoxic spleen presumably undergo similar degeneration. Although anemia improves following splenectomy, reticulocytes increase to 50–70%. This **paradoxical reticulocytosis** is due to increased reticulocyte survival once the adverse metabolic environment of the spleen is removed. The distal glycolytic block in PK deficiency causes a two- to threefold increase in red cell 2,3-DPG (to 10–15 mmoles/liter of red cells); this minimizes some adverse effects of the anemia since 2,3-DPG enhances oxygen release from hemoglobin (see lecture 9).

C. Glucose phosphate isomerase deficiency

Glucose phosphate isomerase (GPI) deficiency is the second most common glycolytic disorder that produces hemolysis. Because products of HMP shunt metabolism are recycled through GPI, defects in this enzyme, like those of G-6-PD, lead to some oxidant sensitivity. The specific cell injury leading to hemolysis is not known.

IV. HEMOLYSIS DUE TO DEFECTS IN RED CELL NUCLEOTIDE METABOLISM

A. Pyrimidine-5′-nucleotidase deficiency

Deficiency of pyrimidine-5′-nucleotidase is the third or fourth most common enzyme deficiency leading to hemolysis. This enzyme functions to degrade pyrimidine nucleotides to cytidine and uridine, which can diffuse out of the cell. Lacking this activity, red cells accumulate partially degraded messenger and ribosomal RNA, which produces prominent **basophilic stippling** of up to 5% of the red cells on blood smears. Interestingly, the basophilic stippling of lead poisoning is apparently produced by a similar mechanism since pyrimidine-5′-nucleotidase is markedly inhibited by lead. Patients with the inherited (autosomal recessive) deficiency of this enzyme have a chronic, moderately severe hemolytic anemia. The mechanism of hemolysis is unknown, but may in part be due to inhibition of the HMP shunt by high concentrations of pyridine nucleotides. Splenomegaly is common, but splenectomy produces little discernible benefit.

SELECTED REFERENCES

Reviews

Arese, P., and De Flora, A. Denaturation of normal and abnormal erythrocytes II. Pathophysiology of hemolysis in glucose-6-phosphate dehydrogenase deficiency. *Semin. Hematol.* 27(1990): 1–40.

Beutler, E. Minireview: the molecular biology of hematologically significant enzyme defects. Molecular biology of enzyme defects. *Acta Haematol.* (*Basel*) 80(1988): 181–184.

Beutler, E. Glucose-6-phosphate dehydrogenase: new perspectives. *Blood* 73(1989): 1397–1401.

Beutler, E. Glucose-6-phosphate dehydrogenase deficiency. In Williams, W. J., Beutler, E., et al., eds. *Hematology*, 4th ed. New York: McGraw-Hill, 1990, pp. 591–606.

Beutler, E. Hereditary nonspherocytic hemolytic anemia: pyruvate kinase and other abnormalities. In Williams, W. J., Beutler, E., et al., eds. *Hematology*, 4th ed. New York: McGraw-Hill, 1990, pp. 606–612.

Beutler, E. The genetics of glucose-6-phosphate dehydrogenase deficiency. *Semin. Hematol.* 27(1990): 137–164.

Beutler, E., and Yoshida, A. Genetic variation of glucose-6-phosphate dehydrogenase: a catalog and future prospects. *Medicine* (*Baltimore*) 67(1988): 311–334.

Nagel, R. L., and Roth, E. F., Jr. Malaria and red cell genetic defects. *Blood* 74(1989): 1213–1221.

Saltman, P. Oxidative stress: a radical view. *Semin. Hematol.* 26(1989): 249–256.

Stern, A. Drug-induced oxidative denaturation in red blood cells. *Semin. Hematol.* 26(1989): 301–306.

Tanaka, K. R., and Zerez, C. R. Red cell enzymopathies of the glycolytic pathway. *Semin. Hematol.* 27(1990): 165–185.

Valentine, W. N., and Paglia, D. E. Erythroenzymopathies and hemolytic anemia: the many faces of inherited variant enzymes. *J. Lab. Clin. Med.* 115(1990): 12–20.

Wainscoat, J. S., and Fey, M. F. Assessment of clonality in human tumors: a review. *Cancer Res.* 50(1990): 1355–1360.

Original articles

Bellingham, A. J., Lestas, A. N., et al. Prenatal diagnosis of a red-cell enzymopathy: triose phosphate isomerase deficiency. *Lancet* 2(1989): 419–421.

Beutler, E., Dunning, D., et al. Erythrocyte glutathione S-transferase deficiency and hemolytic anemia. *Blood* 72(1988): 73–77.

Beutler, E., Kuhl, W., et al. Molecular heterogeneity of glucose-6-phosphate dehydrogenase A^-. *Blood* 74(1989): 2550–2555.

Chiu, D., and Lubin, B. Oxidative homoglobin denaturation and RBC destruction: the effect of heme on red cell membranes. *Semin. Hematol.* 26(1989): 128–135.

Goldberg, D. E., Slater, A. F. G., et al. Hemoglobin degradation in the malaria parasite *Plasmodium falciparum*: an ordered process in a unique organelle. *Proc. Natl. Acad. Sci. USA* 87(1990): 2931–2935.

Halperin, J. A., and Nicholson-Weller, A. Paroxysmal nocturnal hemoglobinuria. A complement-mediated disease. *Complement* 6(1989): 65–72.

Platt, O. S., and Falcone, J. F. Membrane protein lesions in erythrocytes with Heinz bodies. *J. Clin. Invest.* 82(1988): 1051–1058.

LECTURE 16

Blood Groups I. Chemistry and Physiology

W. Hallowell Churchill, Jr.

EDITOR'S COMMENT

The individuality of human blood was not fully appreciated until 1901 when Karl Landsteiner found that red cells could be separated into three different groups by testing sera. From this modest start, the individual characteristics of red cells have been so expanded it is now quite improbable that any two people, other than identical twins, would have the same combination of red cells surface markers. In other words, individuals have unique combinations of these molecules. Blood groups depend on antigenic substances on the red cell surface that are present in certain members of the species but absent in other members of the same species. These antigens are usually detected with antibodies that cause red cells to agglutinate. With minor exceptions, the blood groups are constant throughout life and are inherited according to mendelian laws. The nature of the major blood group antigens is slowly being unraveled—and this lecture gives a useful and compact summary of present knowledge. Aside from its obvious importance as background for the practical aspects of transfusion therapy discussed in lecture 17, the systems we call blood groups raise interesting biologic questions. What, in fact, is the biologic utility of these remarkable polymorphic systems? What are some of these "blood group substances" doing in cells other than red cells or, for that matter, in lima beans and other plants? Since it is doubtful that evolution produced blood group substances in anticipation of blood transfusion technology, one can only wonder what mechanisms of natural selection account not only their universal presence in animal blood, but for their diversity and complexity.

I. INTRODUCTION

Blood group antigens and their associated antibodies are important not only in clinical medicine but also in anthropology, human genetics, and forensic science.

A. Definitions

Blood groups are determined by antigenic structures on the surface of red cells and are detected by reactions with specific antibodies. The antigenic phenotype is under genetic control and remains relatively constant throughout life. A blood group **system** is defined by antigens that are regulated either by allelic genes or closely linked genes.

Table 16.1
Survey of Major Red Cell Blood Group Systems

System	Important antigens[a]	Year discovered	Discoverer(s)	Antibody source[b]
ABO	A_1, A_2, *B*, *H*, A_3, A_m, A_x	1900–1902	Landsteiner	*1*
MNSs	*M*, *N*, *S*, *s*, U, M^g, Mi^a, Hu, He Mt^a, Vw, M_2, N_2, S_2	1927	Landsteiner and Levine	*2*
P	P_1, p^k, P_2, (Tj^a)	1927	Landsteiner and Levine	*2*
Rh	*D*, *C*, *E*, *c*, *e*, C^w, E^w, ce, Ce,	1939–1941	Levine	*3*
	G, CE, cE, D^u, C^u, E^u, LW	1940	Landsteiner and Wiener	*4*
Lutheran	Lu^a, Lu^b	1945	Callender and Race	*5*
Kell	*K*, *k*, Kp^a, Kp^b, Js^a, Js^b	1946	Coombs et al.	*3*
Lewis	Le^a, Le^b	1946	Mourant	*1*
Duffy	Fy^a, Fy^b, Fy3, Fy4, Fy5	1950	Cutbush and Mollison	*5*
Kidd	Jk^a, *Jkb*	1951	Allen and Diamond	*3*
Wright	Wr^a, Wr^b	1953	Holman	*3*
Diego	Di^a, Di^b	1955	Layrisse et al.	*3*
Cartwright	Yt^a, Yt^b	1956	Eaton et al.	*5*
Xg	Xg^a	1962	Sanger et al.	*5*
Dombrock	Do^a, Do^b	1965	Swanson et al.	*5*
Colton	Co^a, Co^b	1967	Heisto et al.	*5*

a. The most important antigens in each system are in italics.
b. Numbers refer to source of original antibody, as follows: *1*, naturally occurring isohemagglutinin of normal human serum; *2*, serum from rabbits immunized with human red cells; *3*, serum from mother of baby with erythroblastosis fetalis; *4*, serum from rabbits immunized with rhesus monkey red cells; *5*, serum from subjects given transfusion with incompatible blood.

B. Known blood groups

The number of red cell blood groups now exceeds 400. Table 16.1 lists some of them with the dates of their discovery. Note that the rate of detection of new blood group systems greatly increased after the development of the Coombs test in 1945.

C. Antibodies: sources and properties

1. Normal humans

Antibodies to some blood group antigens occur in the serum of individuals who lack the antigen and have had no prior exposure to it. Such antibodies are referred to as **natural isohemagglutinins**. The major ones are directed against surface antigens such as the ABO, Ii, and P systems, the specificity of which is controlled by oligosaccharides. It is presumed that these antibodies are elicited by similar sequences on microbial surfaces. These antibodies are usually IgMs. They are effective hemolysins because they efficiently fix complement. Occasionally, IgG antibodies specific for these antigens also appear. Isohemagglutinins with ABO specificity are always clinically significant. In other blood group systems such as P or Ii, clinical significance may depend more on the thermal amplitude of the antibody than on the actual titer.

2. *Immunized animals*

If animals are immunized with **human red cells**, they may form antibodies to certain of the xenogeneic blood group antigens. This is an important source of blood group antisera. Initially these sera are carefully absorbed with human red cells to establish specificity. Recently developed antigen-specific **monoclonal antibodies**, which do not require such absorption, may soon replace the blood group antigens now raised in animals.

3. *Immunized humans*

The third major source of the blood group antibodies are donors who have been allogenically immunized either by (1) prior blood transfusion or (2) previous pregnancies. Such antibodies, sometimes called **immune antibodies**, are elicited by prior exposure to red cell antigens and are commonly IgGs. It is often difficult or provoke an immune response in animals to the particular antigens for which an antibody is desired. Hence antibody is still being harvested from allogeneically immunized humans.

The prevalence in Caucasians of immune red cell antibodies other than the most common one, anti-D, is shown in table 16.2. Together with anti-D, the antibodies shown in table 16.2 are those most likely to cause clinical problems for the transfusionist. The prevalence of these antibodies provides a measure of antigenic potency that is based on comparisons of the frequency of a particular antibody and the calculated frequency of possible immunizations (i.e., the chance of a positive donor as encountering a negative recipient). Thus, for Kell, the probability of an immunizing combination is 3.5 times less than with Duffy (Fy^a), but anti-Kell is 2.5 times more common that anti-Fy^a. Therefore Kell must be 9 times more potent than Fy^a. Similar calculations can be used to rank the other impor-

Table 16.2
Prevalence of Immune Red Cell Antibodies Other Than D (or CD or DE)

Antibody	%
E	32.7
K (or k)	28.7
c	19.2
Fy^a or Fy^b	11.2
Jk^a or Jk^b	4.3
Ce	2.5
C (or Ce)	0.7
S (or s)	0.2
Others	0.5

tant blood group antigens. However, as yet there is no good structural explanation for the relative antigenic potencies observed. Fortunately many blood group antigens have no opportunity to establish their antigenic potency because their incidence is so high that the probability of an immunizing event is very low.

D. Methods of detection

1. Agglutination by specific antibody

Under physiologic conditions of pH and ionic strength, normal red cells repel each other owing to their negative surface charge, or **zeta potential**. The charge, which is largely attributable to sialyl residues, serves to keep the cells in suspension with a minimum intercellular distance of about 250 Å. Reaction of red cells with antibody causes visible agglutination if the antibody is capable of bridging the distance between adjacent cells. Such antibodies are most often IgM.

The older nomenclature (i.e., saline antibodies, complete agglutinins) was developed before it was understood that difference in size and number of binding sites explained why IgM antibodies function more efficiently than IgG antibodies as agglutinins in saline.

2. Enhancement of agglutination by antibody

a. REDUCTION OF ZETA POTENTIAL

In many cases weak agglutination must be enhanced to be detected. Antibodies that fail to produce agglutination with red cells in saline have been called **incomplete** antibodies. This is a misnomer because lack of agglutination is due to the number of antibodies on the cell surface and to the immunoglobulin class (usually IgG) and not to the fact that the antibodies are incomplete in some sense. In such a situation, several techniques are available for enhancing the aggregation by reducing the zeta potential and thus shortening the intercellular distances. Zeta potential can be reduced by the additon of colloid (albumin, polyvinylpyrrolidone, or dextran) to the suspending medium or by removal of the negative charge from the red cell surface by treating cells with neuraminidase or proteolytic enzymes such as papain or ficin. Use of enzyme-treated cells may enhance weak reactions and facilitate identification of antibodies that might otherwise be missed.

b. INSERTION OF ANTIBODY RED CELL BRIDGES

Agglutination may be produced or enhanced by the addition of Coombs reagent (i.e., antiglobulin antibody) to a suspension of washed red cell antigens. As described in lecture 13, Coombs reagent may have specificity for IgG or complement (usually C3b and C3d) or any of its components. Coombs reagents do not have specificity against IgM or IgA and hence will not detect antibody of these classes on red cell surfaces.

3. Use of lectins

Antibody-like substances with specificity for red cell surface carbohydrates can be extracted from a variety of plant seeds of mollusks. These reagents are useful in identifying such blood group antigens as A, B, H, M, and N. Two pounds of lima beans could provide enough anti-A lectin for all the blood grouping of an entire year in the United States.

4. Automated techniques

Solid-phase antibody and antigen immobilization techniques can be used to automate blood grouping, crossmatching and, to a lesser extent, antibody identification. These offer greater sensitivity, automated endpoints that can be read without human intervention, and greater speed. Such technology is mainly used in high-volume regional blood centers. As yet, little progress has been made in adapting this technology to hospital blood banks.

E. Genetics

Inheritance of blood group antigens is according to mendelian laws. Heredity is generally autosomal codominant, i.e., there is an expression of both alleles in the heterozygous individual. A notable exception to the usual mode of inheritance is the case of Xg^a, which is X linked. Some systems, notably ABO, Rh, and MNSs, encompass more than two alleles. Most systems, however, involve two common alleles; remaining alleles are usually rare.

1. Linked genes

Owing to the normal crossing over of homologous chromosomes at meiosis, most of the genetic loci—even those on the same chromosome—show independent inheritance. If two loci are near each other, however, crossing over is diminished, and the genes appear to be inherited together through successive generations, or linked.

The MNSs and Kell systems, for example, constitute groups of closely linked loci. Whether the Rh system represents multiple loci or multiple epitopes of a single polymorphic system has been argued since discovery of this system. The Fisher-Race and Weiner nomenclature for the Rh system are based respectively on these two opposing genetic interpretations.

2. Interaction with other genes

The expression of some blood groups depends on the interaction of genes at several different loci. For example, in the Lewis system expression of

Table 16.3
Chromosome Assignments of Some Blood Group Loci

Locus	Chromosome
ABO	9
Rh	1
Fy	1
Chido, Rogers	6
MNSs	4
Xg	X
Sc	1

Le^b requires the presence of alleles from two other genes. H gene is required to make the necessary substrate, the H chain. The Se gene of the Se/se secretor system, is needed to convert the H chain to the Le^b antigen by adding a second fucose. Absence of either H or Se will prevent the expression of Le^b gene. Multigene control of a blood group antigen can confuse family studies unless the effects of all genes are considered.

3. Loci of blood group genes on chromosomes

Loci of some blood group genes are known. These are summarized in table 16.3. In some cases blood group loci are linked with genetic diseases. For example, the rare nail-patella syndrome is linked to the ABO locus; hereditary elliptocytosis is linked to the Rh locus.

4. Occurrence of blood group antigens

A and B antigens are ubiquitous and are found in animal tissues, plants, and bacteria. Rh antigens are present only on the red cells of primates. In any individual, A, B, H, Le^a, Le^b, P, and I may be present in many tissues, whereas other blood group antigens are probably limited to the red cells (and, in the case of MN, Kell, and Diego, to the neutrophils as well). In some instances, distribution of blood group antigens on solid tissues is important in planning organ transplantation. For example, ABO compatibility is required in kidney and liver transplantation but not in bone marrow transplantation. This difference is probably due to the lack of ABH antigens on bone marrow stem cells.

II. ABO SYSTEM

A. Historical notes

The ABO system, clinically the most important, was the first blood group discovered. In 1900 Landsteiner obtained blood from six colleagues. On mixing serum from one individual with washed red cells from another in all possible combinations, he noted agglutination with some combinations but not with others. He was thus able to classify individuals on the basis

Table 16.4
The ABO System Defined by Anti-A and Anti-B

Blood groups	Antigens on red cells	Antibodies in serum
O	None	Anti-A and anti-B
A	A	Anti-B
B	B	Anti-A
AB	A and B	None

Table 16.5
Subdivisions of A Antigen and Anti-A Serum

		Reactions with	
Group	Antigens	Anti-A	Anti-A_1
A_1	AA_1	+	+
A_2	A	+	−

of antigens on their red cells and agglutinins in their serum. In subsequent work Landsteiner recognized that the pattern of reactions could be explained by two antigens, which he designated A and B. In this analysis, O signified the state of not having A or B. He also noted a reciprocal relation between the presence of antigen and agglutinin. The Landsteiner scheme is summarized in Table 16.4.

B. Subdivisions of A antigen

A antigen and anti-A are complex. Anti-A serum from a group B donor contains two types of antibodies, anti-A and anti-A_1 (see table 16.5). If certain A or AB cells (A_2 or A_2B) are used to absorb such antiserum, reactivity with A_2 or A_2B cells is lost, but the antiserum continues to react with certain other A or AB cells (A_1 or A_1B). On the other hand, anti-A absorbed with A_1 or A_1B cells removes all reactivity. Thus all A cells have a common A antigen, but A_1 or A_1B cells have an additional antigen (A_1).

About 80% of group A bloods have the A_1 phenotype; the remainder are A_2. Occasionally, an A_2 individual becomes immunized against A_1 antigen but these antibodies are clinically significant only if they react at 37°C. Such a patient must be transfused with group O red cells.

Until recently, it was uncertain whether the differences between the A_1 and the A_2 phenotype were quantitative or qualitative. Recent studies demonstrate that the A_1 phenotype has unique oligosaccharides.

Other subgroups of A and B exist. They have fewer antigen sites per cell but the details of the structural differences remain unknown. These subgroups are rare. Because of the decreased expression of A or B, the chance of these subgroups being mistyped as group O cells is increased. Aside from this risk, these subgroups are of no clinical importance.

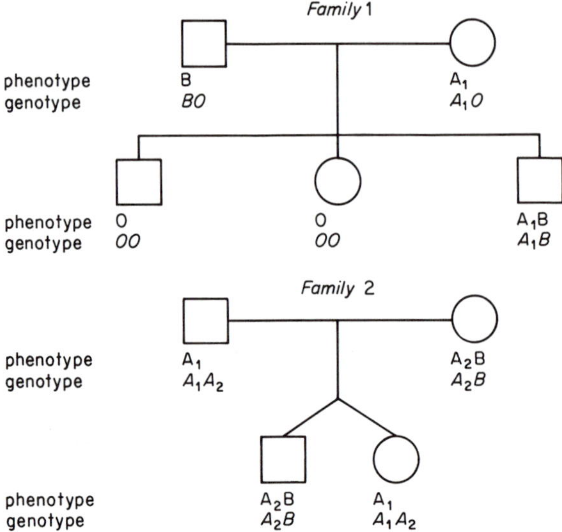

Fig. 16.1
Illustration of the usefulness of family studies in the elucidation of phenotypes. **Family 1** (upper diagram), ambiguous phenotypes of father and mother (B and A_1) are shown to be associated with genotypes BO and A_1O by demonstration of two type O children. **Family 2** (lower diagram), ambiguous phenotypes of father and daughter (A_1) are shown to be associated with genotypes A_1A_2 by demonstration of phenotypes A_2B in mother and twin son. (From R. R. Race and R. Sanger, *Blood Groups in Man*, 6th ed. Oxford: Blackwell, 1975.)

C. Genetics

1. Phenotypes and genotypes

A child receives one of four genes from each parent: A_1, A_2, B_1, or O. Six phenotypes are possible because the A antigen associated with group A_2 is also present on group A_1 cells.

There are, however, ten possible genotypes. Group A_1 may have three genotypes (A_1A_1, A_1O, A_1A_2). Group A_2 can have either A_2A_2 or A_2O genotypes. Group B can have either BB or BO genotypes.

Finally, for the phenotypes A_1B, A_2B, and OO, the genotypes correspond to the phenotypes.

2. Determination of genotypes

To determine which of several genotypes is responsible for an ambiguous phenotype, appropriate studies must be performed on members of a family. Figure 16.1 illlustrates such studies in two families in which ambiguous ABO phenotypes are resolved by studies of family members.

D. H antigen

As shown in figure 16.2, the surface oligosaccharide that constitutes the H antigen is the precursor of the A and B antigens. A is formed by adding

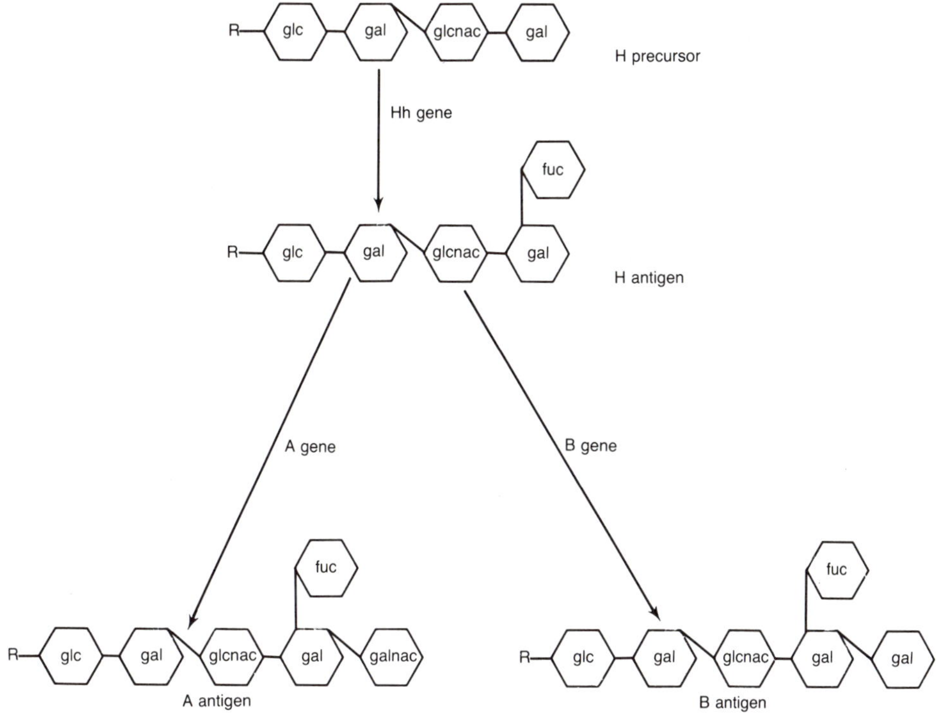

Fig. 16.2
Synthesis of ABH antigens. H antigen is formed by the addition of L-fucose to the terminal galactose of the H precursor. Addition of *N*-acetylgalactosamine (galnac) to H yields the A antigen, while addition of galactose forms the B antigen. Individuals homozygous for h gene lack the fucosyl transferase required to make H antigen and thus have the Bombay phenotype. (From W. H. Churchill and S. R. Kurtz, eds. *Transfusion Medicine*. Boston: Blackwell Scientific Publications, 1988.)

N-acetylgalactosamine (GalNac) to the terminal galactose of the H antigen. For the B antigen, galactose is added to the terminal galactose of the H chain. It follows that O cells, in which conversion to A or B has not occurred, will have the most H antigen. Conversely, cells with the largest number of converted sites (A_1 cells) will have the least amount of H antigen. Thus antibodies with H specificity are less likely to react with A and B cells than they are to react with O cells.

In the rare variant called **Bombay**, the H precursor cannot be converted to H antigen. These cells lack H antigen, and hence A or B phenotype cannot be expressed, even if the suitable genotype is present. Despite the lack of A, B, and H groups, these cells survive normally. However, patients with Bombay blood invariably have anti-H and thus can be transfused only with Bombay bloods.

E. Chemistry of antigens

1. Effect of branching in surface carbohydrates

The chemistry of ABH antigens—and of other blood groups in which specificity is controlled by surface carbohydrates (Lewis, Ii, and P antigens)—was elucidated in studies of soluble blood group substances and, more recently, of red cell glycosphingolipids. The glycosphingolipids are linked through glucose to ceramide (*N*-fatty acyl sphingosine). Depending on the sequence of sugars supporting the terminal blood group antigen, these glycosphingolipids are subclassified as lactosyl ceramides (Galβ1-4Glcβ1 → cer), globoside series of ceramides (Galα1-4Galβ1-4Glcβ1 → cer), or as the ganglioside ceramides (GalNAcβ1-Galβ1-4Glcβ1-cer).

Carbohydrate sequences with blood group activity are also linked to proteins. These sequences can be linked through *N*-acetylglucosamine (GlcNAc) to the amino group of asparagine or *N*-acetylgalactosamine to the oxygen group of serine or threonine.

A second level of heterogeneity depends on the length and extent of branching of the oligosaccharides. The internal sequence GlcNAc-Gal becomes progressively more branched with cell maturation. This process has been demonstrated with the Ii antigens (see below) and also in maturing squamous epithelium. Increased complexity of branching has been observed in both glycolipids and glycoproteins, which have blood group activity.

A third level of heterogeneity is caused by the subterminal disaccharide in A and B antigens. Four types have been observed. The terminal sequence for type 1 H chain is Gal β1-3GlcNAcβ1-R; for type 2 the sequence is Gal β1-4GlcNAcβ1-R. Only recently recognized, type 3 has a repetitive A antigen sequence in which several sequences of GalNAcα1-3Galβ1-3GalNAcα1-R appear. Finally type 4, the globo- or gangliosphingolipids, have as the subterminal sequence Galβ1-3GalNAcβ1-R.

There are significant differences in the distribution and specificity of each of the chain types:

- Type 1 chains are found in the soluble blood group antigens and on endodermally derived tissues.
- Type 2 chains are found on red cell antigens synthesized on the cell surface and on ectodermally derived tissues.
- Type 3 chains are in general attached by O linkage to proteins. The repetitive A antigen sequence is thought to contribute to the unique specificity of the A_1 antigen.
- Type 4 chains are only found in the glycosphingolipids.

The immediate precursor of the H chain lacks the terminal Fuc (fucose). Bombay blood lacks the **glycosyl transferase** needed to convert the H precursor in the H antigen by the addition of Fuc).

2. *Role of gene products in determining specificity*

Although specificity of these antigens is controlled by the surface carbohydrate oligosaccharide, the gene product in each case is a glycosyl transferase that adds appropriate sugars to the carbohydrate chain. Thus assay of specific glycosyl transferases can establish genotype. In Group O it had been thought that gene product is not expressed; however, recent evidence suggests that a protein antigenically similar to the glycosyl transferase in A and B genotype is present but without function. Rather than lacking a gene, Group O individuals may have an abnormal nonfunctional glycosyl transferase.

III. OTHER CARBOHYDRATE ANTIGENS

A. Lewis system

The Lewis antigens are made from the same precursors as the ABH antigens except that they are exclusively type 1 chains. The site of synthesis is unknown. Soluble plasma antigens are absorbed after synthesis onto red cell surfaces. These antigens develop in the postnatal period so that the final phenotype is not apparent in the first 2 years. In Caucasians about 72% are Le^{a-b+}, 22% are Le^{a+b-}, and 6% are Le^{a-b-}, In black populations as many as 40% are the double-negative phenotype.

Expression of these antigens depends on the interaction of the H gene, the Se gene, and the Le gene. Individuals with the Le gene make an antigen called Le^a, which resembles H substance, differing only in the position of its Fuc. If an individual lacks the secretor (Se) gene, Le^a is found in body fluids and absorbed onto red cells. If Se is present, H substance is also present in body fluids, and it is converted to Le^b by the adition of a second Fuc, so that all Le^a is converted to Le^b. These individuals characteristically have the phenotype Le^{a-b+}.The following combinations are possible:

Le gene	Se gene	Phenotype
+	+	Le^{a-b+}
+	−	Le^{a+b-}
−	+ or −	Le^{a-b-}

B. P system

These antigens were recognized by antisera developed in rabbits. They are glycosphingolipids and originate on a ceramide dihexose (Gal–Gal–ceramide). In the rare individual unable to add sugars beyound the initial two, a p antigen is said to be present. Addition of another Gal yields an antigen called p^k. Subsequent addition of GalNAc converts p^k to P antigen, which is the antigen against which Donath-Landsteiner antibody is directed (see lecture 13). P_1 antigen is synthesized by a different route in which the type 2 H-chain precursor is converted to P_1 by addition of Gal. The most common antibody against these antigens is anti-P_1. It is naturally occurring and causes hemolytic reactions only if it is reactive at 37°C. On the other hand, individuals with a p or p^k phenotype have antibodies against determinants of most red cells; hence, they are difficult to transfuse.

C. Ii system

Most cold antibodies have specificity against the Ii antigen system (see table 13.3). These antigens are found in red cells and nonhematopoietic tissues. Fetal and red cells and their precursors have i. Red cells do not fully develop I until age 2 years. The transition from i to I is mediated by an enzyme under the control of a separate gene, tentatively called Z, the absence of which causes persistence of i. Z is responsible for converting straight-chain i sequences to a more complex branched-chain I sequence. Both I and i are made up of either branched- or straight-chain sequences of galactose *N*-acetylglucosamine (Gal–GlcNac) in recurring sequences. These sugars are also part of the subterminal sugars of the H chain. Hence blood group active carbohydrates sometimes have IH specificity as well as A and B specificity.

I and i cannot be considered alleles because the transition from i to I is accomplished by the action of a separate enzyme.

Most sera have low titers of clinically insignificant anti-I antibodies. Significant hemolysis is usually due to anti-I antibodies of high titer and wide amplitude. Rarely, anti-i antibodies cause hemolysis. The hemolysis in infectious mononucleosis is an example.

IV. THE SIALOGLYCOPROTEINS: MNSs AND U ANTIGENS

A. Clinical features

These three antigen pairs are controlled by three separate, closely linked genes. M and N antibodies are usually naturally occurring and rarely clinically significant. Unlike most other naturally occurring antibodies, anti-M is usually IgG rather than IgM. Dialysis patients may acquire an anti-N if exposed to dialysis equipment sterilized with formaldehyde. M and S tend to segregate together, as do N and S. U antigen is always present except in Ss individuals, in whom U is absent about three-quarters of the time. These individuals may acquire an anti-U antibody that can cause transfusion reactions and hemolytic disease of the newborn.

B. Antigen structure and genetics

After SDS polyacylamide gel electrophoresis, staining with PAS stain reveals four sialoglycoproteins, which are called α, β, γ, δ sialoglycoproteins (SGPs). α SGP, also termed glycophorin A, is associated with MN activity, and β SGP, or glycophorin B, is associated with Ss and U activity.

Glycophorin A has been fully sequenced (see figure 14.3). Its mol. wt. is 31,000. About 70 amino acids extend beyond the membrane; 20 are in the lipid bilayer and 40 are in the cell cytoplasm. The N-terminal portion is glycosylated with a tetrasaccharide whose structure is NANA–Gal–GalNac–Ser/Thr, where NA denotes neuraminic or sialic
|
NANA
acid. These are identical for both M and N; however, amino acid sequencing shows that M activity correlates with serine in position 1 and glycine in position 5. Thus MN antigens are probably the result of differences in interaction of the oligosaccharides with polypeptides that display the genetically controlled differences. Similar studies have associated glycophorin B with Ss and U activity. The genes controlling these antigens are autosomal.

C. Contribution of oligosaccharide on sialoglycoproteins to polyagglutination: T, T^k, and Tn antigens

Removal of terminal sialic acids (NAs) of the major oligosaccharide exposes Gal–GalNac. This disaccharide reacts with most adult sera because of a naturally occurring antibody called **anti-T**. Hence these cells are called **polyagglutinable**. The most common cause of so-called **T activation** is exposure in vivo or in vitro to bacterial neuraminidase. **T^k activation** occurs when a similar process exposes GlcNac, presumably by the action of another bacterial product, β-endogalactosidase, on ABH and I oligosaccharides. **Tn activation** results from exposure of GalNac through lack of the two terminal sugars. This persistent defect is due to a stem cell mutation. Tn activation has been observed in patients with acute myelocytic leukemia.

V. Rh SYSTEM

A. Historical notes

In 1939, Levine and Stetson described and antibody in the serum of a mother of a stillborn fetus and noted that this antibody reacted with the red cells of her husband and about 80% of ABO-compatible donors. Independently Landsteiner and Weiner reported in 1940 that antisera prepared in rabbits against the blood of the rhesus monkey reacted with the red cells of about 85% of Caucasian New Yorkers.

Although initially thought to have the same specificity, which was termed Rh (for rhesus), these antisera were later shown to differ. The rabbit antisera detect a specificity LW that can be separated from the Rh specificity. The complexity of the Rh antigen system was soon demonstrated by the identification of many other related specificities in this system.

Table 16.6
Frequencies of Rh Gene Complexes in England

Gene complex		
Fisher-Race nomenclature	Wiener nomenclature	Frequency
CDe	R^1	0.4076
cde	r	0.3886
cDE	R^2	0.1411
cDe	R^0	0.0257
C^wDe	R^{1w}	0.0129
cdE	r^u	0.0119
Cde	r^1	0.0098
CDE	R^z	0.0024

Source: R. R. Race and R. Sanger, *Blood Groups in Man*, 6th ed. Boston: Blackwell Scientific Publications, 1975.

B. Nomenclature: relation to genetic models

1. Fisher-Race theory

The nomenclature is confused because two parallel systems are used interchangeably. The Fisher-Race system postulates three closely linked genes designated **Cc**, **Dd**, and **Ee**. In this system the Rh antigen is renamed D; the allele for d has never been identified. However, antisera have been developed against the C, c, E, and e. The term **Rh positive** refers only to the presence of the D antigen, also called Rh or Rh factor. **Rh negative** denotes absence of D but does not denote absence of other antigens of the Rh system (C, c, E, or e). Studies of families have shown that all possible combinations of these phenotypes can be identified, but some are more common than others (table 16.6). Products of the three closely linked genes segregate together.

2. Weiner system

The Weiner system assumes that there is one gene with multiple specificities and that each of the three-letter complexes in the Fisher-Race system is the product of a single gene symbolized by a single letter and superscript (table 16.6).

In converting from Weiner to Fisher-Race nomenclature, R signifies presence of D and r absence of D, which is symbolized d. Superscript 1 or prime (′) implies presence of C and e; superscript 2 or double prime (″) implies presence of c and E. Thus, R^1 = CDe; R^2 = cDE; r′ = Cde; r″ = cdE, r = cde, etc. Other rules are given in textbooks.

3. Rosenfield system

This system avoids commitment to a specific genetic theory and identifies antigents by number—for example, D = Rh 1, C = Rh 2, E = Rh 3, c = Rh 4, and e = Rh 5.

Each of these systems has some advantages. The Weiner system is convenient shorthand for gene complexes that in the Fisher-Race system would require 3 letters to specify; the Rosenfield system lends itself to computerization.

Current information about these antigens has still not established whether the Weiner or Fisher-Race mode is correct (see below).

C. Compound antigens

Some isoantibodies have specificity for what appears to be a combination of two known antigens, such as c and e. Such **compound antigens** can be recognized only if the genes are part of the same haplotype. The main use of these antisera is in genetic studies.

D. Weakened antigens

Some individuals have a weakly reactive D antigen, which is called D^u. Formal terminology would be Rh^+, D^u variant, even though it would appear to be Rh negative without special techniques. For purposes of transfusion, the D^u variant is equivalent to Rh^+. Genetically Rh^+, D^u variant recipients are Rh^+ and are unlikely to be sensitized by administered Rh^+ blood.

The chemical basis for the weakened D antigen is not understood. One theory postulates that the normal D antigen is made up of four components and that weakened antigen is due to the absence of some of these components. Another theory proposes that the presence of C, d on the haplotype opposite the D causes this effect.

E. Deleted antigens: Rh null cells

Rare individuals lack part or all of the common Rh antigens. In Fisher nomenclature, partially deleted cells lack one or more of the antigens (-D-); fully deleted cells (---) are called **Rh null cells** and lack all evidence of Cc, D, or Ee antigens. Unlike cells lacking ABH antigens, red cells lacking Rh antigens have many abnormalities, including shortened survival, stomatocytic morphology, and impaired transport of sodium and potassium ions.

The Rh null syndrome is caused either by a gene that blocks conversion of Rh precursor to Rh antigens or, in some cases, to absence of an Rh structural gene. In the latter instance, heterozygotes express only a single Rh haplotype.

These partially and fully deleted cells are valuable reagents for studying the specificity of warm-type antibodies found in immunohemolytic anemia (see lecture 13).

F. Rh antigen structure

The D antigen depends on membrane phospholipids for expression and is thought to be an integral membrane protein.

There is still disagreement about the structure of the D antigen. Plapp has suggested that partial purification could be achieved by SDS gel electrophoresis and affinity chromatography with Rh immune globulin. The isolated antigen had features of a proteolipid. It specifically blocked the interaction of anti-D on red cells. He also found an antigen on the inside of Rh negative cells that reacted with anti-D.

Two other groups have recently studied the D antigen. Both found a Mr 30,000 integral membrane protein, which could be isolated only from Rh positive cells and was attached to the red cell cytoskeleton. How these observations relate to the work of Plapp is not clear. However, extension of such studies may eventually resolve the conflicting genetic views embodied in the Fisher-Race and Weiner nomenclatures.

VI. OTHER CLINICALLY SIGNIFICANT SYSTEMS

A. Kell system

The Kell antigen system rivals the Rh system in its complexity and clinical importance. Appearing in response to prior immunization, anti-Kell antibodies have caused hemolytic transfusion reactions and hemolytic disease in newborns. Anti-kell is a common antibody, but because about 90% of bloods are Kell negative, it is easy to find blood to use in patients with anti-Kell. The main antigen pairs, **K-k**, **Kp^a-Kp^b**, and **Js^a-Js^b**, are controlled by three closely linked loci or three subloci of a single gene. Unlike the situation in the Rh system, not all expected combinations have been encountered. The incidence of these antigens also varies according to race (table 16.7).

The autosomal loci of these genes are unknown. Little is known of antigen biosynthesis, but investigation of the uncommon McLeod phenotype (k Kp^b Js^b) suggests two steps in the synthetic process of these

Table 16.7
Racial Distribution of Kell Antigen

	% of bloods positive	
Antigen	Caucasians	Blacks
K	9.0	3.5
k	99.8	>99.9
Kp^a	2.0	< 0.1
Kp^b	99.9	>99.9
Js^a	< 0.1	19.5
Js^b	>99.9	98.9

antigens. Synthesis of the precursor of Kell antigen, Kx, is controlled by a locus on the X chromosome. A second autosomal gene, whose location is unknown, then converts this precursor to the normal Kell antigens.

McLeod cells are acanthocytes with reduced survival in vivo. Normal Kell antigens are present in decreased amounts, and antibody may develop against Kx (the precursor substance) and Km (a high incidence antigen associated with the usual Kell antigens). Leukocytes normally display Kx antigen, but Kx is absent in patients with the X-linked chronic granulomatous disease (see lecture 19). Both McLeod syndrome and chronic granulomatous disease exist separately or together with Kx lacking involved cell lives.

There is little structural information about Kell system antigens. Treatment with sulfhydryl reagents such as dithiothreitol reduces expression of Kell antigens. A Kell-reactive protein has been isolated from red cell membranes. Molecular weight was estimated to be 90,000.

B. Duffy system

Distribution of the relatively simply Duffy phenotypes in Caucasians and blacks is shown in table 16.8. These antigens are degraded by proteolysis. Fy^a has been partially purified and is thought to be 35,000 to 45,000 daltons. Structural information about other Duffy antigens is not yet available.

Double-negative phenotype red cells, Fy (a−b−), are totally resistant to invasion by *Plasmodium vivax*. Hence selective pressures may be responsible for the high incidence of this phenotype in blacks. The genes are located on chromosome 1. Individuals of double-negative phenotype lack Fy3, which travles with Fy^a and Fy^b. They may acquire antibody against Fy3, which reacts with all Fy(a) or Fy(b) positive cells. Transfusion of incompatible blood into Duffy-sensitive individuals can cause severe hemolysis.

C. Kidd system

The Kidd system behaves like a two-allele system with a silent allele of infrequent occurrence. In Caucasians the incidence of $\mathbf{Jk^a}$ is 77% and of

Table 16.8
Racial Distribution of Duffy Antigen

	% of bloods positive	
Phenotypes	Caucasians	Blacks
Fy (a+ b−)	17	9
Fy (a+ b+)	49	1
Fy (a− b+)	34	22
Fy (a− b−)	–	68

Jk^b 72%. The double-negative phenotype is rare and occurs mainly in Chinese and South American Indians. Jk^a and Jk^b are always associated with another antigen, Jk^3, which is also lacking on the double-negative phenotype. Hence these individuals may make an antibody against Jk^3.

Immunization to Kidd is caused mainly by transfusions. Kidd antibodies are evanescent warm-active incomplete antibodies that may not be detected in red cell antibody screens. Consequently they often cause delayed transfusion reactions, which may be severe. A reliable transfusion history is the best way to prevent such reactions.

D. Lutheran system

This system parallels the Kidd system. There are two common alleles, **Lu**^{a} and **Lu**^{b}, and a silent one. Lu^a is found in 8% of Caucasians and Lu^b in more than 99%. The double-negative phenotype is caused by either a dominant inhibitor gene or a recessive silent allele. The phenotype caused by dominant inhibitor displays small amounts of Lu^a and Lu^b and hence does not make antibody against Lu^3, an antigen that travels with Lu^a and Lu^b. On the other hand, double negatives with the silent allele do make anti-Lu^3 and thus may become difficult transfusion problems. In additon, two other closely liked allelic pairs and several high incidence antigens have been identified. Fortunately the latter are usually of little clinical importance.

The autosomal location of Lu genes has not been identified, but it is closely linked to the Se/se gene of the ABH system. Antigen structure is unknown.

E. Xg^a blood group

This antigen is controlled by a gene on the X chromosome. It is not clinically significant but is of interest as a marker for X chromosomes that appear to escape inactivation by the Lyon mechanism. This is in contrast with Xk, which *is* inactivated. Thus, McLeod females can have a mixture of McLeod and normal red cells.

VII. USES OF BLOOD GROUPING DATA

A. In clinical medicine

1. Pretransfusion testing

Prior to transfusion, blood is typed and crossmatched (by methods described in lecture 17) to establish ABO and D compatibility. Typing for other antigens is omitted unless the recipient is known to be sensitized to them. Justification of this policy is that it is easier to provide antigen-negative blood for individuals who become sensitized (10–15% of multitransfused patients) than it is to match blood more extensively with the recipient's phenotype prior to sensitization.

2. *Hemolytic disease of the newborn*

The relationship between blood groups and transplacental hemolytic disease of the newborn and other acquired hemolytic anemias is discussed in lectures 13 and 17.

B. In genetics

Blood groups are important for chromosome mapping because their inheritance can be traced serologically, and sometimes they can be localized quite precisely. For example, the Rh locus is on the short arm of chromosome 1 and is part of the linkage group that can be easily separated from the Duffy locus. Distribution of blood groups of large populations is useful in the study of population movement and origins of different ethnic groups.

C. In forensic medicine

1. *Identification studies*

Demonstration of blood groups in fresh or even dried blood or other materials (such as semen) is indispensable in establishing the human origin of the specimen and in identifying the individual from whom it came.

2. *Paternity testing*

In cases of disputed paternity, blood grouping of mother, child, and putative father can either exclude paternity or give a statistical probability that an accused man is the father. It is almost always possible now, by the use of many genetic markers, to establish when a man is not the father of a child.

SELECTED REFERENCES

Reviews

Anstee, D. J. The blood group MNSs: active sialoglycoproteins. *Semin. Hematol.* 18(1981): 13–31.

Clausen, H. and Hakamori, S. ABH and related histo-blood group antigens; immunochemical differences in carrier isotypes and their distribution. *Vox San.* 56(1989): 1–20.

Huestis, D. W., Bove, J. R., et al. *Practical Blood Transfusion*, 4th ed. Boston: Little, Brown, 1988.

Issitt, P. D. The Rh blood group system, 1988: Eight new antigens in nine years and some observations on the biochemistry and genetics of the system. *Transf. Med. Rev.* 3(1989): 1–12.

Levene, C., Levene, N. A., et al. Red cell polyagglutination. *Transf. Med. Rev.* 2(1988): 176–185.

Marcus, D. M., Kundu, S. K., et al. The P blood group system: recent progress in immunochemistry and genetics. *Semin. Hematol.* 18(1981): 63–71.

Mollison, P. L., Engelfriet, C. P., et al. *Blood Transfusion in Clinical Medicine*, 8th ed. Boston: Blackwell Scientific Publications, 1987.

Tippett, P. Chromosomal mapping of blood genes. *Semin. Hematol.* 18(1981): 4–12.

Original articles

Agree, P., Saboori, A. M., et al. Purification and partial characterization of the Mr 30,000 integral membrane protein associated with the erythrocyte Rh(D) antigen. *J. Biol. Chem.* 262(1987): 17497–17503.

Bloy, C., Blanchard, D., et al. Human monclonal antibody against Rh(D) antigen: partial characterization of the Rh(D) polypeptide from human erythrocytes. *Blood* 69(1987): 1491–1497.

Hadley, T. J., David, P. H., et al. Identification of an erythrocyte compound carrying the Duffy blood group Fy^a. *Science* 223(1984): 597–599.

Jaber, A., Blanchard, D., et al. Characterization of the blood group Kell (Kl) antigen with a human monclonal antibody. *Blood* 73(1989): 1597–1602.

Mojena, M., and Boscá, L. Identification of an anti-A and anti-B blood group glycosyltransferase antibody after incompatible bone marrow transplant. *Blood* 74(1989): 1134–1138.

Plapp, F. V., Kowalski, M. M., et al. Partial purification of Rho(D) antigen from Rh positive and negative erythrocytes. *Proc. Natl. Acad. Sci. USA* 76(1979): 2964–2968.

Redman, C. M., Huima, T., et al. Effect of phosphatidylserine on the shape of McLeod red cell acanthocytes. *Blood* 74(1989): 1826–1835.

Sinor, L. T., Brown, P. J., et al. The Rh antigen specificity of erythrocyte proteolipid. *Transfusion* 24(1984): 179–180.

Suyama, K., and Goldstein, J. Enzymatic evidence for differences in the placement of Rh antigens within the red cell membrane. *Blood* 75(1990): 255–260.

Wallas, C., Simon, R., et al. Isolation of a Kell-reactor protein from red cell membranes. *Transfusion* 26(1986): 173–176.

Yamamoto, F., Clausen, H., et al. Molecular genetic basis of the histo-blood group ABO system. *Nature* 345(1990): 229–233.

Yoshida, A., Yanaguchi, Y. F., et al. Immunologic homology of human blood glycosyltransferases and the genetic background of blood group (ABO) determination. *Blood* 54(1979): 344–350.

LECTURE 17

Blood Groups II. Transfusion Therapy

W. Hallowell Churchill, Jr.

EDITOR'S COMMENT

Blood transfusion remains a critical part of the management of many diseases. Yet despite advances in the technology of procurement, processing, storage, and serologic testing, risks remain for transfusion recipients. These consist mainly of the possible transmission of infectious diseases via the blood of an apparently healthy donor. Hepatitis and AIDS are the most serious risks and in large measure account for the widespread recent use of autologous blood and for the surprising recent decrease in the use of blood and blood products. Transfusions of whole blood and red cells reached a peak of 12.2 million units in 1986 and then declined to 11.6 million units in 1987 and continued to decline in 1988. The use of platelet transfusions (6.4 million units in 1987) also slowed. The proportion of platelets transfused as platelets from single donors grew from 11% in 1980 to 25% in 1987. Donations of autologous blood increased sharply from less than 30,000 units in 1982 to 370,000 units in 1987. This is equivalent to 3% of homologus blood collections. Apparently, this unprecedented decline in transfusions, coupled with the continued importation of packed red cells from Europe and the offsetting effect of autologous predeposits, has forestalled the shortages of blood that could have resulted from declining homologous blood collections. All of these changes reflect the AIDS epidemic.

I. HISTORICAL NOTES

Transfusion into human beings of calf blood was first attempted in 1667 by Dennis. The resulting hemolytic transfusion reaction, which was described magnificently, quickly caused this procedure to be banned. No further effort at transfusion therapy was initiated until 1818 when Blondell attempted to transfuse women hemorrhaging during childbirth. Little progress was made until 1900 when recognition of the ABO blood groups permitted matching of major blood groups and 1914 when development of anticoagulants allowed preservation of donated blood in vitro. Since that time transfusion therapy has advanced to the point that each year millions of units of blood are now being drawn and fractionated into components so that products from one unit may be reliably used by more than one recipient.

II. BLOOD COLLECTION

A. General aspects

Recruitment of blood donors is carried out by local, regional, and national organizations, all of which face the problem that only about 5% of eligible donors actually donate even though the need for safe blood is widely publicized. Voluntary donors are a safer source of blood than paid donors. Studies suggest that altruism, replacement of blood used by a friend, and peer pressure are all important motivating factors, whereas fear of needles and the overall process of blood donation are important deterrents.

Blood donation is a routine and relatively painless process taking about 45 minutes. Side effects are minimal. Most prospective healthy donors between the ages of 17 and 66 can be accepted. They are rejected only when (1) their blood may be hazardous to a recipient or (2) medical problems might make donation hazardous.

B. Specialized methods

1. Autologous donation

The safest procedure is an **autologous donation** in which the recipient is given his or her own blood. This eliminates the possibility of transfusion reaction or transmission of blood-borne disease. The availability of anticoagulants, which permit a shelf life of up to 49 days, and the preservation of blood by freezing for longer periods make "banking one's own blood" an option for many patients undergoing elective surgery. The main problems are the logistics of storing the blood and returning it to the donor at surgery. Donors with hematocrits as low as 34 can be accepted (ordinary donors must have hematocrits of at least 38), but the number of donations may be limited by the donor's marrow response to phlebotomy (bleeding). There may also be added costs, especially if the blood must be frozen. None of these obstacles is significant compared to the cost of blood-transmitted hepatitis and/or acquired immunodeficiency syndrome (AIDS), which is a risk with heterologous donations.

2. Directed donation

Directed donations are made with the intent that the products go to a specific recipient. This is an old idea that before the AIDS epidemic saw little application. Current public demand for directed donation is based not on the small number of specific medical indications, but rather on fear of blood-borne infections. Presently, donors selected by the recipient are safer than those selected from anonymous voluntary donors.

The evidence supporting this assumption is thus far unconvincing. AIDS and hepatitis are both sexually transmitted and available studies show no evidence of greater safety. The prevalence of markers for blood-borne infections is the same in directed donors as in first-time anonymous donors, though slightly lower than in repeat donors. This result is not surprising since two-thirds of directed donors are first-time donors.

Directed donation also has disadvantages.

- Donors are no longer anonymous and recipients will know the source of transfusion.
- Individuals under pressure to donate may not want to be candid about their medical histories.
- Such a system is more expensive than voluntary donation.
- Hence, more resources are used for a product not yet shown to have greater safety than for blood donated to meet the community blood needs.

Despite the lack of proven benefit, public demand for directed donation is so great that this service is now available in most blood banks.

3. *Apheresis donation*

Cell separators now available can, by continuous or discontinuous centrifugation techniques, selectively remove large numbers of platelets or white cells from a single donor in about 2 hours. These components are essential during cancer or leukemia chemotherapy and other disorders. Donors undergoing apheresis suffer no significant side effects.

III. PREPARATION AND STORAGE OF BLOOD

A. Component preparation

A **unit of whole blood** contains 450 ml of blood plus 63 ml of an anticoagulant-preservative. Whole blood can be separated into various components by a series of differential centrifugations. Packed **red cells** with a hematocrit of about 70 (termed **packed cells**) are made by centrifugations of whole blood and removal of platelet-rich plasma. **Platelet concentrate** is then prepared by centrifugation of this fraction and resuspension of the platelets in about 40 ml of citrated plasma. The remaining platelet-poor plasma, if frozen within 6 hours of collection, retains all of the coagulation factors and is called **fresh frozen plasma** (FFP). Cryoprecipitate is obtained from FFP by collecting the fraction which is still insoluble when FFP has just been thawed and is still close to 0°C. These cold-insoluble proteins include factor VIII, fibrinogen, fibronectin, and von Willebrand's factor.

The plasma remaining after the cryoprecipitate has been removed is then used to prepare a derivative, **5% albumin**. When blood is left unfractionated, the platelets and certain labile plasma factors (factor VIII and factor V) rapidly lose activity. Consequently, in order to obtain maximum benefit from each unit, most blood collected is immediately converted into components.

B. Blood preservation and storage

Storage conditions are designed to minimize hemolysis, loss of red cell 2,3-DPG and ATP, and accumulation of extracellular K^+ and NH_3, all of which reflect the "storage lesion" of banked blood. Shelf life is determined by assays of in vivo survival. To be acceptable, 70% of red cells must survive at least 24 hours after transfusion. Improved anticoagulant-preservatives, which contain additional adenine, glucose, and mannitol, have increased shelf life from 21 days for ACD (acid citrate dextrose) anticoagulant-preservative or CPD (citrate phosphate dextrose) to 42 days for the latest formulations, which are called Adsol or Nutricel.

Both of these newer formulations have the advantage that the nutrients required to prolong red cell shelf life remain within the red cells and are not found in the plasma. Because extra saline is also added to the red cells, the final hematocrit is lower, usually in the range of 50%. This change means that red cell flow is better than with red cells suspended in CPD-A (CPD plus added adenosine) but a larger volume load is also being given.

After treatment with a cryoprotective agent such as glycerol, red cells can be preserved indefinitely in the frozen state (at −80°C). This approach is particularly useful for the preservation of rare blood types and the preparation of red cells with more than 95% of the white cells removed.

IV. PRETRANSFUSION TESTING

A. Of donor unit

After collection, the donor unit is typed to determine ABO group and Rh and screened for the presence of red cell antibodies and markers of blood-borne infections. Anti–red cell antibodies in the donor plasma are excluded to avoid infusing donor plasma which might react with recipient red cells. The list of required tests to exclude transfusion-transmitted diseases now includes:

- Tests for hepatitis B surface antigen (HBsAG)
- Antibody to hepatitis B core antigen (Anti-HBc)
- Antibody to human immunodeficiency virus (anti-HIV)
- Antibody to human T-cell lymphotropic virus (anti-HTLV-1) and elevation in alanine aminotransferase (ALT)

Each of these tests is done to reduce the risk of transmitting blood-borne infections such as hepatitis B, non-A, non-B hepatitis (NANB), HIV, and HLTV-1. Anti-HBc and ALT testing are included because donations that are positive by these criteria have an increased likelihood of transmitting NANB hepatitis. Only when the initial testing is complete can the unit be made available for transfusion.

B. Of recipient

1. Drawing the blood specimen

A blood specimen must be drawn from the intended recipient within 72 hours of transfusion, properly labeled with the patient's name, date, and time, and initialed by the phlebotomist. Mislabeling of patient specimens is the most dangerous error that can occur. Blood banks have no means of detecting the error unless they have the patient's blood type on file.

2. Typing

ABO and Rh group of the recipient is determined by testing both red cells with known antisera (forward typing) and his or her serum with red cells of known ABO phenotype (reverse typing). If forward and reverse typing results do not agree, the discrepancy must be resolved prior to transfusion. Possible explanations include subgroups of A and B, agammaglobulinemia, neonatal sera, laboratory error, cold antibodies, and polyagglutinable cells (see lecture 16). When the type has been established, transfusion of ABO-compatible blood without further testing would bring the risk of incompatibility to about 3%. This is the approximate probability that the recipient will have, in addition to ABO isohemagglutinins, antibodies against other red cell antigens.

C. Antibody screen

Recipient serum is screened for anti-red cell antibodies by incubation with cells of known phenotype that include the clinically important red cell antigens. These must be present in the homozygous state because occasional antibodies are not detected by heterozygous cells. After incubation, cells are washed and tested for antibody by addition of the Coombs reagent. If this procedure is negative, recipient serum is said to be free of anti–red cell antibodies. Under these circumstances the chance of incompatibility on subsequent cross-match is about 0.5%.

D. Crossmatch: the final check

A **major crossmatch** is carried out by incubating the recipient's serum with donor red cells and testing for agglutination in both saline and in media designed to enhance agglutination (see lecture 16). Cells are then washed and tested for antibody by the addition of Coombs serum. Occasionally the major crossmatch will reveal incompatibility when the antibody screen was negative.

Incompatibility when the antibody screen is negative is so rare that many blood banks have given up the requirement for using the Coombs serum in the final phase of the crossmatch in individuals with negative antibody screens and no prior history of forming antibodies to red cell antigens. In patients with a low likelihood of needing blood during surgery, preoperative testing is often limited to a type and screen because, if blood is needed urgently, it can be released after an abbreviated crossmatch. Such a policy has the advantage of limiting unnecessary crossmatches without causing any significant change in the risk to the patient.

In an emergency, type-specific blood can be obtained in about 5 minutes, while an antibody screen followed by a Coombs crossmatch requires about 50 minutes. If the antibody screen is already known to be negative, blood can be released in about 10 minutes. Availability of fresh frozen plasma depends on the time required to thaw the product—about 45 to 60 minutes. Consequently urgent volume expansion must be accomplished with a crystalloid or 5% albumin.

V. TRANSFUSION THERAPY

The major immediate goals of transfusion therapy are these:

- Maintenance of oxygen transport
- Maintenance of adequate hemostasis
- Volume replacement

Their goals are best achieved by transfusion of the specific components needed to replace particular deficits. At present there is almost no indication for the use of unfractionated whole blood. Whole blood offers no advantage over component therapy in the maintenance of hemostasis.

A new dimension was added to transfusion therapy with the development of mechanical devices capable of separating specific cell components from the blood of a single donor. These instruments utilize the principle of differential centrifugation. Red cells sediment faster than leukocytes, platelets, or plasma. The principle is applied either by **intermttent flow centrifugation** or **continuous flow centrifugation** to collect a therapeutic dose of platelets or leukocytes from a single normal donor. Separators utilize sterile plastic systems that in most cases are completely disposable.

A. Red cell concentrates (packed cells)

Red cell concentrates are useful for the vast majority of red cell transfusions. The hematocrit of transfused concentrates depends on the anticoagulant used. For blood suspended in CPD-A, it is between 70–80% with the flow being relatively slow in comparison to blood suspended in Adsol, with an hematocrit of about 50%.

Conversion of whole blood to packed red cells removes both the plasma, which during storage has accumulated excess K^+, NH_3, and hemoglobin as well as most of the white cells in the buffy coat.

Packed cells are preferred for patients with chronic anemia. These cells can also be used for replacement of acute blood loss in conjunction with appropriate volume expanders.

B. "Leukopoor" blood

In patients with febrile transfusion reactions—usually the result of donor leukocytes interacting with recipient antileukocyte antibodies—it is important to reduce the number of leukocytes in the transfused blood as much as possible.

Several methods are available which remove about 90% of the leukocytes. Frozen deglycerolized red cells lose about 95% of the leukocytes and also have the advantage of being washed extensively during the deglycerolization process. Their main disadvantage is increased cost and short 24-hour shelf life once the unit is thawed.

C. Platelets

1. Products

Platelet concentrates are prepared from recently donated units of blood by differential centrifugation. A slow-speed centrifugation separates the platelets and plasma from the red cells. The platelet-rich plasma is collected and then recentrifuged at a higher speed to concentrate the platelets in about 40 ml of plasma. A typical platelet concentrate, prepared in this manner from whole blood, contains 5.5×10^{10} platelets. Ordinarily, a pool of six platelet concentrates is given in each transfusion.

A therapeutic dose of platelets can be obtained from a single donor by using a cell separator. These machines automatically separate the platelets and return the red cells and plasma to the donor. This process takes about 2 hours and yields about 5×10^{11} platelets.

In comparison to platelet concentrates, single-donor platelets have the following advantages: exposure to one donor instead of six means a lower risk of transfusion-transmitted diseases and reduced exposure to HLA antigens on platelets and donor leukocytes contained in the platelets; possibly some delay in alloimmunization to platelet antigens; and, if properly selected, greater effectiveness in alloimmunized recipients. Disadvantages include greater cost and increased difficulty in obtaining donors. Both factors limit the availability of this product.

2. Indications

Before transfusing platelets, one should consider:

- The patient's platelet count
- Whether thrombocytopenia is due to decreased platelet production or increased destruction (see lecture 28)
- Whether platelet function is normal or abnormal

Bleeding patients with platelet counts below 100,000 should receive platelet transfusions. Their effectiveness will depend on whether the thrombocytopenia is due to decreased production or increased destruction. When thrombocytopenia is due primarily to increased destruction as in idiopathic thrombocytopenic purpura (ITP), an instance of immunothrombocytopenia (see lecture 28), circulating platelets tend to be "young" or immature and hemostatically more effective than the older platelets in the thrombocytopenia of marrow depression secondary to chemotherapy.

In patients with abnormal platelet function, the need for platelet transfusion depends on the underlying disorder. For example:

- The endogenous platelets of patients recently treated with aspirin are irreversibly abnormal, but transfused platelets that have not been exposed to aspirin should function normally.
- In contrast, platelets transfused into uremic patients are exposed to the same environmental stresses as endogenous platelets and thus will be of little value.

Bleeding post-coronary bypass patients are a special case because their platelets have an acquired functional defect that is reversible. Platelet transfusion are helpful even when the platelet count is well over 100,000. Because there is no reliable way to predict in which of these patients dysfunctional endogenous platelets will cause bleeding, and because the incidence of bleeding in such patients is low, platelet transfusions should be used only after bleeding has developed and not used prophylactically.

3. *Evaluation of clinical results*

Responses to transfused platelets are influenced by such host factors as fever, sepsis, splenomegaly, and alloimmunization or drug-induced antibodies. Response is best evaluated by effects on bleeding and platelet count 1 hour and 24 hours after transfusion. In an adult of average size, an increment at 1 hour of 10,000 per 5.5×10^{10} platelets transfused (six units) should be anticipated. At 18–24 hours, the increment should be 15,000–20,000. Meager post-transfusion increments should prompt a search for possible host factors that might be modified. Of such factors, alloimmunization is most difficult to deal with. Options include use of HLA-matched platelets and gamma globulin infusions (the effectiveness of which is still under study).

4. *Complications*

Complications of platelet transfusions parallel those of red cell transfusions, including transmission of blood-borne infections, febrile and urticarial reactions, alloimmunization, and rarely hemolytic reactions (if ABO incompatible plasma is given with platelets).

- Febrile and urticarial reactions can be controlled by providing, respectively, leukopoor or washed platelets.
- Newer methods of platelet preparation significantly delay onset of alloimmunization.

- Because platelets are contaminated by red cells, alloimmunization to red cell antigens may occur. In Rh-negative women with childbearing potential, it is important to give Rh-negative platelets. If Rh-positive platelets are used, Rh-immune globulin (RhoGAM®) may prevent sensitization (see below).
- Hemolysis from infusion of ABO-incompatible plasma occurs only when the plasma contains an unusually high titer of A and B isoagglutinins. This problem is avoided by donor selection and by use of ABO-compatible platelets when available. This complication is so rare there is no reason to require that transfused platelets be ABO compatible.

D. Granulocytes

Leukocyte transfusions have been under investigation for several years. A number of techniques exist whereby a therapeutic dose of granulocytes ($\sim 10^{11}$ white cells) may be obtained from a normal donor. These cells are collected with the aid of mechanical cell separators. In selected patients who are severely leukopenic, have Gram-negative sepsis, and some prospect of marrow recovery, granulocyte transfusion appears to have some value. However, much work remains to be done before this becomes standard therapy.

Granulocyte transfusions may also transmit blood-borne infections and cause febrile and urticarial reactions. Hemolytic reactions are avoided by appropriate crossmatching. Severe leukoagglutinin reactions may occur, especially if amphotericin is being administered. Such reactions can be minimized by crossmatching donor leukocytes with recipient serum.

E. Fresh frozen plasma (FFP)

FFP is plasma frozen within 6 hours after donation. All of the clotting factors maintain their stability in the frozen product. FFP is extremely useful in replacing clotting factors in patients with deficiencies in one or more clotting factors. It also provides volume expansion but should not be used for this purpose alone because derivatives such as 5% albumin are just as effective and carry no risk of blood-borne infection or citrate toxicity. The main disadvantage of FFP is the large volume of plasma required to replace clotting factors and the risk of transfusion reactions.

F. Cryoprecipitate

Cryoprecipitate is the cold-insoluble material left in the sediment when a unit of FFP thaws. Cryoprecipitate is rich in factor VIII (antihemophilic factor), factor I (fibrinogen), fibronectin, factor XIII, and von Willebrand's factor. Assuming that one unit is the amount of factor activity in 1 ml of FFP, a bag of cryoprecipitate contains 80–100 units of factor VIII. In addition, there is about 20–30% of the factor XIII and fibronectin initially present and at least 150 mg fibrinogen.

Cryoprecipitate is the only available concentrated form of fibrinogen. Hence it is used in the treatment of acquired hypofibrinogenemia and congenital or acquired dysfibrinogenemia. It is also used in the treatment of factor XIII deficiency and von Willebrand's disease. Its role in the treatment of mild factor VIII deficiency is changing because of the availability of factor VIII concentrates of greater purity and reduced risk of transmitted infections.

G. Albumin

Human serum albumin is fractionated from pooled plasma and serum by the Cohn fractionation procedure (cold alcohol precipitation). The albumin is rendered hepatitis-free by heating to 60°C for 10 hours. Standard terminology notwithstanding, it is not actually salt poor. Albumin is extraordinarily useful as a safe and effective volume expander. It has the added advantages of long shelf life at room temperture and absence of transfusion reactions.

H. Clotting factor concentrates

Concentrates rich in factor VIII or factor IX may be prepared by precipitation and lyophilization from pooled plasma. Lyophilized factor VIII concentrates have the advantage of being more concentrated than factor VIII in cryoprecipitate. These are derived from pools of 2000 donors. Hence, the risk of transmitted blood-borne infections has in the past been nearly 100%. However, recent improvements in the preparation of these concentrates have eliminated this risk. Unfortunately, these improvements have made these products more expensive.

Improved factor VIII concentrates are the treatment of choice for a new patient who has either moderate or severe hemophilia A. Whether or not patients already exposed to older products would benefit from switching to more purified preparations is still unclear.

Factor IX concentrates also contain factors II, VII, and X. In addition, some preparations contain activated factors (particularly VIII). Highly purified factor IX is also available. Factor IX preparations are used in treatment of patients with hemophilia B and of some patients with factor VIII inhibitors (see lecture 29). Because of the decrease of activated components, liver disease that decreases the clearance of clotting factors may lead to multiple thromboses.

Development of genetically engineered factor VIII and factor IX is under way. When these products are available, the indications for the partially purified concentrates will obviously be modified.

VI. HAZARDS

A. Acute hemolytic transfusion reactions

Hemolytic transfusion reactions are the most serious and dreaded complication of transfusion therapy. They are caused by the immunologic destruction of donor red cells by antibody in recipient serum. The antibody-antigen reaction triggers a variety of systems in the plasma proteins that activate a host of vasoactive substances. Symptoms include fever, chills, back pain, chest pain, facial flushing, hypotension, nausea, vomiting, hemoglobinemia, hemoglobinuria, diffuse bleeding, and renal shutdown. Although the reactions may be caused by any red cell blood group, the most serious are due to ABO reactions. The usual cause of these reactions is a clerical error, such as failure to identify adequately the recipient or inaccurate labeling of patient specimens for typing and crossmatch.

B. Delayed hemolytic transfusion reactions

These reactions occur 3–14 days following a transfusion and are associated with immunologic destruction of the donor cells by a specific blood group antibody. They occur in patients who have been previously sensitized to a blood group antigen but do not have detectable antibody at the time of compatibility testing. The immune system is stimulated to produce a secondary response resulting in the rapid production of high levels of specific antibody. Clinically, patients have a positive direct antiglobulin test and evidence of hemolysis. The direct antiglobulin test ultimately becomes negative as the incompatible units are hemolyzed and the indirect antiglobulin test becomes positive. These reactions are usually distinguishable from immunohemolytic anemia by serologic testing and can best be avoided by a careful transfusion history.

C. Transfusion-transmitted diseases

Transfusion-transmitted diseases occur when a blood donor with a clinically inapparent infection is not detected by postdonation laboratory screens. In the United States the most important of these diseases are viral hepatitis, AIDS, and cytomegalovirus infections. Strategems to reduce these infections include donor selection and education, postdonation laboratory screening, and decreased use of allogeneic blood products.

1. Hepatitis

Viral hepatitis remains the most common serious transfusion hazard. Four viruses have been implicated:

- **Hepatitis A** is rare because there is only a brief period of viremia and no carrier state.

- **Hepatitis B** was the most common cause prior to development of a sensitive and specific test for the virus (HBsAg). Screening of all donated units for this antigen has reduced the number of new cases to less than 10% of all new patients with post-transfusion hepatitis.
- The fulminating hepatitis associated with **Delta virus** only occurs in patients already infected with hepatitis B virus because Delta virus is defective and requires the presence of a DNA virus such as hepatitis B to replicate.
- Patients in whom infection with A, B, or Delta virus have been excluded are considered to have **non-A, non-B hepatitis** (NANB hepatitis). The risk of NANB infection is hard to estimate. Most studies put it between 1 and 5% of all blood transfusions. The recently introduced screening for elevation in alanine aminotransferase or for anti-HBc may lower these estimates.

Progress in this field was delayed by failure to identify the viruses responsible for post-transfusion hepatitis and by the absence of a specific test for donors with NANB hepatitis.

The clinical consequences of NANB hepatitis are considerable. If 7 of 100 blood recipients are infected, 3.5 of 100 will develop a mild chronic disease reflected by modest elevation of liver enzymes; 10% of these, or 3.5 of 1000, will develop cirrhosis, and of those, about 25% may die from liver disease (0.9 of 1000). This will continue to be an important reason to limit use of allogeneic blood until the virus(es) are identified and specific screening tests developed.

2. HIV infection

That HIV can be transmitted by blood products was suspected by 1984, and soon thereafter proven by ELISA and Western blot assays for antibody to HIV. In March 1988, 3.8% of all AIDS cases were attributed to transfusion-associated HIV infection.

This risk has been substantially lowered by donor education concerning risk factors, postdonation confidential exclusion of donor units if a donor fails to mention risks prior to donation, and the development of sensitive screening assays for antibody to HIV. A practical method of identifying integrated virus or viral antigen that could also be used as a screening technique is not yet available. Lack of a direct assay for virus makes it possible for a recently infected donor to be missed because detectable antibody has not yet appeared. The magnitude of this risk is not yet known.

D. Other complications

1. Febrile, nonhemolytic reactions

Febrile, nonhemolytic reactions, usually mediated by antileukocyte antibodies, present with fever, malaise, and flulike symptoms in the absence of hemolysis. They may be distinguished from hemolytic reactions by routine serologic studies and can usually be prevented by using leukopoor products.

2. *Urticaria*

Urticarial reactions, or hives, are caused by reactions of patients' antibodies with donor plasma proteins. These can often by controlled with antihistamines and do not usually require stopping the transfusion.

3. *Anaphylaxis*

Rarely an acute anaphylactic reaction develops when an IgA-deficient recipient is exposed to IgA during transfusion. The gene for IgA deficiency is relatively common (1 in 600). It is not understood why only few carriers of this gene develop anaphylactic reactions. If an IgA-deficient individual requires transfusion, this complication should be anticipated and IgA-deficient products should be used whenever possible.

4. *Other immunologic reactions*

Other rare immunologically mediated complications of transfusion include:

- Post-transfusion purpura
- Graft-versus-host disease
- Transfusion-induced lung disease

Use of irradiated blood products can completely prevent transfusion-induced graft-versus-host disease. Thus, prevention of this rare, but often lethal, complication requires recognition of which recipients (other than bone marrow transplant patients) are so immunocompromised they are susceptible to graft-versus-host disease.

Transfusion-induced lung diseased presents with signs of normal pressure pulmonary edema. It results from leukoagglutination in the lung, usually caused by infused donor leukoagglutinins and rarely by recipient antibodies reacting with donor leukocytes.

The pathophysiology of post-transfusion purpura is poorly understood and is probably not prospectively preventable (see lecture 29).

VII. HEMOLYTIC DISEASE OF THE NEWBORN

Hemolytic disease of the newborn (HDN) is a disease in which the life span of a fetus's red cells is diminished by the action of specific antibodies derived from the mother and transferred to the fetus across the placenta. In its most severe form, death may occur in utero. This illness is also known as **erythroblastosis fetalis**, a name that relates to the presence of markedly increased numbers of nucleated red cells in the blood of the fetus. If the infant is born alive, it may suffer from **hydrops fetalis**, an illness characterized by massive edema of the fetus presumed secondary to anemia, hypoalbuminemia, and cardiac failure. Hydropic infants frequently do not survive.

The discovery of the Rh blood group system between 1939 and 1941 led to the identification of the specificity of the antibody responsible for most cases of HDN, that is, anti-D(Rh_o). Less commonly, antibodies against other antigens of the Rh system or other blood groups such as Kell or antigens of the ABO system have been implicated. The common denominator in all cases is presence in the fetus of a red cell antigen that is not part of the mother's phenotype and against which she has become sensitized. Much progress has been made in the diagnosis, treatment, and prevention of HDN in the past 50 years, especially those cases that are due to the D(Rh_o) antigen.

A. Pathophysiology

HDN develops because of the transfer of specific antibody from mother to fetus. Only maternal antibodies of the IgG class are transferred across the placenta. Thus only IgG antibodies mediate the disease. Sensitization to fetal antigens occurs in the mother primarily as a result of **fetomaternal hemorrhage**. Fetal erythrocytes may be detected in the maternal circulation as early as 8 weeks after conception. However, sensitization is most likely to occur at the time of delivery of the infant since that is the time of the largest fetomaternal hemorrhage. Once sensitized, a mother is at risk for the development of hemolytic disease in subsequent pregnancies.

HDN from ABO antigens occurs in group A or group B children of group O mothers. Since group O mothers have anti-A and anti-B of the IgG class without fetomaternal sensitization, this disorder may develop during the first pregnancy.

The disease affects the fetus in several ways. The fetus is **anemic** with varying degrees of complications, the most serious of which is cardiac failure. In its most severe form, hydrops fetalis, the fetus is massively edematous and may succumb rapidly. The fetus compensates for the destruction of red cells by increasing **extramedullary erythropoiesis** that affects vital organs. Thus, the liver, spleen, and marrow enlarge owing to the presence of erythropoietic cells. This may lead to a decrease in liver function. Finally, the destruction of large quantities of red cells leads to **hyperbilirubinemia**. The newborn is not biochemically equipped to handle the excess load of bilirubin, at least in part because of inadequate activity of bilirubin-conjugating enzymes at birth. The elevated bilirubin in the postnatal period may then be associated with **kernicterus**. This complication is characterized by brain damage resulting in death from neurologic impairment caused by bilirubin toxicity.

B. Prenatal diagnosis

The prenatal diagnosis of HDN is often suggested by the patient's history. A history of previously affected offspring should alert one to the possibility of HDN. However, many severely affected infants are born in the absence of any previous history. Simple Rh typing of mother and father and screening of the mother's serum for atypical red cell antibodies should be helpful in defining potentially affected fetuses. **Amniocentesis** is the procedure by which amniotic fluid is aspirated (see lecture 11) and analyzed for bilirubin pigment. Increased concentrations of bilirubin in the amniotic fluid are correlated with increased red cell destruction of fetal red cells. The concentrations of bilirubin can be correlated with the prognosis of the fetus, and appropriate steps can then be taken to prevent development of severe disease.

C. Treatment

1. Prenatal

Severe disease may be treated by intrauterine transfusion of blood into the fetus between the 20th and 33rd weeks of gestation. Blood compatible with the mother's serum is injected into the peritoneal cavity of the fetus. The blood is absorbed across the peritoneum and the transfused blood will not be immunologically destroyed by the maternal antibody. This procedure may be repeated if necessary. Premature induction of labor may be contemplated if the fetus is approximately 33 weeks or older. At birth, the transfer of maternal antibody ceases, and soon after birth the hemolytic rate begins to decline.

2. Postnatal

A number of options exist for the postnatal therapy of an infant with HDN. **Exchange transfusion** is the single most effective means of treating both the anemia and the hyperbilirubinemia of the disease. In the usual practice, two units of blood compatible with the mother's are slowly exchanged with the infant's blood. This has the effect of raising the hemoglobin, washing out the offending antibody, and washing out the high level of bilirubin. The process may be repeated if necessary.

In less severe cases, infants may be treated with phototherapy, which has the effect of lowering the serum bilirubin. The infusion of albumin (which binds bilirubin) and the treatment of mothers with barbiturates (which induces higher levels of bilirubin-conjugating enzymes) are less commonly employed.

D. Prophylaxis of Rh disease

One of the major achievements of modern medicine is the development of an effective means of prevention of alloimmunization to the $D(Rh_0)$ antigen. Sensitization to the D antigen may be prevented by the passive injection of 300 μg of IgG anti-$D(Rh_0)$, that is, Rh immune globulin (RhoGAM®), to an Rh negative mother of an Rh positive infant within 72 hours of delivery. If the mother has not been previously sensitized to the $D(Rh_0)$ antigen, the passive injection of antibody will prevent immunization. Likewise, patients undergoing therapeutic abortions are also at risk for sensitization to the D(Rh_o) antigen. All Rh-negative women undergoing abortion should receive a dose of Rh immune globulin to prevent sensitization to the D(Rh_o) antigen. The widespread use of this technique has dramatically reduced the incidence of Rh sensitization and Rh HDN in recent years.

SELECTED REFERENCES

Reviews

Berkman, S. A. Infectious complications of blood transfusion. *Blood Rev.* 2(1988): 206–210.

Colman, N. Introduction: Closing the window on AIDS. *Transfusion Med. Rev.* 3(1989): 1(Suppl 1).

Churchill, W. H., and Kurtz, S. R., eds. *Transfusion Medicine*. Boston: Blackwell Scientific Publications, 1988.

Forbes, B. A. Acquisition of cytomegalovirus infection: an update. *Clin. Microbiol. Rev.* 2(1989): 204–216.

Heyward, W. L., and Curran, J. W. The epidemiology of AIDS in the U.S. *Sci. Am.* 259(1988): 72–81.

Hoyer, L. W. Molecular pathology and immunology of factor VIII (hemophilia A and factor VIII inhibitors). *Hum. Pathol.* 18(1987): 153–161.

Kunicki, T. J., and Beardsley, D. S. The alloimmune thrombocytopenias: neonatal alloimmune thrombocytopenic purpura and posttransfusion purpura. *Progr. Hemost. Thromb.* 9(1989): 203–232.

Lee, C. A., and Kernoff, P. B. A. Viral hepatitis and haemophilia. *Br. Med. Bull.* 46(1990): 408–422.

Lee, D., and Napier, J. A. ABC of transfusion. Autologous transfusion. *Br. Med. J.* 300(1990): 737–740.

Menitove, J. E. Current risk of transfusion-associated human immunodeficiency virus infection. *Arch. Pathol. Lab. Med.* 114(1990): 330–334.

Murphy, M. F., and Waters, A. H. Platelet transfusions: the problem of refractoriness. *Blood Rev.* 4(1990): 16–24.

Plapp, F. V., Sinor, L. T., et al. The evolution of pretransfusion testing: from agglutination to solid-phase red cell adherence tests. *Crit. Rev. Clin. Lab. Sci.* 27(1989): 179–209.

Popovsky, M. A., and Moore, S. B. Diagnostic and pathogenetic considerations in transfusion-related acute lung injury. *Transfusion* 25(1985): 573–577.

Slichter, S. J. Platelet transfusion therapy. *Hematol. Oncol. Clin. North Am.* 4(1990): 291–311.

Surgenor, D. M., Wallace, E. L., et al. Collection and transfusion of blood in the United States, 1982–1988. *N. Engl. J. Med.* 322(1990): 1646–1651.

Underwood, J. C. E. Hepatitis C virus and transfusion transmitted liver disease: review. *J. Clin. Pathol.* 43(1990): 445–447.

Vyas, G. N. Symposium on transfusion-associated infections and immune response. *Transfusion Med. Rev.* 2(1988): 193.

Original articles

Goodnough, L. T., and Brittenham, G. M. Limitations of the erythropoietic response to serial phlebotomy: implications for autologous blood donor programs. *J. Lab. Clin. Med.* 115(1990): 28–35.

Charache, S. Editorial: Problems in transfusion therapy. *N. Engl. J. Med.* 322(1990): 1666–1668.

Cohen, N. D., Muñoz, A., et al. Transmission of retroviruses by transfusion of screened blood in patients undergoing cardiac surgery. *N. Engl. J. Med.* 320(1989): 1172–1176.

Goodnough, L. T., Rudnick, S., et al. Increased preoperative collection of autologous blood with recombinant human erythropoietin therapy. *N. Engl. J. Med.* 321(1989): 1163–1168.

Gould, S. A., Sehgal, L. R., et al. The efficacy of polymerized pyridoxylated hemoglobin solution as an O_2 carrier. *Ann. Surg.* 211(1990): 394–398.

Graf, H., Watzinger, U., et al. Recombinant human erythropoietin as adjuvant treatment for autologous blood donation. *Br. Med. J.* 300(1990): 1627–1628.

Mojena, M., and Boscá, L. Identification of an anti-A and anti-B blood group glycosyltransferase antibody after incompatible bone marrow transplant. *Blood* 74(1989): 1134–1138.

Sarnaik, S. A., Chang, C.-H., et al. Transfusional iron overload in sickle cell anemia: relationship between liver iron, magnetic resonance imaging findings, and hepatic fibrosis. *Ann. NY Acad. Sci.* 565(1989): 460–462.

Schorn, T. F., and Knospe, W. H. Fatal delayed hemolytic transfusion reaction without previous blood transfusion. *Ann. Intern. Med.* 110(1989): 241–242.

Wolfe, L. C. Oxidative injuries to the red cell membrane during conventional blood preservation. *Semin. Hematol.* 26(1989): 307–312.

Yamamoto, F., Clausen, H., et al. Molecular genetic basis of the histo-blood group ABO system. *Nature* 345(1990): 229–233.

LECTURE 18

Leukocytes I. Physiology

William S. Beck

EDITOR'S COMMENT

Unlike the red cell, which performs its functions within the blood, the granulocyte uses the bloodstream mainly as a transport vehicle to take it to sites outside of the vascular tree—where it "does its thing." For many reasons, knowledge of these complex and fascinating cells has trailed behind our understanding of the red cell. Its time has come, however, and granulocyte research has expanded rapidly in the last decade into basic investigations of motility, phagocytosis, chemotaxis (all functions that make granulocytes kin with protists), as well as metabolism, life span, and the physiology of granulopoiesis and its regulation (which was discussed in lecture 1). This lecture begins a three-lecture sequence on granulocytes and other white cells, their physiology, special functions, and pathophysiology.

I. INTRODUCTION

We use the terms **leukocyte** and **white cell** to refer to any of the nucleated cells normally present in blood, whose major function is defense against foreign invaders. The terms are usually not used to refer to fixed cells of the RES or free tissue macrophages (discussed in lecture 2), though these cells share many properties with circulation blood leukocytes.

A. Types of leukocytes

The different types of leukocytes may be classified in several ways:

- By the type of **defense function**—phagocytosis in the case of **phagocytes** (i.e., granulocytes and monocytes), antibody production and cellular immunity in the case of **immunocytes** (i.e., lymphocytes and plasma cells).
- By the **shape of the nucleus** (polymorphonuclear or mononuclear).
- By the **site of origin** (myeloid or lymphoid).
- By the presence of absence of **specific-staining granules** (granulocytes or nongranulocytes). The granulocytes in turn are classified by the nature of their specific-staining granules, which are neutrophilic, eosinophilic, or basophilic.

Table 18.1
Normal Values of Blood Leukocyte Concentration

Cell type	Mean (cells/mm^3)	Mean (%)	95% confidence limits (cells/mm^3)
Neutrophils	4300	55.3	1800–6700
Lymphocytes	2710	34.8	1400–3930
Monocytes	500	6.4	140–860
Eosinophils	230	3.0	0–570
Basophils	40	0.5	0–120

Source: Modified from D. Boggs, *Semin. Hematol.* 4(1967): 359.

B. Normal leukocyte count

Table 18.1 summarizes the reported values for the concentration for various keukocyte types in the venous blood of 105 normal male students, according to Boggs. Note that the majority of blood leukocytes are neutrophils in the normal adult. Lymphocytes predominate in infants and young children.

C. Historical notes

The classic staining researches of Paul Ehrlich (1878 et seq.) led to important advances in the knowledge of leukocytes. Prior to Ehrlich's discovery of polychromatic and supravital stains, granulocytes had been observed and counted, and their capacity for motility and phagocytosis had been recognized—but their morphology and classification were unexplored. The main elements of our understanding of the maturation sequence came from the work of Pappenheim (1914).

II. GRANULOCYTES

A. Morphologic aspects of granulopoiesis

1. Maturation stages

Figure 18.1 summarizes the highlights of granulopoiesis. Six maturation stages are recognized: myeloblast → promyelocyte → myelocyte → metamyelocyte → band form → mature polymorphonuclear granulocyte.

At shown in figure 18.1, the myeloid maturation sequence is characterized by progressive decrease in nuclear size, the early presence of nucleoli and their subsequent disappearance, late nuclear indentation and segmentation, characteristic changes in chromatin character, early appearance of azurophilic granules, and later appearance of specific-staining granules. Myeloblasts are easily recognized but may by difficult to distinguish from lymphoblasts. **Auer rods**, when present, indicate that the cell is a myeloblast or monoblast. They are not seen in lymphoblasts. These curious

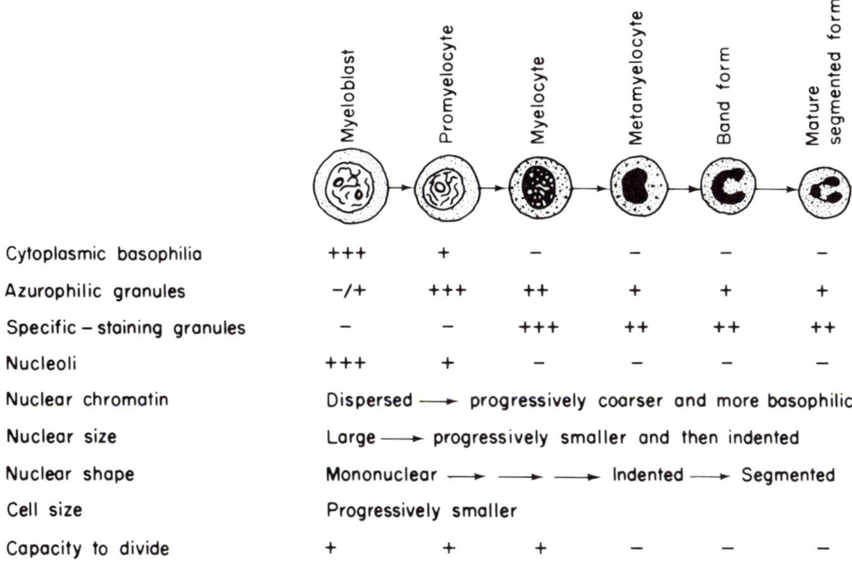

	Myeloblast	Promyelocyte	Myelocyte	Metamyelocyte	Band form	Mature segmented form
Cytoplasmic basophilia	+++	+	–	–	–	–
Azurophilic granules	–/+	+++	++	+	+	+
Specific – staining granules	–	–	+++	++	++	++
Nucleoli	+++	+	–	–	–	–
Nuclear chromatin	Dispersed ⟶ progressively coarser and more basophilic					
Nuclear size	Large ⟶ progressively smaller and then indented					
Nuclear shape	Mononuclear ⟶ ⟶ ⟶ Indented ⟶ Segmented					
Cell size	Progressively smaller					
Capacity to divide	+	+	+	–	–	–

Fig. 18.1
Stages of myeloid cell maturation.

structures appear to arise from clumped azurophilic granule material. They are seen only in leukemia (see lecture 22).

2. *Granules*

The granules visible in stained smears are lysosomes that contain the hydrolytic enzymes and antibacterial agents required for the digestion of phagocytized particles. Two types of granules are distinguishable:

- **Primary**, or **azurophilic granules**, coarse reddish-purple granules, 0.8 μm in diameter, that appear first at the promyelocyte stage (and are peroxidase-positive)
- **Secondary**, or **specific-staining granules**, neutrophilic, eosinophilic, or basophilic granules, 0.5 μm in diameter, that appear first at the myelocyte stage (and are peroxidase-negative)

Azurophilic granules are formed chiefly in promyelocytes and their numbers per cell decrease after that stage. Their intense staining properties are diminished in later maturation stages owing to an increased concentration of acidic glycoproteins, which bond to basic protiens that would otherwise take stain. Granules also have a distinctive appearance on electron microscopy (figure 18.2). Note in the figure that the Golgi complex is prominent in the promyelocyte. Intense granule synthesis takes place at that stage, and there is evidence that synthesis of both types of granules occurs in the Golgi complex at different stages. The two types of granules appear to come from opposite faces of the Golgi: specific-staining granules from the distal or convex face, azurophilic from the proximal or concave face.

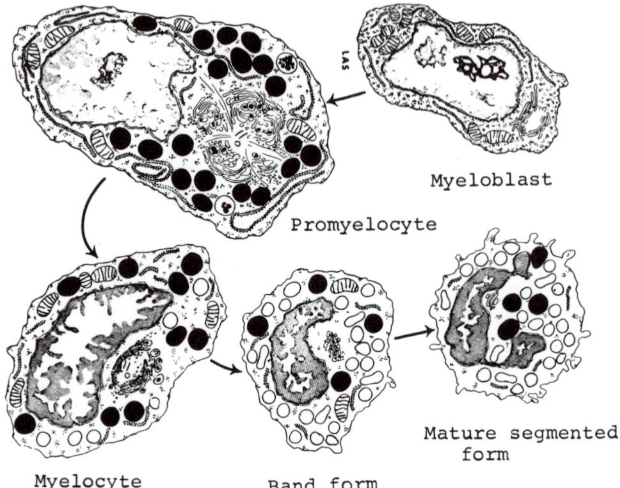

Fig. 18.2
Diagram of maturation stages of granulopoiesis as observed by electron microscopy. Dense lysosomes are primary or azurophilic granules. Lighter lysosomes are secondary or specific-staining granules. Note that both types of granules are found in the mature cell. (From D. F. Bainton and M. G. Farquhar, *J. Cell. Biol.* 28[1966]: 277.)

Azurophilic granules contain (in addition to lysosomal hydrolytic enzymes) neutral proteases, myeloperoxidase, glycosyl aminoglycans, acid phosphatase, cationic bactericidal proteins, defensins, and lysozyme.

Specific-staining granules contain lysozyme, apolactoferrin, cobalamin-binding protein, and other components to be discussed below. Alkaline phosphatase, once thought to be in specific-staining granules, is now localized on the plasma membrane.

3. *Acquired and hereditary anomalies*

A number of defects of granulocyte morphology are recognized. Although rare, they are interesting for the insight they may give into the mechanisms of maturation. (Functional anomalies of granulocytes are discussed in lecture 19).

a. DÖHLE BODIES

Döhle bodies are common and easily recognized abnormalities of neutrophil cytoplasm. In stained smears, they are single or multiple gray-blue cytoplasmic inclusion bodies that are usually seen along the outer edge of mature neutrophils but may occur in earlier forms. They were first described by H. Döhle in 1911 in patients with scarlet fever and were thought by him to be pathognomonic. They were later found in severe infections, pregnancy, burns, cancer, and many other conditions. As noted below, they occur also in certain hereditary anomalies. Döhle bodies are thought to be ribosome-containing remnants of endoplasmic reticulum retained from promyelocyte cytoplasm.

b. MACROPOLYCYTES

Acquired hypersegmented neutrophils occur in megaloblastic anemia (see figure 5.2B). Neutrophil hypersegmentation may also be inherited as a benign autosomal dominant trait.

c. PELGER-HÜET ANOMALY

This hereditary abnormality is characterized by failure of normal nuclear segmentation. In typical heterozygotes two-lobed nuclei are seen in the majority of mature granulocytes and eosinophils ("pince-nez" cells). Nuclear chromatin is also condensed. Homozygotes have round nuclei. The disorder, a simple autosomal dominant trait, is benign and occurs in 1 in 6000 people. A similar acquired disorder, known as pseudo-Pelger-Hüet anomaly, occurs in the course of myeloproliferative conditions and virus infections. It may be due to an abnormality of chromatin synthesis. A similar abnormality occurs in rabbits.

d. ALDER-REILLY ANOMALY

This rare hereditary anomaly is part of a clinical complex arising from discordered polysaccharide metabolism that causes a defect of cytoplasmic maturation. Specific-staining granules fail to develop and coarse, lilac-staining azurophilic granules remain. Nuclear maturation and configuration is normal. In some cases all granulocytes (as well as monocytes and lymphocytes) may be affected. In others normal and abnormal cells are present.

e. CHÉDIAK-HIGASHI SYNDROME (CHS)

This disorder of humans and cattle is associated with hereditary gigantism of azurophilic granules of all cells of the myeloid series, ocular and skin hypopigmentation, and giant melanosomes. Giant lysosomes are present in many body tissues. Granulocyte function is defective, with abnormal lysosome fusion in phagocytosis (see lecture 19). Chemotaxis is also impaired. Hence patients suffer severe recurrent infections. Platelets lack dense granules, and platelet function is defective (see lecture 28). Recent data suggest that CHS is also associated with defective microtubular proteins.

f. MAY-HEGGLIN ANOMALY

This is a rare autosomal dominant trait manifested by giant platelets and large basophilic bodies in granulocytes. The condition is usually benign, although some patients have a bleeding tendency associated with thrombocytopenia and/or qualitative platelet defect.

B. Cytokinetics

For many reasons, knowledge of granulocyte (or neutrophil) kinetics has lagged behind that of erythrokinetics. Aside from their scientific importance, questions relating to granulocytic kinetics frequently arise at the bedside—most commonly in the interpretation of high and low white counts. The diagnostic procedures available in this area range from the simple and available to generally unavailable research-type techniques.

The white cell count and differential count are the most widely used clinical guides to the level of neutrophil production, although they provide no quantitative information on rate of neutrophil production or destruction, the status of marrow reserves, or possible abnormalities in cell distribution. Nonetheless, they provide helpful data and are indispensable in following the effects of many ongoing disorders or of cytotoxic chemotherapy.

The following discussions concern methods of assessing neutrophil life span, rates of granulopoiesis, and granulocyte turnover.

1. *Life span*

Methods used to determine granulocyte life span employ in vitro or in vivo labeling techniques.

a. IN VITRO LABELS

In the in vitro methods, leukocytes are removed from the subject, labeled, and returned to the blood. Thus, only circulating cells are labeled. Diisopropylfluorophosphate-^{32}P ([^{32}P]DFP), or the ^{3}H derivative, attaches covalently to a serine residue of a cell protein. Use of this technique revealed two important facts. Upon reinfusion of labeled cells, half of the radioactivity seems to disappear from the blood (figure 18.3A). This observation led to the realization that the total blood granulocyte pool (TBGP) includes two subpools: the circulating granulocyte pool (CGP) and the marginal granulocyte pool (MGP; figure 18.3B). The MGP consists of intravascular cells that have marginated along the walls of small capillaries and venules. The leukocyte count, as determined in venous blood samples taken from the axial stream, measures only the CGP. Cells are continually and rapidly exchanged between the two intravascular pools. Certain factors to be described shift cells from one pool to the other. The exponential decline in radioactivity of the CGP (figure 18.3A) indicates that cells are

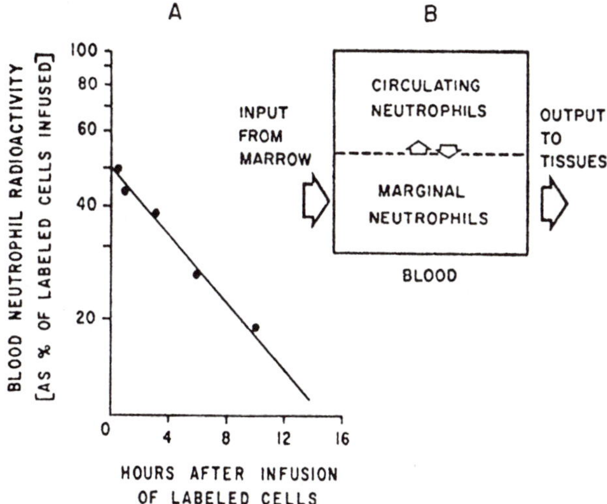

Fig. 18.3
Major conclusions from leukocyte life-span studies employing an in vitro label. *A*, Time-course of disappearance of [^{32}P]DFP-labeled neutrophils in a normal subject. *B*, Model of blood neutrophil kinetics. (From D. Boggs, in C. E. Mengel, *Hematology: Principles and Practice*. Chicago: Year Book, 1972.)

removed from the circulating pool in random fashion with a half-life of about 6.7 hr (normal range, 4–10 hr). Hence, the CGP turns over 2.5 times per day, and the average time that a cell spends in the blood is about 10 hr. The average number of neutrophils entering and leaving the blood each day in normal adults is 167×10^7/kg body weight. In a 70-kg man, this equals 1.1×10^{11} neutrophils/day. Since 10^{10} neutrophils have a packed volume of about 5 ml (see figure 20.3), volume of the daily output is about 55 ml. By use of [^{32}P]DFP, Cartwright et al. obtained the results in table 18.2 in normal male volunteers.

b. IN VIVO LABELS

In methods employing in vivo labels, cells take up a systemically administered radioactive substance. Procedures are of two types: (1) those that label early granulocyte precursors and (2) those that label all stages. Since early precursor cells are actively dividing, DNA labels (inorganic ^{32}P or [^{3}H]dThd) are used to tag them. Labeled DNA provides a stable marker for the studies of granulocyte kinetics.

The time course of radioactivity in blood granulocytes following injection of inorganic ^{32}P (figure 18.4) indicates that a 5- to 8-day delay occurs before labeled granulocytes enter the blood. Such data also show that the mean age of granulocytes (from myeloblast to death) is 9–10 days and that granulocytes entering the blood quickly move off into the tissues. When [^{32}P]DFP is given systemically, it labels all granulocyte precursors. Thus,

Table 18.2
Blood Neutrophil Values in Normal Subjects

Parameter	Mean	95% confidence limits
Total blood granulocyte pool (TBGP), 10^7 cells/kg	70	14–160
Circulating granulocyte pool (CGP), 10^7 cells/kg	31	11–46
Marginal granulocyte pool (MGP), 10^7 cells/kg	39	0–85
Granulocyte turnover rate (GTR), 10^7 cells/kg/day	163	50–340
Half-disappearance time ($T_{1/2}$), hr	6.7	4–10

Source: From G. E. Cartwright, J. W. Athens, and M. M. Wintrobe, *Blood* 24(1964): 780.

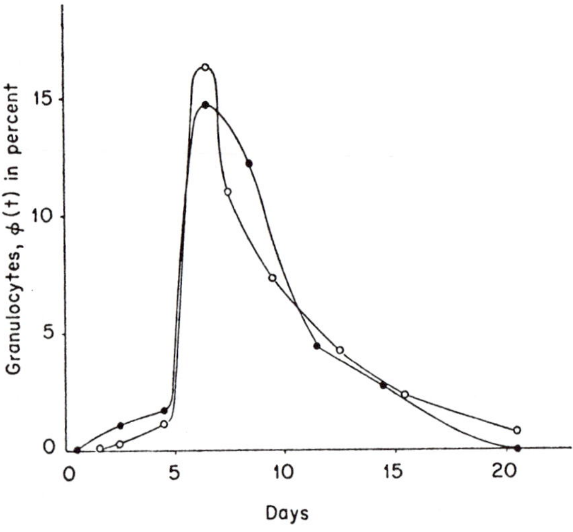

Fig. 18.4
Time course of blood granulocyte radioactivity after in vivo labeling with inorganic ^{32}P in two subjects. (Modified from J. Ottesen, *Acta Physiol. Scand.* 32[1954]: 75.)

for a time, cells emerging from the bone marrow are already labeled. From detailed studies of the time course of radioactivity in blood granulocytes, this methodology provides futher confirmation of a half-life of 7 hr and a 9- to 10-day interval between early precursor and adult neutrophil.

2. *Rate of granulopoiesis*

The clinician commonly attempts to gauge rates of neutrophil production by determining the cellularity and E/M ratios of bone marrow aspirates or biopsies (see lecture 1). However, this approach is subject to many errors. For example,

- Erythroid hyperplasia accompanying myeloid hyperplasia may hide the latter by keeping the E/M ratio in the normal range.
- The absence of mature forms in marrow may signify either true "maturation arrest" (see lecture 20) or, more commonly, the depletion of marrow reserves in the wake of intense demand for neutrophils or peripheral destruction.

3. *Normal production of granulocytes*

One view of granulocyte kinetics postulates a series of concatenated stem cell (i.e., α cell) compartments (figure 18.5). The diagram illustrates two important transitions: the myelocyte → metamyelocyte transition and the marrow granulocyte → blood granulocyte transition, in which labeled marrow cells become labeled blood cells. An earlier transition (initial pluripotential stem cell → maturation series) is equally important, but is less accessible experimentally.

a. MYELOCTYE → METAMYELOCYTE TRANSITION

In the myelocyte → metamyelocyte transition, cells labeled in the proliferating (DNA-synthesizing) compartment move into the nonproliferating compartment as a consequence of serial divisions of myelocytes. Myelocyte divisions are thought to cease after a time, possibly due to accumulation of cytoplasmic inhibitors. There is evidence favoring three models of the myelocyte → metamyelocyte transition: an $\alpha \rightarrow 2\alpha$ model, an $\alpha \rightarrow 2n$ model, and an $\alpha \rightarrow \alpha,n$ model (These models are explained in lecture 1.) The scheme in figure 18.5A views the transition as an $\alpha \rightarrow \alpha,n$ model.

Myelocyte production is probably in excess of that represented by the myelocytes entering the metamyelocyte compartment. Excess myelocytes presumably die in the marrow. Hence, a significant amount of ineffective granulopoiesis may occur normally. This model, which remains to be validated, suggests that marrow provides granulocytes quickly on demand, first by dumping cells from the marrow granulocyte reserve into the circulation and second by increasing production at the myelocyte level. The latter would have no effect on the blood granulocyte count until after completion of the metamyelocyte and band stages.

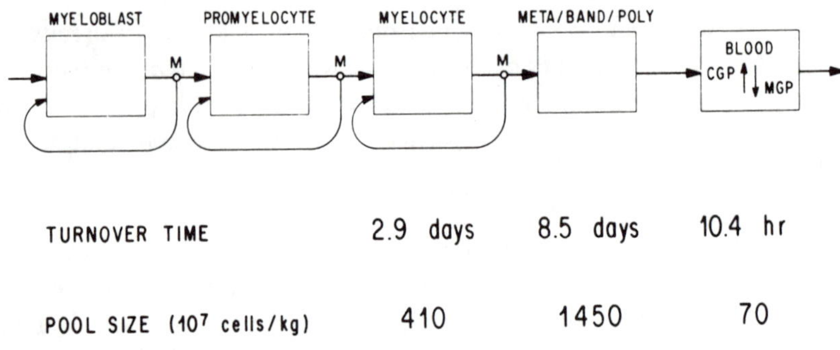

A

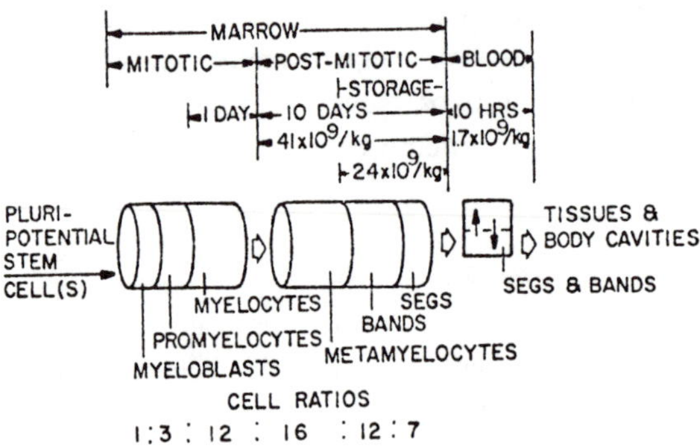

B

Fig. 18.5
Current models of granulopoiesis. *A*, Model according to Cartwright. M denotes a mitotic division. (Modified from G. Cartwright et al., *Blood* 24[1964]: 780.) *B*, Model according to Boggs (From D. Boggs, *Semin. Hematol.* 4[1976]: 359.)

b. MARROW GRANULOCYTE RESERVE

The term **marrow granulocyte reserve** was first used to denote the mature granulocytes that were promptly released from marrow in response to **leukapheresis**, an experimental procedure in which massive numbers of circulating granulocytes are removed. In a clinical context, the reserve is the readily mobilizable granulocyte pool released from marrow in response to an administered test dose of endotoxin.

This procedure employs Pyrexal®, a purified pyrogenic lipopolysaccharide from *Salmonella abortus equi.* Following intravenous injection of Pyrexal®, the granulocyte count first drops (in 1–2 hr) owing to margination and sequestration. Then it rises by 3000–5000 mature cells within 4–5 hr owing to a reverse shift *and* to an outpouring of marrow reserves. A smaller response and/or a significant "shift to the left" indicates a decreased granulocyte reserve. When reserves are depleted, the marrow becomes devoid of mature granulocytes. This marrow pattern is often mistakenly called "maturation arrest." Etiocholanolone administration produces a comparable increase in white count, without the preceding decrease.

The reserve, which is shown diagrammatically as the postmyelocyte compartments in figure 18.5, has been estimated to contain 400–1600 cells × 10^7/kg. If normal daily granulocyte consumption is 167 cells × 10^7/kg, the reserve would represent a 4- to 10-day supply.

c. RELEASE FROM MARROW

The blood granulocyte count is nearly constant in normal subjects. This constancy is achieved in part by two regulatory feedback loops—a slow one that controls entrance of stem cells into the granulopoietic pathway and a fast one that controls release of stored granulocytes from marrow into blood. Cyclic changes in the blood granulocyte count (cyclic netropenia) may occur when the two loops are operating dyssynchronously.

d. HUMORAL CONTROL REVISITED

As noted in lecture 1, differentiation of pluripotent stem cells into presursor cells committed to granulopoiesis is influenced by various **colony-stimulating factors** (CSFs), a major source of which is a membrane fraction of blood leukocytes or cells of the mononuclear phagocyte series. The several CSFs are also present in modest amounts in serum and urine and various other tissues.

The model in figure 18.6 suggests a scheme for control of both granulocytes and monocytes. It suggests that low CSF levels favor monocyte production and high levels favor granulocyte production. More will be said on monocytes and their production in lecture 19.

e. FATE OF GRANULOCYTES

The rate of egress of granulocytes from blood into tissues is another factor that determines the granulocyte count. Granulocytes apparently leave the blood on a random basis, though a few may disappear when senescent. The disposition of neutrophils is not known with certainty. In normal subjects, many appear in bronchial and intestinal secretions.

Some information on the rate of peripheral granulocyte destruction can be gleaned from serum levels of such distinctive granulocyte components as **muramidase**, also called **lysozyme** (see below), and **transcobalamin I** or **III**, the cobalamin-binding proteins described in lecture 5. In the presence of high white counts with rapid cell turnover, the levels of both compounds rise. Muramidase is notably increased by high monocyte turnover. Unfortunately, both tests give only sketchy correlations with the results of precise kinetics studies.

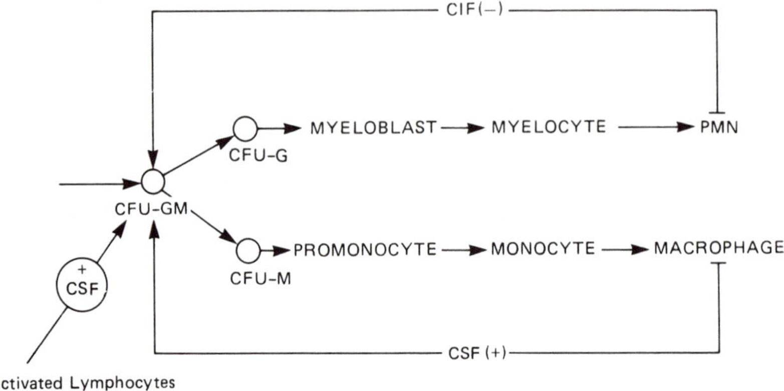

Fig. 18.6
Neutrophils and monocytes are derived from a progenitor cell, which can be identified in culture as a cell that gives rise to colonies containing neutrophils and monocytes or macrophages. This cell, the CFU-GM, differentiates into CFU-G and CFU-M, which give rise to fully differentiated neutrophils and monocytes/macrophages, respectively. The CSFs that cause proliferation of these progenitors are elaborated by stimulated lymphocytes, macrophages, and endothelial cells. CIFs, or colony-inhibiting factors, are putative agents that prevent the proliferation of neutrophil and macrophage progenitors and may be derived from mature neutrophils. (Compare with figures 1.1 and 1.2.)

C. Biochemistry

1. Commonplace features

Granulocytes posses most of the major anabolic and catabolic pathways and cell constituents of other body cells, among which are lipids of diverse types, glycogen, sialic acid, amino acids, nucleic acids, trace metals, and other components. They contain the major coenzymes and actively reduce folic acid. As noted in lecture 5, they contain a cobalamin-binding R-protein. When found in the plasma, it is known as transcobalamin III.

2. Distinctive features

In addition, granulocytes have many unusual biochemical features, among them a rich endowment of lysosomes and associated hydrolytic enzymes, a relatively high content of zinc, and an inability to perform the early steps of de novo purine synthesis. Apolactoferrin, a powerful iron-binding protein in granulocyte lysosomes, may inhibit the growth of iron-requiring bacteria by chelating iron.

Some of the following biochemical features are helpful in clinical diagnosis.

a. AEROBIC GLYCOLYSIS

Granulocytes depend largely on aerobic glycolysis for their energy supply. The tricarboxylic acid cycle occurs in these cells, but, as would be anticipated from the paucity of mitochondria, it is relatively feeble. There is a modest Pasteur effect. These metabolic features became a center of controversy following Warburg's early demonstration that many types of cancer cells possess a higher rate of aerobic glyoclysis and a weaker Pasteur effect than normal cells. He concluded that these changes were both diagnostic criteria and causal mechanisms of the neoplastic state. With the discovery of exceptions—normal tissues with similar characteristics (e.g., retina, kidney medulla, jejunal mucosa, and leukocytes) and tumors without them (e.g., minimal deviation hepatomas)—it become clear that the "cancer pattern" of metabolism lacks specificity.

b. HMP SHUNT PATHWAY

The hexose monophosphate (HMP) shunt pathway is active in circulating leukocytes. As will be discussed in lecture 19, this pathway is stimulated during phagocytosis.

c. ALKALINE PHOSPHATASE

Leukocyte alkaline phosphatase (LAP), an enzyme closely associated with neutrophilic membranes, is readily measured by a quantitative chemical method or a semiquantitative histochemical method. LAP is of interest because activity levels are distinctively altered in disease, as will be discussed later. The leukocytes of chronic myelocytic leukemia are low in LAP. In contrast, those of physiologic leukocytosis, myeloid metaplasia, and polycythemia vera are usually high in LAP. LAP levels are increased by pituitary-adrenal activity, the increase appearing only in newly formed cells.

d. MYELOPEROXIDASE

The enzyme, which accounts for the green color of pus and is sometimes called verdoperoxidase, catalyzes the following reactions:

$$H_2O_2 \rightarrow [O] + H_2O, \qquad AH_2 + [O] \rightarrow A + H_2O,$$

where AH_2 is an oxidizable substrate such as benzidine or guaiac. The physiologic role of myeloperoxidase will be discussed in lecture 19. Its presence in cells has been used as an indicator that they are members of the myeloid series.

e. LYSOZYME (MURAMIDASE)

Lysozyme (muramidase) is a powerful hydrolase that is associated with the lysosomes of granulocytes and monocytes. Its level is especially high in leukemic granulocytes and monocytes. When these cells break down in large numbers, serum and urine lysozyme levels become elevated.

f. CATHEPSINS AND PLASMINOGEN

Granulocyte cathepsins and other proteases participate in the digestion of fibrin. Granulocyte plasminogen may participate in the initiation of fibrinolysis.

g. SURFACE ADHESION MOLECULES

The role of granulocytes in host defense is discussed in Lecture 19. It should be noted here, however, that a distinctive feature of granulocyte biochemistry and biophysics is their rich endowment with **surface adhesion molecules**, members of the **integrin** gene family, which have been identified by monoclonal antibody methods. Among those of great current interest are the so-called CD11/CD18 molecules, which consist of three surface membrane heterodimeric glycoproteins that are expressed only in leukocytes. Their importance in host defense and in noninfectious acute inflammatory reactions is now well established (see lecture 19).

D. Physiologic functions

1. Phagocytosis

The main functions of granulocytes—chemotaxis, phagocytosis, and microbial killing—are discussed in lecture 19.

2. Granulocytes and the plasma kinins

The plasma kinin system consists of a group of polypeptides of low molecular weight (**kinins**). Granulocytes leak a substance that, in the presence of the coagulation factor called Hageman factor (see lecture 27), yields active **kallikrein**, which converts plasma **kininogen** (an α_2 globulin) to one of the prototype kinins, **bradykinin**. Kinins increase vascular permeability, cause local vasodilatation and pain, are chemotactic, and may be responsible for margination of granulocytes along walls of small vessels early in inflammation. This may be one of the several mechanisms for attracting granulocytes to sites of injury or bacterial invasion. Granulocytes are attracted to sites of kinin production, where initially they promote further kinin production. As they accumulate and break down, they eventually destroy kinin. Thus inflammation has two phases: (1) kinin causes local effects (pain, vasodilatation, capillary permeability, and chemotaxis); and (2) then granulocytes accumulate as local kinin concentration decreases.

Corticosteroids are believed to exert their anti-inflammatory effect by stabilizing lysosome membranes and preventing release of chemotactic and cytotoxic substances and inhibiting migration of cells to inflammatory sites.

3. Pyrogens and fever

Pyrogen, the fever-producing substance, is believed to be a cationic protein arising from granulocyte and monocyte lysosomes. More of it is present in exudate granulocytes than in circulating granulocytes. Granulocyte pyrogen is probably not the only cause of fever since fever occurs in diseases (like acute lymphocytic leukemia) in which granulocytes are lacking.

E. Antibodies to neutrophils and other granulocytes

1. Heterologous antibodies

Antigens on neutrophils include those shared with other body cells, notably the HLA antigens, and those specific for neutrophils. It has been known since the time of Metchnikoff (1899) that injection of leukocytes into animals of another species elicits antisera that may have relatively little species specificity. For example, guinea pig anti-bovine leukocyte serum may be active as well against rabbit leukocytes. Nevertheless, such antibodies appear cell-type specific. Thus, an antineutrophil serum may have little effect on monocytes or basophils. Such results indicate marked antigenic differences among leukocyte types.

2. Alloantibodies

Leukocyte alloantibodies have been described that are related to a system of leukocyte antigens resembling the blood group antigens of erythrocytes (lecture 16). Leukocyte and erythrocyte systems are unrelated, however. Many different leukocyte antigens are now known. Leukocyte alloantibodies are agglutinins. They gain importance because they provide (1) a source of possible severe immune reactions after pregnancy with fetomaternal leukocyte incompatibility (with resulting neonatal alloimmune neutropenia if maternal antibodies elicited by paternal antigens cross the placenta); (2) a cause of the febrile nonhemolytic transfusion reactions occurring after multiple transfusions; and (3) a reason for poor survival of transfused granulocytes.

3. Autoantibodies

Leukoagglutinins are occasionally found in sera of leukopenic subjects who never received a transfusion and who therefore are said to have idiopathic autoimmune neutropenia. They are also found in hematologically normal subjects.

The area is controversial because of the uncertain relation to leukopenia in individual patients and the difficulties of distinguishing autoantibodies and alloantibodies.

4. Antinuclear antibodies

Serum may contain antibodies to nuclear material. A number of antibodies of this type have been found with specificity for DNA, whole nucleoprotein, or other nuclear constituents. Antibody to nucleoprotein is the basis of the **LE (lupus erythematosus) cell test**.

5. Drug-induced antibodies

Although many drugs appear to cause immune neutropenia, the laboratory evidence of an immune mechanism is often sketchy. The famous example of aminopyrine neutropenia is discussed in lecture 20.

F. Eosinophils

Eosinophils are easily recognized by their characteristic staining pattern. Their large granules are rich in a distinctive type of peroxidase. On electron microscopy, they display a crystalloid core that contains the **major basic protein** (MBP) of eosinophils, a functionally important protein of mol. wt. 10,800. When large numbers of eosinophils disintegrate in secretions or exudate, the crystalloids remain intact and may come together to form large particles known as **Charcot-Leyden crystals**.

Until recently, the functions of eosinophils were unknown. There has been a recent upsurge of interest and it is now agreed that the eosinophil is highly specialized offshoot of the granulocyte series. Eosinophils (and basophils) appear to participate in virtually every form of immunologic tissue injury, yet detailed mechanisms remain unclear.

Two attributes appear to distinguish eosinophils from neutrophils and other leukocytes: (1) an ability to inactivate mediators released from mast cells (see below) and thereby modulate or damp down reactions associated with IgE-mediated degranulation of mast cells, e.g., the anaphylactic reaction and immediate hypersensitivity (in the vicinity of which eosinophils accumulate); and (2) an ability to control parasitic infestations. For example, recent work has shown in vitro that isolated eosinophils, unlike neutrophils, kill schistosomula, the larvae of *Schistosoma mansoni*, in an antibody-dependent, complement-independent process. This reaction is largely due to the release of MBP onto the surface of the parasite.

The major clinical conditions associated with **eosinophilia** (i.e., elevated eosinophil count) are listed in table 18.3. It is noteworthy that many of them are allergic states (e.g., extrinsic or allergic bronchial asthma, allergic rhinitis) and parasitic infections. They also accumulate at extravascular sites following multiple antigenic stimulation. Corticosteroids sharply decrease their numbers. This effect was the basis for an early assay of glucocorticoid effects.

Table 18.3
Clinical Conditions Often Associated with Eosinophilia

Category	Examples
Drug reactions	Iodide sensitivity, penicillin sensitivity
Allergic reactions	Asthma, angioneurotic edema, hay fever, serum sickness, vasculitis
Parasitic infestations	Amebiases, malaria, hookworm, tapeworm, ascariasis, filariasis, trichinosis
Skin diseases	Exfoliative dermatitis, pemphigus, dermatitis herpetiformis
Neoplasms	Metastatic carcinoma of lung, ovaries, and stomach, Hodgkin's disease, chronic myelocytic leukemia
"Hypereosinophilic" syndromes	Polyarteritis nodosa, eosinophilic granuloma, chronic eosinophilic pneumonia, Loeffler's syndrome
Infections	Brucellosis, tuberculosis, fungus infection, leprosy

G. Basophils

Basophils, the least common blood granulocytes, are members of the **mast cell** family. They contain all of the blood histamine, and they degranulate in allergic reactions in which antigen-antibody reactions of the following type occur (pollen + antipollen IgE). Basophilic granules also contain heparin, hyaluronate, and serotonin. Degranulating mast cells release chemotactic agents (see lecture 19) that attract neutrophils and eosinophils. The latter may then contribute to local control of the disturbance. Basophils also play a role in the deposition of immune complexes in tissues, as well as mediating delayed hypersensitivity reactions. Basophil counts may rise in chronic myelocytic leukemia and other myeloproliferative disorders. They decrease in anaphylactic shock and severe stress. Interestingly, basophils often increase in either bone marrow or blood but not both.

III. MONOCYTES

A. Functions

As discussed briefly in lecture 3, the monocyte is the precursor of fixed and free macrophages in the tissues. Both monocytes and tissue macrophages:

- Ingest and degrade dead and dying cells, bacteria, and foreign particles
- Secrete substances (e.g., M-CSF) that stimulate granulocyte production in the marrow (see lecture 1)
- Remove substances from the lungs (surfactant) to allow air sacs to open more easily
- Participate in the killing of neoplastic cells
- Produce angiotensin and interferon

A more complete list of macrophage functions appears in lecture 19.

B. Monocytosis

The number of monocytes that can be *counted* in normal blood is given in table 18.1. However, a considerably larger number is in the marginal pool. Also the total monocyte oscillates by about 200 cells/mm^3 with a periodicity of 3–6 days. The term **monocytosis** refers to the presence in blood of more than about 800 monocytes/mm^3. Among the disorders often (but not always) associated with monocytosis are:

- Infection (especially tuberculosis, endocarditis, and syphilis)
- Fever of unknown origin
- Various forms of neoplasia and myeloproliferative disorders
- Inflammatory disease (especially bowel disease and rheumatoid arthritis)
- Postsplenectomy state

SELECTED REFERENCES

Reviews

Arnaout, M. A. Structure and function of the leukocyte adhesion molecules CD11/CD18. *Blood* 75(1990): 1037–1050.

Bainton, D. F. Morphology of neutrophils and neutrophil precursors. In Williams, W. J., et al., eds. *Hematology*, 4th ed. New York: McGraw-Hill, 1990, pp. 760–769.

Beck, W. S., and Valentine, W. N. The carbohydrate metabolism of leukocytes: a review. *Cancer Res.* 13(1953): 309–317.

Beris, P. Primary clonal myelodysplastic syndromes. *Semin. Hematol.* 26(1989): 216–233.

Curnutte, J. T., and Babior, B. M. Composition of neutrophils. In Williams, W. J., et al., eds. *Hematology*, 4th ed. New York: McGraw-Hill, 1990, pp. 770–774.

Curnutte, J. T., and Babior, B. M. Metabolism of neutrophils. In Williams, W. J., et al., eds. *Hematology*, 4th ed. New York: McGraw-Hill, 1990, pp. 775–780.

Golde, D. W. Production, distribution, and fate of neutrophils. In Williams, W. J., et al., eds. *Hematology*, 4th ed. New York: McGraw-Hill, 1990, pp. 795–801.

Huizinga, T. W. J., Roos, D., et al. Neutrophil Fc-gamma receptors: a two-way bridge in the immune system. *Blood* 75(1990): 1211–1214.

Kishimoto, T. K., Larson, R. S., et al. The leukocyte integrins. *Adv. Immunol.* 46(1989): 149–182.

Original articles

Bainton, D. F., Friedlander, L. M., et al. Abnormalities in granule formation in acute myelogenous leukemia. *Blood* 49(1977): 693–704.

Beck, W. S., and Valentine, W. N. Biochemical studies on leukocytes. II. Phosphatase activity in chronic lymphatic leukemia, acute leukemia, and miscellaneous hematologic conditions. *J. Lab. Clin. Med.* 38(1951): 245–253.

Hurley, W. L., and Finkelstein, E. Identification of leukocyte surface proteins. *Methods Enzymol.* 184(1990): 429–432.

Valentine, W. N., and Beck, W. S. Biochemical studies on leukocytes. I. Phosphatase activity in health, leukocytosis, and myelocytic leukemia. *J. Lab. Clin. Med.* 38(1951): 39–55.

LECTURE 19

Leukocytes II. Phagocytosis and its Disorders

Thomas P. Stossel

EDITOR'S COMMENT

The remarkable ability of granulocytes to leave the bloodstream rapidly and efficiently and to move to inflammatory sites, there to engulf and destroy invading bacteria, reflects a cluster of phenomena that raises profound questions of mechanism and of evolutionary biology in light of the fact that many of these functions were invented by our unicellular protist ancestors. Granulocyte research has a rich history that began with Metchnikoff and passed through temporary glory with the studies of Otto Warburg in the 1920s on the metabolism of tumor cells. These cells have been difficult to isolate from blood without exposing them to injury and have been even more difficult to work with in view of their sticky tendency to adhere to glass tubes. Most of these problems have been ingeniously solved and much is now known of the mechanisms of granulocyte function. Predictably, most of these systems are subject to mutational and acquired defects. Thus a whole new set of leukocyte disorders is based on defects of individual components of the motility, phagocytosis, and chemotaxis systems.

I. INTRODUCTION

Although leukocytes were discovered late in the eighteenth century, their relevance to human physiology was not appreciated until a century later, when Metchnikoff showed that they are involved in host defense against bacterial infection and in inflammation in general.

The structure, metabolism, and life cycle of neutrophils were discussed in lecture 18. In this lecture, we shall discuss another of the major phagocytic leukocytes, the monocyte, and survey aspects of the physiology of all phagocytic leukocytes that are related to their defensive functions. We shall also review qualitative disorders of these functions.

II. PHAGOCYTIC LEUKOCYTES

A. Neutrophils

As noted in lecture 18, the cytoplasm of neutrophils is filled with glycogen and granules, most of which stain poorly with Wright's stain. The granules are membrane-bound structures that resemble lysosomes. A small fraction of the total granule population contains all of the cell's content of the enzyme, myeloperoxidase, which as discussed below is relevant for its bactericidal activity. It should be noted here that myeloperoxidase-containing granules are synthesized early in neutrophil development—during the promyelocyte stage. Therefore, these granules are counted among the primary or azurophilic granules (see lecture 18). The rest of the granules, synthesized during the myelocyte stage, are the secondary or specific-staining granules.

Only when neutrophils are mature are they capable of directed locomotion and ingestion of bacteria. Finding and killing bacteria invading the tissues are the major activities of neutrophils.

B. Monocytes and macrophages

1. Properties of monocytes

This cell has a lobulated nucleus with reticular chromatin strands. The monocyte is sometimes difficult to distinguish from an atypical large lymphocyte. Compared to most lymphocytes, its cytoplasm has a distinct grey hue in Wright's-stained smears, whereas lymphocyte cytoplasm stains various shades of blue. Maroon granules are occasionally present. The monocyte has fewer myeloperoxidase-containing granules than the neutrophil. It subsists primarily on aerobic glycolysis.

2. Life cycle

Monocytes arise in the bone marrow, where they mature more rapidly than neutrophils, the entire maturation process requiring approximately 24–36 hr. The monocyte sojourns in the blood for about 24–36 hr and then enters the tissues, where it may persist for long periods of time. It differentiates throughout its life span; as it does so, its size increases and its properties change. It is now recognized that monocytes are precursors of tissue macrophages, which are differentiated mononuclear phagocytes that reside in the tissues (see lecture 3).

3. Properties of macrophages

The transformation of monocyte to macrophage is accompanied by fundamental changes in cell structure and metabolism. As they become macrophages, the cells increase in size, lose their peroxidase-containing granules, and produce large quantities of lysosomes filled with acid hydrolases. The transformation is also associated with an increase in mitochondria and an increasing dependence for energy on tricarboxylic acid cycle activity—unlike their monocytic precursors, which depend primarily on glycolysis.

Although macrophages are present in all tissues, they are especially dense in "filter" organs—liver, spleen, lung and lymph nodes—where, perched on endothelial cells and reticulum fibers, they constitute a sentry network (see lecture 3). This network, historically termed the RES (for reticuloendothelial system) is now properly designated the **mononuclear phagocyte system**.

Mononuclear phagocytes (monocytes and macrophages), like neutrophils, can ingest and kill bacteria (particularly pyogenic bacteria) during all phases of their life cycle.

Macrophages, especially those previously activated by exposure to products of antigen-primed T lymphocytes, particularly interferon-γ, are more efficient in killing and ingesting bacteria than monocytes.

However, the mononuclear phagocyte has many other functions.

- Macrophages because of their long life are responsible for the digestion of bacteria killed by neutrophils.
- They are actively pinocytic and probably play a role in normal serum protein catabolism.
- They clear and digest senescent blood cells (see lecture 12).
- They have biosynthetic capacities and produce enormous quantities of lysozyme (muramidase) as well as cytokines (e.g., M-CSF) and proteins of the complement and fibrinolytic systems.
- In various specific locations, they may have properties unique to their site and as yet undetermined local functions.
- They are important for antigen presentation to lymphocytes and together with lymphocytes are involved in immune responses that include programming lymphocytes for antibody formation and containment, if not killing, of so-called facultative intracellular parasites, viruses, protozoa, certain fungi, and mycobacteria.

III. MOTILE ACTIVITIES

Phagocytes must find and ingest invading microorganisms. Cytoplasmic rearrangements must occur during ingestion. These activities are similar in neutrophils and mononuclear phagocytes and are here described together.

A. Chemotaxis

The interaction between microorganisms and tissues results in the elaboration of many substances that attract phagocytes in the process known as **chemotaxis**. Among them are the following:

- A **low-molecular-weight fragment, C5a**, which is derived from the cleavage of the complement protein C5, the cleavage occurring by activation of the "classic" or "alternative" complement pathways (see lecture 13) or by direct proteolytic attack since bacteria and damaged tissue liberate nonspecific proteases.
- ***N*-formyl oligopeptides**, potent chemotatic factors which are molecules liberated from bacteria and mitochondria.

- Metabolic products of arachidonic acid, especially **leukotriene B_4** (LTB_4), which exists in inflammatory fluids.

Many other agents can attract phagocytes in vitro. Chemotactic factors must form a gradient in order to be effective. Neutrophils respond more rapidly than monocytes. Phagocytes have surface receptors for C5a and *N*-formyl oligopeptides, and these receptors are specific and distinct. The dose-response characteristics for chemotactic responses to these agents correlate well with the binding properties of the chemotactic factors to their respective receptors on the phagocyte membranes. The immediate responses activated by the binding include activation of transmembrane calcium fluxes, metabolic phospholipid turnover, and the phosphorylation of intracellular proteins by protein kinases.

Chemotaxis may be assessed semiquantitatively in humans by means of the **Rebuck skin window**, which is prepared by abrading a small skin area on the volar forearm. A clean cover slip is placed over the lesion, covered with cardboard, and taped in place. The cover slip is removed and replaced at 2, 8, and 24 hr. Cover slips stained with Wright's stain show an orderly chemotactic response. The 2-hr slip normally shows mainly neutrophils; the 8-hr slip shows about 50% monocytes; and the 24-hr slip shows monocytes that have been transformed into macrophages. The skin-window response usually reflects the level of circulating neutrophils.

B. Recognition

Having arrived at the invaded site, the phagocytes must recognize what to ingest. It is clear that many microorganisms resist recognition by virtue of their capsules. Serum interacts with these microorganisms to coat them with substances called **opsonins** (from a Greek word meaning "to prepare for dining") that render them attractive to phagocytes. The major opsonins are the following:

- Antibodies of the IgG class that in some instances can coat objects and cause them to be ingested
- More commonly a combination of either IgG or IgM antibody plus complement components that cause two sequential fragments of the third component of complement (C3) to be deposited on the surface of bacteria or other objects, which then elicit recognition

These opsonins interact with specific receptors on the phagocyte plasma membrane. In the case of IgG, the receptors recognize the Fc portion of the antibody molecule. Fc receptors of which there are two separate types (FcRI, FcRII, and FcRIII) trigger ingestion, whereas C3b and C3bi receptors (known as CR1 and CR3, respectively) are more involved with binding of phagocytes to objects. CR3 is particularly important in mediating the adhesion between phagocytes and surfaces that is necessary for locomotion and phagocytosis.

C. Locomotion and ingestion

The response of phagocytes to chemotactic agents by directed locomotion and to recognizable particles by ingestion results in increased rates of energy metabolism. This fact suggests that energy in the form of ATP is involved in these activities. Also associated with locomotion and ingestion is the formation of large pseudopodia by the assembly of actin into filaments. These filaments are cross-linked into a gel state by an actin-binding protein called **filamin** and contracted by myosin in the presence of calcium and ATP. Therefore, chemotactic factors and recognition factors activate locomotion and ingestion by influencing the interactions of contractile proteins, regulated by signal messengers generated at the plasma membrane.

D. Degranulation

During ingestion, pseudopods flow around the bacteria being eaten and encase them within membrane-bound phagocytic vacuoles. The cytoplasmic granules fuse with these vacuoles and secrete their contents into them, simultaneously disappearing from the cytoplasm. Hence, degranulation occurs. The mechanism by which pseudopods fuse at their tips to form the phagocytic vacuole or the fusion mechanism of the granules with the vacuole is unknown.

IV. BACTERICIDAL ACTIVITIES

A. Oxygen-dependent mechanisms

During ingestion neutrophils and mononuclear phagocytes actively metabolize oxygen to produce reactive products that are toxic to ingested bacteria. The activation of mononuclear phagocytes by interferon-γ elaborated by lymphoid cells, a consequence of which is heightened ability of macrophages to kill intracellular parasites, involves the induction of these oxygen-metabolizing mechanisms in the macrophage. The oxidase that catalyzes this reaction is a b-type cytochrome for which pyridine nucleotides (e.g., NADPH) provide the necessary reducing power. The oxygen metabolites are the following.

1. Superoxide anion

Superoxide anion (O_2^-) is the first reduction product of oxygen. It is a highly reactive substance that is further reduced to hydrogen peroxide, especially at acid pH. It is also available for reoxidation to oxygen in the presence of a suitable agent. Such an agent is nitroblue tetrazolium (NBT), a redox dye that concomitantly becomes reduced to a blue formazan. Measurement of the reduction of NBT to formazan provides a method for detecting activation of oxygen metabolism during ingestion.

2. *Hydrogen peroxide*

Hydrogen peroxide (H_2O_2) is the product of oxygen metabolism that is probably most important for bactericidal activity by phagocytes. Hydrogen peroxide can react with superoxide to produce the highly reactive **hydroxyl radical** ($OH\cdot$) as:

$$O_2^- + H_2O_2 \rightarrow O_2 + OH^- + OH\cdot$$

The antibacterial action of hydrogen peroxide is potentiated by the enzyme myeloperoxidase, which is delivered into the phagocytic vacuole by degranulation. Halides are cofactors of this potentiation, chloride most likely being the physiologically relevant participant. The reaction of hydrogen peroxide, myeloperoxidase, and chloride produces toxic **hypochlorous acid** (HOCl) and also toxic **chloramines**. Macrophages lack myeloperoxidase but may have other ways for potentiating the effects of hydrogen peroxide.

B. Detoxificaton of oxygen metabolites

These highly reactive substances are detrimental to both microbes and animal cells. Control of them is achieved in phagocytes by (1) **localization** of superoxide and hydrogen peroxide to **the phagocytic vacuole**; (2) the enzyme **superoxide dismutase**, which rapidly converts superoxide diffusing from vacuole to cytoplasm into hydrogen peroxide in the following reaction:

$$2O_2^- + 2H^+ \rightarrow H_2O_2 + O_2;$$

(3) the enzyme **catalase**, which destroys hydrogen peroxide in the cytoplasm; and (4) **reduced glutathione** (GSH), which in destroying hydrogen peroxide activates the series of coupled enzymatic reactions shown in figure 19.1. Note that GSH-mediated hydrogen peroxide catabolism regenerates NADPH, a possible substrate for oxidase-mediated hydrogen peroxide production.

C. Oxygen-independent mechanisms

A number of oxygen-independent factors are damaging to various types of ingested bacteria. One is the **acid pH** of the phagocytic vacuole. Another

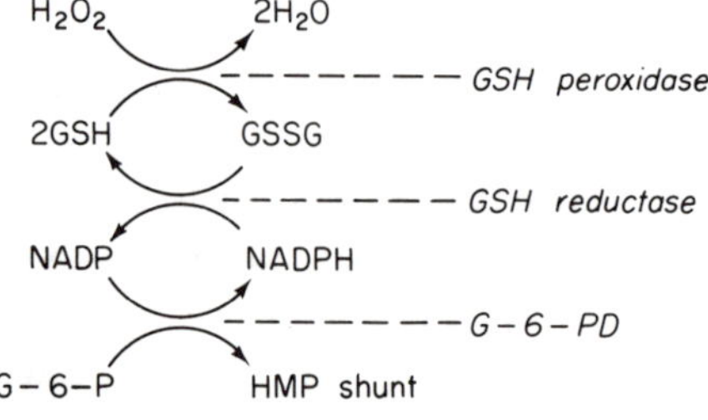

Fig. 19.1
Sequence of reactions by which hydrogen peroxide is detoxified.

is **lysozyme**, which hydrolyzes the mucopeptide cell wall of a few microbial species. **Bactericidal proteins** called **defensins** delivered to the phagocytic vacuole during degranulation can kill bacteria by altering the permeability of their membranes.

V. QUALITATIVE DISORDERS OF PHAGOCYTIC FUNCTION

Any of the mechanisms of phagocytic action can go awry, and many examples of such disorders have been reported. When a functional impairment is serious, affected patients suffer from recurrent pyogenic infections. In some instances, the type and severity of infection can be clearly explained by the defect; in others, the correlation is not so clear. A classification of phagocytic disorders is presented in table 19.1.

A. Disorders of chemotaxis and opsonization

Since synergistic activity of anibody and complement components leads to elaboration of chemotactic factors and coating of bacteria with opsonins,

Table 19.1
Some Disorders of Phagocytosis

	Cells affected		
Function affected	Neutrophil	Mononuclear phagocytes	Both
Mobilization	Neutropenia		Marrow ablation
Chemotaxis	Neutrophil actin dysfunction Deficiency of CD11/CD18 adhesion molecules		Antibody deficiency states Complement disorders
Opsonization			Antibody deficiency states Complement disorders
Ingestion	Neutrophil actin dysfunction Complement receptor deficiency	Macrophage ablation, bypass, diversion	Corticosteroid therapy
Degranulation	Neutrophil granule deficiency		Chédiak-Higashi syndrome
Oxygen metabolism			Chronic granulomatous disease Myeloperoxidase deficiency

it is not surprising that recurrent infections are associated with deficiencies of relevant serum proteins or the presence of agents that prevent complement activation. Thus, patients with antibody deficiency syndromes and complement disorders often have recurrent bacteremias, meningitis, and sinopulmonary infections. The offending organisms are usually high-grade encapsulated pathogens, streptococci, pneumococci, neisseria, *Haemophilus influenzae*, and species of *Pseudomonas*. Specific examples of these deficiency states include:

- Congenital agammaglobulinemia
- Acquired agammaglobulinemia or hypogammaglobulinemia (sometimes associated with multiple myeloma or lymphoproliferative disorders, in which immunoglobulin may be plentiful but useful antibody is depleted)
- Genetic deficiency of C3
- Acquired deficiency of C3 and other complement proteins in systemic lupus erythematosus, advanced liver disease, and immune complex diseases

B. Disorders of locomotion and ingestion

In the following examples, phagocytes are unable to respond to chemotactic factors or opsonins.

1. Patients receiving corticosteroids

Neutrophils from patients treated daily with corticosteroids in sufficient doses are impaired in their ability to migrate into inflammatory lesions and to ingest. Monocytes and macrophages from steroid-treated humans or animals also have defective ingestion capacities. The detailed mechanism of steroid action is unknown. These facts are clinically significant because they may explain why(1) steroid-treated patients or patients with Cushing's syndrome are susceptible to pyogenic infection and (2) steroids reduce inflammation and can reduce the clearance of antibody-coated cells as in immunohemolytic anemia (see lecture 13) or idiopathic thrombocytopenic purpura (see lecture 28).

2. Deficiency of adhesion molecules and of complement receptors

These rare genetic diseases are autosomal recessive disorders associated with absence of the CD11/CD18 granulocyte adhesion molecules discussed in lecture 18. Neutrophils stick poorly to surfaces. Granulocytes lacking complement receptors fail to respond to C3-coated bacteria.

3. Neutrophil actin dysfunction

This is a very rare autosomal recessive genetic disorder in which the patient's neutrophils fail to locomote or ingest because the cytoplasmic actin of neutrophils fails to polymerize into filaments.

4. Chédiak-Higashi syndrome

This congenital (autosomal recessive) disorder is associated with (1) neutropenia; (2) giant lysosomal granules in leukocytes (and other cells) that do not fuse normally with phagocytic vacuoles; and (3) defective chemotaxis in neutrophils and monocytes (although ingestion is normal) with recurrent pyogenic infections. Apparently cells cannot mobilize themselves to respond to a chemotactic gradient. Most patients succumb after entering an accelerated phase, an ill-defined febrile state associated with pancytopenia and massive hepatosplenomegaly. This was also discussed in lecture 18.

5. Macrophage disorders

The infections encountered in the following group of diverse disorders are similar to those seen in patients with humoral disorders.

a. BYPASS

Cirrhosis of the liver can produce shunting of portal blood around the macrophage-rich liver. Cirrhosis is also associated with complement deficiencies. Cardiac shunts may cause systemic venous blood to bypass lung macrophages.

b. ABLATION

Splenectomy is associated with a small but finite risk of serious sepsis (see lecture 3).

c. DIVERSION

Diseases in which macrophages are heavily engaged in ingesting damaged erythrocytes, for example, sickle cell anemia or thalassemia major, are associated with an increased incidence of infection. Adult patients with sickle cell anemia also have asplenia (see lecture 10).

C. Disorders of bactericidal activity

1. Chronic granulomatous disease

This congenital disease is inherited either as an X-linked or autosomal recessive trait. Neutrophils and monocytes do not metabolize oxygen to superoxide or hydrogen peroxide. In most cases, this failure is due either to inactivity or lack of the oxidase(s) that metabolizes oxygen or to deficiencies in the mechanism that activates the oxidase. In rare instances, neutrophils totally lacking G-6-PD cannot metabolize oxygen since the reduced pyridine nucleotide substrates of the oxidase(s) are not regenerated.

There are several consequences of the failure of phagocytes to metabolize oxygen. First, affected phagocytes do not kill certain microorganisms that are catalase-positive and thereby capable of destroying hydrogen peroxide produced by their own metabolic processes. Common catalase-positive organisms include *Staphylococcus aureus*, most gram-negative enteric organisms, and many fungi. Catalase-negative organisms, for example, streptococci, pneumonocci, and certain *Haemophilus* species, accumulate hydrogen peroxide in the narrow confines of phagocytic vacuoles that in synergy with granule-derived myeloperoxidase cause their death—in a sense, a form of suicide. Patients with chronic granulomatous disease suffer from recurrent skin, bone, and visceral infections with catalase-positive organisms.

Since affected neutrophils do not metabolize oxygen, metabolic reactions caused by the presence of oxygen metabolites are not activated during ingestion; for example, NBT is not reduced and HMP shunt activity is not increased. The failure to find enhancement of these reactions during ingestion is diagnostic of the disease. Mothers of boys with the X-linked form of the disease have a defective population of cells, in accordance with the Lyon hypothesis. The low oxidase activity of phagocytes of patients with X-linked chronic granulomatous disease can be increased by interferon-γ therapy.

2. *Myeloperoxidase deficiency*

This is a rare autosomal recessive disorder in which neutrophils and monocytes (but not eosinophils) totally lack myeloperoxidase. Some patients with myeloproliferative disorders develop an acquired partial myeloperoxidase deficiency. The phagocytes have a bactericidal defect demonstrable in vitro since they lack an agent that potentiates the bactericidal activity of hydrogen peroxide. The defect is less severe than that of chronic granulomatous disease phagocytes. Moreover, most "patients" with myeloperoxidase deficiency are not unduly susceptible to infection. The disorder is important because it provides a model for demonstrating the role of myeloperoxidase in antimicrobial activity.

D. Phagocytes as mediators of inflammation

During ingestion of microbes, phagocytes may spill potent toxins into the surrounding medium. Proteases and the oxygen metabolites, in addition to injuring neighboring cells, can cleave serum proteins to generate chemotactic factors, thereby propagating the reaction. Therefore phagocytes have the capacity to be detrimental as well as helpful to the host. Tissue damage in diverse diseases such as acute glomerulonephritis, rheumatoid arthritis, silicosis, and gout may be phagocyte mediated. It is even possible that the oxidants generated by phagocytes alter genes in normal cells, thus predisposing them to mutations and cancer.

E. Clinical approach

1. Diagnosis

The type of disorder can be inferred from the history and documented by (1) measurements of levels of serum immunoglobulins and complement; (2) assay of neutrophil migration and ingestion; and (3) assay of neutrophil oxygen metabolism.

2. Therapy

Therapy occasionally can be specific—for example, gamma globulin in antibody deficiency states. Usually it involves only vigilance and aggresive therapy of specific infections.

SELECTED REFERENCES

Reviews

Anderson, D. C., and Springer, T. A. Leukocyte adhesion deficiency: an inherited defect in the Mac-1, LFA-1, and p150, 195 glycoproteins. *Annu. Rev. Med.* 38 (1987): 175–194.

Baggiolini, M., and Wymann, M. P. Turning on the respiratory burst. *TIBS* 15(1990): 69–72.

Becker, E. L. The short and happy life of neutrophil activation. *J. Leukocyte Biol.* 47(1990): 378–389.

Boyle, M. D. P., Lawman, M. J. P., et al. Measurement of leukocyte chemotaxis *in vivo*. *Methods Enzymol.* 162(1988): 101–114.

Cannistra, S. A., and Griffin, J. D. Regulation of the production and function of granulocytes and monocytes. *Semin. Hematol.* 25(1988): 173–188.

Devreotes, P. N., and Zigmond, S. H. Chemotaxis in eukaryotic cells: a focus on leukocytes and Dictyostelium. *Annu. Rev. Cell Biol.* 4(1988): 649–686.

Ford-Hutchinson, A. W. Leukotriene B_4 in inflammation. *CRC Crit. Rev. Immunol.* 10(1990): 1–12.

Gallin, J. I., Goldstein, I., and Snyderman, R. *Inflammation. Basic Principles and Clinical Correlates*. New York: Raven Press, 1988.

Hemler, M. E. VLA proteins in the integrin family: structures, functions, and their role on leukocytes. *Annu. Rev. Immunol.* 8(1990): 365–400.

Johnston, R. B. Jr. 1988. Monocytes and macrophages. *N. Engl. J. Med.* 312(1988): 747–752.

Orkin, S. H. Molecular genetics of chronic granulomatous disease. *Annu. Rev. Immunol.* 7(1989): 277–307.

Sha'afi, R. I., and Molski, T. F. P. Role of ion movements in neutrophil activation. *Annu. Rev. Physiol.* 52(1990): 365–379.

Stossel, T. P. The molecular biology of phagocytes and the molecular basis of nonneoplastic phagocyte disorders. In G. Stamatoyannopoulos, A. W. Nienhuis, P. Leder, and P. W. Majerus, eds. *The Molecular Basis of Blood Diseases*. Philadelphia: Saunders, 1987, pp. 499–533.

Stossel, T. P., Chaponnier, C., et al. Nonmuscle actin-binding proteins. *Annu. Rev. Cell Biol.* 1(1985): 353–402.

Wilkinson, P. C. Chemotactic factors: an overview. *Methods Enzymol.* 162(1988): 127–131.

Original articles

Bagby, G. C., Jr. Commentary: regulation of granulopoiesis. The lactoferrin controversy. *Blood Cells* 15(1989): 386–399.

Berkow, R. L., and Dodson, R. W. Tyrosine-specific protein phosphorylation during activation of human neutrophils. *Blood* 75(1990): 2445–2452.

Burkhardt, R., Jaeger, K., et al. Chronic myeloproliferative disorders: prognostic importance of new working classification. *J. Clin. Pathol.* 43(1990): 357–364.

Clark, R. A., Malech, H. L., et al. Genetic variants of chronic granulomatous disease: prevalence of deficiencies of two cytosolic components of the NADPH oxidase system. *N. Engl. J. Med.* 321(1989): 647–652.

Clark, R. A., Volpp, B. D., et al. Two cytosolic components of the human neutrophil respiratory burst oxidase translocate to the plasma membrane during cell activation. *J. Clin. Invest.* 85(1990): 714–721.

Cronstein, B. N., Daguma, L., et al. The adenosine/neutrophil paradox resolved: human neutrophils possess both A_1 and A_2 receptors that promote chemotaxis and inhibit O_2^- generation, respectively. *J. Clin. Invest.* 85(1990): 1150–1157.

Curnutte, J. T., Scott, P. J., et al. Functional defect in neutrophil cytosols from two patients with autosomal recessive cytochrome-positive chronic granulomatous disease. *J. Clin. Invest.* 83(1989): 1236–1240.

Ezekowitz, R. A. B., Dinauer, M. C., et al. Partial correction of the phagocyte defect in patients with X-linked chronic granulomatous disease by subcutaneous interferon gamma. *N. Engl. J. Med.* 319(1988): 146–151.

Howard, T., Chaponnier, C., et al. Gelsolin-actin interaction and actin polymerization in human neutrophils. *J. Cell Biol.* 110(1990): 1983–1991.

Lee, J., Gustafsson, M., et al. The direction of membrane lipid flow in locomoting polymorphonuclear leukocytes. *Science* 247(1990): 1229–1233.

Royer-Pokora, B., Kunkel, L. M., et al. Cloning the gene for an inherited human disorder—chronic granulomatous disease—on the basis of its chromosomal location. *Nature* 322(1986): 32–38.

Segal, A. W. The electron transport chain of the microbicidal oxidase of phagocytic cells and its involvement in the molecular pathology of chronic granulomatous disease. *J. Clin. Invest.* 83(1989): 1785–1793.

Unanue, E. R., and Allen, P. M. The basis for the immunoregulatory role of macrophages and other accessory cells. *Science* 236(1987): 551–557.

Unkeless, J. C. Function and heterogeneity of human Fc receptors for immunoglobulin G. *J. Clin. Invest.* 83(1989): 355–361.

Weiss, S. J. Tissue destruction by neutrophils. *N. Engl. J. Med.* 320(1989): 365–376.

LECTURE 20

Introduction to the Disorders of Leukocytes

William S. Beck

EDITOR'S COMMENT

This lecture is a survey of many of the disorders involving granulocytes, which range from purely reactive disorder, such as physiologic leukocytosis on one end of the spectrum to proliferative disorders, such as leukemia and myeloid metaplasia, on the other end. This lecture moves from one end of the spectrum to the other, but leaves the proliferative disorders for later lectures. Along the way it digresses into the many disorders associated with leukopenia (too few white cells).

I. DISEASES OF GRANULOCYTES

A number of themes recur in this necessarily brief survey of the diseases of granulocytes:

- The fact that a disorder makes a prominent display of an elevated or decreased leukocyte count does not imply that other formed elements are uninvolved.
- Some of the disorders to be discussed closely resemble one another (or evolve into one another), and diagnostic acumen may be needed to sort them out.
- In general, the disorders to be discussed may be divided into those involving an essentially physiologic response (or reaction) to an outside insult and those involving "spontaneous" abnormal proliferation.
- Pathophysiologic mechanisms of major granulocyte disorders parallel those of red cell and platelet disorders in many cases.

We shall begin our review of the several categories of granulocyte disorders at the "reactive" end of the spectrum and work toward the "proliferative" end. (The qualitative granulocyte disorders of phagocytic function were discussed in lecture 19.)

A. Leukocytosis

1. Neutrophilic leukocytosis (neutrophilia)

Physiologic **leukocytosis** is the classic instance of reactive behavior by leukocytes. It is a normal response to a noxious stimulus. The term is usually applied when the leukocyte count exceeds 10,000/mm^3. **Granulocytosis** refers to an increase in circulating neutrophilis, bands, and, less frequently,

Table 20.1
Major Causes of Neutrophilia

Acute	Chronic
Infections Bacterial, mycotic, rickettsial, spirochetal, and certain viral infections **Inflammation or tissue necrosis** Burns, electric shock, trauma, infarction, gout, vasculitis, antigen-antibody complexes, complement activation **Drugs, hormones, and toxins** Epinephrine, etiocholanolone, endotoxin, corticosteroids, venoms **Physical agents** Cold, heat, exercise, convulsions, pain, labor, anesthesia, surgery **Emotional stimuli** Panic, rage, stress	**Inflammation or tissue necrosis** Chronic inflammatory reactions, such as rheumatic fever, rheumatoid arthritis, gout, vasculitis, myositis, nephritis, colitis, pancreatitis, dermatitis, thyroiditis, infarction **Infections** Persistence of infections causing acute neutrophilia **Neoplasms** Gastric, bronchogenic, breast, renal, hepatic, pancreatic, uterine, and squamous cell cancers, lymphoma, melanoma, multiple myeloma **Drugs, hormones, and toxins** Continued exposure to agents that cause acute neutrophilia; lithium **Metabolic and endocrine disorders** Uremia, eclampsia, thyroid storm, hyperadrenocorticalism, acidosis **Hematologic disorders** Rebound from agranulocytosis, chronic hemolysis or hemorrhage, asplenia, myeloproliferative disorders

metamyelocytes. By common usage, the term does not imply an increase in other granule-containing cells (eosinophils or basophils). The term **neutrophilia** is somewhat less ambiguous, denoting an increase only in neutrophils. Granulocytosis is perhaps the most commonly encountered disorder in clinical medicine. Its principal causes are listed in table 20.1.

a. MECHANISMS

The system of granulocyte production and release, described in lecture 18, is remarkable for its capacity not only to maintain uniformity (despite minor diurnal variations) of the blood granulocyte count in normal subjects but to pour out granulocytes in the presence of infection or stress. A demand for granulocytes imposed by peripheral bacterial invasion is met at first by the egress into the tissue of cells from the MGP. Release of bone marrow reserves is then accelerated. Finally, there is an increased rate of myeloid cell proliferation in the marrow. These additions of new circulating granulocytes are reflected in the blood by a "shift to the left"—that is, a rise in the ratio of nonsegmented to segmented neutrophils. The mechanism of transmission of information to the marrow from the periphery is unknown.

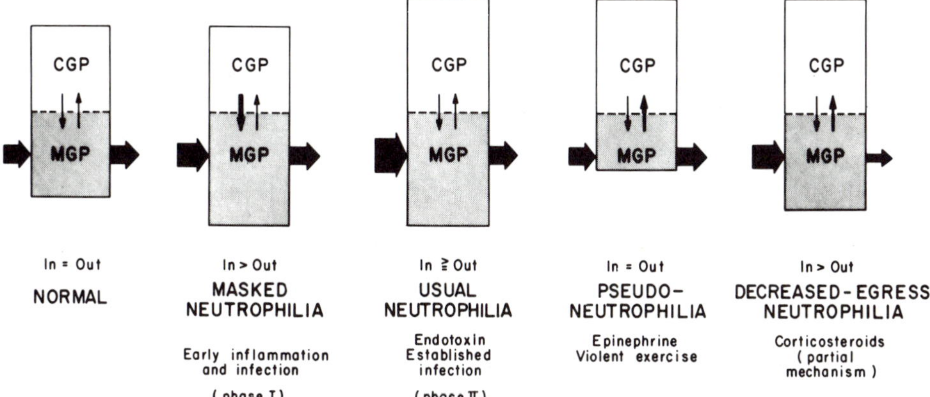

Fig. 20.1
Mechanisms of neutrophilia.

b. PHASES

Labeling studies show that leukocytosis of infection or inflammation has at least three phases (figure 20.1).

In the **phase of early infection**:

- Release of granulocytes by marrow increases (hence, blood granulocytes "shift to the left").
- Circulating cells marginate, so that MGP rises before CGP.
- If egress of cells to tissue exceeds input from marrow, the leukocyte count may decrease (as discussed below under neutropenia).
- Since circulating cells are marginating, infused cells labeled with [^{32}P]DFP are diluted by newly released unlabeled cells. Half-life at this time is short, perhaps 2 or 3 hr (normal, 7 hr). Because TBGP is increased in this phase without an increase in leukocyte count, the picture may be termed **masked neutrophilia**.

In the **phase of established infection**:

- Pools equilibrate, so that CGP equals MGP.
- Input from marrow comes to equal output to tissues, though for a time it may exceed output.
- The number of granulocyte precursors in marrow increases markedly. During this phase the half-life of circulating leukocytes is normal.

In the **phase of recovery**:

- Release of cells from marrow decreases sharply.
- Half-life of circulating granulocytes is prolonged because no new unlabeled cells are being admixed with labeled cells.
- The "shift to the left" disappears.
- The leukocyte count subsides to normal.

An alternative third phase (to be discussed below) occurs in overwhelming infection. Although the myeloid portion of the marrow has become grossly hyperplastic, reserves are exhausted and neutropenia (i.e, decreased neutrophil count) results. Neutropenia in the course of infection is a poor prognostic sign.

c. CLINICAL FEATURES

Abnormal clinical features associated with leukocytosis include:

- "Shift to the left" in blood leukocytes.
- Toxic granulations and Döhle bodies.
- Fever, due to pyrogenic leukocyte products.
- Elevation of LAP (figure 20.2)

2. *Other mechanisms of leukocytosis*

a. PSEUDONEUTROPHILIA

Kinetic studies show that cells from the MGP may reenter the CGP en masse in response to certain vasodynamic states (e.g., violent exercise, epinephrine). The leukocyte count thus may be quickly doubled, the rise

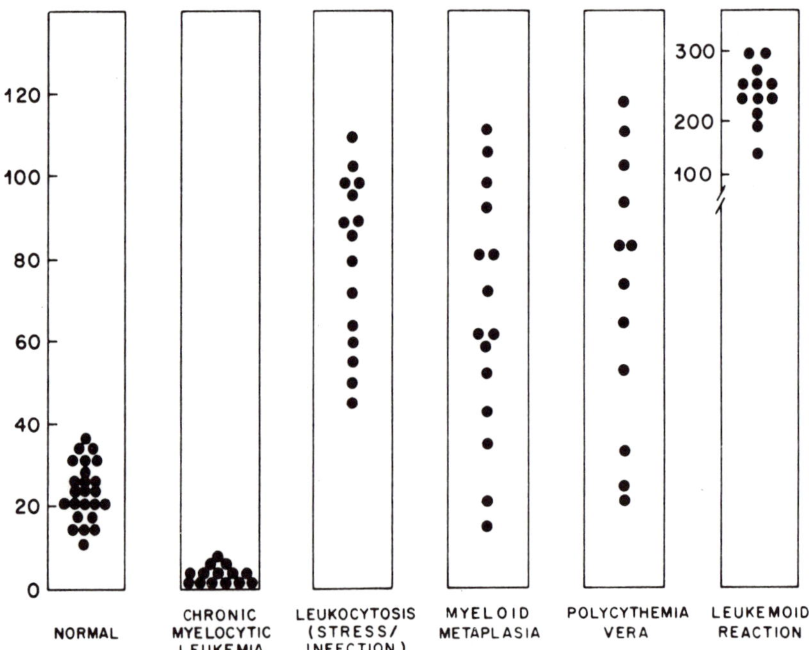

Fig. 20.2
Leukocyte alkaline phosphatase in health and disease. Ordinate: P (in mg) liberated (from β-glycerophosphate) per 10^{10} leukocytes per hour.

being independent of increased granulopoiesis as indicated by the fact that it is not prevented by cytotoxic drugs or radiation. The leukocyte count rises by this mechanism in stressful situations (e.g., paroxysmal tachycardia, intense emotion, anesthesia). The pattern is termed **pseudoneutrophilia** because input, output, and TBGP remain normal.

b. DECREASED-EGRESS NEUTROPHILIA

Administration of pharmacologic doses of corticosteroids produces neutrophilia by the following two mechanisms: (1) increasing the release of granulocytes from marrow; and (2) decreasing the egress of granulocytes from blood. Skin-window studies show that in inflammation, corticosteroids decrease the number of leukocytes in inflammatory exudates relative to controls. This partially accounts for the rise in leukocyte count that accompanies stress and steroid administration. These findings also explain in part the seriousness of bacterial infections that accompany steroid therapy in certain patients. Also, it suggests that steroids may be inappropriate therapy in neutropenia simply because they sometimes raise the leukocyte count.

c. ASPLENIA

Moderate neutrophilia invariably follows loss of the spleen due to surgery or disease. It is presumably the result of persistent circulation of neutrophils that normally are transiently detained in the spleen rather than increased granulopoiesis.

B. "In-between" conditions

1. Leukemoid reaction

A leukemoid reaction is an excessive (but reactive) outpouring of leukocytes with the appearance of immature forms (blasts, myelocytes, metamyelocytes)—hence the term **leukemoid** and the need to distinguish the leukemoid reaction from leukemia. It occurs in response to infectious, toxic, inflammatory, or neoplastic disorders. It may be acute or chronic, or rarely lymphocytic. There is evidence that high levels of GM-CSF and other myeloid growth factors are produced by the cells accumulating in these disorders.

Major associated diseases are severe or chronic infection, especially in children; severe hemolysis; and various solid tumors (especially of breast, kidney and lung, and metastatic cancer). The total leukocyte count is typically 50,000–100,000/mm^3. The cells display prominent toxic granulations, and the LAP is extremely high. The high LAP and lack of the so-called Philadelphia (Ph^1) chromosomes are usually adequate to distinguish leukemoid reactions from chronic myelocytic leukemia (CML), as discussed in lecture 22.

Hyperleukocytosis is a variant in which an excessive leukocytosis occurs that is unaccompanied by immature forms. Its causes are similar to those of leukemoid reaction.

2. *Leukoerythroblastic reaction*

The term **leukoerythroblastic reaction** denotes a blood picture that resembles leukemoid reaction as regards the leukocytes but which includes the presence of substantial numbers of nucleated red cells and abnormalities in the size and shape of mature red cells. It should be noted that one may observe a few nucleated red cells (perhaps 2–3/100 white cells) in any patient with brisk reticulocytosis due, for example, to hemolysis. But patients with leukoerythroblastic reaction may have many nucleated red cells (i.e., 40–80/100 white cells) and relatively few reticulocytes.

The picture most commonly signifies **myelophthisis**, that is, invasion of bone marrow by foreign elements (see lecture 4). Common invaders are metastatic cancer (especially breast cancer), fibrosis, angiitis, granulomas of miliary tuberculosis, and leukemic cells. A leukoerythroblastic-like reaction (in which the blood contains many nucleated red cells and immature leukocytes, albeit with reticulocytosis) may occur in severe hemorrhagic or hemolytic anemias, especially in children. This form of leukoerythroblastosis occurs in the severe hemolytic anemia of the newborn, erythrobastosis fetalis (see lecture 17).

3. *Leukostasis*

Elevation of the white count, one of the most common abnormalities of clinical medicine, always requires further investigation. However, in addition to serving as a sign of illness, it is sometimes itself a cause of serious morbidity. This occurs when white counts are so extremely elevated, they impair blood flow in small vessels, especially in the brain. This disorder, **leukostasis**, can cause death and the appearance of neurological signs in a leukemic patient always justifies urgent therapy, including **leukapheresis** (removal of white cells by blood centrifugation followed by reinfusion of leukocyte-depleted blood).

Interestingly, leukostasis is far more common in myeloid leukemias than in lymphoid leukemias. This is attributable to the relatively larger size of myeloblasts (figure 20.3).

C. Neutropenia

1. *Definitions*

Leukopenia means depression of the leukocyte count. **Neutropenia** (and its near synonym *granulocytopenia*) denotes a total neutrophil (or granulocyte) count of $< 1{,}500/mm^3$. The absolute neutrophil count is the product of total leukocyte count and percentage of neutrophils in the differential count. **Agranulocytosis** means severe granulocytopenia ($< 500/mm^3$). As noted below, this term has acquired a special connotation.

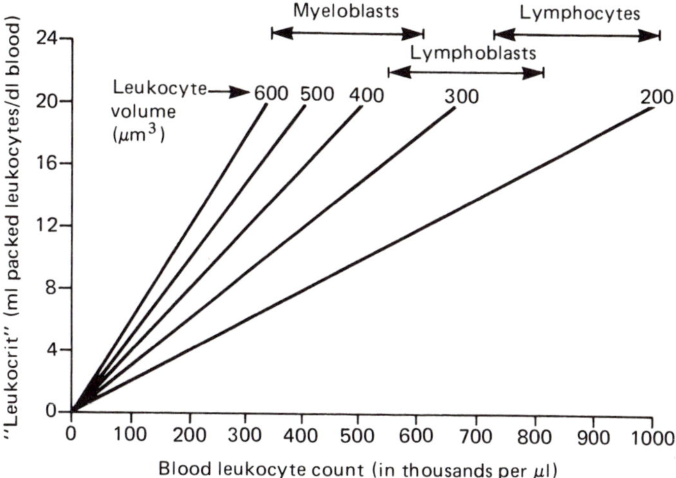

Fig. 20.3
Data showing differences in the volume of various leukocyte types. (Courtesy of Dr. Samuel E. Archer.)

2. *Major causes*

Like anemia and thrombocytopenia, neutropenia has many causes. Though it is useful to draw analogies between the causal mechanisms of the three situations, techniques currently available for the routine study of patients with neutropenia are often imprecise or unavailable. For example, one cause of neutropenia is analogous to a cause of immunohemolytic anemia, but procedures for the detection of leukocyte antibodies are not as reliable as the Coombs test. Similarly, we lack a leukokinetic parameter that is comparable in reliability to the reticulocyte count in the area of erythrokinetics. For these reasons, understanding of neutropenia is inferior to that of anemia, and it is often more difficult to elucidate the basis of a given case of neutropenia.

In general, the classifications of anemia and thrombocytopenia are applicable to neutropenia. Neutropenia can arise from decreased production of neutrophils by marrow or accelerated removal from blood. Accelerated removal, in turn, can be due to nonimmune or immune mechanisms. Often neutropenia, anemia, and thrombocytopenia occur together (pancytopenia). The following are the major categories of neutropenia.

a. REDUCED GRANULOPOIESIS

In this broad category, neutropenia is due to diminished neutrophil production in marrow. Granulopoiesis is inadequate to maintain a normal level of neutrophils, which are leaving the blood at a normal rate (figure 20.4). Major underlying causes are:

- The several varieties of aplastic anemia (see lecture 4)

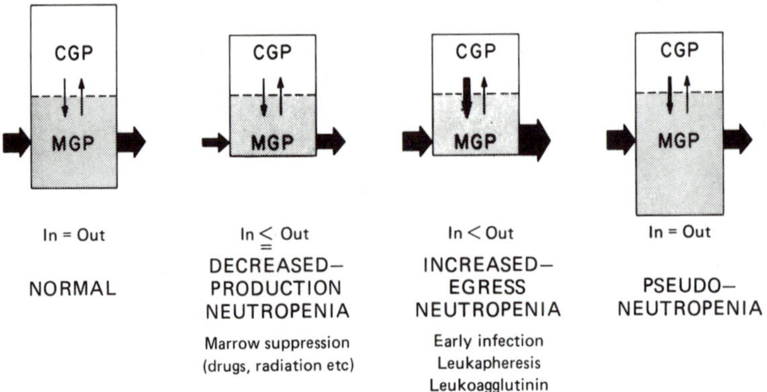

Fig. 20.4
Mechanisms of neutropenia.

- Myelophthisis from invading cancer cells, fibrosis, granulomas, and so forth (see lecture 4)
- Cytotoxic chemotherapeutic agents that by intention or nonintention depress production of granulopoietic cells
- Ineffective granulopoiesis, such as occurs in megaloblastic anemia (see lecture 5)

In all of these instances, marrow failure results in decreased inflow of neutrophils. Eventually, there is decreased outflow. Blood neutrophils may show moderate immaturity. Marrow storage and marginal granulocyte pools are decreased, and the mobilization of neutrophils at inflammatory sites is impaired. Neutrophil survival is normal.

The main therapeutic approach to decreased-production neutropenia is to eliminate underlying or causal factors where possible. Lithium carbonate, which stimulates granulopoiesis (and causes neutrophilia in normal subjects), is sometimes used in the treatment of neutropenia and is currently under evaluation.

b. REDUCED GRANULOCYTE SURVIVAL

In the second major category of neutropenias, egress of neutrophils to tissues exceeds inflow from marrow (figure 20.4) or, alternatively, abnormal neutrophil destruction is taking place. Major causes are:

- Early infection before inflow from marrow increases
- Leukapheresis
- Drug-induced leukoagglutinin (agranulocytosis)
- Complement-induced granulocyte aggregation, a recently recognized complication of hemodialysis
- Hypersplenism as in leukemia, lymphoma, Felty's syndrome, and LE, though in these disorders multiple factors may be depressing the leukocyte count (see lecture 3)

In these situations, increased utilization or destruction of neutrophils in blood results in increased total and effective granulopoiesis in marrow. Some immature neutrophils may enter the blood, with promyelocytes and blasts occasionally being observed. Blood neutrophil survival is short. Half-life after [^{32}P]DFP labeling may be as short as 20–100 min. Thus, this test may help distinguish reduced granulocyte production from reduced survival. The bone marrow contains an increased number of myeloid cells with increased immaturity. Serum leukotoxic substances and leukoagglutinins may be demonstrable. Serum lysozyme may be elevated. Neutrophilia resulting from a drug-induced antibody will be further discussed below.

c. PSEUDONEUTROPENIA

In pseudoneutropenia, circulating (CGP) cells transfer to the MGP. As a result of increased margination—the opposite of epinephrine-induced demargination—neutrophil count decreases, although the TBGP is normal. Leukokinetics are otherwise normal. Usually, these are temporary shifts due to hypersensitivity, viremia, hemolysis, or hemodynamic abnormalities. They may also be permanent and may account for some of the constitutional or familial forms of benign neutropenia mentioned in the next section.

3. *Other mechanisms of neutropenia*

a. PERIODIC OR CYCLIC NEUTROPENIA

This curious genetic disorder (autosomal dominant with variable expression) usually begins in infancy and persists for decades. Neutropenia lasting a few days develops every 21–30 days. During the neutropenic period (which lasts 3–6 days), fever, stomatitis, vaginitis, proctitis, and skin infections—sometimes severe—may develop, and the total monocyte count often rises. Bone marrow during neutropenia shows myeloid hypoplasia. The cause is unknown, but it is probably related to mild marrow hypoplasia that causes dyssynchrony of the two feedback loops that separately regulate granulocyte production and release (see above). The monocytosis occurring during episodes of neutrophilia may reflect operation of the regulatory system diagrammed in figure 18.6. Many mild cases probably escape detection. Recent efforts to treat these patients with GM-CSF have been moderately encouraging but the myeloid precursors respond abnormally to GM-CSF in vitro.

b. CHRONIC FAMILIAL NEUTROPENIAS

A benign autosomal-dominant neutropenia was described by Glänsslen. An autosomal-recessive type associated with consanguinity was described by Kostmann. In this disorder, neutrophil counts are persistently low, and many patients die in early childhood of sepsis. A servere familial neutropenia of infacy was described by Hitzig.

c. CHRONIC IDIOPATHIC NEUTROPENIA

An apparently acquired disorder occurs in which patients have low neutrophil counts ($< 1{,}000/mm^3$) but few infections. Good exudation ordinarily occurs in skin-window preparations.

d. OTHER SYNDROMES

Many other neutropenic syndromes have been described, among them neutropenia associated with agammaglobulinemia and dysglobulinemia; neutropenia associated with pancreatic insufficiency; alymphocytic neutropenia; chronic neutropenia with constitutional defects; and the "normal" genetically determined neutropenia of people of African ancestry.

4. Drug-induced neutropenia

We take special notice of drug-induced neutropenia because it is increasing in frequency. Drugs can cause neutropenia by at least two major mechanisms that should be distinguished in a given patient.

a. DRUG-INDUCED DEPRESSION OF GRANULOPOIESIS

The first mechanism is drug-induced depression of granulopoiesis, which can be caused by:

- Cytotoxic radiomimetic agents (e.g., nitrogen mustard) that do irreparable direct damage to marrow.
- Chemotherapeutic antimetabolites (e.g., cytosine arabinoside) that reversibly block cell division.
- Phenothiazine and like drugs that impair DNA synthesis in some patients.
- Agents like chloramphenicol that idiosyncratically produce marrow aplasia (see lecture 4). The phenothiazines and an ever-growing list of comparable agents (antithyroid drugs, anticonvulsants, antibiotics, etc.) are especially frequent offenders.

When recovery begins, many promyelocytes and early myelocytes may appear, and a brisk monocytosis may herald the return of granulocytes to the blood.

b. DRUG-INDUCED LEUKOAGGLUTININ

In 1922, Schultz drew attention to a syndrome of unknown etiology occurring mainly in middle-aged women in which sepsis and death followed severe sore throat, fever, prostration, and agranulocytosis. The syndrome was shown in 1934 to be associated with ingestion of aminopyrine (Pyramidon®), a widely used aromatic analgesic. About 1% of users developed neutropenia, usually within 7–10 days of the first dose. Sometimes it appeared immediately. When usage of aminopyrine decreased, the disorder became less common.

Aminopyrine-induced neutropenia has been called agranulocytosis, agranulocytic angina, pernicious leukopenia, and Schultz's syndrome. It is usual today to reserve the term **agranulocytosis** for this symptom complex. In this usage, agranulocytosis becomes a specific variety of "neutropenia."

The mechanism of aminopyrine-induced agranulocytosis parallels those of quinidine-induced thrombocytopenia (see lecture 28) and certain drug-induced Coombs-positive hemolytic anemias (see lecture 13). A complex between drug and leukocyte protein becomes antigenic. Antibody is elicited that is active only against the complex. In the absence of drug, the antibody remains in the plasma in inactive form. Subsequent administration of drugs to a sensitized individual activates antibody on the neutrophil surface. The result is massive leukoagglutination with pulmonary sequestration and removal of granulocytes from the circulation. Compensatory myeloid hyperplasia then occurs in the marrow. Continued drug administration leads to marrow exhaustion. Peripheral leukocyte destruction accounts for the high fever. In contrast to the situation in marrow-failure neutropenia, bone marrow shows normal erythropoiesis, normal numbers of megakaryocytes, and myeloid hyperplasia, although the more mature forms (myelocytes, metamyelocytes, bands, and polys) are missing. This pattern has been erroneously termed **maturation arrest**. Actually it is a depletion phenomenon resulting from increased peripheral destruction of granulocytes. In only a few cases has a drug-dependent antibody been clearly demonstrated. However, the recently developed staphylococcal slide test for detection of antineutrophil antibodies promises to clarify these cases in the future. This test can demonstrate opsonizing antibodies in the majority of drug-induced immunoneutropenias.

Therapy of aminopyrine neutropenia is unsatisfactory. Some cases are fatal, some become chronic, and some enter remission. The major therapeutic maneuver is withdrawal of the offending drug. Leukocyte transfusion may be helpful in certain cases.

5. *Consequences of neutropenia*

The major critical consequence of neutropenia is infection. The most dramatic illustration of this tendency is seen in acute drug-induced agranulocytosis. At first, there are few symptoms, but within a day or two patients develop sore throat, chills, fever, necrosis of oral mucous membranes, and bacteremia. When severe neutropenia results from leukocyte destruction, fever is due to pyrogen. Serum muramidase is commonly elevated. However, susceptibility to infection occurs with neutropenia of any cause. Vulnerability to infection becomes serious when the neutrophil count falls below $1000/mm^3$ and very serious when below $500/mm^3$. An exception, as noted above, is chronic, idiopathic, benign neutropenia in which neutropenia rarely leads to infection.

D. Myeloproliferative disorders

1. Introduction

We turn now to a group of disorders in which proliferation of blood cells is not a reaction to some external insult, so far as we know. Rather, there is purposeless proliferation by one, several, or all of the marrow cell lines—granulocytes, erythrocytes, and platelets. If it be allowed that fibroblasts (or fibrocytes) are normal marrow elements, these also may proliferate to produce myelofibrosis.

The term **myeloproliferative disorder** was introduced by Dameshek to designate a group of disorders that had previously been considered separate entities. Although based on meager evidence, the concept gave recognition to certain provocative facts.

- A marrow cell line is almost never singly affected. For example, abnormal erythrocyte proliferation is the most prominent feature of polycythemia vera. However, leukocytes and platelets almost invariably proliferate in this disease.
- Many of these disorders tend to evolve into one another. Polycythemia vera may eventually "turn into" myelofibrosis, myeloid metaplasia, or even leukemia.
- There are intimate phylogenetic and embryologic relations among the hematopoietic tissues.

Since hematopoietic tissues derive from pluripotential cells of mesenchymal origin, it is reasonable to postulate a proliferative or neoplastic abnormality that, once under way, can proceed in one direction or another depending on factors now unknown. Recent work confirms that the myeloproliferative disorders are clonal diseases that are frequently associated with **myelofibrosis**, a reactive process that is *not* clonal.

Although the concept of myeloproliferative disorders is clinically and heuristically useful, one should remember that until the underlying causes of these disorders are known, the concept is little more than an intellectual convenience.

2. Clinical features

a. GENERAL PATTERN

All of the myeloproliferative disorders can display hyperplasia, dysplasia, or metaplasia of the bone marrow, blood cells, spleen, and other organs. Although the well-known specific disorders, to be discussed briefly below, have characteristic clinical pictures, they all display in some measure

Table 20.2
Cell Lines Involved in Specific Myeloproliferative Disorders

Disorder	Red cells	Granulocytes	Megakaryocytes, platelets	Fibroblasts, reticulum cells
Polycythemia vera	++++	+/+++	++/+++	++
Chronic myelocytic leukemia	±	+++	+/++	−
Myeloid metaplasia	+	++/+++	++	++
Thrombocythemia	−	−	++++	−
Erythremic myelosis	++++	−	+	−

- Signs of hypermetabolism (e.g., tissue wasting, intermittent fevers)
- Hyperuricemia
- Little or no tendency for spontaneous remission

b. SPECIFIC DISORDERS

Table 20.2 lists the several disorders that comprise the myeloproliferative syndrome group and indicates the hematopoietic cell lines primarily affected in each. Thus, it is seen that the major manifestation of polycythemia vera (to be discussed in lecture 26) is hyperplasia of red cell elements. However, the other cell lines are also involved. Prominent features of myeloid metaplasia and myelofibrosis (to be discussed below) are hyperplasia of fibroblasts and metaplasia of spleen, liver, and other tissues. In chronic myelocytic leukemia (one of several varieties of leukemia to be discussed in lecture 22), the major manifestation is hyperplasia of granulocytic element. Hyperplasia of platelet elements predominates in thrombocythemia (to be discussed in lecture 28). In erythremic myelosis (Di Guglielmo's syndrome), the major manifestation is hyperplasia and dysplasia of red cell elements. When leukocyte elements become involved later, the disorder is called **erythroleukemia**.

3. *Myeloid metaplasia*

a. INTRODUCTION

It is appropriate to consider myeloid metaplasia in this lecture because granulocyte proliferation dominates the picture. (The other myeloproliferative disorders will be discussed in later lectures.) The disease complex consists of a leukoerythroblastic blood picture (i.e., immature white cells, marked changes in red cell size and shape, and presence of nucleated red cells), myeloid metaplasia (and thus extramedullay hematopoiesis) in spleen and liver, which may become very large, and variable degrees of myelofibrosis.

b. SIGNIFICANCE OF MYELOID METAPLASIA

Myeloid metaplasia is a histologic pattern in which an extramedullary tissue comes to resemble bone marrow. Most commonly, the tissue is one that was active in hematopoiesis in embryonic life, that is, spleen, liver, and lymph nodes (see lecture 3). When tissues undergo myeloid metaplasia, they resume hematopoiesis. This occurs in at least two circumstances. One, the most common, is an increased demand for blood cells that cannot be met by marrow hyperplasia alone. This often occurs in young children following severe and continuing hemorrhage or hemolysis. It also occurs in certain chronic severe anemias in the adult (e.g., thalassemia). Here myeloid metaplasia is reactive. In the second circumstance, a myeloproliferative disorder is present. This kind of myeloid metaplasia is nonreactive. Its cause is unknown, and for that reason it is sometimes called idiopathic or agnogenic myeloid metaplasia. It often accompanies myelofibrosis. Some workers have held that myeloid metaplasia is a compensatory and reactive consequence of the marrow failure of myelofibrosis. The evidence, however, is against this view. Marrow is often hypercellular (and not fibrotic) in the presence of severe myeloid metaplasia of the spleen and liver. Thus the latter should be viewed as part of a generalized myeloproliferative process. It is more likely that the myelofibrosis (a nonclonal process) is a reaction to the primary myeloid metaplasia.

c. CLINICAL FEATURES

Myeloid metaplasia is a disorder of insidious onset in older patients. Its major features are

- Characteristic red cell changes in blood smears with many "teardrop" forms.
- Splenomegaly that is often massive.
- Anemia.
- Usually elevated platelet and leukocyte counts.
- Immature leukocytes.
- Hyperuricemia (with gout and renal stones).
- Hypermetabolism.
- High incidence of aneuploidy in involved tissues.
- Elevated leukocyte alkaline phosphatase (see figure 20.2). The LAP is diagnostically useful because the morphologically similar immature leukocytes of chronic myelocytic leukemia are low in LAP.

When there is doubt whether splenomegaly is due to myeloid metaplasia, a scan with ^{59}Fe is useful in demonstrating that erythropoiesis is taking place in the spleen. Needle biopsy of spleen or liver may reveal myeloid metaplasia.

d. PATHOLOGY OF MYELOFIBROSIS

Two grades of fibrosis are recognized in bone marrow. One is **reticulin** fibrosis. At least in its early stages, it is simply an exaggeration of a pattern present in normal marrow. It occurs in many disorders (benign and malignant) and is of little diagnostic value, though it has been recommended as a prognostic marker in acute leukemia. The other is **collagen** fibrosis, which is also seen in many (though fewer) conditions. They include

- Carcinomatous and lymphomatous marrow infiltration
- Bone diseases (e.g., osteopetrosis, Paget's disease)
- Various immunologic connective tissue disorders
- Myeloproliferative disorders

The myelofibrosis of myeloproliferative disease usually accompanies myeloid metaplasia. Diagnosis requires a marrow biopsy. The process may be patchy or widespread. When widespread, marrow may be unobtainable by aspiration.

e. THERAPY

Therapy is palliative and generally unsatisfactory. Nonetheless, the course is relatively prolonged compared to that of the leukemias. Radiation and alkylating agents may diminish the enlarged spleen, leukocytosis, and hypermetabolism. Splenectomy may be indicated if the spleen is massive or if it is causing intolerable red cell sequestration. The anemia is occasionally benefited by androgen therapy.

II. DISEASES OF LYMPHOCYTES

A. Lymphocytopenia

Lymphocytopenia, though uncommon, is most often associated with corticosteroid therapy. AIDS, Hodgkin's disease, and various chronic diseases (e.g., tuberculosis, LE, sarcoidosis). Little is known of the factors that control the circulating lymphocyte count.

B. Lymphocytosis

Absolute **lymphocytosis** occurs in the various lymphoproliferative malignant disorders and in a number of benign disorders, including pertussis and various virus infections including the severe mononucleosis syndromes and acute infectious lymphocytosis.

1. Infectious mononucleosis

Infectious mononucleosis (IM) is often but not always, a self-limited benign illness that can be caused by a number of viruses, including Epstein-

Barr virus (EBV), cytomegalovirus (CMV), HIV, herpes simplex virus, and several others.

a. EPSTEIN-BARR VIRUS (EBV)

The discovery that EBV is the cause of classic IM occasioned surprise because the same agent is responsible for African (not American) Burkitt's lymphoma (see lecture 23). EBV is ubiquitous in the population. By immortalizing B-lymphocytes, EBV infection allows the virus to persist in latent form. Most people encounter the virus in early childhood and carry it without symptoms. Of individuals not exposed to EBV until adolescence, half develop IM.

For EBV to induce oncogenic transformation, a second cellular event is required. In Burkitt's lymphoma, this involves a translocation of one of the *c-myc* alleles from chromosome 8 to chromosome 14. In a clonal population of infected lymphocytes, only 1 in 10^{3-6} cells produce virus. The latently infected cell is not oncogenically transformed, but does not produce several viral transcripts. During latent infection, the virus produces six viral nuclear proteins and two viral membrane proteins. In the viral lytic cycle, it is estimated that one hundred or more viral antigens are expressed. Interestingly, EBV genomes have been detected in the Reed-Sternberg cells of Hodgkin's disease (see lectures 23, 24) and in the skin lesions of immunocompromised patients.

b. CLINICAL PICTURE

Typically, IM displays the following features:

- In EBV mononucleosis, a rising titer of serum **heterophile antibody**, which is removed by absorption with beef cells. This does not occur in CMV mononucleosis.
- Other immunologic abnormalities, such as cold agglutinins, false-positive serology for syphilis, cryoglobulins, antinuclear factor, and so forth. Presumably these reflect lymphocyte activation by viruses.
- Characteristic atypical lymphocytes in stained blood smears that have been variously known as **virocytes** and **Downey cells**. This occurs in *all* mononucleosis syndromes; hence, the name.
- Splenomegaly and often hepatomegaly.
- Lymphadenopathy.
- Pharyngitis.
- A propensity for involving diverse organs—liver, myocardium, testes, and so forth. These involvements account for occasional fatalities.

2. Acute infectious lymphocytosis

This benign self-limited disorder of unknown cause is associated with an increase in circulating small lymphocytes (sometimes to 100,000/mm^3), occurrence in clusters, and diverse symptomatology. Lymphadenopathy and splenomgaly do not occur. A virus similar to Coxsackie A has been suggested as a possible cause.

SELECTED REFERENCES

Reviews

Betts, R. F. Mononucleosis syndromes. In Williams, W. J., Beutler, E., et al., eds. *Hematology*, 4th ed. New York: McGraw-Hill, 1990, pp. 955–962.

Bowden, R. A., and Meyers, J. D. Prophylaxis of cytomegalovirus infection. *Semin. Hematol.* 27 Suppl. 1(1990): 17–21.

Campion, G., Maddison, P. J., et al. The Felty syndrome: a case-matched study of clinical manifestations and outcome, serologic features, and immunogenetic associations. *Medicine (Baltimore)* 69(1990): 69–80.

Cheeseman, S. H. Infectious mononucleosis. *Semin. Hematol.* 25(1988): 261–268.

Cheson, B. D. The myelodysplastic syndromes: current approaches to therapy. *Ann. Intern. Med.* 112(1990): 932–941.

Emanuel, D. Treatment of cytomegalovirus disease. *Semin. Hematol.* 27 Suppl. 1(1990): 22–27.

Koeffler, H. P. Myelodysplastic syndromes. *Semin. Hematol.* 23(1988): 284–295.

Smith, R. E., Chelmowski, M. K., et al. Myelofibrosis: a concise review of clinical and pathologic features and treatment. *Am. J. Hematol.* 29(1988): 174–180.

Spector, S. A. Diagnosis of cytomegalovirus infection. *Semin. Hematol.* 27 Suppl. 1(1990): 11–16.

Original articles

Demory, J. L., Dupriez, B., et al. Cytogenetic studies and their prognostic significance in agnogenic myeloid metaplasia: a report on 47 cases. *Blood* 72(1988): 855–859.

Falk, R. J., Terrell, R. S., et al. Anti-neutrophil cytoplasmic autoantibodies induce neutrophils to degranulate and produce oxygen radicals *in vitro*. *Proc. Natl. Acad. Sci. USA* 87(1990): 4115–4119.

Ganz, T., Metcalf, J. A., et al. Microbicidal/cytotoxic proteins of neutrophils are deficient in two disorders: Chédiak-Higashi syndrome and "specific" granule deficiency. *J. Clin. Invest.* 82(1988): 552–556.

Hartman, K. R., Mallet, M. K., et al. Antibodies to actin in autoimmune neutropenia. *Blood* 75(1990): 736–743.

Kobayashi, M., Yumiba, C., et al. Abnormal responses of myeloid progenitor cells to recombinant human colony-stimulating factors in congenital neutropenia. *Blood* 75(1990): 2143–2149.

Manoharan, A. Myelofibrosis: prognostic factors and treatment. *Br. J. Haematol.* 69(1988): 295–298.

Medsger, T. A., Jr. Tryptophan-induced eosinophilia-myalgia syndrome. *N. Engl. J. Med.* 322(1990): 926–928.

Migliaccio, A. R., Migliaccio, G., et al. Hematopoietic progenitors in cyclic neutropenia: Effect of granulocyte colony-stimulating factor in vivo. *Blood* 75(1990): 1951–1959.

Paul, C. C., Keller, J. R., et al. Epstein-Barr virus transformed B lymphocytes produce interleukin-5. *Blood* 75(1990): 1400–1403.

Ríos, A., Cañizo, M. C., et al. Bone marrow biopsy in myelodysplastic syndromes: morphological characteristics and contribution to the study of prognostic factors. *Br. J. Haematol.* 75(1990): 26–33.

Salama, A., Schütz, B., et al. Immune-mediated agranulocytosis related to drugs and their metabolites: mode of sensitization and heterogeneity of antibodies. *Br. J. Haematol.* 72(1989): 127–132.

Van der Weide, M., Sizoo, W., et al. Myelodysplastic syndromes: analysis of morphological features related to the FAB-classification. *Eur. J. Haematol.* 41 (1988): 58–61.

Visani, G., Finelli, C., et al. Myelofibrosis with myeloid metaplasia: clinical and haematological parameters predicting survival in a series of 133 patients. *Br. J. Haematol.* 75(1990): 4–9.

Weiss, L. M., Movahed. L. A., et al. Detection of Epstein-Barr viral genomes in Reed-Sternberg cells of Hodgkin's disease. *N. Engl. J. Med.* 320(1989): 502–506.

Wright, D. G., LaRussa, V. F., et al. Abnormal responses of myeloid progenitor cells to granulocyte-macrophage colony-stimulating factor in human cyclic neutropenia. *J. Clin. Invest.* 83(1989): 1414–1418.

LECTURE 21

Malignant Disease: Some General Principles

Stuart E. Lind

EDITOR'S COMMENT

An event of importance to hematology has been the increasing coalescence of hematology and medical oncology. As a result, many teaching hospitals now have a hyphenated Division of Hematology-Oncology. It was a natural evolution, since many of the patients seen by hematologists have malignant disorders—leukemias and lymphomas. Similarly, oncologists using cytotoxic drugs find bone marrow toxicity is the factor limiting such therapy. Thus it is constantly necessary to monitor blood counts in regulating drug dosages. It is also a fact that many nonhematologic malignancies—breast cancer, prostatic cancer, and others—metastasize to bone marrow and there induce a complex of hematologic changes that need intelligent analysis. Are they due to the cancer or its therapy? For the first time, we include an introductory lecture summarizing certain general aspects of malignant disease, both hematologic and solid tumors, as background for the lectures that follow on hemato-oncology.

I. INTRODUCTION

All physicians, especially hematologists, confront malignant disease, and the care of cancer patients is more challenging than that of many other types of patients. Hence, it seems worthwhile to articulate some general principles underlying the current approaches to cancer patients. Most of the points to be made apply both to the hematologic malignancies (discussed in lectures 22–26) and to solid tumors, once the province of oncology and now increasingly of hematology-oncology. Their special importance to the hematologist also stems from the fact that cancer and its therapy can both have serious hematologic sequelae. Indeed, the tolerance of bone marrow is usually a major factor limiting cancer therapy.

II. BASIC CONCEPTS

A. What is cancer?

Cancer, or malignant disease, is a state of unregulated cell growth, often accompanied by abnormal, or atypical, cellular differentiation. The many conditions subsumed by the term cancer are harmful to patients in three major ways:

- They compromise the function of some or many organs or organ systems.
- They alter the patient's metabolic and nutritional status to such an extent that overwhelming infection or some other abnormality occurs.
- They prompt medical intervention, which further alters the structure and/or function of tissues and organs, which may increase the likelihood of death.

B. Natural history

Knowledge of the natural history of a particular type of cancer permits useful predictions of the probable clinical course—and helps the physician to decide when new symptoms reflect a disease complication or a different disease process. It also suggests which problems can be attributed to disease and which to therapy. Although there are many types of cancer, the natural history of many are similar.

C. Metastases

Malignant tumors display uncontrolled growth at their sites of origin and they metastasize to other organs where they establish new foci that continue to grow. An important part of a tumor's natural history concerns its tendency to **metastasize** and the often characteristic pattern of metastases. The process of metastases includes several phases:

- First, cells detach from their neighbors. This may be due to **surface adhesion molecules** (e.g., thrombospondeis that are qualitatively or quantitatively abnormal, or the release of agents such as proteases that promote cellular disaggregation.
- Metastasizing cells then enter the bloodstream. Tumors rarely invade arteries or arterioles, but commonly enter veins, venules, and capillaries. This may be due to such mechanical factors as vessel diameter, the presence of smooth muscle cell layers, or to differences in the molecular structure of vessel walls. Some tumor cells secrete proteases that attack components of the vascular basement membrane such as collagen, laminin, and fibronectin.
- Blood-borne tumor cells eventually lodge in small blood vessels, or attach to endothelium or exposed subendothelium. Some are thrombogenic, activating platelets or the coagulation cascade. Surface interactions with platelets or fibrin strands may play a role in the metastatic process.
- Tumor cells then leave the blood vessel, probably by the same mechanisms that allowed them to enter it. In the extravascular space, the cells must survive inflammatory and/or immune responses of the host.
- **Angiogenesis** is necessary for a tumor metastasis to grow beyond a certain size. Compounds capable of inhibiting this process, now under study, may soon be tested as antimetastasis agents.

D. Tumor heterogeneity

Although a certain pattern of metastases is generally associated with a given cancer, autopsy evidence shows that many patients with histologically identical tumors may depart from the pattern and either develop no metastases in a commonly involved organ or have metastases in unusual sites. Thus, there are biologic differences, or **intertumor heterogeneity**, among tumors of a given histology.

In addition, **intratumor heterogeneity** exists. For example, immunohistochemical staining of breast carcinomas indicates that some cells within a tumor mass may express large amounts of estrogen receptor while others contain little, though all are morphologically similar.

Animal studies suggest that many tumors are composed of cells displaying **behavioral heterogeneity** as well. For example, if a standard number of tumor cells derived from the mouse B16 melanoma line is injected into a mouse, metastases will develop in many organs, including the lungs. If tumor nodules in the lungs are dissected free, dissociated into single cell suspensions, and injected into another mouse, metastases will again be found in many organs, but a higher percentage will be found in the lungs. If this process is carried out repeatedly, the pattern of metastases will change. Eventually, the majority of metastases will be in the lungs. Such data suggest that tumor cell composition may change with time.

III. PRINCIPLES OF THERAPY

Therapy for cancer is generally considered **curative** or **palliative**. Although cure is always hoped for, the physician must temper therapeutic aggressiveness with a realistic appraisal of the probability that cure is possible. The clinical staging of a patient is an essential element in that calculation.

A. Importance of staging

All patients with cancer are obviously not the same, nor are all patients with a given type of cancer. In an attempt to delineate factors underlying differing survival patterns, physicians have developed various staging systems. In the past, such systems were established for each type of cancer. More recently, attempts have been made to establish a common terminology among the systems by focusing on three features common to many tumors:

- Size of the primary tumor
- Absence of presence of lymph node metastases
- Absence or presence of more distant metastases

These factors, along with special rules for each tumor, place most patients in one of four stages (designated by Roman numerals):

- In **stage I**, the primary tumor is usually small and localized (i.e., it has not metastasized).
- In **stage II**, tumor involves local or regional lymph nodes.
- In **stages III** and **IV**, tumor has spread into surrounding structures or to distant sites.

Clinical staging is based on physical and laboratory examinations. **Pathologic staging** is based on examination of tissues removed at surgery. Pathologic staging is considered the more definitive staging method.

B. Goals of therapy

1. Cure

In the past, attempts at curative therapy usually involved surgical removal of a tumor, sometimes with the regional lymph nodes. Because surgery often required removal of varying amounts of normal tissue with resulting deformity or loss of function, attempts were made to replace surgical extirpation of certain cancers with radiation therapy or chemotherapy. For some cancers, surgery remains the mainstay of treatment. For others, notably the hematologic malignancies, radiation therapy and chemotherapy are the dominant treatment modalities, though surgery still has some role.

2. Palliation

When staging indicates that a cancer is too advanced to be cured, the physician generally selects from the three major treatment modalities (surgery, chemotherapy, radiation therapy) in a manner designed to:

- Minimize discomfort
- Prolong life
- Alleviate the consequences of obstruction of a hollow viscus (e.g., radiation therapy aimed at an occluded bronchus or surgery to bypass a compromised common bile duct)

C. Chemotherapy

It is beyond the scope of these lectures to present detailed chemotherapeutic protocols (dosage schedules, and so forth). Such information is available in textboods and journals of hematology and oncology.

1. Cancer drug development

New drugs are constantly being developed and made available for clinical use. Under the aegis of the National Cancer Institute and other agencies, this highly organized process involving many stages or phases begins with drug synthesis or isolation from natural products, screening of agents in tissue culture systems, and animal testing. Promising agents then move to phased clinical trials.

- **Phase I** clarifies pharmacokinetics and determines maximum tolerable doses in various patient groups.
- **Phase II** assesses drug efficacy in common malignancies and observes toxicity. To qualify as a response, a tumor must either disappear completely for at least 1 month (a complete response, or **CR**) or shrink by 50% or more for at least 1 month (a partial response, or **PR**).
- **Phase III** compares efficacy and toxicity of promising agents with recognized agents.

2. *Some general principles*

The following brief statements of basic principles should provide background for later lectures.

- Cancer therapeutic agents are drugs intended to destroy cancer cells. This distinguishes them from the many drugs that suppress symptoms but have no effect on tumor cells.
- The goal of chemotherapy is to eliminate or destroy cancer cells—ideally, all of them, but realistically, only a few log units at a time. The clonal origin of many cancers implies that they arise from a single cell as the result of some agent or event: mutation, oncogenic virus, or chemical carcinogenesis. Hence, cure may require the elimination of every cell—a daunting challenge. Many believe that if chemotherapeutic agents could reduce the number of tumor cells significantly (if not totally), other factors such as host immune responses might eliminate the remainder.
- There are certain tactical differences between the chemotherapy of solid tumors and that of disseminated malignancies such as leukemia, lymphoma, and multiple myeloma. In a sense, the chemotherapy of solid tumors focuses largely on the treatment of metastases.
- In many ways, cancer chemotherapy parallels the chemotherapy of infectious diseases. Agents are needed that are preferentially taken up by target cells and that damage them without seriously damaging host cells. The most useful agents in cancer chemotherapy have high target cell specificity and display satisfactory ratios of target cell toxicity to host cell toxicity. The effectiveness of each drug depends to a large extent on how it is used (i.e., dose, administration schedules based on pharmacokinetics, and so on).
- Drugs used in the treatment of cancer are of many chemical types (e.g., alkylating agents, antimetabolites); they are either of natural origin (e.g., vincristine, *L*-asparaginase) or products of organic synthesis (e.g., methotrexate, fluorouracil); and they attack various phases of cellular metabolism (e.g., DNA synthesis, mitosis).
- Many drugs are more effective when used in various combinations. This has led to the acronymic programs described in later lectures (e.g., MOPP, BACOP), in which each letter signifies a drug (see table 23.7). Most of these programs require complex administration schedules that

are constantly evolving. Many are designed in an empirical manner without particular reference to biochemical principles. Drugs that seem to work best in combination include those known to be partially effective when used alone and those of diverse type and mechanism. Often drug combinations are given in a cyclical or pulsed fashion with scheduled intervals that permit bone marrow or gastrointestinal recovery (see below).

- Administration of high-dose chemotherapy, far in excess of marrow tolerance, has been made possible in some cases by autologous bone marrow transplantation (ABMT). In this procedure, patient marrow is removed and stored before chemotherapy and reinfused afterward. Many problems remain to be solved, but successes have been achieved in both hematologic malignancies and solid tumors. The use of hematopoietic growth factors such as GM-CSF and M-CSF (see lecture 1) is now being evaluated. Perhaps their use will permit earlier recovery from high-dose chemotherapy.

3. Drug resistance

Acquired resistance of cancer cells to drugs is the major reason for the failure of chemotherapy. The following points are important.

- Drug resistance develops by a number of mechanisms, including: (1) loss of the ability of the cancer cell to take up the drug or to activate it; (2) acquisition of an ability to inactivate it; (3) increases in the concentration of a target enzyme through gene amplification; (4) increased use by a target cell of an alternative metabolic pathway; and (5) repair of drug-induced lesions.
- A perplexing problem has been the tendency of tumor cells, in vivo and in vitro, to develop simultaneous resistance to multiple unrelated drugs of natural origin. Recent work attributes this phenomenon to an ATP-dependent **multidrug transport protein** known as **P-glycoprotein** or **P170**, which is encoded by the **MDRI** gene. The multidrug transporter extrudes a large variety of drugs from cells. Using DNA-mediated and retroviral transfers, investigators have conferred the multidrug resistance phenotype on many drug-sensitive cells. Current work seeks agents (such as verapamil and quinidine) that can potentially inhibit this system and reinstate drug sensitivity.

4. Drug toxicity

Although all chemotherapeutic agents are potentially toxic, it is important to judge that potential realistically. Toxic effects are both **immediate** and **delayed**.

a. IMMEDIATE

Suppression of hematopoiesis is common and dosage schedules are commonly designed to avoid serious neutropenia or thrombocytopenia. Most agents cause neutrophil and platelet counts to fall within 7–14 days. Generally, counts return to normal within 1–2 weeks. Some drugs cause a delayed drop in these counts. These are given less frequently to avoid cumulative bone marrow toxicity. Other rapidly dividing cells (e.g., buccal and gastrointestinal mucosa, hair follicles) are sensitive to these agents, and stomatitis, diarrhea, nausea, and alopecia commonly accompany their use. Hypersensitivity reactions also occur with many drugs.

b. DELAYED

These include various neuropathies. Though not life-threatening, they may seriously compromise quality of life. Chemotherapy also impairs gonadal and sexual function. Several drugs, especially alkylating agents, occasionally lead to development of second malignancies, especially leukemia. Distinguishing late drug toxicities affecting lung and kidney from other diseases is difficult but important.

D. Radiation therapy

Ionizing radiation damages cells by producing free radicals that interact with cell membranes and macromolecules. Failure of radiation therapy to eradicate a tumor is often due not to tumor radioresistance but to the fact that adequate doses cannot be administered without injury to normal tissues. Furthermore, normal tissues vary in their tolerance to radiation.

Tissues tend to "remember" radiation exposure, a fact which limits the treatment of a given anatomic region. If an organ such as the spinal cord has received its maximal tolerated dose (i.e., 4400 cGrey), additional treatment several years later with even a small dose (e.g., 1000 cGrey) will result in the same loss of cell function that would follow 5400 cGrey given in a single course.

IV. HEMATOLOGIC EFFECTS OF CANCER

In addition to the hematologic toxicity of chemotherapy, there are many adverse direct effects of malignant disease on blood, bone marrow, and lymphoid tissues.

A. Lymphoid system

Lymph nodes and the spleen may be enlarged by infiltrating tumor cells. Marked splenomegaly occurs in myeloproliferative disease and some lymphomas and may cause anemia or thrombocytopenia (see lecture 3). Enlarged lymph nodes may compromise lymphatic and/or venous drainage, causing edema in an extremity, body wall, or head and neck (the **superior vena cava syndrome**). Infection can occur if there is a break in the skin.

B. Red cells

As discussed in lecture 4, anemia is common with cancer patients. Major mechanisms of anemia are the following (see table 4.5):

- Most commonly the anemia is hypoproliferative (with low reticulocyte count), often with the characteristics of the anemia of chronic disease (see lecture 7).
- Myelophthisis due to bone marrow metastases are common in some cancers, such or breast, prostate, lung cancer, lymphoid malignancies (see lecture 4). Though metastases may "replace" normal marrow elements, it is more likely they alter the microenvironment or regulation by growth factors. They themselves may secrete suppressive factors. Hence, they may suppress marrow growth in a "chemical" rather than a "mechanical" fashion. Tumor metastases in marrow are often associated with nucleated red cells in the blood, immature white cell precursors, and elevated white count in the blood (the **leukoerythroblastic reaction**).
- Anemia can result from folate deficiency (see lecture 6) or iron deficiency secondary to bleeding (see lecture 7).
- Coombs-positive immunohemolytic anemia occurs occasionally (see lecture 13).
- Microangiopathic hemolytic anemia with schistocytes in the blood (see lecture 14) commonly results from chronic disseminated intravascular coagulation (DIC) accompanying acute nonlymphocytic leukemia and mucin-producing adenocarcinomas (see lecture 29). It occurs in the absence of DIC if the pulmonary microvasculature is partially occluded with tumor cells. If thrombocytopenia is also present, the patient may be thought to have thrombotic thrombocytopenic purpura (TTP) (see lecture 28).

C. White cells

The white count is commonly affected by leukemias and myeloma, but rarely by lymphomas. A leukemoid reaction (see lecture 20) may be the initial clue to the presence of a tumor, but most cancer patients have normal white counts. As noted above, neutropenia commonly follows chemotherapy or radiation therapy.

D. Platelets

The platelet count is commonly elevated in myeloproliferative diseases (see lectures 20, 26). It may also rise in apparent "reaction" to a tumor, or as a result of iron deficiency caused by bleeding from a gastrointestinal neoplasm. The platelet count is usually depressed by hematologic malignancies, but not by other types of cancer unless accompanied by DIC. Splenomegaly (see above) may also lower the platelet count.

SELECTED REFERENCES

Reviews

Antman, K., Eder, J. P., et al. High-dose chemotherapy with bone marrow support for solid tumors. In DeVita, V. T., Jr., Hellman, S., et al., eds. *Important Advances in Oncology 1987*. Philadelphia: J. B. Lippincott, 1987, pp. 221–235.

Beahrs, O. H., et al. *Manual for Staging of Cancer* [*American Cancer Society*], 3rd ed. Philadelphia: J. B. Lippincott, 1988.

Boivin, J.-F. Second cancers and other late side effects of cancer treatment: a review. *Cancer* 65 Suppl. (1990): 770–775.

Boone, C. W., Kelloff, G. J., et al. Identification of candidate cancer chemopreventive agents and their evaluation in animal models and human clinical trials: a review. *Cancer Res.* 50(1990): 2–9.

Carter, S. K., Glatstein, E., et al. *Principles of Cancer Treatment*. New York: McGraw-Hill, 1982.

DeVita, V. T., Jr. Principles of chemotherapy. In DeVita, V. T., Jr., Hellman, S., et al., eds. *Cancer: Principles and Practice of Oncology*. Philadelphia: J. B. Lippincott Co., 1982, pp. 132–155.

Endicott, J. A., and Ling, V. The biochemistry of P-glycoprotein-mediated multidrug resistance. *Annu. Rev. Biochem.* 58(1989): 137–171.

Fischer, D. S., and Knobf, M. T. *Cancer Chemotherapy Handbook*, 3rd ed. Chicago: Year Book Medical Publishers, 1989.

Gottesman, M. M., and Pastan, I. The multidrug transporter, a double-edged sword. *J. Biol. Chem.* 263(1988): 12163–12166.

Hagen, U. Biochemical aspects of radiation biology. *Experientia* 45(1989): 7–12.

Hellman, K., Carter, S. K., et al. *Fundamentals of Cancer Chemotherapy*. New York: McGraw-Hill, 1987.

Juranka, P. F., Zastawny, R. L., et al. P-glycoprotein: multidrug-resistance and a superfamily of membrane-associated transport proteins. *FASEB J.* 3(1989): 2583–2592.

Muggia, F. M. (editor) *Cancer Chemotherapy: Concepts, Clinical Investigations, and Therapeutic Advances*. Boston: Kluwer Academic Publishers, 1989.

Upton, A. C. Principles of cancer biology: etiology and prevention of cancer. In DeVita, V. T., Jr., Hellman, S., et al., eds. *Cancer: Principles and Practice of Oncology*. Philadelphia: J. B. Lippincott Co., 1982, pp. 33–58.

Van der Bliek, A. M., and Borst, P. Multidrug resistance. *Adv. Cancer Res.* 52(1989): 165–204.

Young, R. C. Mechanisms to improve chemotherapy effectiveness. *Cancer* 65 Suppl. (1990): 815–822.

Original articles

Feldman, M., and Eisenbach, L. What makes a tumor cell metastatic. *Sci. Am.* 259(1988): 60–87.

Kodish, E., Lantos, J. D., et al. Ethical considerations in randomized controlled clinical trials. *Cancer* 65 Suppl. (1990): 2400–2404.

Marx, J. L. How cancer cells spread in the body. *Science* 244(1989): 147–148.

McManaway, M. E., Neckers, L. M., et al. Tumour-specific inhibition of lymphoma growth by an antisense oligodeoxynucleotide. *Lancet* 335(1990): 808–811.

LECTURE 22

The Leukemias

David C. Harmon

EDITOR'S COMMENT

The diseases we call leukemias are characterized by neoplastic proliferation of one or more of the blood-forming cellular elements. If left untreated, all forms of leukemia are ultimately fatal, although survival varies from days and weeks to decades. The major advances in recent years have consisted in newer methods of tracking cell lineages employing antibody-defined cell surface markers and deepening understanding of various chromosomal translocations and their interesting relations with oncogenes. Frustratingly, therapy is still based largely on witches' brew drug combinations given with the credulous aim of exterminating all leukemic cells. Remarkably, it works in some cases. On the horizon, bone marrow transplantation looms as the harbinger of the future.

I. INTRODUCTION

A. Definition

The leukemias are neoplasms of the hematopoietic system that are variously related to the myeloproliferative disorders and lymphomas. In leukemia ("white blood") uncontrolled proliferation of a malignant clone of one cell line eventually replaces marrow, at the expense of other cell lines, with resulting cytopenias. Immature lymphocytes and myeloid cells predominate in **acute lymphocytic** and **acute myelocytic leukemias**, respectively. In the **chronic leukemias** more mature lymphoid or myeloid cell accumulate. Tissue invasion by abnormal cells eventually causes organ dysfunction and death.

B. Incidence

1. Frequency

Leukemia accounts for 4% of all cancers in the United States with 10 new cases, 5 acute and 5 chronic, arising per 100,000 people each year. Among children acute leukemia comprises nearly half of all malignancies.

2. Age of onset

Despite the relative rarity of pediatric cancer, half of the acute leukemias arise during childhood. **Acute lymphocytic leukemia** (ALL) is most commonly a disease of children, accounting for 80% of all childhood leukemias. The incidence of **acute myelocytic leukemia** (AML), which accounts for 20% of childhood leukemia, increases with age and is the most common adult leukemia. **Chronic lymphocytic leukemia** (CLL) is almost never seen in children and uncommonly before age 40 but then steadily increases in incidence with age. **Chronic myelocytic leukemia** (CML) has a peak incidence in middle age but may occur at any age.

II. ETIOLOGY

When studied with sensitive techniques, virtually all leukemias display chromosomal abnormalities (gains, losses, and translocations) in all cells of the malignant clone. Their patterns are nonrandom.

A. Chromosomal alterations

Specific cytogenetic abnormalities are gradually being associated with specific types of leukemia—for example, the **Philadelphia chromosome**, abbreviated **Ph**^{1} and symbolized (t9; 22) (q34; q11), is associated with CML. Such alterations underlie current theories of malignant transformation and uncontrolled proliferation. Although detailed mechanisms require elucidation, it is believed that various agents operate at a number of "hot spots" within the genetic material to derepress genes responsible for proliferation or to cause failure of feedback regulation.

B. Oncogenes

Activation of cellular oncogenes and overproduction of their products is a key step in some types of neoplastic transformation. Chromosome abnormalities may accomplish this step by bringing oncogenes with transforming ability under the transcriptional control of genes active in that specific cell type. For example, in B cell ALL (B-ALL), CLL, and some B cell lymphomas such as Burkitt's, the genes for κ light chain (2p12), λ light chain (22q11), or μ heavy chain (14q32) are often at break points where they may be brought into association with oncogenes such as *myc* (on chromosome 8). The surface immunoglobulin of the malignant lymphocyte expresses the light chain type of the affected gene in such cases. It remains to be seen what role oncogenes play in leukemogenesis. However, the transfer of *c-abl* to chromosome 22 in CML produces a fusion product with the *bcr* region that encodes a novel protein with increased tyrosine kinase activity. The p210 protein has transforming activity in model systems and could be the first step in leukemic transformation.

C. Host factors

Host factors may include increased susceptibility of the chromosomes themselves to alterations or of the organism to agents that cause genetic damage. Such host factors include the following.

1. Heredity

The identical twin of a patient with acute leukemia has a 25% chance of developing acute leukemia, while a fraternal twin has little excess risk.

2. Congenital chromosome abnormalities

Leukemia occurs relatively frequently in association with aneuploid chromosomes (e.g., Down's syndrome, Klinefelter's syndrome, Turner's syndrome) and with defective repair of chromosome breaks (Fanconi's anemia, Bloom's syndrome) or chromosomal fragments.

3. Immune deficiency

Immune deficiency, whether cell-mediated (ataxia telangiectasia) or humorally mediated (X-linked agammaglobulinemia), may predispose to leukemia.

4. Chronic marrow dysfunction

Preleukemia or **myelodysplastic syndrome** is a clonal hematopoietic stem cell disorder with abnormal maturation and ineffective hematopoietic stem cell disorder with abnormal maturation and ineffective hematopoiesis that terminates in acute leukemia. Abnormal cell morphology and nonrandom cytogenetic abnormalities characterize many cases (e.g., trisomy 8, monosomy 7). In practice, it is difficult to differentiate preleukemia from other chronic marrow disorders that are associated with cytopenias but do not invariably terminate in leukemia (e.g., aplastic anemia, Kostmann's syndrome, refractory sideroblastic anemias, and so on). Paroxysmal nocturnal hemoglobinuria is a clonal disorder with a tendency to develop into acute leukemia, while the myeloproliferative disorders typically undergo a process of clonal evolution with increasingly aberrant chromosomes and abnormal maturation that ends in leukemia.

D. Environmental factors

1. Radiation and chemicals

Ionizing radiation from radiation therapy and atomic bombs can cause chromosome damage and is followed by marked increases in the incidence of acute and chronic myelocytic leukemia. Radiomimetic antitumor agents (especially Alkeran®) also have strong links to leukemia. Statistical associations implicate benzene and some environmental chemical pollutants as well. Carcinogens may act preferentially on specific DNA sites as suggested by the frequency of abnormalities of chromosomes 6 and 7 among chemotherapy-induced leukemia. Chronic immunosuppressive therapy may also increase susceptibility to leukemia (see below).

2. Viruses

Since retroviruses cause some animal leukemias, research has focused on **C-type RNA tumor viruses** in humans. Virus-encoded reverse transcriptase has been found in human lymphoblasts. Significantly, antibody to human T cell leukemia virus (HTLV) has been found in most patients with a rare form of leukemia that occurs in geographic clusters. DNA sequences of this virus have been detected in the cells of the leukemic T cell clone but not in the normal B cells of affected patients. The Epstein-Barr virus also has a close association with lymphoproliferative diseases but is not yet a proved cause of leukemia.

III. PATHOPHYSIOLOGY

A. Abnormal growth in vitro

In vitro cultures of leukemic bone marrows demonstrate abnormal growth patterns. Typical findings are a low cloning efficiency, a tendency to abortive colonies, and an increased percentage of light density CFU-GMs. Most colonies still respond to CSF, though a variety of abnormalities are described. Some preleukemic marrows follow similar patterns. To date no single pattern has emerged that typifies leukemia.

B. Failure of maturation

The crucial problem is the failure to undergo maturation and to produce functional end cells. Hence, in addition to showing morphologic immaturity, leukemic cells (especially in acute cases) may lack enzymes, have altered surface antigens, produce fetal hemoglobin, or perform poorly in functional assays.

C. Growth advantage of leukemic clones

Since they are immature, leukemic cells are likely to stay in the marrow and remain capable of dividing, producing more and more nonfunctional cells that eventually "pack" the marrow. Their presence may inhibit growth of normal cells, perhaps by chalones or by physical and nutritional competition. As a population the neoplastic clone has a growth advantage over normal cells even though the individual stem cells may actually divide more slowly.

D. Cytokinetics

The leukemic cell cycle generation time is ordinarily longer than normal due to an S-phase that is prolonged to 2 to 3 times normal. The cell death rate is high. Nonetheless the growth fraction is such that in acute leukemia, the tumor doubling time may be as short as 4 days. Since the diagnosis of leukemia can be made only when the total body burden exceeds 10^9 leukemic cells (approximately 1 g), a *minimum* of about 120 days (or 3–4 months) must pass between the time of the first malignant transformation and the time diagnosis. When the number of leukemic cells exceeds 10^{12}, the acute leukemias displace normal-functioning bone marrow and prove rapidly fatal. Because only 10 doublings are necessary for 10^9 cells to become 10^{12}, only a brief time (i.e., 10×4 days) is needed for maximally severe symptoms to evolve. This is not true of the chronic leukemias, in which slower cell division is occurring, greater numbers can be tolerated, and symptoms may be of several years' duration. Complete clinical remission occurs whenever the number of leukemic cells can be reduced to fewer than 10^9. Although the body might still contain up to 10^9 cells, ordinarily none might be detectable in blood or bone marrow. Cure can be said to occur only when all leukemic cells are gone.

E. Metabolic complications

Because of ineffective hematopoiesis and resulting high nucleic acid turnover, **uric acid production** increases. Nephrotoxic levels may accumulate, especially following the tumor cell lysis caused by chemotherapy. Massive cell lysis can also cause **hyperkalemia**, while poorly understood renal tubule toxins (possibly lysozyme) occasionally cause **hypokalemia**.

F. Causes of death

Marrow replacement by leukemic cells causes **anemia**, **thrombocytopenia**, and **granulocytopenia**. Bleeding presents a major threat, but infection is the major killer. Opportunistic organisms often infect leukemic patients because of diminished immunity.

IV. CLASSIFICATION

On the basis of clinical history and light microscopy alone, most leukemias can be easily divided into lymphocytic or myelocytic and acute or chronic and their respective prognoses and therapies established. The French-American-British (FAB) system assigns a letter and a number to each of the morphologic subtypes (in brackets below); however, the use of newer approaches is refining basic understanding and clinical approach.

A. Acute

1. **Acute lymphocytic leukemia** (ALL)
   a. Childhood: null cell, B cell, T cell [usually homogenous-L_1]
   b. Adult: null cell, B cell, or T cell [usually heterogenous-L_2]
   c. Burkitt's [L_3]
2. **Acute nonlymphocytic leukemia** (ANLL)
   a. Acute myelocytic leukemia (AML) [M_1 without or M_2 with maturation]
   b. Acute promyelocytic leukemia (APL) [M_3]

c. Acute myelomonocytic leukemia (AMML) [M_4]
d. Acute monocytic leukemia (AMoL) [M_5]
e. Erythroleukemia [M_6]
f. Megakaryoblastic leukemia [M_7]

B. Chronic

1. **Chronic lymphocytic leukemia** (CLL): B cell, T cell, hairy cell
2. **Chronic myelocytic leukemia** (CML)

C. Methods used in classification

Laboratory techniques may help in distinguishing the major types and subtypes of leukemia.

1. Light microscopy

Criteria for distinguishing the blast cells of ALL and ANLL are presented in table 22.1. Morphologic subtypes of ANLL are described in the FAB system. The more mature cells of CLL and CML are usually easily recognized.

2. Electron microscopy

Electron microscopy occasionally can reveal granules missed by light microscopy.

3. Histochemistry

Histochemical staining (table 22.2) brings out patterns useful in differentiating the acute leukemias.

4. Enzymes

In addition to histochemical stains, enzyme assays on blood and urine can detect lysozyme (muramidase) with the same pattern of expression as in table 22.2 and with levels correlating with the white blood cell count. **Terminal deoxynucleotidyl transferase** (TdT), a unique DNA polymerase,

Table 22.1
Morphologic Distinction of Acute Leukemia Blast Cells

Characteristic	ALL	ANLL
Size	Small	Larger
Shape	Round	Irregular
Cytoplasm	Dark blue rim	Pale blue, (granular)
Nucleus	Central, round	Eccentric, irregular
Nucleoli	Faint	"Punched out"
Auer rods	Absent	Present in 50%

Table 22.2
Histochemistry of Acute Leukemias

FAB class of leukemia	M1	M2,3	M4	M5	L1,2,3
Peroxidase or Sudan Black	+	+++	++	+/−	−
Esterase	+	++	+++	+++	−/+
Lysozyme (muramidase)	−	+	++	+++	−
Periodic acid-Schiff (PAS)	−/+	+/−	+/−	+/−	+++/−

Table 22.3
Cell Surface Markers

	Null ALL	Pre B-ALL	B-ALL	CLL	T-cell ALL	ANLL
Surface Ig	−	−	+	+	−	−
Cytoplasmic Ig	−	+	−	−	−	−
I^A	+	+	+	+	−	+
CALLA	+/−	+/−	+/−	−	−	−
T-series	−	−	−	rare +	+	−
My series	−	−	−	−	−	+

Note: See lecture 24.

randomly adds deoxynucleotide units to the 3′-OH terminus of DNA without needing a template. Blasts from 95% of patients with ALL are TdT positive, while fewer than 5% of patients with ANLL have blasts positive for TdT. Some patients with CML evolving into acute leukemia have TdT-positive blasts, and these often look and behave like lymphoblasts.

5. *Cell surface markers*

As discussed in lecture 24, immunologic methods reveal different surface antigens that depend on cell lineages (table 22.3). Surface immunoglobulin (SIg) characterizes all B cells, and in a malignant clone, only one light chain type is expressed. The finding of only one light chain type does not prove monoclonality or malignancy, but in a clinical setting it is often interpreted in that way. The nature of the **common acute lymphocytic leukemia antigen** (CALLA) remains unknown. Empirically it helps distinguish leukemias from other disorders even though it lacks complete specificity. T-series antigens are becoming better understood as monoclonal antibodies are being applied (e.g., the interleukin receptor). Myeloid (My) antigens are just now being explored.

6. *Chromosomes*

Presumably the several leukemias ultimately derive from the multitude of chromosomal alterations that cause neoplastic transformation. Only a handful of these are established (table 22.4).

Table 22.4
Major Nonrandom Chromosomal Alterations in the Leukemias

Abnormality*	Disease
Philadelphia chromosome:	
t(9;22 (q34;q11) *bcr-abl* p210	CML (95% of cases)
Philadelphia chromosome variants:	
(q22, __) *bcr-abl* 210	CML (5% of cases)
t(9;22) upstream altered *bcr-abl* p190	ALL (poor prognosis)
t(9;22) and other changes	AML [M1] (poor prognosis)
t(8:21) (q22;q22)	AML [M2] (good prognosis, Auer rods +)
t(15;17) (q22;q11–12)	APL [M3] (60–100% of cases)
inv16 (p13q22) or t(16;16) (p13;q22)	AMML [M4] (eosinophilia)
del(5q) or del(7q)	ANLL (postchemotherapy)
t(4;11) (q21;q23)	B-ALL
t(8;14) (q24;q32) *c-myc* (μ heavy)	
t(2;8) (p12;q24) *c-myc* (κ light)	
t(8;22) (q24; q11) *c-myc* (λ light)	
t(8:14) (q24;q11) (α-chain T cell receptor)	T-ALL
Many other abnormalities in T-ALL	

*The following rules govern the designation of cytogenetic abnormalities: Chromosome arms are designated by a p (short arm) or q (long arm) following the chromosome number. Band numbers are placed to the right of p or q; e.g., 9p13 is band is on the short arm of chromosome 9. Deletions are represented by del or − (minus); e.g., del 5q or 5q− denote deletions of the long term of chromosome 5. Translocations are denoted by t; e.g., t(8;14) (q24;q32) is a translocation of portions of chromosome 8 (break at q24) and chromosome 14 (break at q32). Inv denotes a rearrangement in which two breaks occur in the same chromosome with rotation of the intervening segment. The break points are noted in parentheses after the chromosome number, as in inv16(p13q22).

7. *Genetic probes*

Although not yet in widespread use, DNA probes using techniques like the polymerase chain reaction may permit sensitive and specific detection of gene rearrangements. For example, the *bcr-abl* fusion gene or its products would point to CML.

V. ACUTE LEUKEMIAS

A. Acute lymphocytic leukemia

1. *Clinical features*

ALL usually presents abruptly with signs and symptoms of only a few weeks' duration.

a. SIGNS OF MARROW DEPRESSION

Bruising, bleeding, fever, pallor, and fatigue with shortness of breath relate to aspects of marrow dysfunction: thrombocytopenia, neutropenia, and anemia. A packed, expanding bone marrow can cause bone pain.

b. SIGNS OF ORGAN INFILTRATION

Splenomegaly and hepatomegaly are commonly found. Lymphadenopathy occurs less often.

c. CNS INVOLVEMENT

A special form of tissue infiltration, central nervous system (CNS) involvement presents in three ways:

- Meningeal leukemia (arachnoidal infiltration can produce headache, nausea, vomiting, lethargy, paresis of legs, enuresis, visual disturbances, papilledema, cranial nerve palsies, seizures, and coma.
- Leukostatic thrombi (more common in AML) occurs when circulating blasts exceed 100,000/mm^3 and can lead to intracerebral hemorrhage.
- Subarachnoid hemorrhage due to thrombocytopenia.

2. *Laboratory features*

a. BLOOD

Anemia is present in more than 90% of patients. The initial white cell count is variable. In nearly half the cases the white count is normal or low; it is above 20,000 in 33% and above 100,000 in 20%. Thrombocytopenia is typically present. Since blasts may or may not be seen in the blood smear, bone marrow aspiration and biopsy are essential for diagnosis.

b. BONE MARROW

The bone marrow is largely replaced by lymphoblasts, which account for 50–100% of all marrow cells even when the circulating white cell numbers and the percentage of abnormal forms in the blood are low. The typical lymphoblast contains a round nucleus with diffuse chromatin and one or two nucleoli and scant basophilic cytoplasm without granules. In many cases it is impossible to distinguish lymphoblasts from myeloblasts.

c. OTHER TESTS

Since blood cell morphology alone sometimes fails to distinguish lymphoblasts from myeloblasts, the following tests are performed on the first marrow sample:

- Terminal deoxynucleotidyl transferase (TdT) is positive in virtually all patients with ALL and negative in ANLL.
- Periodic acid-Schiff (PAS) stain, which detects intracellular glycogen, is more often positive in ALL than ANLL.
- Myeloperoxidase stain is negative in ALL and usually positive in ANLL.
- Nonspecific esterase stain is negative in ALL and often positive in ANLL.
- Electron microscopy can change the diagnosis to ANLL by detecting microgranules. Surface marker studies help distinguish lineage and prognosis (see table 22.3).
- Chromosomes: sometimes ALL evolves from CML. A Ph^1 chromosome can suggest such lineage. It also implies a poorer prognosis.

3. Therapy

Treatment can be viewed in terms of tactics and strategy. Tactics are the means of attaining given strategic ends and vary in different institutions using different drugs, dosages, and scheduling. Strategy, however, has become constant over the last decade and falls under four headings: (1) remission induction; (2) CNS prophylaxis; (3) maintenance chemotherapy; and (4) cessation of treatment.

a. REMISSION INDUCTION

Induction aims at bringing the total leukemic cell number below the level of detectability (approximately 10^9) with the use of **prednisone** (a corticosteroid) and **vincristine** (a mitotic spindle inhibitor) and sometimes an **anthracycline** (a DNA intercalator). **Asparaginase**, which deprives lymphoblasts of an amino acid more essential to them than to normal cells, consolidates remission. Complete remission is achieved in 95% of children and 75% of adults.

b. CNS PROPHYLAXIS

Leukemic cells will have entered the CNS by the time of diagnosis in 70% of patients. Because of the pharmacologic blood-brain barrier, the cells are free to divide in spite of effective bone marrow chemotherapy. Thus, they are said to be in a "sanctuary." The resulting **meningeal leukemia**, or "leukemic meningitis," becomes apparent several months later and strikingly reduces the chance of cure. Effective prevention can be provided by administration of **methotrexate** (a folic acid antagonist) directly into the spinal fluid. Because intrathecal administration introduces the drug into the brain ventricles only in small quantities, prophylactic cranial radiation or a high dose of intravenous methotrexate sufficient to cross the blood-brain barrier may also be useful. Such therapy is undertaken as soon as the bone marrow is in remission.

c. MAINTENANCE CHEMOTHERAPY

Extended treatment aimed at reducing the number of leukemic cells from 10^9 to 0 takes 2 to 3 years in most patients. Effective drugs include **methotrexate** and **6-mercaptopurine** (a purine analogue) with pulses of vincristine, prednisone, and other agents. During this phase chronic bone marrow suppression of a modest degree is necessary to ensure effective drug activity.

d. CESSATION OF TREATMENT

Current data suggest that there is no advantage to continuing chemotherapy beyond $2\frac{1}{2}$–3 years. Even when bone marrow and spinal fluid remain visibly disease free, testicular biopsy occasionally may reveal another sanctuary of disease requiring radiation therapy. Otherwise treatment is terminated, and the patient is followed closely. The major complication of treatment is immunosuppression with increased susceptibility to bacterial, fungal, viral, or parasitic infections. Improved supportive care therefore adds to the cure rate.

4. Prognosis

By following these simple strategic goals, more than 60% of children and over 80% of "good risk" patients are apparently cured. Factors affecting the prognosis adversely are: (1) age (< 2 or > 9 years); (2) male sex; (3) WBC greater than 20,000/mm^3; (4) presence of mediastinal mass; (5) CNS disease; (6) T, B, or pre-B cell disease; and (7) Ph^1 chromosome. The largest group (65–75% of patients) has null-cell, CALLA-positive disease, which has a good prognosis. A small group with T-cell disease combines most of the other adverse prognostic factors and has a dramatically poorer outlook. Adults do not fare as well as children, but results of more aggressive therapy protocols are promising. Almost all relapses occur within 5 years. Though treatable, relapsed ALL is still much harder to cure. Bone marrow transplantation may improve the outlook. In vitro monoclonal antibody treatment offers a way to "clean up" marrow for autotransplantation.

B. Acute nonlymphocytic leukemia

As noted above, this family is subdivided into various categories on the basis of blood cell morphology and biochemical studies; however, their distinctness from ALL places them together.

1. Clinical features

Onset is usually abrupt as in ALL with similar symptoms and clinical findings. Occasionally in an elderly patient, a smoldering leukemia makes a slow appearance over several months or years. Splenomegaly, lymphadenopathy, and CNS disease are less common than in ALL. An unusual form of tissue infiltration, gum involvement, occurs in the monocytic variety. Soft tissue masses called **chloromas** are sometimes seen.

2. Laboratory features

a. AML

Diagnosis rests on a finding of excess nonlymphoid blasts in the bone marrow aspirate and on laboratory studies described above. A typical myeloblast has an irregular nucleus with loose or finely dispersed chromatin, two or more nucleoli with a punched-out appearance, and a moderate amount of light-blue cytoplasm. Usually blasts are accompanied by promyelocytes but by few cells intermediate in differentiation. This is termed a **leukemic hiatus**. **Auer rods**, or **bodies** (needle-like red cytoplasmic inclusions consisting of lysosomal material), are pathognomonic for ANLL but are seen in fewer than 50% of patients. In general, the more granules that are visible on Wright's stain, the more strongly positive will be the peroxidase and esterase stains.

b. MYELOMONOCYTIC AND MONOCYTIC LEUKEMIAS

The leukemic cells in myelomonocytic leukemia combine features of myelocytes and monocytes. They are faintly positive or negative for peroxidase, but histochemical, serum, and urine lysozyme are usually greatly elevated. In a few cases the blast nuclei are clearly monocytoid.

c. PROMYELOCYTIC LEUKEMIA

Characteristic cells are uniformly and densely filled with granules that stain intensely for peroxidase and often with Auer rods in large numbers. Procoagulant material released from these granules, especially after treatment accelerates cell lysis, initiates disseminated intravascular coagulation (DIC) (see lecture 29) and a severe hemorrhagic diathesis, distinctive of promyelocytic leukemia. Coagulation factors are consumed, and fibrin split products accumulate in the serum. Aggressive replacement of clotting factors and platelets is often necessary, and heparin therapy may be required. A specific chromosome translocation (15, 17) can be found in 50% of cases. The white count is often low. Prognosis may be better than for most ANLL.

d. ERYTHROLEUKEMIA

In its early stage this disorder (also known as Di Guglielmo's disease) is characterized by erythroid dysplasia and ineffective erythropoiesis (see lecture 6). As it progresses, the red cell precursors become bizarre and multinucleated. It finally reaches an erythromyelocytic phase marked by increasing number of dysplastic promyelocytes and myeloblasts, along with a population primitive blast cells difficult to classify. Eventually most cases evolve into AML.

e. OTHER LEUKEMIAS

Eosinophilic, basophilic, and megakaryocytic leukemias are rarely encountered leukemias in which immature eosinophils, basophils, or megakaryocytes predominate. Eosinophilic leukemia is difficult to distinguish from the hypereosinophilic syndromes (see lecture 20).

3. Therapy

As with ALL, therapy follows certain widely accepted strategic consideration.

a. REMISSION

Current regimens use **cytosine arabinoside** (a cycle-specific antimetabolite) and **daunorubicin** (an anthracycline antibiotic) given aggressively to induce complete marrow aplasia. In 75% of patients normal marrow regenerates within 3–6 weeks. The supportive care of patients in a prolonged phase of marrow aplasia requires meticulous attention to antibiotics and blood product replacement and can be undertaken only in major medical centers. Remission must be confirmed by the demonstration of normal bone marrow recovery.

b. MAINTENANCE CHEMOTHERAPY

With aggressive maintenance chemotherapy, 5-year disease-free survivals are achieved in approximately 25% of patients. It has not yet been determined at what point therapy can safely be terminated, nor has it been shown that specific CNS treatment is essential. Bone marrow transplantation using HLA-identical siblings produces prolonged disease-free survivals in about 50% of recipients when done during first remission in patients under age 30. Since there is only 1 chance in 4 that a sibling will share HLA identity with a patient, however, marrow transplantation now can be offered to only a small number of leukemic patients. The procedure consists of withdrawing 10^{10} marrow cells by aspiration from the donor and administering them intravenously to a recipient who has been immunosuppressed by total body irradiation and massive chemotherapy. Treating the patient's own marrow in vitro with chemotherapy or immunotherapy can also make autologous transplants worthwhile.

VI. THE CHRONIC LEUKEMIAS

A. Chronic myelocytic leukemia

1. Clinical features

CML is the least common of the major leukemias. Some would group it with the myeloproliferative disorders (see lecture 20). Often it is discovered on routine physical or blood examination during a preclinical phase that lasts 1–3 years. Fullness in the upper abdomen, due to an enlarged spleen, may be the presenting complaint. As disease advances, an enlarged spleen is found in 80–90% of patients. Symptoms due to hypermetabolism include easy fatigue, low-grade fever, night sweats, and weight loss. Bones are often tender. Sometimes accumulation of leukemic cells form masses in the skin and elsewhere called chloromas. Eventually, as in other leukemias, bleeding, anemia, and infection cause disability and death.

2. Laboratory features

a. BLOOD

Leukocytosis is characteristically present with a white count in the range of 50,000–500,000/mm^3. High white counts may be recognized early from the size of the buffy coat in the hematocrit tube. Every 1% of leukocyte hematocrit is roughly equivalent to 15,000 white cells/mm^3. On blood smears neutrophils, metamyelocytes, and myelocytes predominate while some blasts appear. A greater frequency of eosinophilic and basophilic granulocytes helps distinguish CML from benign leukocytosis or leukemoid reaction. Early in the course of CML, moderate anemia is common. Red cells may display anisocytosis but seldom significant pokilocytosis as in myeloid metaplasia (where "teardrop"-shaped cells are common). Occasional normoblasts, polychromatophilic cells, and basophilic stippling of red cells may be seen. Platelet levels are usually normal or increased, sometimes to levels above 1,000,000/mm^3, although their function is often abnormal.

b. BONE MARROW

The marrow shows marked granulocytic hyperplasia with a predominance of metamyelocytes, myelocytes, and frequently increased numbers of megakaryocytes. Bone marrow cells usually resemble those in the blood so that marrow aspiration is not essential. There is no leukemic hiatus between immature and mature forms as in the acute leukemias. The E/M ratio is strikingly depressed, reaching 1:25 or less.

c. Ph^1 CHROMOSOME

The great majority (95%) of patients have a Ph^1 chromosome. The clone of granulocytes having this abnormality develops a selective advantage and over a period of several years replaces normal myeloid precursors. Ultimately all granulocyte, megakaryocyte, erythroid elements, and perhaps B lymphocytes contain the abnormal chromosome. Fibroblasts do not. Thus the Ph^1 chromosome reflects the presence of a somatic cell mutation. Prognosis of the disease is generally poorer in Ph^1-negative or variant patients, in whom death usually occurs within a year.

d. LEUKOCYTE ALKALINE PHOSPHATASE

A low leukocyte alkaline phosphatase is found in 90% of patients. This distinguishes CML from leukemoid reactions and myeloid metaplasia (see lecture 20).

e. OTHER FEATURES

As in other conditions with high granulocyte counts, serum cobalamin and cobalamin-binding proteins (especially TC III) are markedly increased in CML. Uric acid levels are commonly elevated.

3. Course

A rapidly evolving acute phase, or blastic crisis, occurs within 3–6 years of diagnosis. Over a few weeks or months the granulocytes in the blood become increasingly immature, ultimately terminating in a blastic picture indistinguishable from acute leukemia. Further karyotypic abnormalities often accompany the change. In a third of such patients, the blasts have characteristics (positive TdT and negative peroxidase) and electron microscopic appearance of lymphoblasts. In these cases there is often a dramatic though short-lived response to ALL-type induction treatment with vincristine and prednisone, but as in the more common nonlymphoid form, the patient dies of uncontrolled blastic replacement of the marrow within a few months. Most patients live normal and productive lives for a number of years from the time of diagnosis before going into blast crisis or an accelerated phase with attendant infection and bleeding but without excessive blasts.

4. Therapy

The alkylating agent **busulfan** reduces the leukemia cell burden but rarely eradicates all cells with the Ph^1 chromosome to effect a complete remission. **Hydroxyurea** (an agent that blocks DNA synthesis) and **6-mercaptopurine** also control the disease temporarily, and radiation therapy can shrink refractory splenomegaly. Hyperuricemia can be controlled with **allopurinal**. **Interferon** may have a therapeutic role. Thus far cure has been rare even with aggressive chemotherapy. However, by adding total body irradiation, bone marrow transplantation may produce cures. Surprisingly, there have been occasional reports of the leukemia recurring in the donated marrow.

B. Chronic lymphocytic leukemia

CLL is a disease of the elderly that in many ways resembles diffuse, well-differentiated lymphocytic lymphoma (see lectures 23 and 24). It has a peculiar population distribution: rare in Orientals yet one of the most common forms of leukemia among Western peoples.

1. Clinical features

There is usually generalized lymphadenopathy and moderate splenomegaly, often of many years' duration. The disease characteristically follows an indolent, asymptomatic course, but a certain percentage of cases may become more aggressive. Frequently the patients are asymptomatic. Common complaints include fatigure, weight loss, fever, and night sweats.

2. Laboratory features

Typically, the white count ranges between 20,000 and 150,000/mm^3 and is occasionally over 1 million. The cells are primarily mature lymphocytes with clonal B surface markers (i.e., they have surface immunoglobulin with a single light chain type). A 14q$^+$ abnormality is common, as are breaks around the *bcl-1* gene. In spite of the vast number of cells, there is little crowding of normal bone marrow until years into the course. Thus significant thrombocytopenia, neutropenia, and anemia signify advancing disease. Common complications of CLL are immunologic. Reduction of immunoglobulins and decreased numbers of granulocytes predispose to infection. Antibody response to antigenic challenge is impaired, yet autoantibodies sometimes develop. Immunohemolytic anemia may be overt, with icterus, indirect hyperbilirubinemia, brisk reticulocytosis, spherocytosis, and a positive Coombs test (see lecture 13). Less often idiopathic thrombocytopenic purpura aggravates the thrombocytopenia already produced by diminished platelet production and hypersplenism (see lecture 28). Dermatologic manifestations include leukemia cutis, herpes zoster, generalized erythroderma, exfoliative dermatitis, and severe reaction to smallpox vaccination and insect bites. Patients with CLL have a high incidence of nonleukemic malignancies, such as cancer of the skin, lung, and bowel, which may be evidence favoring the view that malignant disease is prevented or controlled in normal subjects by a process of immunologic surveillance.

3. Therapy

The treatment of CLL is undertaken with prudence. In elderly patients, the disease follows a slow and remarkably benign course, with mortality figures for the untreated CLL patients not differing significantly from population controls. In younger patients (ages 40–60) more aggressive disease often necessitates more aggressive treatment. It is usually wise to treat the patient's symptoms rather than the white count. Alkylating agents such as **chlorambucil** or **cyclophosphamide** are the initial choices. **Prednisone** may be added judiciously, though some argue for more aggressive therapy. Radiation therapy can shrink obstructing lymph nodes or a bothersome spleen. Exciting research centers on immunologic approaches to therapy using interferon or monoclonal antibodies against idiotypic determinants of the surface immunoglobulin.

4. Hairy cell leukemia

Leukemic reticuloendotheliosis (hairy cell leukemia) is a rare but malignant variant of CLL characterized by splenomegaly and pancytopenia. Characteristic cells with hairy projections can be seen on phase microscopy or identified histochemically with tartrate-resistant acid phosphatase. The most effective treatment has been splenectomy, but both **α-interferon** and **deoxycoformycin** have produced striking remissions.

5. T cell CLL

Adult T cell leukemia is a rare variety of CLL closely linked to the human T cell leukemia virus (HTLV) (see lecture 24). First described in Japan and the Caribbean, it presents with lymphadenopathy, skin lesions, and hypercalcemia. Mature-appearing lymphocytes with "knobby" nuclear outlines have surface markers of helper cells but functionally help to suppress mitogen-driven antibody production. Much more aggressive than an immunologically distinct chronic T cell leukemia that presents with neutropenia, HTLV-associated leukemia responds poorly to therapy and follows a more subacute course.

SELECTED REFERENCES

Reviews

Bennett, J. M., Foon, K. A., et al. *Immunologic Approaches to the Classification and Management of Lymphomas and Leukemias.* Boston: Kluwer Academic Publishers, 1988.

Beris, P. Primary clonal myelodysplastic syndromes. *Semin. Hemtol.* 26(1989): 216–233.

Butturini, A., Keating, A., et al. Autotransplants in chronic myelogenous leukaemia: strategies and results. *Lancet* 335(1990): 1255–1258.

Champlin, R., and Gale, R. P. Acute lymphoblastic leukemia: recent advances in biology and therapy. *Blood* 73(1989): 2051–2066.

Cheson, B. D., Lacerna, L., et al. Autologous bone marrow transplantation: current status and future directions. *Ann. Intern. Med.* 110(1989): 51–65.

Green, P. L., and Chen, I. S. Y. Regulation of human T cell leukemia virus expression. *FASEB J.* 4(1990): 169–175.

International Workshop on Lymphocytic Leukemia. Chronic lymphocytic leukemia: recommendations for diagnosis, staging, and response criteria. *Ann. Intern. Med.* 110(1989): 236–238.

Jacobs, A. Annotation. Benzene and leukaemia. *Br. J. Haematol.* 72(1989): 119–121.

LeBien, T. W., and McCormack, R. T. The common acute lymphoblastic leukemia antigen (CD10)—emancipation from a functional enigma. *Blood* 73(1989): 625–635.

Santos, G. W. Marrow transplantation in acute nonlymphocytic leukemia. *Blood* 74(1989): 901–908.

Santos, G. W. Bone marrow transplantation in hematologic malignancies: current status. *Cancer* 65 Suppl. (1990): 786–791.

Original articles

Daley, G. Q., Van Etten, R. A., et al. Induction of chronic myelogenous leukemia in mice by the P210$^{bcr/abl}$ gene of the Philadelphia chromosome. *Science* 247(1990): 824–830.

Epner, D. E., and Koeffler, H. P. Molecular genetic advances in chronic myelogenous leukemia. *Ann. Intern. Med.* 113(1990): 3–6.

French Cooperative Group on Chronic Lymphocytic Leukemia. Effects of chlorambucil and therapeutic decision in initial forms of chronic lymphocytic leukemia (stage A): results of a randomized clinical trial on 612 patients. *Blood* 75(1990): 1414–1421.

French Cooperative Group on Chronic Lymphocytic Leukemia. A randomized clinical trial of chlorambucil versus COP in stage B chronic lymphocytic leukemia. *Blood* 75(1990): 1422–1425.

Kurzrock, R., Gutterman, J. U., et al. The molecular genetics of Philadelphia chromosome-positive leukemias. *N. Engl. J. Med.* 319(1988): 990–998.

Mills, K. I., MacKenzie, E. D., et al. The site of the breakpoint within the *bcr* is a prognostic factor in Philadelphia-positive CML patients. *Blood* 72(1988): 1237–1241.

Ohmori, M., Ohmori, S., et al. Myelodysplastic syndrome (MDS)-associated inhibitory activity on haemopoietic progenitor cells. *Br. J. Haematol.* 74(1990): 179–184.

Rambaldi, A., Terao, M., et al. Differences in the expression of alkaline phosphatase mRNA in chronic myelogenous leukemia and paroxysmal nocturnal hemoglobinuria polymorphonuclear leukocytes. *Blood* 73(1989): 1113–1115.

Rowley, J. D. The Philadelphia chromosome translocation: a paradigm for understanding leukemia. *Cancer* 65(1990): 2178–2184.

Rowley, S. D., Jones, R. J., et al. Efficacy of ex vivo purging for autologous bone marrow transplantation in the treatment of acute nonlymphoblastic leukemia. *Blood* 74(1989): 501–506.

Sachs, L. The control of growth and differentiation in normal and leukemic blood cells. *Cancer* 65(1990): 2196–2206.

Saglio, G., Guerrasio, A., et al. Variability of the molecular defects corresponding to the presence of a Philadelphia chromosome in human hematologic malignancies. *Blood* 72(1988): 1203–1208.

Shtalrid, M., Talpaz, M., et al. Philadelphia-negative chronic myelogenous leukemia with breakpoint cluster region rearrangement: molecular analysis, clinical characteristics, and response to therapy. *J. Clin. Oncol.* 6(1988): 1569–1575.

LECTURE 23

The Malignant Lymphomas I. Clinical Aspects

David S. Rosenthal

EDITOR'S COMMENT

The last decade has witnessed a tremendous increase in scientific interest in both Hodgkin's disease and the awkwardly named non-Hodgkin's lymphomas. Progress has followed the discovery of cell surface markers that permit analysis of cell lineages—and, on the clinical side (the focus of this lecture), the search for therapies has greatly intensified. We are still largely dependent on various acronymic combinations of cytotoxic drugs, but with increasing sophistication these are now combined with radiation therapy and in some cases autologous bone marrow transplantation so that more and more cures (defined as 5-year symptom-free survival) are being obtained. Thus we are nibbling away at these disorders. Though we have a long way to go, it is a fact nonetheless that the most impressive advances in the treatment of disseminated cancer have been in the management of leukemias and lymphomas. Indeed, most acute leukemias in young people and many cases of Hodgkin's disease are now curable. Non-Hodgkin's lymphomas constitute a very large and heterogeneous group, and individual types vary greatly in responsiveness and curability. Given the widespread use of old and new surface markers, subclassification improves, as does the likelihood of better regimen selection and more predictable response.

I. INTRODUCTION

A. Definitions

This lecture deals with a group of disorders known as the **malignant lymphomas**. They involve the cells of the **lymphatic system** (discussed in lecture 3) and thus are termed **lymphoproliferative disorders**, a category that also includes the lymphocytic leukemias, ALL and CLL, which were discussed in lecture 22, and Waldenström's macroglobulinemia, which is discussed in lecture 25. Although there are similarities among the various lymphomas, they include a wide spectrum of clinical and histologic patterns. The lymphoproliferative disorders may be subclassified by morphologic appearances but also by their cell of origin (table 23.1).

Because of its characteristic pathology, **Hodgkin's disease** has been separated from the other lymphomas. This fact (and limitations of our knowledge) has led to an unfortunate terminology in which the other lymphoid malignancies are grouped under the term **non-Hodgkin's lymphoma**. Research is active in this area, and new concepts of Hodgkin's disease and

Table 23.1
Classification of Lymphoproliferative Disorders According to B or T Cell Markers

B cell disorders	T cell disorders	Cell type uncertain
Acute lymphocytic leukemia	Infectious mononucleosis	Hodgkin's disease
Poorly differentiated lymphoma	Mycosis fungoides	Histiocytic lymphoma
Hairy cell leukemia	Sézary's syndrome	
Prolymphocytic leukemia	Acute lymphoblastic leukemia (T variant)	
Chronic lymphocytic leukemia	Chronic lymphocytic leukemia (T variant)	
Waldenström's macroglobulinemia		
Cold agglutinin disease		
Heavy chain disease		
Amyloidosis		
Multiple myeloma		

non-Hodgkin's lymphoma are continuously appearing in the literature. The student is urged to consider this changing field critically.

B. Enlarged lymph nodes

One of the major clinical presentations of lymphoma is enlarged lymph nodes. Although lymphadenopathy is always ominous because it may signify malignant disease, it should be emphasized that enlarged lymph nodes are more commonly related to infectious, inflammatory, and other benign disorders. Lymph node enlargement is most commonly a secondary phenomenon—a reaction to a nearby inflammatory process or to a systemic process. Table 23.2 lists the major causes of lymphadenopathy. A careful history and physical examination is most important in evaluating a patient with enlarged lymph nodes. Infectious nodes are usually soft, tender, less than 2 cm in diameter, and located in areas that drain common infections. For example, the anterior and posterior cervical chain of the neck drains the ears and throat. Potentially malignant nodes are generally firm, hard, or rubbery, fixed to underlying tissue, multiple, nontender, greater than 2 cm in diameter, and located in unusual sites—for example, the infraclavicular area. When the diagnosis is uncertain, histologic examination of an enlarged lymph node is essential.

Clinical emergencies may arise when massive lymph node enlargement compresses vital organs. For example, a malignant node may compress the trachea or the venous return to the heart (superior vena caval syndrome) or obstruct urinary flow by extrinsic compression of the ureters. These life-threatening occurrences require immediate therapy.

Table 23.2
Major Causes of Lymph Node Enlargement

Infections
Acute (infectious mononucleosis, toxoplasmosis, cytomegalovirus, generalized dermatitis, common communicable diseases)
Chronic (syphilis, tuberculosis, sarcoidosis)
AIDS
Hypersensitivity reactions and connective tissue diseases
Serum sickness
Rheumatoid arthritis
Systemic lupus erythematosus
Drug pseudolymphoma (diphenylhydantoin)
Primary lymphoproliferative diseases
Hodgkin's disease
Non-Hodgkin's lymphoma
Leukemia (CLL, ALL, blast crisis of CML)
Waldenström's macroglobulinemia
Endocrine disorders
Hyperthyroidism
Hypoadrenocorticalism
Hypopituitarism
Lipidoses
Dermatopathic lymphadenitis
Metastatic cancers
Breast
Lung
Gastrointestinal

II. HODGKIN'S DISEASE

A. Introduction

In 1666 a fatal disease was described in which the lymphoid tissues and spleen appeared as a "cluster of grapes." In 1832 Thomas Hodgkin and later Samuel Wilkes described a disease characterized by gradual progressive enlargement of the lymph nodes "beginning usually in the cervical region and spreading throughout the lymphoid tissue of the body, forming nodular growths in the internal organs, resulting in anemia, and usually, fatal cachexia." The major features of these cases were (1) slow and relentless growth, the disease sometimes lasting many years and (2) characteristic histopathologic pattern (as later elucidated by Reed and Sternberg) that included the distinctive giant cell known as the **Reed-Sternberg cell** (see figure 24.5). Although Reed-Sternberg cells occur in other disorders, pathologists now require that this cell be present before concluding that the diagnosis is Hodgkin's disease. The Reed-Sternberg cell is probably the neoplastic cell, and other cells present are reactive populations of lymphocytes, eosinophils, and plasma cells.

The etiology of Hodgkin's disease is unknown. There has been intense interest, based largely on seroepidemiologic studies in the Epstein-Barr virus (EBV) as a possible oncogenic virus in Hodgkin's disease. However, it is not yet possible to assign a specific role to EBV in this neoplasm. Because of the difficulty in obtaining pure samples of Reed-Sternberg cells, the cell of origin of Hodgkin's disease remains unclear. The Reed-Sternberg cell is not of any lymphoid subset, but has characteristics of the monocyte-macrophage system. The lymphoid tissue surrounding these cells is evidently not made up of malignant cells.

B. Epidemiology

Hodgkin's disease occurs at a rate of 2 per 100,000 population per year in the United States. However, the incidence varies widely according to age, sex, and geography. In the United States and Northern Europe, Hodgkin's disease has a peculiar bimodal age incidence with a high peak occurring between 15 and 35 and a lower peak after the age of 50. There is a slight male predominance.

Recent epidemiologic studies suggest a higher incidence of Hodgkin's disease among high school students in some areas of the United States and in relatives of patients with Hodgkin's disease. However, the statistical validity of these findings has been questioned, and more prospective date will be needed before the existence of clusters or predisposed families can be established.

Several reports suggest that there is an increased incidence or risk of the disease among siblings, especially of the same sex, that may be related to identity of HLA antigens.

C. Clinical features

Hodgkin's disease usually presents with a nonpainful swelling of a lymph node in the neck. Less commonly, the onset may be marked by fever, night sweats, and weight loss. Rarely, patients initially experience severe itching of the skin (pruritus).

Unlike the pattern in other lymphoproliferative disorders, Hodgkin's disease usually spreads contiguously from one lymph node region to another. For example, in a patient with early Hodgkin's disease, there may be involvement of only neck and mediastinal nodes. In patients presenting with more advanced disease, diffuse adenopathy, along with involvement of liver, marrow, lung, or other organs, may be present.

As will be noted below, it is customary to speak of the several **stages** of Hodgkin's disease—and of the process of determining the stage in a given patient's course of disease as **staging**. It is the characteristic contiguous nature of the pattern of spread that makes staging prognostically and therapeutically important.

There is a close relation between the occurrence of symptoms and the course of Hodgkin's disease. Typical symptoms consist of a loss of more than 10% of the body weight (unrelated to dieting), persistent fever not due to infection, and night sweats. Generalized itching (pruritus) may be a related symptom.

D. Histologic classification

The histologic classification currently employed is known as the Rye Conference (1965) classification. This classification, which is discussed in lecture 24, includes four major types: **lymphocyte predominance**, **nodular sclerosis**, **mixed cellularity**, and **lymphocyte depletion**. The natural history of the disease varies with respect to histologic type. Patients who present with nodular sclerosis and lymphocyte-predominance types generally have a much better prognosis than those with mixed cellularity and lymphocyte-depletion types. The histologic features of the four types are discussed in lecture 24.

E. Clinical staging

In addition to the histologic type, prognosis and therapy depend on the extent of disease present at the onset. The four clinical stages of Hodgkin's disease are summarized in table 23.3.

Table 23.3
Modified Definitions of Clinical Stages (Ann Arbor Symposium 1971)

Stage	Clinical features (and terminology)
I	Involvement of a single lymph node region or involvement of a single extralymphatic organ or site
II	Involvement of two or more lymph node regions on the same side of the diaphragm alone or with involvement of limited, contiguous extralymphatic organ or tissue
III	Involvement of lymph node regions on both sides of the diaphragm (which may include the spleen and/or limited contiguous extralymphatic organ or site)
III_1	Involvement limited to spleen, splenic hilar nodes, and high abdominal nodes
III_2	Involvement of para-aortic, pelvic, and iliac nodes in addition to III_1 involvement
IV	Multiple or disseminated foci of involvement of one or more extralymphatic organs or tissues, with or without lymphatic involvement

Note: All cases are further subclassified to indicate the absence (A) or presence (B) of the systemic symptoms: significant fever, night sweats, and/or unexplained weight loss of greater than 10% of normal body weight. Thus, a patient is said to be in stage IIIA or IIIB. The term **clinical stage** (CS) refers to the patient's stage as determined by diagnostic examinations and a single diagnostic biopsy. If a second biopsy or laparotomy is performed, the term **pathologic stage** (PS) is used.

Systematic clinical staging includes the following examinations:

- Physical examination with careful attention to all lymph node areas.
- Various routine laboratory studies.
- Computed tomography (CT) scans of the abdomen and pelvis, supplying information regarding the liver and abdominal nodes.
- A bipedal lymphangiogram, a procedure in which radiopaque dye is injected into lymphatic channels of the feet with resulting visualization of iliac and para-aortic nodes.
- Nuclear medicine studies such as gallium scans.
- In some clinics, laparoscopy is performed following lymphangiography. The liver and spleen are inspected, and the liver is biopsied under direct visualization.
- In most clinics, if the CT scans of the abdomen are negative a so-called staging laparotomy is carried out in which the abdomen is explored and suspicious nodes seen on the lymphangiogram are removed. Splenectomy is performed, and biopsies are performed of both lobes of the liver and the bone marrow. Operative findings often change the therapeutic plan; thus laparotomy is necessary.

Careful and detailed pathologic examination of the spleen can often identify minute areas of Hodgkin's disease. Approximately 20–30% of clinical stages I and II patients will be upstaged to pathologic stage III or IV by surgical staging. Splenic Hodgkin's disease without evidence of disease elsewhere in the abdomen suggests that involvement of various organs (such as the spleen) may occur not only by contiguous extension but by hematogenous spread. Staging laparotomy alters the patient's stage in a third of the cases and, more important, may change the plan for therapy.

F. Laboratory studies

There are no pathognomonic hematologic findings in Hodgkin's disease. Leukocytosis with lymphocytopenia is not uncommon. An elevated erythrocyte sedimentation rate (ESR) will correlate with disease activity, and serial ESR studies may be a useful way to follow the disease process. Eosinophilia and rarely monocytosis are noted. Other hematologic abnormalities such as leukopenia and thrombocytopenia usually appear with advanced disease and are either secondary to bone marrow involvement or previous therapy.

Patients frequently demonstrate defects in delayed hypersensitivity reaction and have negative tuberculin reactions even in the presence of active tuberculosis. This defect in cellular immunity is associated with an increased incidence of infections with unusual organisms, such as *Pneumocystis carinii*, various fungi, and herpes zoster. The impairment of cellular immunity is related in part to active suppression of T lymphocyte function.

G. Course and prognosis

Prognostic factors are the following:

- **Presence or absence of "B" symptoms** (reference is to staging categories, not cell type).
- **Age of the patient**. Older patients tend to do more poorly than younger patients.
- **Type of histology**. Patients with lymphocyte predominance, nodular sclerosis, and mixed cellularity have a more favorable prognosis than those with lymphocyte depletion.
- **Clinical stage**. Patient in stages I and II have a more favorable prognosis than those in stages III and IV (and those in stage III have a better prognosis than those in stage IV).

H. Therapy

Major therapeutic developments that began in the early 1960s dramatically improved the response rate and survival in Hodgkin's disease. Today almost 70% of patients with Hodgkin's disease are long-term survivors. Success has been related primarily to careful staging, understanding of the pattern of spread of this disease, and advances in radiation and chemotherapy.

The therapeutic approach is usually to treat regions of known disease *and* the presumed next potential site of involvement. For example:

- In a pathologically staged IA patient presenting only with cervical adenopathy, the disease can often be cured by a "mantle" irradiation field plus the contiguous area (i.e., the upper abdomen or para-aortic field).
- In a patient with diffuse adenopathy above and below the diaphragm plus fevers and night sweats (stage IIB), the next potential site of involvement would be an extranodal site. Therefore, chemotherapy would be primary therapy.

In general, limited radiation therapy is recommended for early stages of Hodgkin's disease while chemotherapy with or without irradiation for advanced stages. Results of such an approach with 5-year disease-free survival rates are shown in table 23.4

1. Radiation therapy

The concept of intensive, "curative" irradiation therapy for Hodgkin's disease was developed by Gilbert and Peters and later by Kaplan and Johnson. Details of therapy and expected results vary with the stage. Table

Table 23.4
Five-Year Disease-free Survival Rates in Hodgkin's Disease

Stage	Therapy	Five-year disease-free survival (%)
I and IIA	Intensive radiation therapy	85–90
IB, IIB (rare)	Intensive radiation therapy	80–85
IIIA	Intensive radiation therapy or chemotherapy	60–90
$IIIA_1$	Intensive radiation therapy or chemotherapy	60–80
$IIIA_2$	Chemotherapy ± radiation therapy	60–80
IIIB	Chemotherapy ± radiation therapy	60–80
IVA and IVB	Chemotherapy alone	30–50

23.4 summarizes approximate 5-year disease-free survival rates currently associated with various therapeutic programs. Radiation therapy is usually delivered into three major fields—known as the mantle, para-aortic, and pelvic or inverted Y fields (figure 23.1). In total nodal radiation therapy, treatment is given to all three fields, which encompass most of the body's lymph node regions.

2. *Chemotherapy*

Aggressive chemotherapy has also produced long disease-free remissions in advanced Hodgkin's disease. A program developed by DeVita and coworkers, known as MOPP (for the drug combination Mustargen® [nitrogen mustard], Oncovin® [vincristine], procarbazine, and prednisone) has resulted in complete remissions in 60–70%. However, 5-year disease-free survival was obtained in only 50% of these cases. Recently, other combined chemotherapy programs employing Adriamycin®, bleomycin, vinblastine, and dacarbazine (the ABVD regimen) have yielded similar results. The duration of therapy is generally 6–12 months—or at least 2 months after achievement of complete remission.

3. *Complications*

Complications (table 23.5) of **radiation therapy** common to patients of all ages include radiation-induced hypothyroidism, pericarditis, and pneumonitis. In females, pelvic irradiation can lead to sterility and in both sexes varying degrees of myelosuppression. The latter complication varies most with age. Regeneration of marrow activity is quite rapid in patients under age 20, moderately delayed from age 20–40, and severely delayed from age 40–70. The current recommended dose for Hodgkin's disease is 3200–4000 CGy.

Complications of **chemotherapy** include myelosuppression, nausea, vomiting, alopecia, paresthesias, pulmonary fibrosis, and rarely cardiomyo-

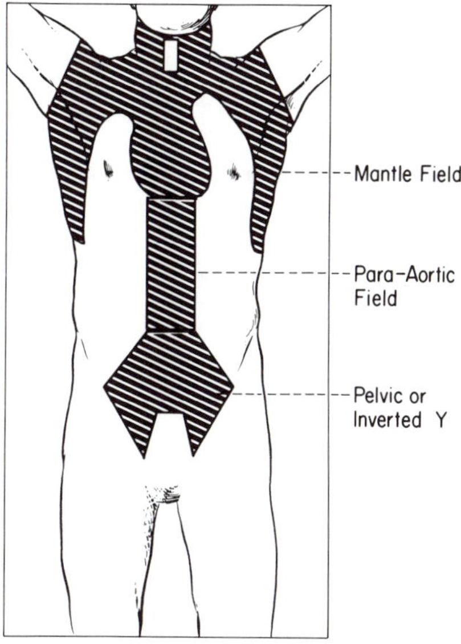

Fig. 23.1
Radiation fields in therapy of Hodgkin's disease. Shaded areas represent the three treatment fields. The **mantle field** is the uppermost field. Lungs and vocal cords are protected by leads blocks; heart and thyroid are within the field. The **para-aortic field**, or middle field, extends from the diaphragm to just above the bifurcation of the aorta. When the spleen has not been removed, this field is extended to include the entire spleen and splenic hilum. The **pelvic** or **inverted Y field** is the lowest field. It encompasses the pelvic and inguinal nodes and includes a large area of bone marrow.

Table 23.5
Complications of Therapy of Hodgkin's Disease

Radiation therapy (RT)
Hypothyroidism
Pericarditis
Pneumonitis
Chemotherapy (CT)
Nausea, vomiting
Alopecia (especially with Adriamycin®)
Sterility in males (especially with alkylating agents) and females
Myelosuppression
Neuropathy (vincristine)
Cardiomyopathy
RT plus CT (combined modality therapy)
Second malignancies, especially acute leukemia and non-Hodgkin's lymphoma

pathy. Sterility is the rule in males and often occurs in females. There is an increased incidence of second malignancies, usually acute leukemia or non-Hodgkin's lymphoma. The frequency of acute leukemia has approached 5–7% in patients receiving protracted courses of alkylating agents or chemotherapy combined with total nodal irradiation. Opportunistic infections such as herpes zoster and *Pneumocystis carinii* are common.

III. NON-HODGKIN'S LYMPHOMA

A. Introduction

This is a heterogenous collection of lymphoid malignancies with some common features and many differences. Unlike Hodgkin's disease they appear to be multicentric in origin with a tendency to spread widely early in the disease. A peripheral blood leukemic phase is not uncommon (figure 23.2A), and there is some evidence that nearly all patients have malignant cells in their blood regardless of the stage of disease.

B. Etiology and incidence

The annual age-adjusted incidence of non-Hodgkin's lymphoma is 2.6–5.8 per 100,000. There is a progressive increase in incidence with age.

As in Hodgkin's disease, the etiology of most types of non-Hodgkin's lymphoma is unknown. However, several situations imply possibly causal relations. For example,

- The incidence of non-Hodgkin's lymphoma rises in immunosuppressed patients (e.g., renal transplant recipients), and in those with hyperfunctioning immune systems (e.g., Sjögren's syndrome).
- Viruses apparently cause specific lymphomas. African Burkitt's lymphoma is associated with EBV infection, and an aggressive T cell leukemia/lymphoma occurring in Japan and the Caribbean islands is associated with HTLV-I infection (see lecture 24).
- Cytogenetic abnormalities are common but less consistent than those in the acute leukemias. The exception is Burkitt's lymphoma, which is usually associated with an 8;14 translocation, or in some patients a variant 8;22 or 8;2 translocation. Interestingly, these translocations all involve the *c-myc* proto-oncogene.
- About 60% of all non-Hodgkin's lymphoma have a $14q^{+}$ marker chromosome. About 35% of nodular B-cell non-Hodgkin's lymphoma have a 14;18 translocation. The significance of these changes is unknown.
- Other cytogenetic studies show that the non-Hodgkin's lymphomas may be biclonal or multiclonal in origin.

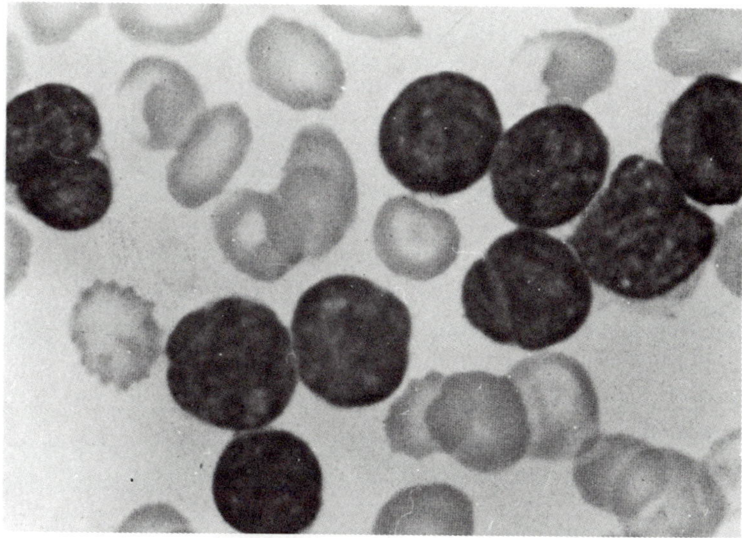

A

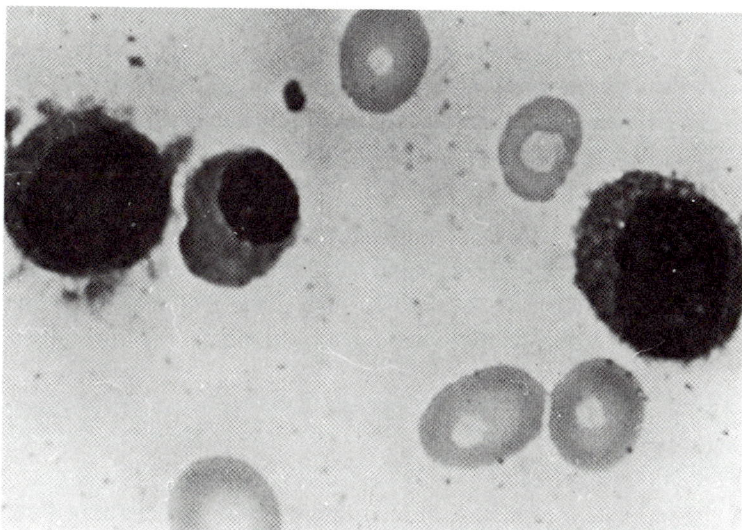

B

Fig. 23.2
Abnormal peripheral blood in lymphoproliferative disorders. A leukemic blood picture may occur during the course of non-Hodgkin's lymphoma. *A*, Cells in this field (× 500) have cleaved or fissured nuclei. *B*, Hairy cells with cytoplasmic projections and cleaved nuclei (× 500).

C. Clinical features

Presenting signs and symptoms are extremely variable and relate to site and extent of disease. Many patients seek investigation of an enlarged node or abdominal mass. Other cases begin with complaints referable to the alimentary tract, for example, a pharyngeal mass, abdominal pain, vomiting, or gastrointestinal bleeding. Systemic manifestations are nonspecific: Fever, sweats, and itching are uncommon; weight loss is common.

Most non-Hodgkin's lymphomas are B-cell malignancies and may be accompanied by hypogammaglobulinemia and autoimmune phenomenon such as immunohemolytic anemia or immunothrombocytopenia.

D. Classification

The classification (see lecture 24) of the non-Hodgkin's lymphomas is a complicated subject that can be approached in three ways:

- **Nodal architecture** (according to Rappaport): nodular (follicular) appearance versus diffuse histology.
- **Degree of cellular differentiation**, that is, well-differentiated lymphocytic versus poorly differentiated versus undifferentiated cell types.
- **Immunologic classification** (according to Lukes), based on whether a malignant lymphoid cell is a B cell, T cell, or undefined. The majority (80%) are of B cell origin.

A recent review demonstrated that non-Hodgkin's lymphomas could be subgrouped into three major categories that had clinical significance: low-grade, intermediate-grade, or high-grade malignancies (table 23.6). This working formulation attempts to combine the three previously used classifications.

E. Clinical staging

The extent of disease at initial presentation is determined on the basis of history, physical examination, blood studies, bone marrow biopsy, adominal CT scan, and nuclear medicine scans. Such studies have demonstrated that less than 15% of patients with non-Hodgkin's lymphoma are in stage I or II when first seen (compared to 30–60% in Hodgkin's disease). Thus most patients have advanced disease from the onset and staging laparotomy is of no benefit.

F. Incidence of leukemia

Unlike Hodgkin's disease, in which leukemia occurs only rarely (and then it may be as a complication of combined intenseive radiation therapy and chemotherapy), leukemia is common in the non-Hodgkin's lymphomas.

Table 23.6
A "Working Formulation" of Non-Hodgkin's Lymphomas for Clinical Use

Category	Abbreviation
Low Grade	
Malignant lymphoma, small lymphocytic	WDL
a. Consistent with chronic lymphocytic leukemia	
b. Plasmacytoid	
Malignant lymphoma, follicular, predominantly small cleaved cell	NPDL
Malignant lymphoma, follicular, mixed small cleaved and large cell	NM
Intermediate grade	
Malignant lymphoma, follicular, predominantly large cell	NH
Malignant lymphoma, diffuse, small cleaved cell	DPDL
Malignant lymphoma, diffuse, mixed small and large cell	DM
Malignant lymphoma, diffuse, large cell*	DH
a. Cleaved cell	
b. Noncleaved cell	
High grade	
Malignant lymphoma, large cell, immunoblastic*	DH
a. Plasmacytoid	
b. Clear cell	
c. Polymorphous	
Malignant lymphoma, lymphoblastic	LB
a. Convoluted	
b. Nonconvoluted	
Malignant lymphoma, small non-cleaved cell	DU
a. Burkitt's	
b. Non-Burkitt's	

*Many authorities now believe that all diffuse large cell lymphomas should be grouped together in the high-grade category.

The leukemic cell type is usually similar to that seen in the involved lymph node.

G. Therapy

Since disease is rarely localized, curative radiation therapy is not possible and chemotherapy is the primary modality (Table 23.7). Aggressive chemotherapy is rarely curative in the low-grade non-Hodgkin's lymphomas but can produce long disease-free intervals (?cure) in the high-grade types.

1. Low-grade non-Hodgkin's lymphoma

Low-grade types, such as nodular, poorly differentiated lymphocytic (NPDL), are frequently slow growing, quick to respond to relatively little chemotherapy or radiation, and asymptomatic patients often require little or no therapy for months to years. Unfortunately, although ex-

Table 23.7
Chemotherapy Programs Used in Non-Hodgkin's Lymphomas

Single agents	Combination programs
Vinca alkaloids: vincristine (Oncovin®) vinblastine (Velban®)	CVP or COP: cyclophosphamide, vincristine (Oncovin®), prednisone C-MOPP: cyclophosphamide plus MOPP
Corticosteroids: prednisone	B-COP: bleomycin plus COP BACOP: Adriamycin® plus B-COP
Alkylating agents: cyclophosphamide (Cytoxan®) chlorambucil (Leukeran®)	M-BACOP: high-dose methotrexate plus BACOP CHOP: COP plus Adriamycin®
Anthracycline: Adriamycin®	
Other drugs: procarbazine methotrexate bleomycin	

tremely sensitive to therapy, there is a high recurrence rate, and very few patients are free of disease for the long term. Statistics for various therapies demonstrate 40–60% 10-year survivors but only 5–15% 10-year disease-free survivors. Currently it is recommended that patients be treated conservatively for symptoms of enlarging or obstructing adenopathy. Eventually this "favorable" subgroup may convert to a "high-grade," "unfavorable," or resistant non-Hodgkin's lymphoma, with death ensuing eventually.

2. *High-grade non-Hodgkin's lymphoma*

High-grade types, for instance, diffuse histiocytic (DH), are aggressive forms whose cells are very immature, have a high growth rate, a short natural history of disease (several months), and resist mild forms of therapy. In patients who achieve a complete remission, however, a significant proportion (40–60%) continue in remission long after stopping chemotherapy and appear to be cured. It is suspected that because these lymphomas are so rapidly growing, they can be cured by aggressive chemotherapies.

H. Unusual clinical problems

1. *Burkitt's lymphoma*

This extranodal lymphoma (usually affecting the jaw) was first described in Uganda by Burkitt. The histology is specific. The disorder is probably caused by an infections DNA virus, specifically the Epstein-Barr virus (discussed above), which is the same agent that causes infectious mononucleosis (see lecture 10). Specific cytogenetic abnormalities have been described involving translocation of 2, 14, 22 with 12. The disease is notably sensitive to chemotherapy.

2. Primary gastrointestinal lymphoma

This disorder, common in Mediterranean area, is associated with an IgA gammopathy.

I. Related disorders

1. Mycosis fungoides

Mycosis fungoides is a slowly progressive neoplastic proliferation of T-lymphocytes. The disease presents with skin involvement and may remain confined there for years but in time spreads to other organs. Skin lesions are destructive. Biopsy reveals an indurated plaque with a mixed infiltrate in the upper dermis near the epidermal basement membrane. Histology is classified in lecture 24.

As the disease progresses, nodules and fungating tumors develop in the skin, and histiocytic proliferation spreads to lymph nodes, lung, spleen, liver, bone marrow, and myocardium.

2. Sézary's syndrome

Sézary's syndrome is a rare chronic disorder that is associated with diffuse erythroderma that is progressive and pruritic, exfoliative lesions, and lymphadenopathy. Characteristics of Sézary cells are described in lecture 24. Unlike the abnormal lymphocyte of CLL, which is a B cell, this a T cell. Skin biopsy reveals an upper dermal infiltrate somwhat like that of mycosis fungoides. The T cell in both mycosis fungoides and Sézary's syndrome is usually of the helper subset (T4).

3. Waldenström's macroglobinemia

This IgM gammopathy is a form of non-Hodgkin's lymphoma. It is discussed in lectures 24 and 25.

4. Hairy cell leukemia

This disorder, also known as **leukemic reticuloendotheliosis**, is characterized by pancytopenia, massive splenomegaly, and a diagnostic bone marrow pattern. The marrow aspirate is dry and the biopsy shows myelofibrosis with "hairy cell" infiltration. It is often temporarily controlled by splenectomy alone. The "hairy cells" are immunologically similar to CLL cells, that is, they are B cells in more than 90% of cases and are positive for **tartrate-resistant acid phosphatase** (TRAP) (see figure 23.2B).

SELECTED REFERENCES

Reviews

Armitage, J. O., and Gale, R. P. Bone marrow autotransplantation. *Am. J. Med.* 86(1989): 203–206.

Cheson, B. D., Lacerna, L., et al. Autologous bone marrow transplantation: current status and future directions. *Ann. Intern. Med.* 110(1989): 51–65.

Bennett, J. M., Foon, K. A., et al. *Immunologic Approaches to the Classification and Management of Lymphomas and Leukemias.* Boston: Kluwer Academic Publishers, 1988.

Portlock, C. S. Non-Hodgkin's lymphomas: advances in diagnosis, staging, and management. *Cancer* 65 Suppl. (1990): 718–722.

Rosenberg, S. A. Hodgkin's disease: challenges for the future. *Cancer Res.* 49(1989): 767–769.

Rowley, J. D. Recurring chromosome abnormalities in leukemia and lymphoma. *Semin. Hematol.* 27(1990): 122–136.

Samuels, B. L., and Ultmann, J. E. Lymphomas—current progress and future directions. *Perspect. Biol. Med.* 32(1989): 513–525.

Original articles

Bermudez, M. A., Grant, K. M., et al. Non-Hodgkin's lymphoma in a population with or at risk for acquired immunodeficiency syndrome: indications for intensive chemotherapy. *Am J. Med.* 86(1989): 71–76.

Bookman, M. A., Lardelli, P., et al. Lymphocytic lymphoma of intermediate differentiation: morphologic, immunophenotypic, and prognostic factors. *JNCI* 82(1990): 742–748.

Colombat, P., Gorin, N.-C., et al. The role of autologous bone marrow transplantation in 46 adult patients with non-Hodgkin's lymphomas. *J. Clin. Oncol.* 8(1990): 630–637.

Fenaux, P., Lai, J. L., et al. Burkitt cell acute leukaemia (L3 ALL) in adults: a report of 18 cases. *Br. J. Haematol.* 71(1989): 371–376.

Formenti, S. C., Gill, P. S., et al. Primary central nervous system lymphoma in AIDS: results of radiation therapy. *Cancer* 63(1989): 1101–1107.

Freedman, A. S., Takvorian, T., et al. Autologous bone marrow transplantation in B-cell non-Hodgkin's lymphoma: very low treatment-related mortality in 100 patients in sensitive relapse. *J. Clin. Oncol.* 8(1990): 784–791.

Gobbi, P. G., Dionigi, P., et al. The role of surgery in the multimodal treatment of primary gastric non-Hodgkin's lymphomas: a report of 76 cases and review of the literature. *Cancer* 65(1990): 2528–2536.

Lavey, R. S., Eby, N. L., et al. Impact on second malignancy risk of the combined use of radiation and chemotherapy for lymphomas. *Cancer* 66(1990): 80–88.

McManaway, M. E., Neckers, L. M., et al. Tumour-specific inhibition of lymphoma growth by an antisense oligodeoxynucleotide. *Lancet* 335(1990): 808–811.

Pals, S. T., Horst, E., et al. Expression of lymphocyte homing receptor as a mechanism of dissemination of non-Hodgkin's lymphoma. *Blood* 73(1989): 885–888.

Petersen, F. B., Appelbaum, F. R., et al. Autologous marrow transplantation for malignant lymphoma: a report of 101 cases from Seattle. *J. Clin. Oncol.* 8(1990): 638–647.

Sparano, J., Ramirez, M., et al. Increasing recognition of corticosteroid-induced tumor lysis syndrome in non-Hodgkin's lymphoma. *Cancer* 65(1990): 1072–1073.

Preijers, F. W. M. B., De Witte, T., et al. Autologous transplantation of bone marrow purged in vitro with anti-CD7-(WT1-) ricin A immunotoxin in T-cell lymphoblastic leukemia and lymphoma. *Blood* 74(1989): 1152–1158.

Veerman, A. J. P., and Pieters, R. Drug sensitivity assays in leukaemia and lymphoma. *Br. J. Haematol.* 74(1990): 381–384.

LECTURE 24

The Malignant Lymphomas II. Pathology

Nancy L. Harris

EDITOR'S COMMENT

This lecture lays out the maturation stages of lymphoid and mononuclear cells, emphasizing their characteristic surface markers and morphology. It then argues that the various lymphomas and leukemias are in fact proliferations or expansions of different stages along the developmental sequence. For example, molecular biology has now revealed the B or T cell origin of lymphoid neoplasms, thus permitting their classification as distinct maturational stages of B or T cell development. By the ordered sequence of IgG rearrangement, it has become clear that acute lymphocytic leukemia and the lymphoid blast crisis of chronic myelocytic leukemia are developmental stages of B cell precursors and that the IgG rearrangment pattern unique to each tumor serves as a marker with which to follow its course and search for low levels of residual tumor after therapy. Pursuing this theme, Dr. Harris offers a complete and valuable classification of these complex disorders.

I. INTRODUCTION

Malignant lymphomas are neoplasms of the cells that consitute the immune system. Although they usually arise in lymph nodes, they may occur in extranodal sites as well. Whereas normal immunologic responses involve many types of cells (i.e., they are histologically **polymorphous**), neoplasms ordinarily involve proliferation of a single cell type (i.e., they are **monomorphous** or **clonal**). In normal immunologic responses, cellular proliferation occurs in an orderly fashion in certain compartments of the lymphoid tissues. Lymphomas, in contrast, do not respect these compartments. Thus the diagnosis of lymphoma is based on two major observations: (1) **cellular composition** and (2) **architectural pattern**. These two features distinguish reactive from neoplastic lymphoid proliferations. Lymphomas are generally classified according to the normal cell counterpart that appears to be proliferating.

Understanding lymphomas is enhanced by understanding the normal immune system. The development of immunologic markers for different subtypes of lymphoid cells has facilitated diagnosis, classification, and correlation of neoplastic lymphoid cells with their normal counterparts. Since lymphomas appear to represent clones of lymphocytes arrested at particular stages of differentiation, studies of lymphoma cells have helped in elucidating the normal pathways of lymphocyte differentiation.

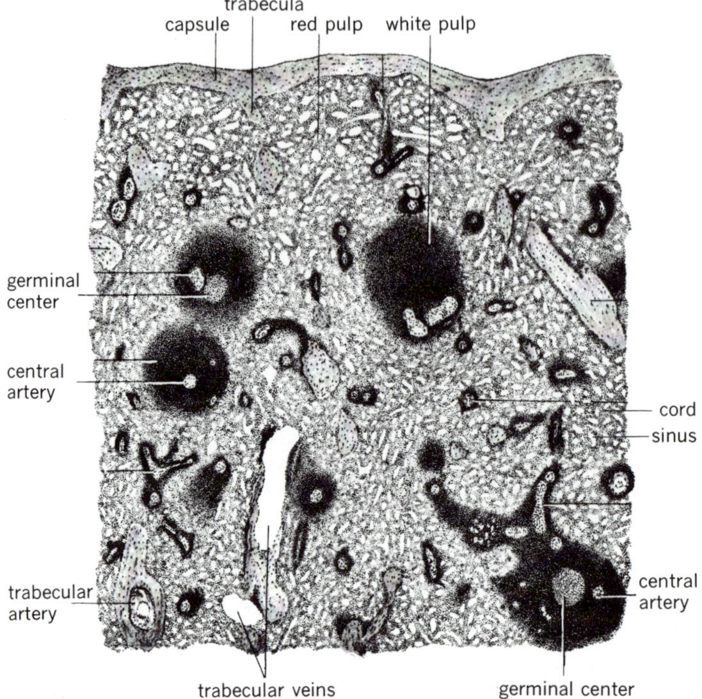

Fig. 24.1
Normal lymph node architecture. The cortex contains follicles with germinal centers. These are B cell regions. The paracortex just under the capsule contains predominantly T cells. The medulla and its cords contain a mixture of T and B cells and plasma cells, and the medullary sinuses contain phagocytic histiocytes as well as some lymphocytes. (Compare with figures 3.3 and 3.4.)

II. REVIEW OF THE IMMUNE SYSTEM

A. Architecture of normal lymph node

As noted in lecture 3 (see figure 3.4), the normal lymph node has three compartments (figure 24.1). The **cortex** is the subcapsular zone that contains primary follicles and germinal centers; this is a B cell area. The **paracortex** is the space between and deep to the follicles; this is primarily a T cell area. The **medulla** is between the paracortex and the hilus of the node; it contains the medullary cords (T and B cells, plasma cells) and medullary sinuses (histiocytes).

B. Lymphoid cells

1. Immunologic surface markers

Individual B and T lymphoid cells can be recognized by the presence of surface or cytoplasmic molecules (antigens) that can be detected with antibodies bearing fluorescent or enzymatic labels. At various stages of differentiation, lymphoid cells undergo changes in both morphology and surface antigen expression, which are characteristic for each stage. These features identify both normal and neoplastic lymphoid cells in tissue sections. The constellation of antigens expressed by a cell at a given time is called its **immunophenotype**. Nomenclature for many of the antigens detected by more than one monoclonal antibody has been standardized in the form of **cluster designations** (CD). Antigens relevant to lymphomas are summarized in Table 24.1.

Immunophenotyping can be done on either viable cell suspensions or fresh-frozen or paraffin-embedded tissue sections, using either polyclonal or monoclonal antibodies. Cell suspension analysis is best suited to cells that naturally occur in suspension (i.e., blood cells), while tissue section analysis is preferable for many biopsy specimens. Although some antigens can be detected on formalin-fixed, paraffin-embedded tissue sections of the sort used for routine histologic diagnosis, most lymphocyte-associated antigens detected by currently available monoclonal antibodies do not survive this processing. Thus whenever a biopsy is performed on a lesion suspected of being lymphoma, fresh tissue should be obtained for immunophenotyping studies.

Immunophenotyping studies can be useful in the diagnosis and classification of lymphoid neoplasia in the following circumstances (Table 24.2):

- Distinguishing between benign and malignant lymphoid infiltrates
- Distinguishing between lymphoma and nonlymphoid tumor
- Subclassification of lymphoma
- Subclassification of leukemia

The panel of antigens to be analyzed varies with the specific differential diagnosis (table 24.3).

2. *Genotypic markers*

B cell differentiation involves rearrangements of the genes responsible for immunoglobulin production. Those that encode the constant and variable regions of the immunoglobulin heavy and light chains are located far apart on the chromosomes in germline cells. In order to produce mRNA for an immunoglobulin protein, many thousands of DNA base pairs must be deleted to bring different portions of the immunoglobulin gene together. These rearrangements change the position on the DNA of restriction sites (points at which restriction endonucleases cleave DNA). Thus, fragments produced by digesting B cell DNA with these enzymes will be of a different size than those produced by digesting non-B cell (germline) DNA, and will migrate differently in an electrophoresis gel. When radiolabeled DNA probes (cloned segments of DNA produced by bacteria) that are complementary to specific portions of the immunoglobulin gene are applied to such a gel, they will specifically mark the position of the immunoglobulin gene, which can be demonstrated on an autoradiograph. The exact size, and therefore position on the gel (Southern blot), of each immunoglobulin

Table 24.1
Some Antigens of Interest in the Study of Lymphoid Neoplasms

CD	Other/Names	Antigen mol. wt. (Kd)	Spectrum of reactivity
CD1	T6, OKT6, Leu6, NA1/34	45	Thymocyte/Langerhans
CD2	T11, OKT11, 9.6, Leu5	50	Pan-T (E rosette receptor)
CD3	T3, OKT3, Leu4	19, 29	Pan-T (T receptor related)
CD4	T4, OKT4, Leu3	55	T helper (MHC II cytotoxic)
CD5	OKT1, Leu1	67	Pan-T, rare B
CD6	T12, TU33	120	Pan-T, rare B
CD7	Leu9, TU14, 3A1	41	Pan-T
CD8	T8, OKT8, Leu2	32	T suppressor (MHC I cytotoxic)
CD9	J2, BA2	24	T, B, myeloid
CD10	J5, BA3, VilA1	100	Pre-B, pre-T, GC (CALLA)
CD15	Leu-M1	—	Granulocyte, monocyte, RS cells, epithelial cells
CD19	B4	95	Pan-B (not PC)
CD20	B1	35	Pan-B (not PC)
CD21	B2	145	Restricted B: PB, GC, MZ; FDC
CD22	Leu 14, (To15), SHCL1	135	Pan-B
CD23	Tu1, Blast 2	45	Restricted B: MZ, ?GC, not PB
CD24	BA1	45, 55, 65	Pan B; granulocyte; PC
CD25	TAC, ANTI ILR	55	Activated T + B (Anti-IL2 receptor)
—	TdT		B and T precursors, cortical thymocyte
—	HLA-DR (Ia-like)		B (not PC), activated T (MHC class II antigen)
CD30	Ki-1, Ber H2	—	RS cells, activated T and B cells
CD45	LCA, T29/33, PD7/26	200	Leukocyte common antigen (T, B, M)

Abbreviations: CALLA, common acute lymphoblastic leukemia antigen; CD, cluster designation; FDC, follicular dendritic cells; Gc, germinal center; IL2, interleukin-2; Kd, kilodaltons; MHC, major histocompatibility complex; MZ, mantle zone; PB, peripheral blood; PC, plasma cell; RS, Reed-Sternberg; TdT, terminal deoxynucleotidyl transferase.

Table 24.2
Major Categories of Lymphoproliferative Diseases Now Recognizable by Morphology and Immunologic Markers

Name	Morphologic features	Markers
Hodgkin's disease	Reed-Sternberg cells, reactive cells	Mixed T and B cells, RS cells, CD30+, CD 25+, CD15+, CD45−, Ia+
B cell neoplasms		
B-precursor lymphoblastic lymphoma/leukemia (ALL/LBL)	Lymphoblasts; medium-sized cells, dispersed chromatin, inconspicuous nucleoli, scant cytoplasm	TdT+, CD10+, Cmu+ (Ig gene rearrangement), pan-B+
Burkitt's and Burkitt-like lymphomas	Medium-sized cells, multiplc nucleoli, basophilic cytoplasm, "starry sky," high mitotic rate	SIg+, CD10+, pan-B+
Small lymphocytic lymphoma/B-chronic lymphocytic leukemia (SLL/CLL)	Small lymphocytes	SIgM+D+, CD5+(CLL), pan-B+
Plasmacytoid lymphocytic lymphoma (PLL)	Plasmacytoid lymphocytes, plasma cells, lymphocytes	SIgM+CIg+ (M-component), pan-B+
Centrocytic lymphoma (diffuse small cleaved, intermediate cell)	Small cleaved follicular center cells	SIg+, M+D, CD5+, pan-B+
Germinal center lymphoma (follicular lymphomas)	Mixture of follicular center cells, usually follicular pattern	SIg+, CD10+, pan-B+
Large cell lymphoma (immunoblastic, centroblastic [noncleaved])	Monomorphous large cells, prominent nucleoli, basophilic cytoplasm, high mitotic rate	SIg+(+CIg), pan-B+
Hairy cell leukemia (HCL)	Small lymphocytes, "hairy" cytoplasm	SIg+, pan-B+
Plasmacytoma, multiple myeloma	Plasma cells, plasmablasts	CIg+(G/A), pan-B−, HLA-DR, CD45−
T cell neoplasms		
T-lymphoblastic lymphoma/leukemia (T-ALL/LBL)	Lymphoblasts: medium-sized cells, nuclear convolution, inconspicuous nucleoli	TdT+, pan-T+, CD1, 4, 8+
T-chronic lymphocytic leukemia (T-CLL)	Small lymphoid cells with convoluted nuclei, granular cytoplasm	Pan-T+, CD4+ or CD8+, TdT−, CD1−
Large cell lymphoma (T-LCL, IBL)	Immunoblasts (similar to B-large cell lymphomas)	TdT−, pan-T+, CD4+ or CD8+
Adult T cell lymphoma/leukemia (ATL-L)	Variable proportions of atypical lymphocytes and immunoblasts	Pan-T+, CD4+, TdT−, HTLV-I+
Pleomorphic T cell lymphomas (nonendemic)	Like ATL/L	Pan-T+, CD4+ or CDB+
Mycosis fungoides (MF)	Small and large lymphoid cells with "cerebriform" nuclei	Pan-T+, CD4, TdT−

Abbreviations are defined in the text.

Table 24.3
Clinical Application of Immunophenotyping

Differential diagnosis	Antibody panel
Reactive vs. neoplastic lymphoid proliferations	Immunoglobulin light chains
Lymphoma vs. nonlymphoid tumor	Leukocyte common antigen, immunoglobulin, pan-B and pan-T markers, cytokeratin
Subclassification of lymphomas	Immunoglobulin heavy and light chains, pan-B and pan-T antibodies, TdT, CD10 (lymphoblasts), T/B subset antibodies, CD15, 30, 45 (Hodgkin's disease)
Subclassification of leukemias	TdT, CD10, myeloperoxidase, lysozyme, myeloid antigens, pan-T, pan-B, immunoglobulin

gene fragment is unique to an individual B cell; thus this technique provides not only a specific marker for B cells, but also a true marker for monoclonality.

An analogous process occurs in T cell differentiation, involving the DNA encoding T cell specific surface molecules. These serve as the T cell receptor for antigen and are analogous to surface immunoglobulin (SIg) on B cells. As in the B cell system, the size of restriction fragments of the DNA encoding the T cell receptor gene are specific for a single clone of T cells. Thus T cell receptor gene rearrangement is a specific marker for T cells, and also a true marker for monoclonality in T cells.

In addition to lineage-specific gene rearrangements, specific chromosomal translocations occur in certain lymphoid malignancies. In some cases, translocations involve oncogenes. For example,

- In Burkitt's lymphoma, a translocation involving chromosome 8 snd 14 moves the *c-myc* oncogene into the immunoglobulin heavy chain locus.
- In follicular lymphomas, a putative oncogene, *bcl-2*, is moved from chromosome 18 to the same region of chromosome 14.

Overexpression of these genes in abnormal loci may contribute to neoplastic transformation of the cell.

Genotyping studies have begun to find application in the diagnosis and classification of lymphoid neoplasms. Detection of clonal T cell receptor or immunoglobulin gene rearrangement can confirm T or B cell malignancy. Specific oncogene rearrangements can suggest specific lymphoma subtypes and by polymerase chain reactions can detect early lymphoma relapse.

3. Pathways of lymphocyte differentiation

As shown in figure 1.1, a common stem cell (CFU-LM) is believed to give rise to both lymphoid and myeloid cells (figure 24.2). A common lymphoid stem cell is postulated to give rise to the T and B cell lines. There are two distinct phases of development within both T and B cell lines: **antigen-independent** and **antigen-dependent**.

a. ANTIGEN-INDEPENDENT DIFFERENTIATION

Antigen-independent proliferation and differentiation occur in the primary lymphoid organs—bursa-equivalent (?bone marrow) and thymus—*without* exposure to antigen. This process takes the lymphocyte from a stem cell to a mature, "virgin," or unstimulated T or B cell that is capable of responding to antigen but has not yet been exposed to it.

b. ANTIGEN-DEPENDENT DIFFERENTIATION

Antigen-dependent differentiation and proliferation occur in peripheral lymphoid tissues. On encountering an antigen that fits its surface receptor, the mature T or B cell undergoes **blastic transformation**, proliferates, and differentiates further into an antigen-specific effector cell. Also from this reaction, antigen-specific "memory" is generated—cells that are capable of an accelerated response on reexposure to the same antigen. Thus in both T and B cell systems, there are several stages of development at which proliferation occurs, as well as several resting stages.

In the following sections, each of the two modes of development will be described separately.

c. B CELLS

(1) Antigen-independent differentiation

The following sequence occurs:

- The earliest B cells are bone marrow **lymphoblasts** that contain TdT, have rearranged Ig genes but do not make Ig, and express HLA-DR antigen and CALLA (CD10).
- Later, at the **pre-B cell** stage, cytoplasmic μ heavy chain appears. **Neoplastic counterpart**: "common," "null," or B-precursor acute lymphoblastic leukemia/lymphoblastic lymphoma.
- Still later, at the **"early" B cell** stage, a complete surface IgM molecule is expressed, with either κ or λ light chain. This cell no longer expresses TdT. **Neoplastic counterpart**: ?Burkitt's lymphoma.
- Early B cells mature into **virgin B cells**, small lymphocytes with both SIgM and IgD, and possibly CD5, that are found in primary lymph node follicles and in the blood. **Neoplastic counterpart**: B-CLL, small lymphocytic lymphoma.

Each individual B cell is committed to a single light chain, either κ or λ, and all of its progeny express the same light chain. Reactive, polyclonal

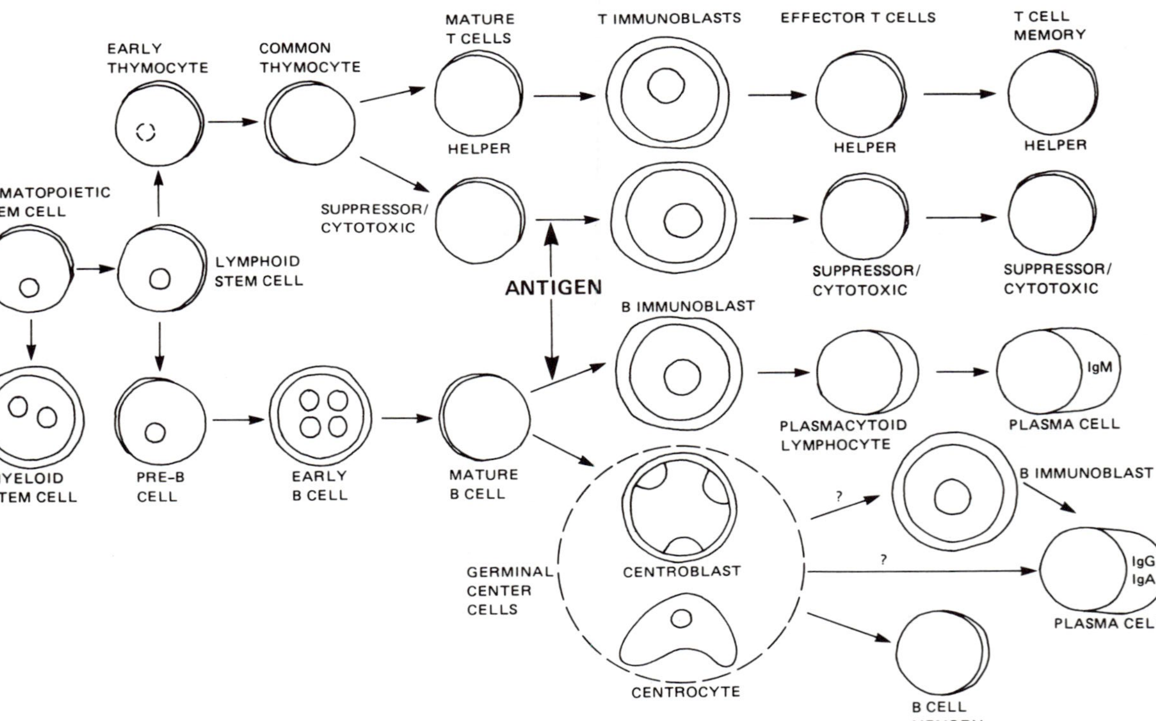

Fig. 24.2A
Hypothetical scheme of lymphocyte differentiation.

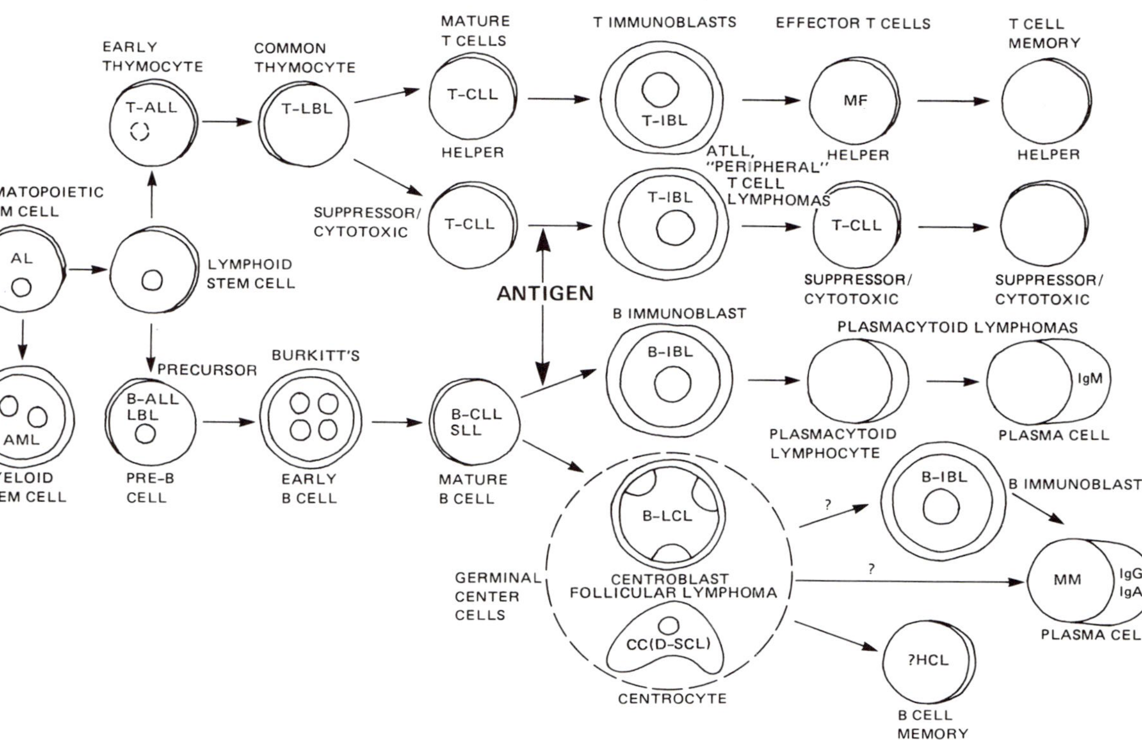

Fig. 24.2*B*
Scheme of lymphocyte differentiation showing lymphoid neoplasms corresponding to each stage (see text for abbreviations).

populations of B cells contain mixtures of cells, some with κ and some with λ light chains. Neoplastic populations are clones of a single precursor cell and express only the light chain of the progenitor cell, either κ or λ, not both. Thus, light chain restriction in a population of B cells indicates monoclonality and, in most cases, neoplasia.

(2) Antigen-dependent differentiation

Antigen-dependent B cell differentiation can take two forms.

- In the early **primary response**, the virgin B cell transforms into an **immunoblast**, a large proliferating cell with a prominent central nucleolus and abundant, basophilic cytoplasm. **Neoplastic counterpart**: large cell lymphoma, immunoblastic. These cells mature into **plasma cells**, which lose surface antigens, including pan-B cell antigens, HLA-DR, and leukocyte common antigen, as cytoplasmic IgM accumulates and proliferation ceases. These cells produce the IgM of the early immune response. This reaction occurs in the paracortex and medulla of lymph nodes. **Neoplastic counterpart**: plasmacytoid lymphocytic lymphoma.
- In the **late primary** or **secondary immune response**, the B cell encounters antigen presented on the processes of dendritic cells of the primary follicle. The germinal center reaction gives rise to a better-fitting IgG antibody. The switch from IgM to IgG (or IgA) production involves heavy chain class switching that occurs in individual B cells. These cells continue to express the same light chain (κ or λ). IgD is lost on blastic transformation. Germinal center B cells continue to express pan-B antigens, leukocyte common antigen, and HLA-DR; CD5 may be expressed by some cells.

The earliest cells seen in germinal centers are large cells with round clear nuclei, one to three peripherally located nucleoli, and a narrow rim of basophilic cytoplasm. These are termed **enteroblasts** or large **noncleaved follicular center cells. Neoplastic counterpart**: large cell lymphoma, centroblastic or noncleaved type.

Later in the germinal center reaction, cells with irregular, cleaved nuclei appear. These are termed **centrocytes** or **cleaved follicle center cells. Neoplastic counterpart**: centrocytic or diffuse cleaved cell lymphoma. Follicular lymphomas contain both centroblasts and centrocytes in varying proportions. The precise pathways and relationships between different follicle center cells, immunoblasts, and plasma cells are not understood.

With differentiation of the mature plasma cell, there is sequential loss of surface immunoglobulin, pan-B cell antigens, HLA-DR antigen, and CD45, and cytoplasmic IgG or IgA accumulates. These **plasma cells** produce the better-fitting IgG antibody of the later primary or secondary immune response. **Neoplastic counterpart**: multiple myeloma, plasmacytoma (see lecture 25).

d. T CELLS

(1) Antigen-independent differentiation

The following stages occur:

- The earliest T cells are bone marrow and thymic **lymphoblasts** that express TdT and CD2; at the cortical thymocyte stage they express CD1 and both CD4 and CD8, and variably express pan-T cell antigens. **Neoplastic counterpart**: T-lymphoblastic lymphoma/acute lymphoblastic leukemia.
- **Virgin T cells** are small lymphocytes that are found in the thymic medulla, lymph nodes, or blood. They lack TdT and CD1 and express either CD4 or CD8, not both, as well as pan-T cell antigens. **Neoplastic counterpart**: ?T-chronic lymphocytic leukemia.

(2) Antigen-dependent differentiation

The following stages occur.

- On encountering antigen, mature T cells transform into **immunoblasts**, large cells with prominent nucleoli and basophilic cytoplasm, which may be indistinguishable from B immunoblasts. T immunoblasts, in contrast to T lymphoblasts (thymocytes), are TdT and CD1 negative, strongly express pan-T cell antigens, and express either CD4 or CD8, not both, as well as HLA-DR. Antigen-dependent T cell reactions occur in the paracortex of lymph nodes and the periarteriolar lymphoid sheath of the spleen. **Neoplastic counterpart**: T-immunoblastic lymphoma.
- T-immunoblasts differentiate into **antigen-specific effector cells** of either CD4 or CD8 type, which may help or suppress the function of B cells or other T cells, and are cytotoxic toward certain types of cells. **Neoplastic counterpart**: mycosis fungoides/Sézary syndrome [CD4], adult T cell lymphoma/leukemia [CD4], other "peripheral" T cell lymphomas.

III. FEATURES OF LYMPHOMAS

As noted in lecture 23, lymphomas are divided into Hodgkin's disease and the non-Hodgkin's lymphomas. With the use of a combination of morphologic features, clinical information, and immunologic studies, we can now recognize at least 13 types of lymphomas, as well as Hodgkin's disease. Non-Hodgkin's lymphomas differ from one another as much as they do from Hodgkin's disease and thus are distinct entities. The different classification schemes lump and split these entities in a variety of ways, and the current state of the art has not produced an ultimately satisfactory lymphoma classification. In the United States, lymphomas are classified for clinical purposes according to the NCI "Working Formulation" (see table 23.6).

Hence we will simply list the lymphomas that can be recognized at present. These are given in summary form in table 23.6.

The following sections summarize morphologic and clinical features of each disease and attempt, to the extent possible, to place each in a scheme of lymphocyte differentiation, as shown in figure 24.2. The lymphomas are listed in order of their putative positions along the B and T cell differentiation pathways. Lymphomas and lymphoid leukemias are discussed together; the distinction between them is artificial, since many lymphomas can have a leukemic phase, and diseases usually classified as leukemia may not have circulating malignant cells in all cases.

A. Hodgkin's disease

1. Immunology and cell of origin

The malignant cell of Hodgkin's disease is believed to be the **Reed-Sternberg cell** and its mononuclear variants. Its lineage remains obscure. Some believe it arises from either the lymphocyte or the histiocyte/macrophage line, but definitive evidence is lacking.

The neoplastic-appearing cells of all but lymphocyte-predominant Hodgkin's disease lack specific T and B cell markers, as well as the leukocyte common antigen. They express HLA-DR, the granulocyte associated antigen CD15, and CD30, an "activation" antigen. Recently, rearrangements of both T cell receptor and immunoglobulin genes have been reported in selected cases of Hodgkin's disease and in cell lines derived from tumors. In lymphocytic predominant Hodgkin's disease, the atypical cells express B lineage antigens. The infiltrating lymphocytes consist of T cells with an "activated" phenotype, and polyclonal B cells. No single marker is diagnostic of Hodgkin's disease. Hence, the diagnosis rests primarily on morphologic criteria.

2. Morphology

The morphology of Hodgkin's disease differs strikingly from that of non-Hodgkin's lymphomas, which usually consist of a relatively uniform population of neoplastic lymphoid cells. In Hodgkins's disease the neoplastic cells comprise a minority of the cells in the infiltrate, the bulk of which is usually made up of reactive lymphocytes, histiocytes, fibroblasts, eosinophils, and plasma cells. The diagnosis of Hodgkin's disease rests on finding Reed-Sternberg cells in the appropriate cellular background. Diagnostic Reed-Sternberg cells are large cells (25–50 μm in diameter) with bilobed or double nuclei, with at least two prominent inclusion-like nucleoli (figure 24.3). The symmetrical double nuclei, each with its nucleolus, give the cell a characteristic "owl's eye" appearance. Mononuclear cells with similar nucleoli are also found. These are also believed to be malignant; however, since they are not reliably distinguishable from benign immunoblasts, they are not in themselves diagnotic of Hodgkin's disease.

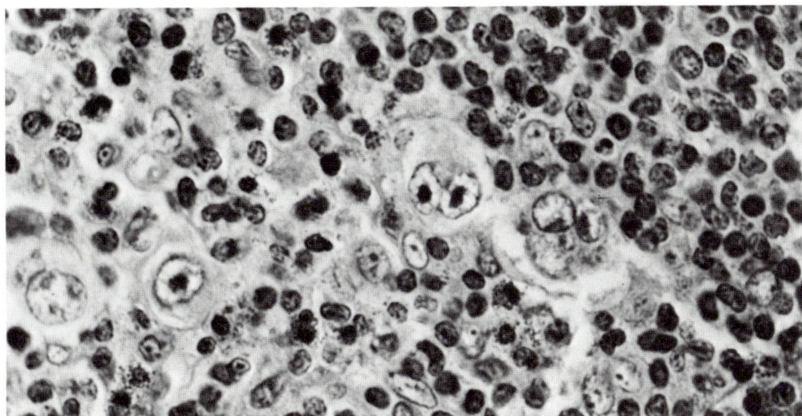

Fig. 24.3
Reed-Sternberg cell. The bilobed nucleus and double nucleoli give the cell an "owl-eye" appearance.

Table 24.4
Histologic Classification of Hodgkin's Disease

Type	Histologic characteristics	Prognosis	Approximate median survival (yrs)
Lymphocytic predominance	Lymphocytes, histiocytes	Most favorable	8
Nodular sclerosis	Fibrous bands, lacunar cells	Favorable	4
Mixed cellularity	Eosinophils, plasma cells	Intermediate	2.5
Lymphocytic depletion	Predominance of Reed-Sternberg cells, diffuse fibrosis	Least favorable	1.5

3. Classification

As shown in table 24.4, four histologic types of Hodgkin's disease are recognized by the relative proportions of Reed-Sternberg cells, lymphocytes, other inflammatory cells, and fibrosis.

- **In lymphocytic predominance**, lymphocytes are numerous, and Reed-Sternberg cells are hard to find.
- In **mixed cellularity**, Reed-Sternberg cells are easily found, and the infiltrate contains numerous eosinophils and plasma cells, in addition to lymphocytes.
- In **lymphocytic depletion**, Reed-Sternberg cells and atypical mononuclear cells constitute the predominant cells, and there is diffuse fibrosis.
- In **nodular sclerosis**, a special type of Hodgkin's disease most common in young adults, dense, fibrous bands divide the tumor into nodules (figure 24.4). It is also characterized by a particular multinucleated variant of the Reed-Sternberg cell, called the **lacunar cell**.

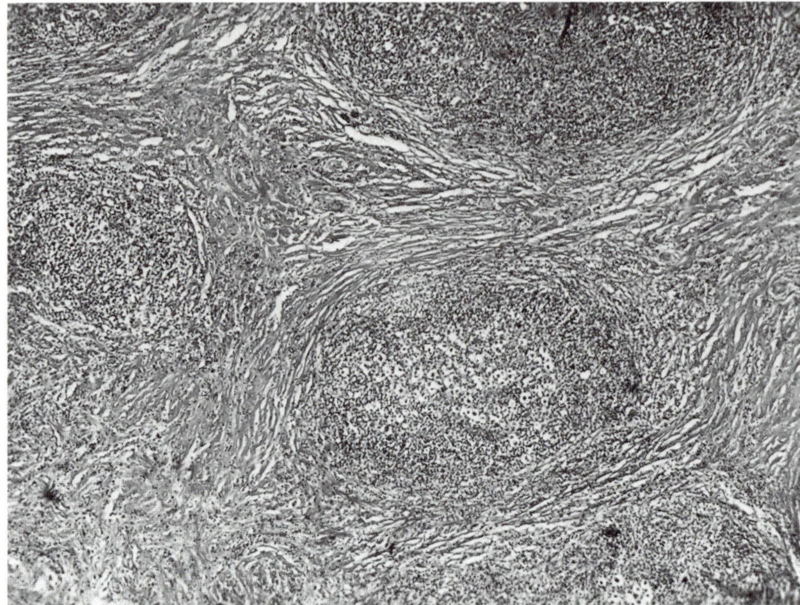

Fig. 24.4
Hodgkin's disease, nodular sclerosis type. Fibrous bands divide the tumor into nodules.

4. Clinical correlations

Prior to advances in therapy, the prognosis of Hodgkin's disease was related to the histologic type, with lymphocytic predominance the most indolent and mixed cellularity and lymphocytic depletion more aggressive. Improvements in the therapy have obscured these differences. In current practice the major determinant of treatment and survival is the stage of the disease at diagnosis. For this reason there is little current controversy about subclassification.

With increased survival due to improved therapy, two recent complications have been seen: acute nonlymphocytic leukemias (ANLL) and non-Hodgkin's lymphomas. The ANLL appear related to the use of combined modality therapy (radiation therapy plus chemotherapy with alkylating agents). The non-Hodgkin's lymphomas—usually Burkitt-like or immunoblastic—may result from the immunosuppressed state associated with either Hodgkin's disease or cytotoxic therapy.

B. B cell neoplasms

1. B-precursor lymphoblastic lymphoma/leukemia (ALL/LBL)

In childhood ALL, 80% of cases lack either surface immunoglobulin or the E-rosette receptor. About 30% of these so-called null lymphoblastic leukemias have cytoplasmic μ chains (Cμ) and are therefore pre-B cells. More recently the majority of both Cμ+ and Cμ− ALL have been shown to react with monoclonal antibodies to B cells and to display immunoglobulin gene arrangement. Therefore the cells of most "null" ALL are primitive B cell precursors, which are TdT positive. Neoplasms of null and pre-B cell types usually present with diffuse bone marrow involvement and an elevated leukocyte count (common in children, infrequent in adults). Occasionally neoplasms of these cells present as a solitary tumor of bone or other sites. These are termed **null lymphoblastic lymphomas**.

2. *Burkitt's tumor and Burkitt-like lymphomas*

a. IMMUNOLOGY AND CELL OF ORIGIN

The position of these tumors in the B cell differentiation pathway is controversial. Cells resembling Burkitt's tumor cells are not readily identified in normal lymphoid tissues. Occasional germinal center cells, particularly in children, may resemble Burkitt's tumor cells. African Burkitt's tumor and non-African cases of similar histology invariably have surface immunoglobulin, usually IgM with κ light chains, but occasionally λ. In contrast to pre-B cell neoplasms. Burkitt's tumor is TdT negative. As noted above, the chromosome translocation (8 : 14) found in the majority of the cases involves translocation of a cellular oncogene (*c-myc*) from chromosome 8 to the Ig heavy chain switch region, located on chromosome 14. Epstein-Barr virus (EBV) genomes can be demonstrated in the tumor cells in most African cases and occasionally in non-African cases.

b. MORPHOLOGY

Burkitt's tumor cells are similar in size to those of ALL—larger than normal circulating lymphocytes but smaller than immunoblasts and large follicular center cells. In typical Burkitt's tumors, the cells are uniform in size and shape; in Burkitt-like lymphomas, there is more variation in cell size and shape. The nuclei are round, with coarsely clumped, dark chromatin, multiple (two to five) nucleoli that tend to be central, and abundant cytoplasm that is basophilic on Giemsa stain. The cells are cohesive, and the abundant cytoplasm imparts a mosaic or pavement-like appearance to the infiltrate. Sharply defined cell borders are frequently seen. The mitotic rate is high and may exceed 20 per 40× field. A starry-sky pattern is usually present, imparted by numerous benign macrophages that have ingested nuclear debris.

c. CLINICAL FEATURES

Classic Burkitt's tumor is primarily a disease of childhood. In African (endemic) cases there is a predilection for involvement of the jaw and other facial bones. In American (nonendemic) cases, jaw tumors are uncommon. Over half of the cases present with abdominal tumors, most commonly involving the distal ileum and/or mesentery, ovaries, or kidneys. Burkitt's and Burkitt-like lymphomas account for approximately one-third of childhood non-Hodgkin's lymphomas in the United States. The M/F ratio is 2–3:1. A second peak of frequency is seen in older adults. These tumors are usually Burkitt-like. Approximately 10% of nonendemic cases have bone marrow involvement. A few present as acute leukemia with Burkitt's tumor cells (B-ALL). Untreated tumors are rapidly fatal, but the tumor is very sensitive to chemotherapy. Life-threatening tumor lysis syndrome may occur during treatment of patients with bulky disease. In children, if the tumor can be completely resected, the 2-year survival with chemotherapy may be as high as 80%. With bulky disease the survival drops to 40% at 2 years. There is no apparent different in survival between children with Burkitt and Burkitt-like lymphomas. Mortality in adults is higher. Tumors with this morphology are common in patients with the acquired immunodeficiency syndrome (AIDS).

3. Small lymphocytic lymphoma/B-chronic lymphocytic leukemia (B-CLL)

a. IMMUNOLOGY AND NORMAL CELLULAR COUNTERPART

Over 90% of cases of typical CLL are of B cell type, with faint SIg of IgM ± IgD type. The presence of both IgM and IgD in the majority of cases favors the idea that these are virgin B cells, since antigen-stimulated and memory B cells are thought not to have SIgD. In addition to B-lineage antigens, B-CLL cells express the pan-T antigen CD5.

b. MORPHOLOGY

Tissue involvement by small lymphocytic lymphoma is indistinguishable from CLL. A diagnosis of CLL requires peripheral lymphocytosis. Typical CLL produces a diffuse infiltrate in lymph nodes. The predominant cell may be slightly larger than a normal lymphocyte, with clumped chromatin and a round nucleus (figure 24.5A). Many mitotically active large lymphoid cells may be seen in lymph nodes involved with CLL. The number of large cells does not adversely affect prognosis, but a mitotic rate greater than 30 per high power field is associated with a short survival. Bone marrow involvement is common and may be focal or diffuse.

c. CLINICAL FEATURES

As discussed in lecture 22, CLL is predominantly a disease of older adults. It follows a protracted course, with gradual enlargement of lymph nodes and spleen and progressive marrow and organ infiltration. Blastic transformation, common in CML, is a rare but well-documented phenomenon termed **Richter's syndrome**.

B cell lymphomas of small lymphocytes without CLL may also occur. These may involve lymph nodes or extranodal sites, such as the orbit, lung, stomach, and skin, where they may be impossible to distinguish from benign lymphoid infiltrates without special studies to demonstrate monotype SIg. Some may develop CLL; others may not. Lymphomas of small B lymphocytes in extranodal sites are believed to arise from mucosa-associated lymphoid tissue (MALT).

4. Plasmacytoid lymphocytic lymphoma

a. IMMUNOLOGY AND CELL OF ORIGIN

Plasmacytoid lymphocytic lymphomas are tumors of lymphocytes that are capable of secreting Ig, usually IgM. Thus they are analogous to the effector cells of the primary immune response. In suspension the tumor cells have abundant SIgM, in contrast to the faint SIgM of CLL; IgD is lacking; in imprints or sections some cells also have cytoplasmic Ig.

b. MORPHOLOGY

The predominant cell is the small **plasmacytoid lymphocyte**. A varying number of cells have abundant basophilic cytoplasm but lymphocyte-like nuclei. Some cases have typical plasma cells in addition to these plasmacytoid lymphocytes.

c. CLINICAL FEATURES

They occur in the same general age group as CLL. Bone marrow is frequently involved, as are lymph nodes and spleen. Extranodal sites—especially orbit, lung, thyroid, salivary gland, and stomach (MALT)—may be involved. Leukemia may occur but is less common than in nonplasmacytoid lymphomas, and average total lymphocyte count is lower. A monoclonal serum protein, usually IgM, occurs in approximately half the cases (Waldenström's macroglobulinemia). Lymphomas that arise in patients with autoimmune disease—most notably Sjögren's syndrome and Hashimoto's thyroiditis—are characteristically of lymphoplasmacytoid type. Type I or type II cryoglobulinemia and/or Coombs-positive hemolytic anemia may be associated with the paraprotein. Like CLL, the disease may terminate in a large cell lymphoma.

5. Centrocytic lymphoma (diffuse, small cleaved cell)

a. IMMUNOLOGY AND CELL OF ORIGIN

This is a B cell tumor that is usually SIgM +, with or without IgD. Most cases express the CD5 pan-T antigen. The cell of origin is thought to be the small cleaved cell of the germinal center or inner mantle zone.

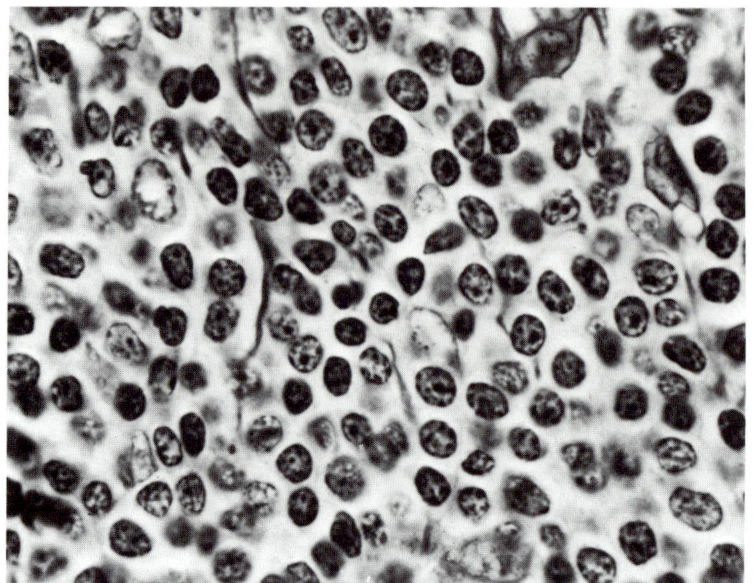

A

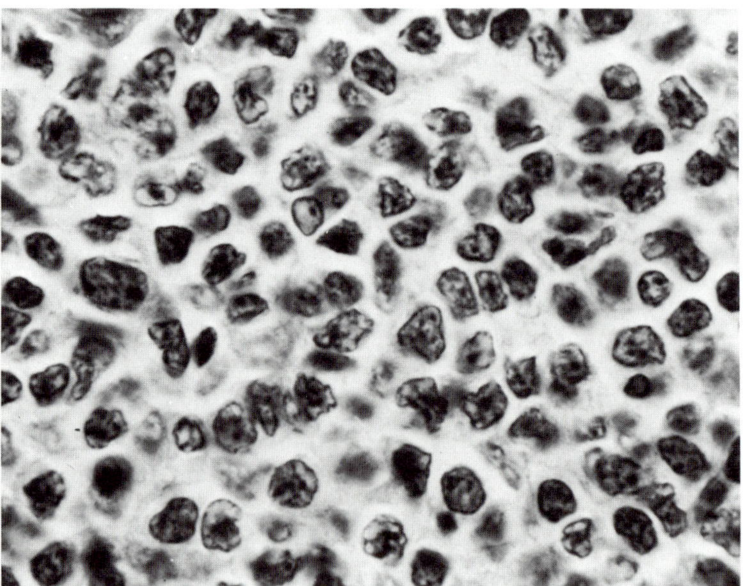

B

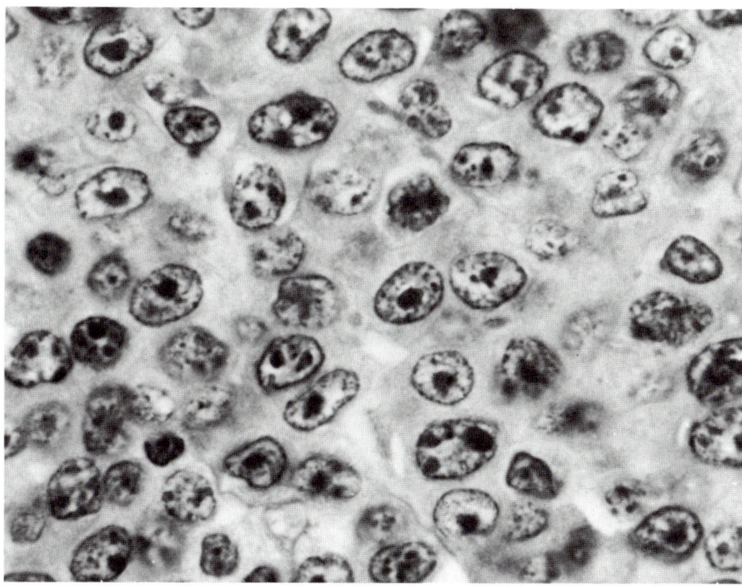

C

Fig. 24.5
Cytologic features of non-Hodgkin's lymphoma. *A*, Small lymphocytic lymphoma; *B*, Small cleaved cell lymphoma; *C*, Large cell lymphoma, immunoblastic. Lymphomas are subclassified on the basis of the size and shape of the nucleus, nucleoli, and cytoplasm.

b. MORPHOLOGY

The tumor is composed exclusively of small cleaved cells (figure 24.5B). In some cases the cells are very small, and some cells resemble small lymphocytes. Large noncleaved cells are rare or absent. The pattern is usually diffuse but may be vaguely nodular. Well-defined follicles as in follicular lymphomas are not seen. Marrow involvement and leukemia are frequent. The tumor in the marrow may be either focal and paratrabecular or diffuse. Marrow and blood involvement by centrocytic lymphoma may be indistinguishable from that by follicular lymphoma.

c. CLINICAL FEATURES

In contrast to follicular lymphomas, centrocytic lymphoma has a high male predominance, an increased frequency of extranodal involvement, and a relatively poor prognosis, with median survival in the range of 2–4 years instead of 7–9. Like follicular lymphomas, patients usually have widespread disease at presentation and a high incidence of peripheral blood involvement. The presence of leukemia does not adversely affect prognosis. The incidence of this tumor is higher in Europe, particularly in Italy than

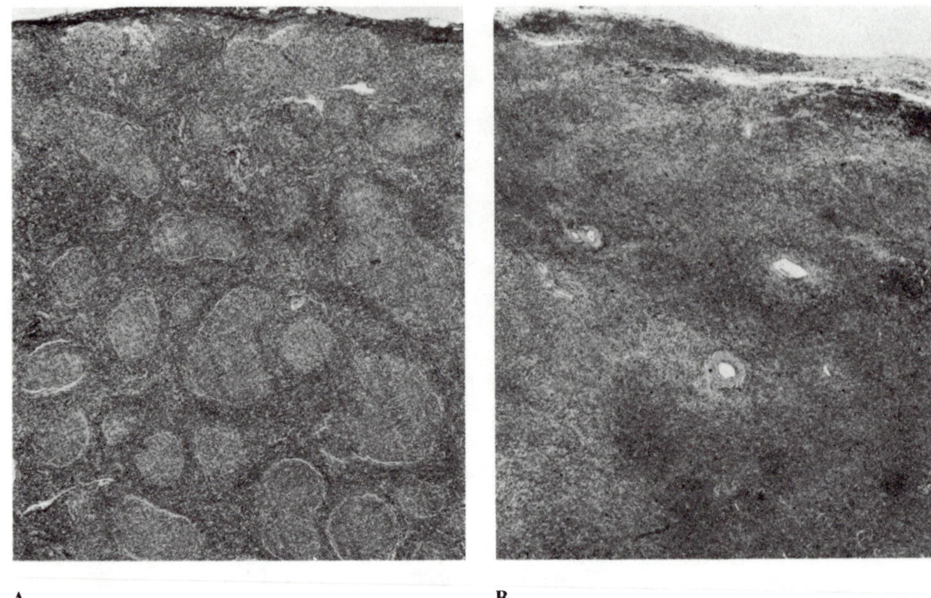

Fig. 24.6
Architectural features of non-Hodgkin's lymphoma. *A*, Follicular lymphoma. *B*, Diffuse large cell lymphoma. Note that the neoplastic infiltrates obliterate the normal nodal architecture. (Compare with figure 24.1.)

in the United States. Synonyms in the U.S. include intermediate lymphocytic lymphoma and diffuse small cleaved cell lymphoma.

6. Follicular lymphomas (nodular lymphomas)

a. IMMUNOLOGY AND CELL OF ORIGIN

Follicular lymphomas are germinal center B cell tumors (figure 24.6A). They are SIg+, having either IgM, IgG, or IgA.

b. MORPHOLOGY

Like germinal centers, follicular lymphomas are composed of a mixture of centrocytes and centroblasts. The predominant cell is usually a centrocyte, which may range in size from small to large. Centroblasts are in the minority but are always present. In most classification schemes, follicular lymphomas are classified according to the predominant cell type. However, 85% or more of the cases are of "small" or "mixed small and large" type; these have a very similar prognosis in most series.

Marrow involvement is frequent; tumor cell aggregates are characteristically paratrabecular. The follicular pattern may not be apparent on marrow biopsy, and the cells may appear smaller than in the node. Thus classification of lymphoma should not be attempted on marrow biopsy alone. The gross appearance of the enlarged spleen is shown in figure 24.7A.

Follicular lymphomas tend to progress to a larger cell type and/or a diffuse pattern. It is not uncommon to see variation in cytologic composition from one nodule to another in the same biopsy or from one biopsy to another in a given patient. If we think of the centroblast as the proliferating cell, which normally matures into centrocytes, then this natural history can be explained as follows. In the usual follicular lymphoma, the tumor cells retain their ability to mature all the way to centrocytes, and these cells tend to form follicles. Thus, only a few centroblasts remain. These are actively dividing. With time the tumor cells either gradually lose their ability to mature or begin to proliferate more rapidly, so that fewer centrocytes accumulate and the relative number of centroblasts increases. Concomitantly the tumor shows less tendency toward nodularity. Clinically the tumor becomes more aggressive, and histologically an increase in large noncleaved cells is seen. The overall picture is interpreted as progression from a follicular small cell or mixed lymphoma to diffuse large cell lymphoma, but in reality it represents only a transition to a more aggressive phase of the original tumor. The fact that in such cases the same immunoglobulin chains can be demonstrated on the original follicular lymphoma and on the subsequent diffuse large cell lymphoma supports this interpretation.

c. CLINICAL FEATURES

Follicular lymphomas are a distinct clinical entity. They consitute 40–50% of adult non-Hodgkin's lymphomas in the United States. The incidence is much lower in Europe. They are rare under age 20. The sex incidence is approximately equal. Patients present with painless adenopathy, which is frequently generalized yet asymptomatic. Involvement of the bone marrow is common at diagnosis, occurring in up to 75% of patients. Follicular lymphoma is a predominantly nodal disease, with less than 20% presenting in extranodal sites. The long natural history (7- to 8-year median survival) appears largely unaffected by treatment.

7. *Large cell lymphoma*

a. IMMUNOLOGY AND CELL OF ORIGIN

Up to 80% of tumors designated histiocytic lymphoma in the Rappaport classification are of B cell origin, as demonstrated by the presence of surface or cytoplasmic immunoglobulin. In addition, many Ig-negative large cell lymphomas react with anti-B cell monoclonal antibodies and have rearranged Ig genes.

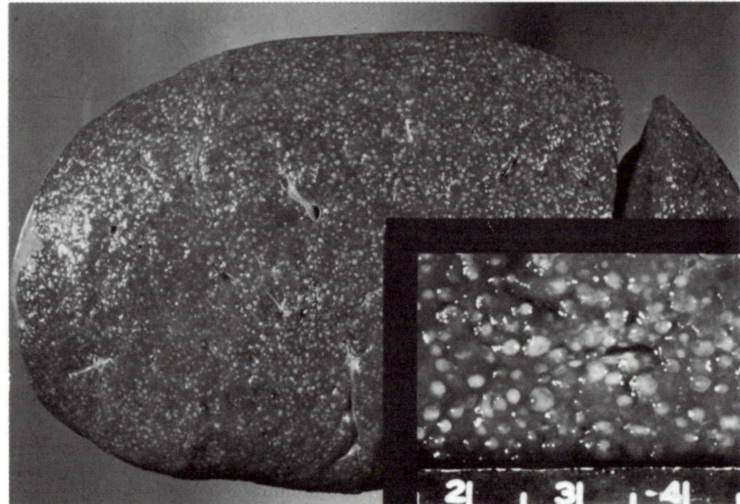

A

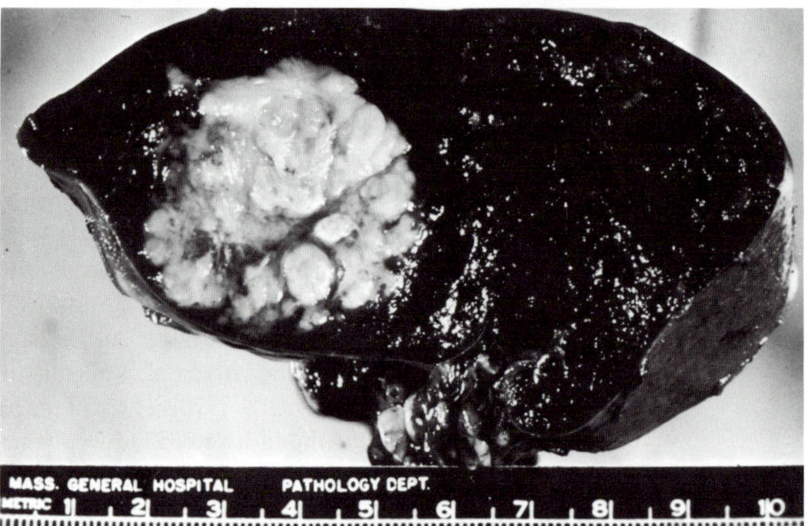

B

Fig. 24.7
Gross features of non-Hodgkin's lymphomas in the spleen. *A*, Follicular lymphoma. *B*, Diffuse large cell lymphoma. The neoplastic cells of the follicular lymphoma "home" to the normal B cell regions of the white pulp, while the large cell lymphoma forms a destructive, invasive tumor mass.

b. MORPHOLOGY

Large cell lymphomas are subclassified according to the predominant cell, which may resemble either a large cleaved or noncleaved follicular center cell or an immunoblast (figure 24.5C). B immunoblastic lymphomas may or may not have plasmacytoid features. The majority of large cell lymphomas are of noncleaved or immunoblastic type, and both types of cells may be present in some cases. The gross appearance of the spleen is shown in figure 24.7B.

c. CLINICAL FEATURES

Diffuse large cell lymphomas (figure 24.6B) are clinically distinct from follicular lymphomas. These tumors constitute 30–40% of adult non-Hodgkin's lymphomas and are thus comparable numerically to follicular lymphomas of small cleaved and mixed cell type. The M/F ratio is greater than 1. The age range is broad, and large cell lymphoma is more common in young adults than is follicular lymphoma. Large cell lymphoma constitutes 25–30% of childhood lymphomas. Patients typically present with a rapidly enlarging, often symptomatic mass at a single nodal or extranodal site. The disease is much more likely to be localized than is follicular lymphoma, and extranodal presentation is more common. Untreated, large cell lymphomas are rapidly progressive and fatal, but if a complete response can be obtained with therapy, long-term disease-free survival (? cure) may be possible (see lecture 23). This is in contrast to follicular lymphomas, which show a continuous slow mortality rate with time regardless of therapy.

8. Hairy cell leukemia

a. IMMUNOLOGY AND CELL OF ORIGIN

Most cases of hairy cell leukemia are SIg+ B cell lymphomas. The presence of tartrate-resistant acid phosphatase in hairy cells is characteristic, but it is neither necessary nor sufficient for the diagnosis. There is no recognized normal counterpart to the hairy cell.

b. MORPHOLOGY

The hairy cell has an oval or bean-shaped nucleus with chromatin slightly less clumped than that of a normal lymphocyte. The abundant, pale cytoplasm has a syncytial appearance in tissue sections; hence nuclei appear widely separated in contrast to the closely packed nuclei of small lymphocytic lymphomas. The bone marrow is almost always involved and because of increased reticulin is not readily aspirated. The spleen is usually involved and may be massive. Tumor involves the red pulp; the white pulp is usually atrophic.

c. CLINICAL FEATURES

Hairy cell leukemia is a disease of adults. As noted in lecture 22, patients present with pancytopenia and may or may not have circulating neoplastic cells. The diagnosis is best made on marrow biopsy. A marked defect in cell-mediated immunity is seen despite normal T cell subsets. Atypical mycobacterial infections as well as other infections are common. The course may be protracted. Long, spontaneous remissions occur. It does not respond to conventional lymphoma chemotherapy. Splenectomy is often followed by prolonged clinical improvement.

9. Plasmacytoma/multiple myeloma

a. IMMUNOLOGY AND CELL OF ORIGIN

The plasma cell of multiple myeloma represents the terminally differentiated B cell of the late primary or secondary immune response, which secretes IgG or IgA rather than IgM. Neoplastic plasma cells in myeloma lack SIg, pan-B and pan-leukocyte markers, and have only cytoplasmic immunoglobulin.

b. MORPHOLOGY

Typical cells resemble mature or immature plasma cells, with no admixture of lymphoid cells. An "anaplastic" stage resembling large cell lymphoma may be a preterminal event.

c. CLINICAL FEATURES

This topic merits extended discussion and is covered in lecture 25.

C. T cell neoplasms

1. T lymphoblastic lymphoma (LBL) and T cell ALL

a. IMMUNOLOGY AND CELL OF ORIGIN

Most cases of lymphoblastic lymphoma are of T cell origin. About 20% of cases of ALL have T cell markers. Both neoplasms represent primitive thymic T cells (cortical thymocytes). Analysis with monoclonal antibodies indicates that the cells of T-ALL are at a more primitive stage of development than those of T-LBL. The cells of both tumors are TdT+, usually form E-rosettes, and react with many monoclonal anti-T cell antibodies.

b. MORPHOLOGY

Involved lymph nodes or thymus contain a diffuse proliferation of small to medium-sized lymphoid cells with finely dispersed chromatin and inconspicuous nucleoli. Some cells have fine nuclear grooves or convolutions. In contrast to Burkitt's tumor, the cytoplasm is scant and only moderately basophilic; the cells appear noncohesive. In imprints the cells are indistinguishable from the lymphoblasts of childhood ALL.

c. CLINICAL FEATURES

Lymphoblastic lymphoma is a disease of adolescents and young adults. It constitutes less than 5% of all non-Hodgkin's lymphomas but up to 40% of childhood lymphomas. Patients are predominantly male and present with rapidly enlarging, symptomatic mediastinal (thymic) masses and/or supradiaphragmatic lymphadenopathy. Untreated, it is rapidly fatal, usually terminating in acute leukemia. CNS involvement is common. Combination chemotherapy may be beneficial, but the prognosis is not as good as that for common ALL.

2. *Chronic lymphocytic leukemia (T-CLL)*

a. IMMUNOLOGY AND NORMAL CELLULAR COUNTERPART

Only 1% of cases of CLL have a T cell phenotype. The majority of these are of the CD4 phenotype, but the CD8 type also occurs. The cells lack TdT and CD1 and express pan-T cell antigens; hence, it is a "mature" T cell phenotype. Functional T cell activity has not been observed in most CD4 cases, but immunoneutropenia has been reported. Cells of the CD8 cases (T-γ) have displayed signs of suppressor activity, e.g., chronic neutropenia. Cells in some cases may correspond to virgin T cells and in others to fully differentiated T effector cells.

b. MORPHOLOGY

T-CLL cells may be indistinguishable from B-CLL, but nuclear irregularity and cytoplasmic granules are seen in many cases of T-CLL. In the spleen, red pulp is predominantly involved. Liver involvement may be prominent, with striking sinusoidal infiltration.

c. CLINICAL FEATURES

T-CLL may be less indolent than typical B-CLL. Cutaneous or mucosal infiltrates are common, perhaps because normal T cells often participate in cutaneous immunologic reactions. Because of the difference in clinical behavior, it is important to distinguish between B-CLL and T-CLL. CD8 proliferations associated with nonimmune neutropenia may have such an indolent clinical course. They may appear not to be neoplastic. However, T cell receptor gene rearrangements and occasional progression to high-grade neoplasia suggest that this is a low-grade malignancy.

3. Large cell lymphomas, T-cell type

a. IMMUNOLOGY AND NORMAL CELLULAR COUNTERPART

Large cell lymphomas, composed of immunoblasts, with T cell markers and T cell receptor gene rearrangement correspond to the proliferative stage of antigen-dependent T cell differentiation. These tumors may express CD4 or CD8 antigens, as well as other markers of post-thymic T cells. They lack TdT and CD1. Many lack one or more normal T cell antigens, such as a pan-T antigen or a subset antigen.

b. MORPHOLOGY

Large cell lymphomas cannot reliably be distinguished from B-large cell lymphomas on morphologic grounds.

c. CLINICAL FEATURES

Too few T-large cell lymphomas have been reported to provide a clear picture of their clinical features. There is no conclusive evidence that large cell lymphomas of T cell type differ in prognosis from those of B cell type. This contrasts with other T and B cell lymphomas of similar general morphology, such as lymphoblastic lymphoma, CLL, and ATL/L. Thus immunophenotyping of large cell lymphomas is not now of clear clinical value.

4. Adult T cell lymphoma/leukemia (ATL/L)

a. IMMUNOLOGY AND CELL OF ORIGIN

In the late 1970s Japanese workers noted that the majority of non-Hodgkin's lymphomas and CLL seen in certain areas of Japan were of T cell type. Since the clinical spectrum includes both nodal disease and blood involvement, this disease is now known as adult T cell lymphoma/leukemia, to distinguish it from childhood T cell ALL. A unique human retrovirus has been identified in cultured cells from both the Japanese patients and also from black patients with a similar disorder from the Caribbean and southeastern United States. Antibody to this **human T cell lymphoma/leukemia virus** (HTLV-I) is found in the blood of patients with the disease in all three areas but is not found in the blood of most normal individuals. Close relatives of patients and individuals residing in southern Japan have an increased incidence of antibodies to HTLV. The virus isolated from human tumor cells causes cord blood T cells to transform into continuously growing cell lines, mimicking the effect of Epstein-Barr virus on B cells. Current evidence supports the conclusion that ATL/L is a true virus-induced neoplasm. The surface marker phenotype is that of mature CD4 + T cells.

b. MORPHOLOGY

The histologic picture of HTLV-associated lymphomas and leukemia is variable. The neoplastic cells range from small lymphocytes to pleomorphic giant cells resembling Reed-Sternberg cells. There are no distinctive histologic features that permit a definite diagnosis of ATL to be made on paraffin-embedded sections alone. The diagnosis rests on the combination of morphology, immunologic studies, and documentation of HTLV infection, in the form of serum antibodies and/or virus identification in tumor cells.

c. CLINICAL FEATURES

Most cases have been reported in southern Japan, the Caribbean, and the southeastern United States. Patients are adults of all ages. The majority are leukemic and have widespread disease involving lymph nodes, liver, and spleen at the time of diagnosis. Skin infiltration and hypercalcemia (due to osteoclast activation) are common. Patients usually respond poorly to therapy and die in 1–2 years.

5. *Pleomorphic T-cell lymphomas*

a. IMMUNOLOGY AND NORMAL CELLULAR COUNTERPART

In numerous reports, lymphomas with T cell markers have been given a variety of names, including peripheral T cell lymphoma, T-immunoblastic sarcoma, node-based T cell lymphoma, T zone lymphoma, Lennert's lymphoma, angioimmunoblastic lymphadenopathy-like T cell lymphoma, and angiocentric lymphoma. Since there is no marker for T cell neoplasms that is analogous to light chain restriction in B cell neoplasms, it is often difficult to be certain whether these cases are true T cell malignancies or tumors of other types that contain many reactive T cells. As noted above, morphology alone cannot reliably define the T cell origin of a lymphoma. In order to make a definite diagnosis of T cell neoplasm, a homogeneous population of morphologically malignant cells must be shown to have a specific T cell marker. Since well-defined and supposed T cell tumors both display heterogeneous nodal infiltrate, this requirement is difficult to meet. New methods for detecting clonal rearrangements of the T cell receptor gene should soon facilitate our understanding of T cell neoplasms.

b. MORPHOLOGY

Most of these tumors fall into the **diffuse, mixed small** and **large cell** categories of the Working Formulation (table 24.4). Some B cell neoplasms of either plasmacytoid lymphocytic or germinal center type may also fall into these categories. Since both of these are fairly well-defined clinical entities, it is important to immunophenotype diffuse mixed lymphomas to distinguish B and T cell types. Often distinguishing between pleomorphic T cell lymphoma and Hodgkin's disease is difficult. Demonstration of T cell receptor gene rearrangememt may prove useful.

c. CLINICAL FEATURES

Patients are typically adults, with widespread nodal and/or visceral disease. T-cell types commonly run a more aggressive clinical course than B cell lymphomas in this category.

6. *Mycosis fungoides/Sézary's syndrome (MF/SS)*

a. IMMUNOLOGY AND CELL OF ORIGIN

The neoplastic cell of MF/SS is a T lymphocyte of the helper subset. A few patients with clinical features indistinguishable from MF have antibodies to HTLV, but most do not.

b. MORPHOLOGY

The characteristic cell of MF is a large lymphocyte with a highly convoluted (cerebriform) nucleus. This cell infiltrates the epidermis, producing microabscesses. In SS the circulating cell is a small cerebriform lymphocyte. As a terminal event a large cell lymphoma may develop; this probably represents a failure of maturation of the large MF cells rather than development of a second neoplasm.

c. CLINICAL FEATURES

Chronically progressive cutaneous disease leads to eventual visceral lymphoma and death. Symptoms are alleviated by various therapies, but the disease is not curable. Recently monoclonal anti-T cell antibodies have been used therapeutically.

SELECTED REFERENCES

Reviews

Bennett, J. M., Foon, K. A., et al. *Immunologic Approaches to the Classification and Management of Lymphomas and Leukemias.* Boston: Kluwer Academic Publishers, 1988.

Clark, E. A. Structure, function, and genetics of human B cell–associated surface molecules. *Adv. Cancer Res.* 52(1989): 81–150.

Facer, C. A., and Playfair, J. H. L., Malaria, Epstein-Barr virus, and the genesis of lymphomas. *Adv. Cancer Res.* 53(1989): 33–72.

Griesser, H., Tkachuk, D., et al. Gene rearrangememts and translocations in lymphoproliferative diseases. *Blood* 73(1989): 1402–1415.

Jaffe, E. S. The elusive Reed-Sternberg cell. *N. Engl. J. Med.* 320(1989): 529–531.

Knecht, H. Angioimmunoblastic lymphadenopathy: ten years' experience and state of current knowledge. *Semin. Hematol.* 26(1989): 208–215.

LeBien, T. W., and McCormack, R. T. The common acute lymphoblastic leukemia antigen (CD10)—emancipation from a functional enigma. *Blood* 73(1989): 625–635.

Parnes, J. R. Molecular biology and function of CD4 and CD8. *Adv. Immunol.* 44 (1989): 265–312.

Reis, M. D., Griesser, H., et al. T cell receptor and immunoglobulin gene rearrangements in lymphoproliferative disorders. *Adv. Cancer Res.* 52(1989): 45–80.

Original articles

Agnarsson, B. A., and Kadin, M. E. The immunophenotype of Reed-Sternberg cells: a study of 50 cases of Hodgkin's disease using fixed frozen tissues. *Cancer* 63 (1989): 2083–2087.

Armitage, J. O., Greer, J. P., et al. Peripheral T-cell lymphoma. *Cancer* 63(1989): 158–163.

Billaud, M., Rousset, F., et al. Low expression of lymphocyte function-associated antigen (LFA)-1 and LFA-3 adhesion molecules is a common trait in Burkitt's lymphoma associated with and not associated with Epstein-Barr virus. *Blood* 75 (1990): 1827–1833.

Deane, M., and Norton, J. D. Detection of immunoglobulin gene rearrangement in B lymphoid malignancies by polymerase chain reaction gene amplification. *Br. J. Haematol.* 74(1990): 251–256.

Ellis, M. E., Diehl, L. F., et al. Trephine needle bone marrow biopsy in the initial staging of Hodgkin disease: sensitivity and specificity of the Ann Arbor staging procedure criteria. *Am. J. Hematol.* 30(1989): 115–120.

Ellison, D. J., Hu, E., et al. Immunogenetic analysis of bone marrow aspirates in patients with non-Hodgkin lymphomas. *Am. J. Hematol.* 33(1990): 160–166.

Gingrich, R. D., Dahle, C. E., et al. Identification and characterization of a new surface membrane antigen found predominantly on malignant B lymphocytes. *Blood* 75(1990): 2375–2387.

Hanson, C. A., Jaszcz, W., et al. True histiocytic lymphoma: histopathologic, immunophenotypic and genotypic analysis. *Br. J. Haematol.* 73(1989): 187–198.

Janier, M., Katlama, C., et al. The pseudo-Sézary syndrome with CD8 phenotype in a patient with the acquired immunodeficiency syndrome (AIDS). *Ann. Intern. Med.* 110(1989): 738–740.

Lenert, P., Kroon, D., et al. Human CD4 binds immunoglobulins. *Science* 248(1990): 1639–1643.

Purtilo, D. T., Grierson, H. L., et al. Detection of X-linked lymphoproliferative disease using molecular and immunovirologic markers. *Am. J. Med.* 87(1989): 421–424.

Ratner, L., Vander Heyden, N., et al. Familial adult T-cell leukemia/lymphoma. *Am. J. Hematol.* 34(1990): 215–222.

Schouten, H. C., Sanger, W. G., et al. Chromosomal abnormalities in untreated patients with non-Hodgkin's lymphoma: associations with histology, clinical characteristics, and treatment outcome. *Blood* 75(1990): 1841–1847.

Simon, R., Durrleman, S., et al. The non-Hodgkin lymphoma pathologic classification project: long-term follow-up of 1153 patients with non-Hodgkin lymphomas. *Ann. Intern. Med.* 109(1988): 939–945.

Sitar, G., Brusamolino, E., et al. Isolation of Reed-Sternberg cells from lymph nodes of Hodgkin's disease patients. *Blood* 73(1989): 222–229.

Tonks, N. K., Charbonneau, H., et al. Demonstration that the leukocyte common antigen CD45 is a protein tyrosine phosphatase. *Biochemistry* 27(1988): 8695–8701.

Trainor, K. J., Brisco, M. J., et al. Monoclonality in B-lymphoproliferative disorders detected at the DNA level. *Blood* 75(1990):

Weiss, L. M., Movahed, L. A., et al. Detection of Epstein-Barr viral genomes in Reed-Sternberg cells of Hodgkin's disease. *N. Engl. J. Med.* 320(1989): 502–506.

Winberg, C. D., Sheibani, K., et al. T-cell-rich lymphoproliferative disorders: morphologic and immunologic differential diagnoses. *Cancer* 62(1988): 1539–1555.

LECTURE 25

Plasma Cell Disorders and the Dysproteinemias

W. Hallowell Churchill, Jr.

EDITOR'S COMMENT

Studies of multiple myeloma have yielded a rich harvest of basic biologic knowledge. It was the study of a monoclonal M component protein that led originally to present understanding of immunoglobulin structure. That in turn led to other major advances in immunology. This disease and its several variants are forms of lymphoma that are marked by the production of so-called paraproteins and in consequence a singular clinical picture: an M-component in the serum immunoelectrophoresis pattern, various bone lesions, and a greater or lesser hyperviscosity syndrome. For that reason, we consider them apart from the other non-Hodgkin's lymphomas. In this lecture, the clinical and scientific depth of this field becomes apparent.

I. NORMAL IMMUNOGLOBULINS

The immunoglobulins of normal blood serum are a heterogeneous group of proteins with antibody activity. The concentrations of immunoglobulins that comprise the normal range reflect the antigen exposure that all of us experience. This normal range differs among different populations and rises with age, most markedly in the first few years of life.

A. Classes

On the basis of certain structural features that are detected by reactivities with antisera prepared against proteins of homogeneous structure, the immunoglobulins have been shown to consist of five major classes of molecules: **IgG, IgA, IgM, IgD,** and **IgE**. Subclasses based on immunologic reactivities have also been found. Thus, a given IgG molecule, for example, may be either IgG1, IgG2, IgG3, or IgG4. There are two such IgA and IgM subclasses. Even within a subclass, molecules are structurally and electrophoretically heterogeneous.

B. Structure

1. Arrangements of H and L chains

IgG molecules consist of two kinds of polypeptides, **H chains** (for heavy) and **L chains** (for light), that are arranged symmetrically with respect to the long axis of the molecules. Thus, each half-molecule has one H and

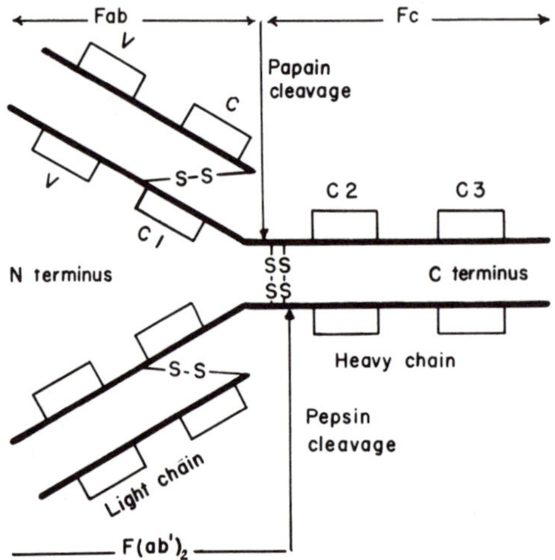

Fig. 25.1
Schematic diagram of structure of IgG molecule.

one L chain (figure 25.1). In any given molecule, the two H chains are structurally identical, as are the two L chains. Papain cleaves IgG molecules near the hinge (interchain disulfide bridge) point. Two kinds of fragments result:

- **Fab** (for **antigen-binding**) **fragments**, consisting of the L chains and about half the H chains.
- **Fc** (for **crystallizable**) **fragments**, which contain the remaining portions of the H chains.

The structure of non-IgG immmunoglobulins generally resembles that of IgG. IgM molecules occur chiefly as pentamers. A portion of IgA is dimeric. The monomer resembles IgG except for the class specificity of the H chain.

2. *Classes, subclasses, and types*

Class specificity resides in the H chain. Each of the major immunoglobulin classes has a distinctive kind of H chain. These are termed γ, α, μ, δ, and ε, the Greek letters corresponding to the Roman letters designating the groups. Four varieties of γ chains occur: γ_1, γ_2, γ_3, and γ_4. These are the basis for the subclasses of IgG. Finally, all L chains are κ or λ; corresponding immunoglobulins are classified as type K and type L. It should be noted that an individual immunoglobulin molecule contains only one class of H chain and one type of L chain.

IgM in its usual pentameric form and the dimeric form of IgA have one **J chain** (mol. wt. 22,000) per polymer. Moreover, in bodily secretions, IgA exists in a special form (**secretory IgA**) that, in addition to a J chain, has a protein moiety (mol. wt. 55,000) called the **secretory component**.

3. Constant and variable portions

When given IgG molecules were compared, it was found that the C-terminal halves of the L chains and the corresponding parts of the H chains have similar amino acid sequences within a given class or subclass. However, the remaining N-terminal portions (V_H and V_L) are **variable** in structure (figure 25.1). The variability is known to be related to antibody specificity. Each light chain has two interchain disulfide bridges, one in V_L, the other in the **constant** region C_L. Similarly, there is an intrachain disulfide bridge in V_H and one in each of the three constant domains, C_H1, C_H2, and C_H3. The various biologic properties of IgG molecules reside in one or another of these domains.

C. Serum concentrations

The bulk (80–85%) of total serum immunoglobulin is IgG. The normal concentrations per deciliter in adults are IgG, 600–1500 mg; IgA, 60–290 mg; IgM, 50–200 mg; IgD, approximately 3 mg; and IgE, only 0.05 mg. The ratios of IgG1:IgG2:IgG3:IgG4 are approximately 70:24:3.5:2.5. The ratio of κ to λ type molecules in the serum immunoglobulins is 2:1. Other properties are summarized in table 25.1.

Table 25.1
Properties of Imunoglobulins

	IgG	IgA	IgM	IgD	IgE
Molecular weight	150,000	180,000 or 390,000[a]	900,000	150,000	200,000
Sedimentation coefficient	7S	7S or 11S[b]	19S	7S	8S
Concentration in plasma (mg/100 ml)	600–1500	60–290	50–200	3	0.05
Biologic half-life (days)	20[b]	6	5	3	2
Complement fixation	+	0	+	0	0
Passive cutaneous anaphylaxis	+	0	0	?	?
Reagenic antibody	0	0	0	0	+
Placental transfer	+	0	0	0	0

a. Secretory IgA.
b. Half-life of IgG1.

II. HYPOGLOBULINEMIA

A decreased serum concentration of the immunoglobulins may result from decreased synthesis (congenital agammaglobulinemia) or increased catabolism and/or loss (nephrotic syndrome or exudative enteropathy). In some instances acquired hypogammagobulinemia is the presenting finding in a patient with a plasma cell dyscrasia.

III. HYPERGLOBULINEMIA

An increased serum concentration of one or more immunoglobulins may result from hyerplasia or neoplasia of B lymphocytes or their derivatives, plasma cells.

A. Type

Hyperglobulinemia is divisible into two types with different clinical and biochemical features: **monoclonal** and **polyclonal gammopathies**.

1. Monoclonal

In the monoclonal type, proliferating plasma cells produce one (or at most a few) structurally homogeneous immunoglobulin molecules. Monoclonal gammopathies involve greatly increased concentrations of one or a few immunoglobulins, which are referred to as **M-components**. A complete M-component belongs to a single immunoglobulin class, subclass, and type and is similar in structure to normal immunoglobulin molecules. Since complete M-components usually have molecular weights of 150,000 or higher, they are largely restricted to circulating plasma and extracellular fluid. They appear in the urine in significant amounts only in the presence of glomerular damage. However, fragments of immunoglobulin molecules (e.g., free light chains or heavy chains) are produced in some patients, and a given patient may have a complete M-component, an incomplete M-component (L chain), or both. Unlike complete M-components, free L chains are found primarily in the urine. They occur in plasma in significant concentrations only in the presence of renal failure or when production is massive. If both complete and incomplete M-components are found in the same patient, the free L chains are usually identical to those in the complete molecule. Of the many M-components of different patients that have so far been studied, no two have been structurally identical. Significantly antibody or antibody-like activity has been found in some M-components. This is evidence that the structural information derived from the study of these monoclonal proteins can be extrapolated to the antibodies produced by normal B cells. However, the most direct evidence supporting the hypothesis that myeloma proteins are similar to immunoglobulins derived from nonmalignant B cells is the observation that antibody response to certain pneumococcal polysaccharides is monoclonal.

2. *Polyclonal*

Polyclonal hypergammaglobulinemia results from the proliferation of plasma cells that produce immunoglobulins which are heterogeneous in class, electrophoretic mobility and antigen specificity. The antigens stimulating the proliferative response are often not identifiable.

B. Laboratory features

Laboratory abnormalities may be divided into (1) those due to hyperglobulinemia per se (rouleaux of red cells, elevated erythrocyte sedimentation rate, increased plasma viscosity, and positive Sia water test); and (2) those tests that distinguish between monoclonal and polyclonal gemmopathies (i.e., electrophoretic and immunodiffusion procedures).

1. *Elevated serum globulin*

Normal serum contains 3.5–4.5 g albumin/dl and 3.0–4.0 g globulin/dl. Increased production of immunoglobulins usually elevates the total serum globulin level.

2. *Erythrocyte sedimentation rate*

An increased sedimentation rate of red cells in plasma reflects the presence of plasma substances that aggregate red cells. The most common cause is an increase in the concentration of fibrinogen; however, hyperglobulinemia of moderate to severe degree can also be a cause. If the abnormal immunoglobulin is a cryoglobulin, however, the sedimentation rate may be retarded by the resulting cryogel.

3. *Sia water test*

The Sia water test is a simple procedure for demonstrating the presence of euglobulins (proteins insoluble at low ionic strenghth). A positive result indicates hyperglobulinemia, which may be polyclonal or monoclonal.

4. *Electrophoretic demonstration of M-component(s)*

Serum electrophoresis is the best screening test for diseases of immunoglobulin-producing cells (figure 25.2). M-components appear on **zone electrophoresis** (paper, agarose, agar, cellulose acetate) as narrow bands with sharp leading and trailing edges (figure 25.2C–E). In contrast the hypergammaglobulinemia of polyclonal gammopathies gives a diffuse pattern (figure 25.2A). On **immunoelectrophoresis** M-components produce a localized distortion or blister of the normal arc of the immunoglobulin class or type to which they belong (figure 25.3). The immunoelectrophoretic patterns of patients with polyclonal gammopathies show an increase in density and length of the normal IgG, IgA, and IgM arcs without local distortions. Zone electrophoresis of serum and of urine (concentrated about 30-fold) is the simplest means of detecting M-components (figure

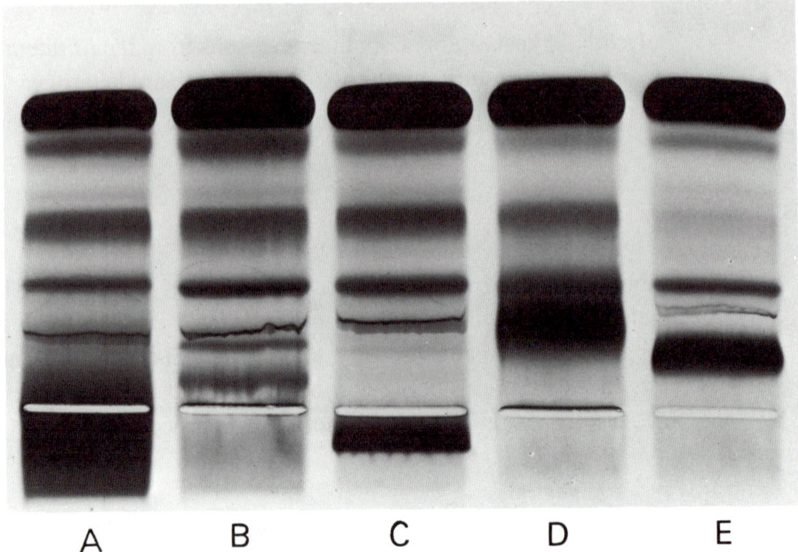

Fig. 25.2
Agarose gel electrophoresis of serum protein: *A*, diffuse hypergamma-globulinemia. *B*, Normal plasma, showing fibrinogen just anodal to origin; *C*, IgG M-component. *D*, IgA M-component. *E*, IgM M-component.

25.2). For positive identification and typing, immunoelectrophoresis using antisera to κ and λ chains and other appropriate monospecific antisera is required. Such procedures also distinguish between free L chains and intact M-components. Protein electrophoresis and immunoelectrophoresis of serum and urine together should be able to identify virtually all monoclonal proteins encountered. If the screening protein electrophoresis is normal, it is most unusual to find a significant abnormality on the immunoelectrophoresis.

5. *Bence Jones proteinuria*

Over 120 years ago Henry Bence Jones reported on the presence of "animal matter" in the urine of a patient with "fragilitas et mollities ossium," later called multiple myeloma. The material precipitated on heating of the urine to 50–60°C and redissolved as the temperature was raised to the boiling point. Later work identified Bence Jones protein as free L chains. The characteristic behavior of free L chains on heating has been used as a screening test for multiple myeloma for over a century; however, the heat test is relatively insensitive and may be falsely negative. Also, excretion of L chains occurs not only in multiple myeloma but in other of the M-component disorders to be discussed below. "Stick tests" for proteinuria (such as Albustix®) are positive only in the presence of albumin and may be negative if only L chains are present.

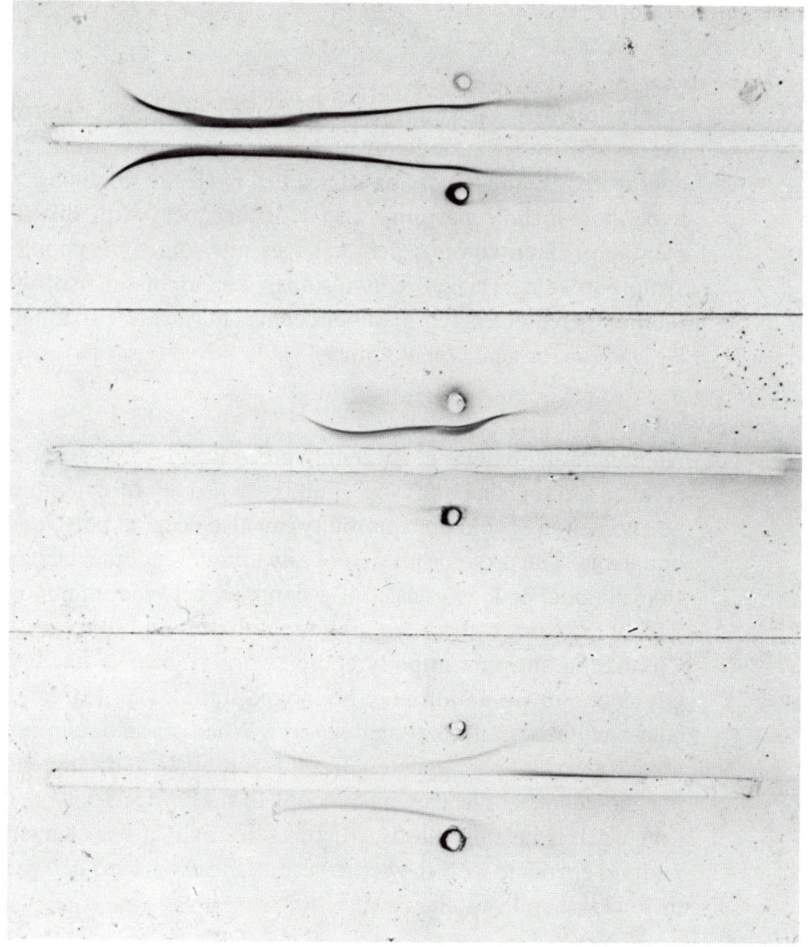

Fig. 25.3
Immunoelectrophoretic appearance of M-components. The anode was at the right. The antisera used to develop patterns were (from top to bottom) anti-IgG, anti-IgM, anti-IgA. All lower wells contained normal serum. Upper wells contained (top to bottom) IgG myeloma serum, serum from a patient with Waldenström's macroglobulinemia, and IgA myeloma serum. Note that M-components produce distortion and thickening of precipitin arcs.

C. Clinical features

1. Hyperviscosity

Hyperglobulinemia of any type, when sufficiently severe, may cause plasma hyperviscosity with sludging of blood in the capillaries. This effect is aggravated by the formation of red cell rouleaux. Sludging may lead to: hyperglobulinemic purpura; visual disturbances with dilation and segmentation of retinal veins, hemorrhages, and sometimes papilledema; CNS symptoms (e.g., vertigo, convulsions); and right-sided congestive heart failure. Increased excretion of light chains may cause proximal renal tubular acidosis, or acute renal failure.

2. Cryoglobulinemia

An immunoglobulin that reversibly precipitates (or gels) in the cold (4°C) is called a **cryoglobulin**. Cryoglobulins are usually M-components, but the phemomenon of cold precipitability can also occur in polyclonal hyperglobulinemia. The proteins may be of any immunoglobulin class, including L chains alone, or may consist of a complex between immunoglobulins of different classes, or between immunoglobulins and other serum proteins. Circulating antigen-antibody complexes may behave like cryoglobulins. Cryoglobulin formation may be looked upon as an extreme example of cold-facilitated molecular aggregation. When cryoglobulin precipitates in vivo, Raynaud's phenomenon, frank thrombosis, and gangrene may occur in exposed areas. Electron microscopy of the cryogels demonstrates variation in gels from amorphous structures to a tight lattice of crystals. Clinical findings correlate with the gel structure, the crystalline gels producing the most peripheral vascular obstruction.

3. Interference with coagulation

M-components may interfere with normal blood coagulation by (1) complex formation with specific clotting factor (e.g., factor VIII); (2) interference with polymerization of fibrin monomer; or (3) coating platelets, thereby inducing a defect in platelet aggregate formation so that a poor primary hemostatic plug is formed despite a normal platelet count (see lectures 27–29). The latter is most common with IgM paraproteins.

4. Anemia, leukopenia, and thrombocytopenia

Coating of blood cells by M-components may accelerate their destruction. Myeloma proteins absorbed onto red cells may cause a positive direct Coombs test. However, the eluate will not show specificity for red cell antigens. In myeloma and related disease, anemia can result from marrow replacement, uremia and folate/or cobalamin deficiency. Increased destruction from hemolysis may also be present. The chronic inflammation which is a frequent cause of polyclonal hypergammaglobulinemia contribute to the anemia by suppressing iron utilization.

D. Classification

A. Polyclonal gammopathies
B. Monoclonal gammopathies
  1. Myeloma
    a. Aggressive variants; anaplastic myeloma
    b. Heavy chain diseases
      1. Gamma (γ) chain disease
      2. Alpha (α) chain disease
      3. Mu (μ) chain disease
    c. Light chain disease
    d. Indolent variants: smoldering myeloma; solitary plasmacytoma
    e. Monoclonal gammopathy of unknown significance
  2. Macroglobulinemia of Waldenström
  3. Amyloidosis
  4. Cryoglobulinemia

IV. POLYCLONAL GAMMOPATHIES

An otherwise normal individual develops diffuse hypergammaglobulinemia about 10–14 days following a sufficient antigenic stimulus. An increase in many or all immunoglobulins may occur reactively in many disorders, among them bacterial pneumonia, abscess, other chronic infections, connective tissue disorders such as rheumatoid arthritis and systemic lupus erythematosus, and chronic hepatocellular disease. Often the antigen causing the polyclonal production of immunoglobulin cannot be identified.

V. MONOCLONAL GAMMOPATHIES

A. Multiple myeloma

Multiple myeloma is the most common disease in which the initial finding is (often) a monoclonal gammopathy. The incidence increases with age. At 50, it is about 7 in 100,000; at 70, about 20 in 100,000. Widespread but patchy marrow involvement by a monoclonal proliferation of plasma cells is the usual finding. The clinical spectrum ranges from very aggressive variants, which, though temporarily controlled by therapy, immediately relapse, to indolent forms that do not require treatment. The goal of initial evaluation and staging is to place patients within this spectrum so that treatment decisions can be made.

1. Diagnostic criteria

Major diagnostic criteria include the following:

- A plasmacytoma outside the marrow.
- Bone marrow plasmacytosis with sheets of plasma cells or an increase in plasma cells to $>30\%$ of all marrow cells.

- A monoclonal gammopathy; for IgG, this means >3.5 g/dl; for IgA, >2.0 g/dl.
- Excretion of >1 g/24 hr of κ or λ light chains.

Any two of these criteria are sufficient to make the diagnosis of myeloma.

There are in addition certain minor criteria which include:

- Lytic bone lesions
- Smaller amounts of the monoclonal protein
- Bone marrow plasmacytosis of <30% and with cells not arranged in sheets
- Evidence that the plasma cells represent a monoclonal expansion
- The presence of reduced amounts of normal immunoglobulins

One or more of these minor criteria together with one of the major criteria listed above is usually sufficient to make the diagnosis of myeloma.

2. *Clinical features*

The clinical picture reflects (1) the infiltration of organs by plasma cells; and (2) abnormalities caused by the monoclonal gammopathy, some of which are summarized in Table 25.2. The peak incidence is between ages 55 and 65, except for light chain disease, which may occur earlier. Except for IgD myeloma in which men exceed women by a 3:1 ratio, the distribution between the sexes is equal. The incidence of different heavy chain types roughly parallels their relative concentration among normal globulins. Light chain distribution is similar to that of normal light chains with 2 κ to every λ light chains. Untreated, the median survival is 18 months. Survival is directly related to the state at onset and other prognostic factors, but with adequate treatment it is generally 3–5 years.

a. BLOOD PICTURE

Almost all patients have a normochromic-normocytic anemia. As noted, this anemia has multiple causes. Moderate leukopenia and thrombocyto-

Table 25.2
Clinical Features of Multiple Myeloma

	IgG myeloma	IgA myeloma	IgD myeloma	Light chain disease
Mean age at diagnosis	56	62	64	52
M/F ratio	1:1	1:1	3:1	1:1
κ/λ ratio	2:1	2:1	1:9	1:35
Incidence of Bence Jones protein (%)	60	70	92	100
Amyloidosis			↑	↑
Extraosseous involvement			↑	

penia are common. The blood smear typically shows rouleaux formation. When marrow is heavily infiltrated, the blood smear may display a leukoerythroblastic reaction (see lecture 20). Rarely, plasma cells appear in the blood (**plasma cell leukemia**). This usually occurs later.

b. BONE MARROW

Aspirated bone marrow containing 10–30% plasma cells is suggestive but not diagnostic unless "sheets" of plasma cells are found. Chronic liver disease can cause marked plasmacytosis that can be distinguished from the monoclonal expansion of myeloma by immunocytochemical studies. The morphology of individual cells is not in itself diagnostic, but classification by morphologic criteria has prognostic value. Because marrow involvement is patchy, several marrow aspirates might be required to assess the extent of marrow involvement.

c. BONE LESIONS

The osteolytic bone disease of myeloma is due to production by myeloma cells and lymphocytes of **osteoclast activating factor** (OAF). Prostaglandins (E_2 and I_2) produced by macrophages and endothelial cells also contribute by regulating OAF production by lymphocytes. Stimulated osteoclasts cause osteolysis without associated osteoblastic changes so that ^{99m}Tc (technetium-99m) bone scans are often negative. Skeletal x-rays thus better assess the extent of bone involvement. Osteolytic lesions heal following treatment in less than a third of patients.

Hypercalcemia is found in 10% of patients. In them, bone disease is usually present. However, the extent of bone disease does not correlate well with calcium levels because impaired renal function is an equally important causal factor for hypercalcemia.

d. RENAL IMPAIRMENT

Many factors contribute to renal impairment in myeloma.

- Hypercalcemia and volume depletion often lead to acute loss of renal function.
- Intravenous pyelography is an occasional cause in volume-depleted patients.
- Light chain excretion is commonly associated with chronic progressive loss of renal function. Some light chains may cause proximal tubular injury with renal tubular acidosis.
- Renal amyloidosis is often associated with massive proteinuria.

Many of these complications are preventable with good medical management, but once renal failure is present, it is rarely reversed.

e. ASSOCIATED IMMUNOGLOBULIN ABNORMALITIES

All but 1–2% of patients have a monoclonal protein that can be identified in the serum and/or the urine. The levels of normal immunoglobulins are usually reduced in multiple myeloma. Why should there be a relative deficiency of normal immunoglobulins in patients with myeloma? It is known that mononuclear cells from patients with myeloma inhibit the pokeweed-driven synthesis of immunoglobulin by normal B cells. This suppressive activity is a property of the adherent mononuclear cell fraction. At least for IgG, increased amounts of IgG monoclonal protein enhance the catabolism of normal IgG. These changes presumably contribute to the known tendency of patients with myeloma to have difficulty with infections. There is no evidence that gamma globulin replacement therapy is of clinical value. However, because 30% of patients respond with protective levels of antibody, immunization with pneumococcal vaccine may provide prophylaxis.

3. Cytokinetics and staging

Because myeloma cells produce a discrete protein, it is possible to make precise estimates of cell mass at different stages. The per-cell production rate of IgG can be established in vitro. Turnover studies establish whole-body catabolic and synthetic rates. Division of the whole-body rate by the per-cell production rate yields estimates of tumor burden that correlates well with prognosis.

- **Good-prognosis**, low tumor burden patients have a hemoglobin of $\geqq 10$ g/dl, normal calcium, no lytic lesions in the bones, and a relatively small monoclonal component (IgG $\leqq 5$ g/dl, IgA $\leqq 3$ g/dl), and urinary light chain $\leqq 4$ g/dl/24 hr).
- **Poor-prognosis**, high tumor burden patients have a hemoglobin $\leqq 8.5$ g/dl, a serum calcium $\geqq 12$ mg/dl, multiple bony lytic lesions, large M-components (IgG $\geqq 7$ g/dl, IgA $\geqq 5$ g/dl), and urinary light chains $\geqq$ 12 g/dl/24 hr.
- Patients with intermediate values have intermediate tumor burdens and intermediate prognoses.

This staging system relies in part on subjective judgments of the extent of bone disease or performance status. Laboratory-based staging systems avoid these elements by relying largely on the labeling index and β_2-microglobulin levels, the only variables that predicted outcome in a recent study. Other approaches seek to predict responses to chemotherapy with clonogenic soft agar tissue culture systems or chromosomal studies.

4. Aggressive variants

Anaplastic myeloma is a rare variant characterized by morphology resembling immunoblastic lymphoma. It can appear de novo or evolve from a more indolent myeloma. Median survival is only a few months. An osteosclerotic variant sometimes associated with marrow fibrosis and peripheral neuropathy is also unresponsive to treatment.

5. *Heavy chain diseases*

These rare variants are associated with excretion of fragments of free heavy chains. The clinical picture varies with the heavy chain class.

a. GAMMA (γ) CHAIN DISEASE

The clinical course is similar to a lymphoma with hepatosplenomegaly and node involvement. Selective uvula swelling is sometimes encountered. Median survival is about a year. An identical heavy chain is found in serum and urine. Structural studies usually reveal amino acid deletions. Renal excretion and/or fast migration may cause the heavy chain fragment to be missed on protein electrophoresis. Normal immunoglobulins are depressed and there is increased susceptibility to infection. Lytic bone lesions are not present. This disorder has been called **Franklin's disease**.

b. ALPHA (α) CHAIN DISEASE

Alpha chain disease is the most common of the heavy chain diseases. Typical cases have abdominal lymphoma with a serum and urine M-component related to the H chain (α type) of IgA (see lecture 23). Patients have been mainly of North African or Eastern Mediterranean origin. Outside the Mediterranean area, α chain disease occurs in a rarer pulmonic form. Peak incidence is in the second and third decades of life, with 50% more males affected than females. In some, early stages of this disease are modified by antibiotics.

c. MU (μ) CHAIN DISEASE

A few cases of CLL have serum M-components consisting only of μ chains. Unlike the situation with other heavy chain diseases, the abnormal protein is not found in the urine. Large vacuolated plasma cells may be found in the bone marrow.

6. *Light chain disease*

Light chain disease is associated with depressed levels of normal immunoglobulins. Bone lesions are more common and the survival shorter than in patients with an intact myeloma protein even when light chain excretion is also present.

7. *Indolent variants*

Certain "smoldering myelomas" have an unusually indolent course.

- Bone marrow plasma cells are $>10\%$, but sheets are not found.
- Light chains may be present.

- Other immunoglobulins are normal or depressed.
- Renal disease and bone lesions are usually absent.
- Plasma β_2 microglobulin levels are lower than in typical myeloma.

Solitary plasmacytomas, more common in males, are found about a decade earlier than in multiple myeloma. About 85% progress to multiple myeloma. In the absence of bone involvement, cure by radiation therapy is likely.

8. *Monoclonal gammopathy of unknown significance*

Monoclonal IgG proteins are often found without other evidence of disease and are seemingly **benign**.

- Hemoglobin and albumin levels are normal.
- M-component is <2 g/dl and does not increase with time.
- Bone marrow plasmacytosis and renal and bone diseases are not present.
- Immunoglobulins are normal.
- A significant number develop myeloma if followed long enough.
- Incidence increases with age and may be as high as 6% in octogenarians.

Small IgM M-components commonly occur in **lymphoproliferative disorders** (CLL and lymphoma). All such patients require careful long-term follow-up.

9. *Therapy*

Drugs effective in myeloma include L-phenylalanine mustard (Alkeran®), cyclophosphamide (Cytoxan®), prednisone, vincristine, BCNU, and Adriamycin®. The standard therapy against which other therapy is compared is still Alkeran® and prednisone.

- Whether multiple-drug chemotherapy is better than standard therapy in the initial management of poor-prognosis patients is still unclear.
- In contrast to initial therapy, therapy of patients who relapse after an initial response is improved by using a combination chemotherapy (vincristine, Adriamycin®, and prednisone).
- Therapy is usually stopped when the M-component is no longer decreasing and the patient is otherwise stable.
- Long-term maintenance therapy is avoided when the patient is stable because of the risk of secondary leukemia.
- Good supportive care is essential in preventing such complications as infection, hypercalcemia, dehydration, hyperviscosity, and spinal cord compression.

B. Macroglobulinemia of Waldenström

This disorder, also known as primary macroglobulinemia, is a neoplastic proliferation of plasmacytoid lymphocytes that may be considered a variant of lymphocytic lymphoma (see lecture 23) in which the abnormal cell is an activated B lymphocyte. Marrow and other organs are infiltrated with immunoglobulin-producing cells, and tissue mast cells are increased.

1. Clinical features

The peak incidence occurs at age 60–70%. There is a slight predilection for males. Survival averages 2–5 years but occasionally is much longer. The clinical picture is determined by the tumor cell infiltration and the effects of IgM. Infiltration usually causes hepatosplenomegaly and lymphadenopathy (which is unusual in multiple myeloma). Bone involvement (in contrast to multiple myeloma) is rare. Neurologic symptoms, such as peripheral neuropathy, are common. Manifestations of the abnormal protein are:

- Presence of an IgM M-component
- Hyperviscosity of the blood
- Retinal hemorrhages and mucosal bleeding
- Bence Jones proteinuria in at least 10% of cases (which is less common than in multiple myeloma)
- Renal disease which is usually glomerular rather than tubular

2. Therapy

As in multiple myeloma, therapy consists mainly of cytolytic agents such as chlorambucil (Leukeran®), cyclophosphamide (Cytoxan®), and L-phenylalanine mustard (Alkeran®). In the face of incipient blindness from retinal hemorrhage, intractable congestive failure, or other severe manifestations of the hyperviscosity syndrome, intensive plasmapheresis may be useful. Unlike the abnormal proteins of multiple myeloma, the IgM of macroglobulinemia is largely within the blood and thus can be substantially diminished by plasmapheresis.

C. Amyloidosis

1. Classification

Patients with amyloidosis have proteins whose secondary structure is a β-pleated sheet rather than an α-helix. This secondary structure accounts for the green birefringent fluorescence under polarized light after Congo red staining. The type of protein is used to classify various amyloidosis syndromes:

- In **primary amyloidosis** and that associated with plasma cell disorders, the protein includes a portion from the variable region of the light chain and the **P-component**. (P-component is found in all types of amyloid and is closely related to the acute phase reactant C reactive protein).
- In **secondary amyloidosis**, the protein has the P-component and **amyloid A**, which is derived from another acute phase reactant called serum amyloid A.

2. *Clinical features*

The following findings are common in primary amyloidosis and amyloidosis associated with plasma cell disorders:

- Light chains often have a κ/λ ratio of 2, the reverse of the normal ratio.
- Clinical findings reflect sites of amyloid deposition. Areas frequently involved include: tongue, cardiac muscle and conduction system, kidney, synovia of joints, liver and spleen, peripheral and autonomic nerves, and small bowel involvement, which may cause malabsorption. Endocrine glands are usually not involved. Diagnosis is made by biopsy of the involved organ, bone marrow examination and protein electrophoresis of the serum and urine.

3. *Therapy*

There is no established therapy for these disorders.

D. Cryoglobulinemia

1. *Classification*

Cryoglobulins are circulating proteins that become insoluble at reduced temperatures. There are three types:

- **Type I** consists of monoclonal proteins, usually in a patient with myeloma.
- **Type II** is a monoclonal antibody, which forms a complex with IgG.
- **Type III** comprises immune complexes in which both components are polyclonal.

2. *Diagnosis*

Diagnosis depends on demonstration of the abnormal protein or immune complex and identification of its components. Precautions are required to ensure that the cryoglobulin does not precipitate during serum protein electrophoresis or immunoelectrophoresis. The clinical picture depends on the precipitation temperature and the structure of the resulting gel.

3. *Therapy*

The approach to therapy depends on clinical severity. In some cases, plasmapheresis can reduce cryoglobulin levels. Treatment of an underlying disease may also be helpful.

VI. SERUM PROTEIN ELECTROPHORESIS

This brief section provides a guide to the interpretation of serum electrophoretic patterns and an assessment of the value and limitations of this simple and widely used technique in the interpretation of clinical problems. Discussion of abnormalities in M-component diseases will not be repeated.

Table 25.3
Proteins Visible on Agarose Gel Electrophoresis

Protein	Function	Concentration in normal serum (mg/dl)	Mol. wt.
Prealbumin	Thyroxine-binding	10–40	70,000
Albumin	Colloid osmotic pressure; transport	3500–5000	69,000
α_1-Antitrypsin	Protease inhibitor	200–400	45,000
α_2-Macroglobulin	Protease inhibitor	150–400	720,000
Haptoglobin	Hemoglobin binding	50–200	85,000
Transferrin	Fe transport	200–400	90,000
β-Lipoprotein	Lipid transport	300–900	>2,000,000
C3	Complement component	100–200	220,000
IgG	Antibody	600–1500	160,000

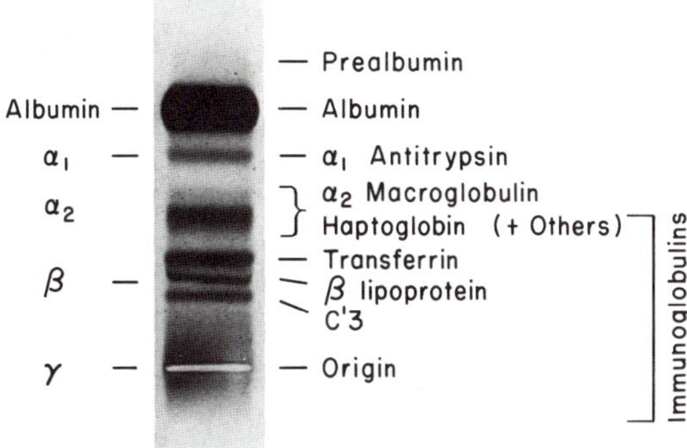

Fig. 25.4
Agarose gel electrophoresis pattern of normal human serum. The anode is at the top and the electrophoresis buffer is pH 8.6, 0.05 M barbital.

A. Proteins in serum

More than 100 serum proteins are known, and the list continues to grow. Many occurring in trace amounts are of great biologic importance. The proteins visible on clinical serum electrophoresis are a small fraction of the number present and represent only those occurring in sufficiently high concentration to form distinct stainable bands (table 25.3). A popular electrophoretic medium is agarose gel; cellulose acetate is also used. Agarose has the advantage of transparency. It also allows distinct separation of transferrin and β-lipoprotein (figure 25.4). If Ca^{2+} is included in the buffer, a slow C3 band can be visualized. If one desires to quantify proteins, chemical or immunochemical techniques must be used. Such methods are now available for 40 to 50 serum proteins.

Table 25.4
Changes in Serum Proteins in Disease

Disease state	Pre-alb	Alb	α_1-at	α_2-glob*	Tf	Lip	C3	IgG
Acute inflammation	↓	↓	↑	↑	↓	±↑	±↑	0
Chronic inflammation	↓	↓	±↑	±↑	↓	±↑	±↑	↑
Obstructive jaundice	0	0	0	0	0	↑	↑	0
Chronic liver disease	↓	↓	±↓	↓	↓	±↓	±↓	↑
Nephrotic syndrome	↓	↓↓	±↓	↑↑	↓	↑↑	0	±↓
Hemolytic anemia	0	0	0	↓	0	0	0	0
Iron deficiency	0	0	0	0	↑	0	0	0
Acute glomerulonephritis	0	0	0	0	0	0	↓	±↑
Lupus erythematosus	↓	↓	↑	±↓	↓	0	±↓	↑

Note: 0 = no change; ↓ = decrease; ↑ = increase; ±↑ = variable increase, etc.
*Changes in α_2-globulin are due mainly to alterations in haptoglobin concentration, except in the nephrotic syndrome, where the increase is due largely to α_2-macroglobulins.

B. Patterns in disease

Table 25.4 summarizes the changes observed on agarose gel electrophoresis of fresh serum from patients with various disease states. Abbreviations in table 25.4 refer to zones and bands described in figure 25.4 and table 25.3. These patterns may overlap in a given patient. For example, the patterns of chronic liver disease and obstructive jaundice often coexist. If a patient with hemolytic anemia also has an inflammatory process, α_1-antitrypsin may be elevated, but haptoglobin does not rise correspondingly. Thus, the α_2-globulin area appears relatively less dense. Changes in lupus erythematosus are variable because the disease is variable in its expression and severity. A low C3 usually indicates severe disease with renal or other parenchymatous involvment. Whether haptoglobin is relatively or absolutely decreased depends on the presence or absence of hemolytic anemia.

1. Acute inflammation

The pattern of acute inflammation is probably the most common in any hospital population. In general, it is nonspecific and occurs in a wide variety of acute inflammatory or necrotic processes, for example, post-surgery, after an acute myocardial infarction, in malignant tumors with necrosis, after pneumonia, or after endotoxin administration. The noted changes occur within a day or two of the insult and persist for 5–7 days, except that C3 does not rise until after the first week and the increase is only moderate.

The pattern of chronic inflammation or necrosis is variable because of varying contributions by continuing acute inflammation and varying antigenic stimulation (the latter resulting in a rise in immunoglobins).

2. *Obstructive biliary disease*

In obstructive biliary disease (or any jaundice with increased conjugated bilirubin), the bilirubin complex binds to albumin and causes a shift in electrophoretic mobility of the albumin toward the anode. Drugs (such as aspirin) can cause the same phenomenon because the altered albumin is more acidic than unaltered albumin.

3. *Chronic liver disease*

In chronic liver disease, α_2-globulin is often decreased because of decreased haptoglobin owing to concomitant hemolytic anemia. The increase in immunoglobulins is particularly marked in the slow β area (because of the marked increase in IgA usually present in this disorder).

4. *Nephrosis*

The nephrotic pattern is one of the most striking of those listed. The increase in α_2-globulin chiefly represents α_2-macroglobulin. In this disorder, there is a general increase in the synthesis of nonimmunoglobulin protein and an increase in the catabolism of all proteins in rough proportion to their molecular weights. The usual cutoff is at about 200,000–300,000. Thus, β-lipoprotein (mol. wt. $>200{,}000$) and α_2-macroglobulin (mol. wt. 720,000) are markedly increased in concentration and most other proteins are reduced. IgG is usually reduced, but if normal, one should suspect preexisting hyperglobulinemia.

5. *Iron deficiency*

The only change in iron deficiency is the increase in transferrin, which is reflected in the rise in total iron-binding capacity (see lecture 7). An artifactual increase in this band may result from extensive hemolysis in vitro since hemoglobin A has the same mobiliy. Small amounts of hemoglobin arising from hemolysis in vitro cause a backward slurring of the α_2-area owing to formation in vitro of hemoglobin-haptoglobin complex.

6. *Acute glomerulonephritis*

In uncomplicated acute glomerulonephritis, the decrease or absence of the C3 band is striking. This persists for up to 4–6 weeks. One must be certain that (1) Ca^{2+} is present in the electrophoresis buffer and (2) the serum sample is fresh. On storage of serum, particularly at elevated temperatures, C3 converts to a large fragment, C3c, that travels just ahead of transferrin. The increase in immunoglobulin often seen in this condition results from the previous streptococcal infection.

7. *Lupus erythematosus*

The pattern in systemic lupus erythematosus usually shows a pronounced increase in slowly migrating IgG. Signs of acute inflammation are also usually present; decreases in α_2-globulin and C3 were discussed above.

8. *Others*

Other situations need only brief mention. Hemoconcentration and hemodilution may be detected by changes in total protein concentration. A decrease in total protein and a general decrease in individual proteins is associated with protein-losing enteropathy. All bands and zones show either an increase or decrease. Specific deficiency states show an absence of single bands or zones (e.g., of albumin, α_1-antitrypsin, transferrin, β-lipoprotein, C3, and the immunoglobulins).

SELECTED REFERENCES

Reviews

Alper, C. A. Plasma protein measurements as a diagnostic aid. *N. Engl. J. Med.* 291(1974): 287–290.

Buzaid, A. C., and Durie, B. G. Management of refractory myeloma: a review. *J. Clin. Oncol.* 6(1988): 889–905.

Durie, B. G. Staging and kinetics of multiple myeloma. *Semin. Oncol.* 13(1986): 300–309.

Fritz, E., Ludwig, H., et al. Prognostic relevance of cellular morphology in multiple myeloma. *Blood* 63(1984): 1072–1079.

Jacobson, D. R., and Zolla-Pazner, S. Immunosuppression and infection in multiple myeloma. *Semin. Oncol.* 13(1986): 282–290.

Kyle, R. A., and Garton, J. P. The spectrum of IgM monoclonal gammopathy in 430 cases. *Mayo. Clin. Proc.* 62(1987): 719–731.

Podell, D. N., Packman, C. H., et al. Characterization of monoclonal IgG cryoglobulins: fine-structural and morphological analysis. *Blood* 69(1987): 677–681.

Sporn, J. R., and McIntyre, O. R. Chemotherapy of previously untreated multiple myeloma patients: an analysis of recent treatment results. *Semin. Oncol.* 13(1986): 318–325.

Stone, M. J. Amyloidosis: a final common pathway for protein deposition in tissues. *Blood* 75(1990): 531–545.

Original articles

Alexanian, R. Localized and indolent myeloma. *Blood* 56(1980): 521–525.

Bataille, R., Grenier, J., et al. Beta-2-microglobulin in myeloma: optimal use for staging, prognosis, and treatment—a prospective study of 160 patients. *Blood* 63 (1984): 468–476.

Bellotti, V., Merlini, G., et al. Relevance of class, molecular weight and isoelectric point in predicting human light chain amyloidogenicity. *Br. J. Haematol.* 74(1990): 65–69.

Bergsagel, D. E., Bailey, A. J., et al. The chemotherapy on plasma-cell myeloma and the incidence of acute leukemia. *N. Engl. J. Med.* 301(1979): 743–748.

Boccadoro, M., Gavarotti, P., et al. Low plasma cell ^{3}H-thymidine incorporation in monoclonal gammopathy of undetermined significance (MGUS), smouldering myeloma and remission phas myeloma: a reliable indicator of patients not requiring therapy. *Br. J. Haematol.* 58(1984): 689–696.

Brouet, J. C., Clauvel, J. P., et al. Biologic and clinical significance of cryoglobulins. A report of 86 cases. *Am. J. Med.* 57(1974): 775–788.

Durie, B. G., Young, L. A., et al. Human myeloma in vitro colony growth: interrelationships between drug sensitivity, cell kinetics, and patient survival duration. *Blood* 61(1983): 929–934.

Greipp, P. R., Katzmann, J. A., et al. Value of beta 2-microglobulin level and plasma cell labeling indices as prognostic factors in patients with newly diagnosed myeloma. *Blood* 72(1988): 219–223.

Greipp, P. R., and Kyle, R. A. Clinical, morphological, and cell kinetic differences among multiple myeloma, monoclonal gammopathy of undetermined significance, and smoldering multiple myeloma. *Blood* 62(1983): 166–171.

Hjorth, M., Hellquist, L., et al. Initial treatment in multiple myeloma: no advantage of multidrug chemotherapy over melphalan-prednisone. *Br. J. Haematol.* 74(1990): 185–191.

Kyle, R. A. Monoclonal gammopathy of undetermined significance. Natural history in 241 cases. *Am. J. Med.* 64(1978): 814–826.

Kyle, R. A,, and Greipp, P. R. "Idiopathic" Bence Jones proteinuria: long-term follow-up in seven patients. *N. Engl. J. Med.* 306(1982): 564–567.

LECTURE 26

The Polycythemias

William B. Castle

EDITOR'S COMMENT

An early draft of this Editor's Comment stated that though retired from his distinguished posts at Harvard Medical School and the Veterans Administration Hospital, Dr. Castle continues to participate in the progress of hematology—and it spoke of our pride in this contribution to our fifth edition. Sadly, Dr. Castle died at the end of the summer of 1990. We will miss him very much and we dedicate this lecture to his memory.

The long list of disorders causing erythrocytosis continues to attract interest and study. The advent of practical assay methods for serum and urine erythropoietin have in the last few years enhanced our ability to distinguish between secondary and primary polycythemias, the former including disorders in which erythropoietin production is either appropriate or inappropriate. Primary polycythemia, a clonal myeloproliferative disorder, continues to elude our basic understanding. It is one of a cluster of stem cell disorders characterized by sustained excessive proliferation of erythroid, myeloid, and megakaryocytic cells in the marrow. Although it is usually well managed by various forms of therapy, each has its disadvantages and the prognosis remains unfavorable after the passage of some years.

I. INTRODUCTION

A. Terminology

The term **polycythemia** denotes a pattern of blood changes that includes a sustained increase in blood hemoglobin concentration (to about 18g/dl or more), red count ($6 \times 10^6/mm^3$ or more), and hematocrit (to 55% or more). The term (and its synonym **erythrocytosis**) is without specific etiologic or diagnostic connotations, polycythemia occurring in a variety of conditions. The increase in red cells and hemoglobin (concentrations) may be unaccompanied by an increase in the total red cell mass (volume). Moreover, in mild hypochromic or microcytic anemia, the red count may be somewhat increased while the hemoglobin concentration is less than normal. Thus the proper distinction between polycythemia and anemia is based strictly on the blood's hemoglobin concentration. In this lecture, **polycythemia** and **erythrocytosis** (a term analogous to **leukocytosis**) are used interchangeably to refer to a nonspecific blood picture. **Absolute polycythemia**, or **absolute erythrocytosis**, is polycythemia in which there is an absolute increase in red cell mass (as determined by ^{51}Cr labeling). **Relative**

erythrocytosis refers to conditions in which the hemoglobin level, red count, and hematocrit are elevated (owing to decrease of plasma volume) but the red cell mass is normal. **Polycythemia vera**, or **erythremia** (a term analogous to **leukemia**), is a myeloproliferative disease in which increased red cell mass is one of several manifestations of panmyelosis.

B. Historical notes

Paul Bert in 1878 predicted that as a "harmonious compensation of Nature," an increase in red cells and hemoglobin would characterize the blood of humans and animals living at high altitudes. In 1890 Viault supposedly confirmed this hypothesis by finding 16×10^6 red blood cells/mm^3 in the blood of Peruvian llamas (mountain sheep). He then demonstrated that although their hemoglobin was partially unsaturated, their blood had a relatively normal oxygen content owing to its increased oxygen-carrying capacity. This finding was later confirmed in humans residing at 15,000 feet above sea level near Lima. In 1892 Vaquez described a patient with polycythemia and cyanosis thought to be secondary to arterial hypoxia from an intracardiac septal defect until autopsy disclosed no such lesion. Consequently, he ascribed the polycythemia to overactivity of the blood-forming organs. This early delineation of the primary form (polycythemia vera or erythremia) attracted the attention of Osler at the turn of the century. Another form of polycythemia, sometimes found in association with certain tumors, was first ascribed to humoral agents from a hypernephroma by Forssell in 1946. Familial polycythemia due to an abnormal hemoglobin with increased affinity for oxygen was first reported by Charache and coworkers in 1966.

II. CLASSIFICATION OF THE POLYCYTHEMIAS

In table 26.1, the polycythemias are divided into those associated with **relative erythrocytosis** (i.e., with normal red cell mass and decreased plasma volume) and those associated with **absolute erythrocytosis** (i.e., with increased red cell mass). Absolute erythrocytosis is divided into those **secondary** to variously induced forms of hypoxia with compensatory erythropoietin elaboration (see lecture 1), those secondary to inappropriate erythropoietin activity, and those due to a **primary**, neoplastic or autonomous increase in erythropoiesis.

III. PATHOPHYSIOLOGY

A. Red cell survival

Whatever the cause, polycythemia is not due to prolonged red cell survival. Erythrokinetic data show that survival is usually normal, though in polycythemia vera a small population of red cells may be short-lived. Increased

Table 26.1
Classification of the Polycythemias

Relative polycythemia (decreased plasma volume)	Water deprivation or febrile dehydration Loss of water and electrolytes: gastrointestinal disease (vomiting or diarrhea); renal disease; adrenocortical insufficiency; stress; Gaisböck's syndrome; vigorous diuretic therapy; etc. Loss of plasma: burns; enteropathy; etc.
Absolute polycythemia	
A. Secondary polycythmia	
1. With compensatory erythropoietin elaboration	With low arterial oxygen saturation Low PO_2 in inspired air: high altitude Low PO_2 in umbilical vein in fetus Ventilation-perfusion imbalance and alveolar hypoventilation: insensitivity of respiratory center; restrictive and/or obstructive pulmonary disease; obesity and/or recumbent posture; kyphoscoliosis; sarcoid; pulmonary fibrosis; berylliosis V-A shunting: intracardiac septal defects; great vessel anomalies; intrapulmonary A-V aneurysm; hemangiomata With normal arterial oxygen saturation Decreased oxygen transport by hemoglobin: methemoglobinemia; carboxyhemoglobinemia; M hemoglobins Increased affinity for oxygen by abnormal hemoglobins: Chesapeake, Rainier, Little Rock, etc. Failure of tissue perfusion: low-output cardiac failure Decreased heme oxygen sensor function: $CoCl_2$ administration
2. With inappropriate erythropoietin elaboration	Renal diseases: hydronephrosis, cysts, hypernephroma Cerebellar hemangioblastoma Hepatoma Adrenal virilizing adenoma Uterine fibroids Thyroid or androgen administration
B. Primary polycythemia	Polycythemia vera (erythremia)

hemoglobin concentration and red cell mass result from a sustained increase in the level of erythropoiesis in the bone marrow. Although the hematocrit and hemoglobin concentration may be nearly double the normal values, they can be sustained by a doubling of the rate of red cell production. Such an increase in marrow activity is distinctly less than the six- to eightfold increase occurring in various chronic hemolytic anemias with short red cell life spans. Absolute reticulocyte counts in polycythemia are therefore only modestly increased.

B. Blood volume and hematocrit

The major determinants of the blood volume are **red cell mass** and **plasma volume**. Normal values for these in males are, respectively, 28.2 ± 4.7 and 39.7 ± 5.3 ml/kg. Because red cells remain confined to the intravascular compartment, the size of the circulating red cell mass can be altered only by variations in the rate of red cell production as long as red cells are destroyed at a fixed rate. Erythropoietic activity of bone marrow is sensitively regulated by the erythropoietin system, but resulting changes in red cell mass occur slowly. Plasma volume is also regulated by homeostatic mechanisms sensitive to pressure, osmolarity, and flow rate, but plasma volume changes occur rapidly because of the ease with which fluid shifts between the intravascular and extravascular compartments. The **hematocrit** is a measure of the volume of red cells per unit volume of blood. The hematocrit of circulating blood varies in different parts of the vascular tree. Thus, the capillary hematocrit, because of the relatively larger amount of plasma adjacent to the proportionately greater vessel wall surface, is lower than the hematocrit of blood in veins or arteries, which in turn is lower than that of blood in spleen and marrow sinusoids. At a given moment, one-fifth of the blood volume is in the capillaries, the low-hematocrit compartment. Hence, the "total body hematocrit" is lower than the "venous hematocrit." This is confirmed when plasma and red cell volumes are measured simultaneously by isotope dilution techniques, the ratio of body hematocrit to venous hematocrit equaling approximately 0.9. This means that true plasma volume exceeds plasma volume calculated from measurements of red cell mass and venous hematocrit. These considerations imply that elevation of the venous hematocrit can result from an increase in red cell mass or a decrease in plasma volume. The two conditions accounting for absolute and relative polycythemia, respectively, cannot be distinguished unless red cell mass is measured.

C. Homeostasis of oxygen transport

Observations in patients with polycythemia vera and in normovolemic and hypervolemic animals have thrown light on the hemodynamic mechanisms that help to maintain the constancy of the blood hemoglobin level.

1. *Viscosity and flow rate*

In normal circumstances, hemoglobin leaving the lung is nearly saturated with oxygen. Measured in vitro in capillary tubes, the **viscosity** of such blood increases exponentially with increases in hematocrit (figure 26.1, curve A). When the **flow rate** through the capillary tube is determined (as reciprocal of viscosity) at various hematocrit levels, flow is seen to decrease as an essentially linear function of hematocrit (figure 26.1, curve B). If flow rate is multiplied by oxygen content (a function of hematocrit), the product provides a relative measure of the rate of **oxygen transport** at different hematocrits for this in vitro system. At low hematocrits oxygen content of the blood is small; at high hematocrits flow rate is small. Consequently oxygen transport is maximal in vitro at intermediate hematocrit values of 45–50%. Were this strictly so in vivo, however, if the hematocrit were to increase even slightly, oxygen transport would decrease, tissue hypoxia would occur, and erythropoietin activity would rise. Thus a vicious cycle or positive feedback loop of ever-increasing hypoxia and polycythemia would be established. But these events do not follow a rise in hematocrit in vivo. In 1929 Campbell found in hypertransfused (and presumably hypervolemic and polycythemic) animals that tissue oxygen tension—determined by analysis of peritoneal or subcutaneous gas pockets—increased whenever the hematocrit increased. Modern experiments in animals confirm the appropriate homeostatic responses of tissue PO_2, respectively, to transfusion polycythemia and blood loss anemia (figure 26.2).

2. *Blood volume and cardiac output*

Despite the increased viscosity of polycythemic blood, polycythemia enhances oxygen transport in vivo. Hence other factors were sought to explain this seeming paradox. These factors were found to be **increased blood volume** and **increased cardiac output**. Blood volume is invariably increased in patients with polycythemia approximately by the amount of the increase of red cell mass. In turn, the venous vascular bed enlarges and peripheral resistance decreases. Since blood pressure remains stable, increased venous return and consequent cardiac output must accompany these peripheral vascular changes. Together the increased cardiac output and the higher hematocrit (oxygen content) result in increased oxygen transport despite the increased viscosity of the blood. Indeed oxygen transport in hypervolemic (polycythemic) dogs is better than in normovolemic dogs, especially at moderately high hematocrits (figure 26.3). This causes an increase in tissue oxygen tension and consequently a decrease in erythropoietin production. On the contrary, there is an increase in erythropoietin production in anemic dogs and humans. This occurs because of the decreased tissue oxygen tension that results from the lowered hemoglobin concentration and despite the opposition of lessened blood viscosity and peripheral vascular resistance (hypoxia) that increase cardiac output and despite the rightward shift of the hemoglobin oxygen dissociation curve due to increased red cell 2,3-DPG (see lecture 9).

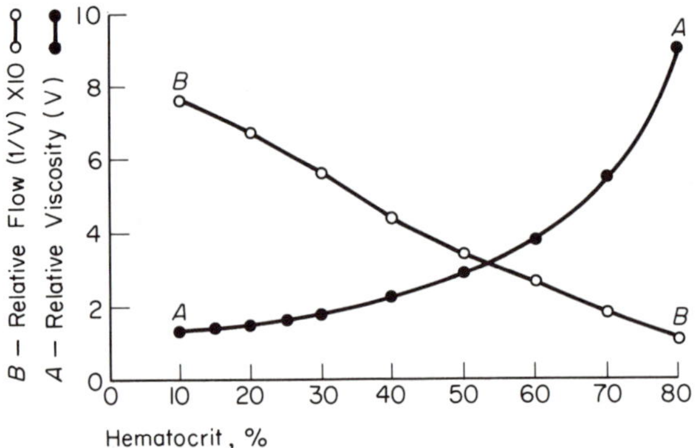

Fig. 26.1
Relation of blood viscosity (curve A) and relative blood flow through a capillary tube (curve B) of human blood of various hematocrits. Curve B is the reciprocal of curve A. In order to employ the same ordinate scale, its values were multiplied by 10. (From W. B. Castle and J. H. Jandl, *Semin. Hematol.* 3[1966]: 193, by permission of Grune & Stratton, New York.)

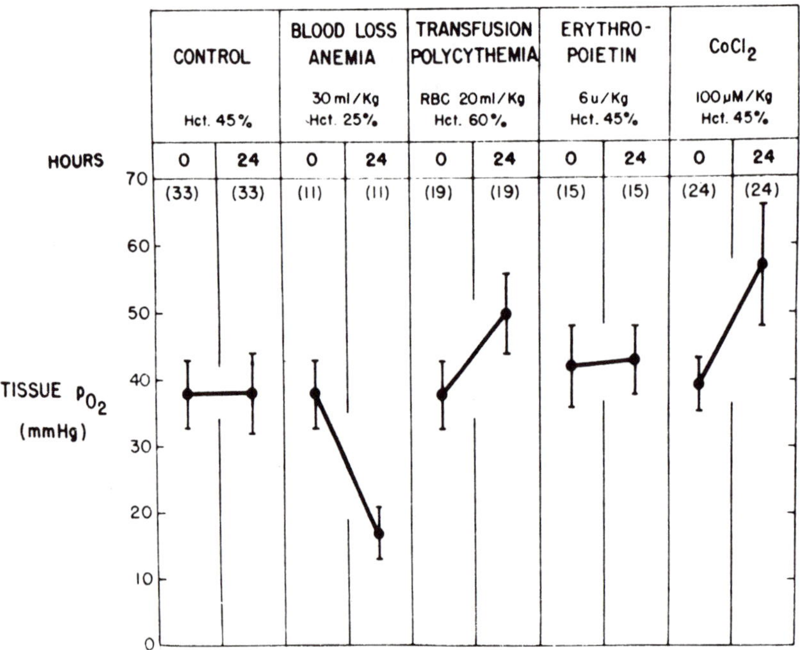

Fig. 26.2
Oxygen tension (mean ±15.0) of air pockets introduced subcutaneously in rats. The effects of bleeding, transfusion, erythropoietin, and cobalt on the oxygen tension are given. As expected, bleeding causes hypoxia, transfusion causes hyperoxia, and erythropoietin has no immediate effect. Cobalt has recently been shown to impair erythropoietin production by blocking the renal oxygen sensor, a heme protein. (From A. J. Erslev and T. G. Gabuzda, *Pathophysiology of Blood.* Philadelphia: W. B. Saunders Co., 1975, p. 25, by permission of W. B. Saunders Co., Philadelphia.)

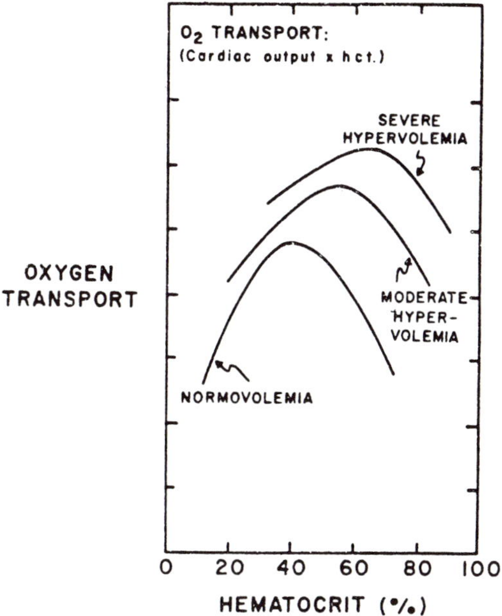

Fig. 26.3
Calculated in vivo oxygen transport in normovolemic and hypervolemic conditions after red cell transfusions in dogs. Oxygen transport increases when red cell mass is increased, because cardiac output and oxygen content of arterial blood are increased. (From J. F. Murray et al., *J. Clin. Invest.* 42[1963]: 1150, and E. B. Thorling and A. J. Erslev, *Blood* 31[1968]: 332, by permission of Grune & Stratton, New York.)

In sum, the constancy of the normal hemoglobin level, a function of the rate of red cell production, depends on the homeostatic effect of tissue oxygen tension. This implies the existence of tissue oxygen sensors in the negative feedback loop that determines erythropoietin production.

3. *Situation in polycythemias*

In polycythemia vera, the increase in blood oxygen content, blood volume, and cardiac output are not in response to a physiologic need for better tissue oxygenation. Consequently, normalization of these is inherently advantageous. In secondary hypoxic polycythemia, however, the arterial blood is unsaturated with oxygen. Nevertheless, the rise in cardiac output increases oxygen transport, though to a lesser extent for a given hematocrit. Thus, some degree of polycythemia is acceptable provided it can be sustained without cardiac strain.

IV. RELATIVE POLYCYTHEMIA

Two types of fluid shifts account for a high hematocrit in the presence of a normal red cell volume: (1) an absolute decrease in plasma volume and (2) a normal total plasma volume accompanied by an abnormal

Table 26.2
Mean Blood Volume Values in Spurious Polycythemia

Subjects	Venous hematocrits (%)	Red cell volume (ml/kg)	Plasma volume (ml/kg)	Hypertension (%)
Normal	47 ± 2.5	28.2 ± 4.1	39.7 ± 5.3	0
Group I	54.2 ± 2.4	32.9 ± 2.2	33.1 ± 3.9	38
Group II	54.6 ± 2.0	27.9 ± 2.4	30.4 ± 5.2	55

Figures are means ± SD. Patients in group I have high normal red cell volumes and slightly low plasma volumes. Patients in group II have low normal red cell volumes and low plasma volumes. Hypertension, more common in group II, probably classifies these as Gaisböck's syndrome or stress polycythemia. (Adapted from N.J. Weinreb and C.-F. Shih, *Semin. Hematol.* 12[1975]: 397.)

distribution of blood in the vascular tree such that the fraction in the low-hematocrit (capillary) compartment is relatively increased.

Both may occur acutely, as in dehydration, burns, and after vigorous diuretic therapy, or they may be chronic as in adrenocortical insufficiency. In some cases the condition is chronic and without obvious cause. Such patients are typically florid and tense middle-aged men, sometimes with moderate hypertension, who complain of headaches, dizziness, and increased sweating. Their heavy smoking habits may produce some carboxyhemoglobin. These obese individuals have short necks and hypoventilate in the recumbent position. Both of these traits may produce hypoxic secondary polycythemia. The hematocrit in these patients rarely exceeds 60%. The blood count is otherwise normal. Other frequent laboratory abnormalities are hypercholesterolemia and/or hyperlipemia and modest hyperuricemia. The cases of hypertension and elevated red cell count described by Gaisböck in 1905 as **polycythemia hypertonica** were probably examples of this condition. This picture was later called **stress erythrocytosis**, but this term inappropriately suggests the presence of an elevated red cell mass. Better terms are **relative erythrocytosis** or **spurious erythrocytosis** since they emphasize that hematologic disease is not present. Indeed the venous hematocrit may be elevated in the case of a high *normal* red cell volume (mass) and a low *normal* plasma volume (table 26.2). Moreover the estimation of red cell mass is subject to less than precise correlations with body weight and surface area.

V. ABSOLUTE POLYCYTHEMIA

A. Secondary polycythemia

Cases of secondary or reactive polycythemia are divided into (1) those in which tissues are hypoxic and a compensatory elaboration of erythropoietin occurs and (2) those in which tissue oxygenation is normal but an inappropriate elaboration of erythropoietin takes place. The properties of erythropoietin, its relation with the kidney, and mode of action are described in lecture 2.

1. With compensatory erythropoietin elaboration

a. WITH LOW ARTERIAL OXYGEN

The low PO_2 of air at high altitudes decreases arterial oxygen saturation. Partial, temporary compensation is provided the newly arrived lowlander by increases in cardiac output and pulmonary ventilation. The latter elevates alveolar PO_2 but initially causes alkalosis and a leftward shift of the oxygen dissociation curve via the Bohr effect (see figure 9.6). Simultaneously, there begins an increase in red cell 2,3-DPG that causes a rightward shift of the dissociation curve that persists after reestablishment of normal blood pH (see lecture 9). In a few days, the reticulocyte count rises, and over a period of several weeks the hemoglobin concentration increases. However, even in the fully acclimated barrelchested Andean native, the PO_2 of polycythemic arterial blood remains decreased despite hyperventilation, and there is mild cyanosis. Despite its augmented oxygen content, the oxygen saturation of the arterial blood is always less than the oxygen-carrying capacity (which is proportional to its hemoglobin content), as shown in table 26.3. Despite the lower PO_2 with which arterial blood enters the capillaries, its increased oxygen content helps to maintain a higher average capillary oxygen tension than would have been the case without the increase in hemoglobin and oxygen capacity.

Most earlier studies were conducted on small groups in high-altitude mining communities (table 26.3). Since many suffered from chronic respiratory disorders including silicosis, results could not be attributed solely to low atmospheric PO_2. Later studies of native Peruvian shepherds and farmers at 14,000 feet above sea level showed mean hemoglobin levels of 17.3 ± 1.5 g/dl and mean hematocrits of $51.4 \pm 3.9\%$. These values resemble those found earlier by Hurtado et al. at an altitude of only 4800 ft

Table 26.3
Arterial Blood in Altitude Polycythemia

		Arterial oxygen		
Altitude (ft × 10^{-3})	Hemoglobin (g/dl)	Capacity (vol %)	Content (vol %)	Saturation (%)
0	16.5	21.4	20.6	96.0
4.8	17.1	22.2	20.9	93.8
12.0	19.4	25.2	22.1	87.6
14.7	21.1	27.5	22.3	81.0
17.4	23.2	30.2	23.0	76.2

Source: From A. Hurtado, C. Merino, and E. Delgado, *Arch. Intern. Med.* 75(1945): 284.

(table 26.3). Clearly the striking polycythemia in the industrial Andean group was due to a combination of high altitude and chronic respiratory insufficiency.

Certain animal species may be genetically adapted to low ambient oxygen levels. California ground squirrels living at an altitude of 12,500 ft have a mean hemoglobin of only 14.3 ± 0.8 g/dl, whereas laboratory rats born and raised at that altitude have mean levels of 19.3 ± 1.5 g/dl. In ground squirrels (and Himalayan sherpas) the leftward shift of the oxygen dissociation curve favors the uptake of oxygen by hemoglobin at high altitude (figure 26.4). Despite the resulting decrease in oxygen unloading in the tissues, the animals were able to perform well at low tissue PO_2 values that killed more than half of the altitude-acclimatized rats in an hour. In both humans and animals such as the Peruvian llama the relatively normal hematocrits at high altitude permit increased oxygen transport without the disadvantage of increased blood viscosity of polycythemia (see figure 26.1).

In the other forms of tissue hypoxia—including those induced by cardiopulmonary disease, arteriovenous shunting, or depression of the respiratory center—erythrocytosis likewise results from reduced arterial oxygen content and tissue PO_2 (figure 26.5). Consequently, in these cases determination of arterial PO_2 is a necessary diagnostic procedure. A patient with significant erythrocytosis due to arterial hypoxia is cyanotic even in a warm room, and his or her arterial blood may be unsaturated to a degree corresponding to that of polycythemic subjects residing at high altitude (table 26.3). In practice, especially in patients with pulmonary disease, the

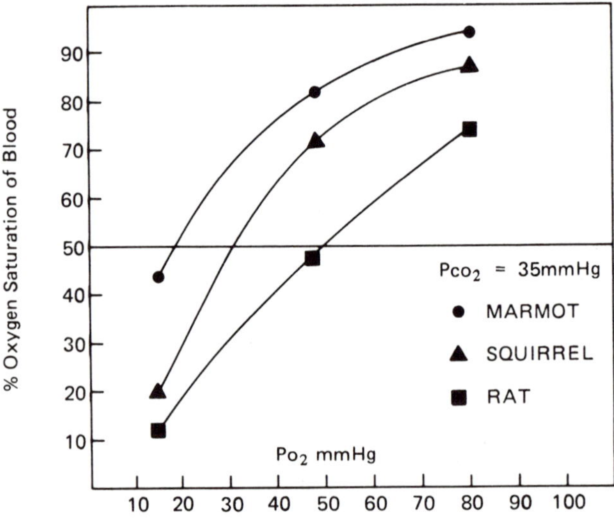

Fig. 26.4
Three-point oxygen-hemoglobin dissociation curves determined for the ground squirrel and marmot native to high altitude and altitude-acclimatized rat. The leftward shift of the native rodent's curves permits higher percentage of oxygen saturation for them at the diminished oxygen tensions of high altitude. (From R. W. Bullard, *J. Applied Physiol.* 20[1966]: 997.)

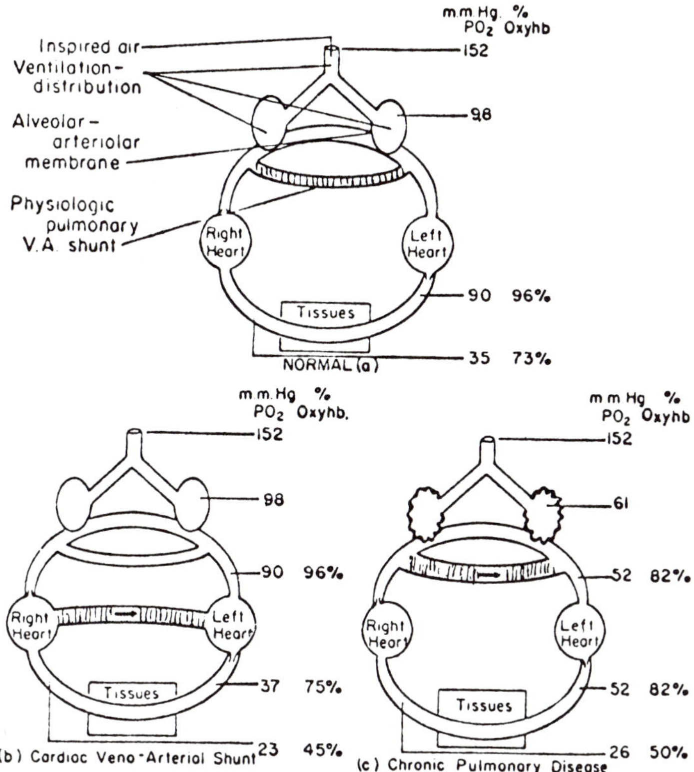

Fig. 26.5
Pathologic physiology of secondary hypoxic polycythemias. In altitude polycythemia, the normal diagram would be modified to show a lower PO_2 in the inspired air with consequent unsaturation of the arterial blood. In hypoventilation polycythemia, as in chronic pulmonary disease, the major abnormality in the transport of oxygen is the lowered PO_2 of the alveolar air. (From M. A. Escobar and F. E. Trobaugh, Jr., *Med. Clin. North Am.* 46[1962]: 253, by permission of W. B. Saunders Co., Philadelphia.)

arterial PO_2 level does not always correlate with the degree of erythrocytosis. It may be **high** relative to the hemoglobin concentration because (1) it was determined after therapeutic improvement in respiratory function; (2) the procedure of arterial puncture may briefly stimulate better ventilation via psychological or reflex mechanisms; or (3) respiration during sleep or recumbency, especially in obese subjects, is less effective than during wakefulness, when the determination is made. It may be **low** relative to the hemoglobin concentration because chronic infection accompanying a pulmonary disorder inhibits the erythropoietin response or renders the marrow less responsive to erythropoietin.

b. WITH NORMAL ARTERIAL OXYGEN

Tissue hypoxia may occur in the presence of normal arterial oxygen saturation in any circumstance that impairs the binding or release of oxygen by hemoglobin. Its well-known association with chronic carbon monoxide exposure is based on the fact that increasing concentrations of blood carboxyhemoglobin shift the oxygen dissociation curve leftward. Perhaps the heavy cigarette smoking of many patients with "stress polycythemia" produces this effect. According to Astrup, continuous cigarette smoking for 2 hr may result in 15% carboxyhemoglobin. Several hemoglobin variants are described in lecture 10 that cause a leftward shift in the oxygen dissociation curves (obvious at PO_2 50) and erythrocytosis. These genetically determined abnormal hemoglobins cause minimal symptoms. They escaped earlier recognition because most of them are electrophoretically normal and saturate normally at PO_2 100. Their high oxygen affinity results from amino acid substitutions that (1) stabilize the oxyhemoglobin form (Chesapeake and Yakima); (2) destabilize the deoxyhemoglobin form (San Diego and Rainier); or (3) inhibit binding of 2,3-DPG (Little Rock). Thus previously reported instances of "benign familial polycythemia" all require reinvestigation as possible manifestations of such hemoglobinopathies. Interestingly, polycythemia does not develop in all individuals with these hemoglobin variants, in some instances because the instability of the variant causes an associated hemolysis. Also, there are rare instances of benign polycythemia in young persons for which no explanation can be offered for the expanded erythropoietic marrow pool. In others autonomous erythroid colony formation is observed in marrow cultured without added erythropoietin, as in polycythemia vera.

Hemoglobin fails to transport oxygen when its iron is oxidized. This condition (methemoglobinemia) may be acquired (lecture 9) or congenital (lecture 10). Patients with congenital methemoglobinemias rarely display more than slight polycythemia, possibly the result of a mild associated hemolytic process. Finally, tissue hypoxia with normal arterial oxygen saturation may result from substances that impair the function of the renal oxygen sensor (a heme protein) that regulates erythropoietin production. These include cobaltous and nickel ions. Thus subcutaneous gas pockets formed in mice injected daily with $CoCl_2$ contain higher oxygen tensions than those of control mice given saline injections (see figure 26.2). Sustained sublethal concentrations of cyanide may have a similar effect because of the action of cyanide on tissue cytochromes.

2. *With inappropriate erythropoietin elaboration*

Appreciation that the effect of hypoxia on erythropoiesis is mediated by a humoral factor, erythropoietin, and development of assay methods for erythropoietin has led to an understanding of many isolated cases of erythrocytosis occurring in the absence of demonstrable tissue hypoxia. The mechanism of erythrocytosis appears to be an exaggeration of erythropoietin production by the tissues that normally produce it or inappropriate secretion by tissues not normally involved in its production.

Renal tissue is involved in the production of erythropoietin, and polycythemia has occurred in association with hydronephrosis and renal cystic disease and in the rejection phase of renal transplants. In these conditions the increased production of erythropoietin is probably analogous to the experimental production of polycythemia in animals by local interference with renal blood or urine flow and consequent stagnant hypoxia of renal tissue. This may also be so with renal tumors.

Polycythemia may also result from an ectopic source of erythropoietin, such as renal or hepatic tumor, cerebellar hemangioblastoma, or large uterine fibroids. During fetal and neonatal life the liver is the primary site of erythropoietin production, but in the adult it contributes only 10%. Renal and hepatic erythropoietins are biologically and antigenically identical. Urinary assays have shown that the increased erythropoietin excretion with tumors is independent of the hematocrit level. Removal of a variety of primary renal tumors has abolished the polycythemia, which has recurred when metastases developed in the opposite kidney (and perhaps elsewhere). The possibility remains that some renal tumors induce increased erythropoietin production by causing local tissue hypoxia and that the subtentorial location of the usual vascular brain tumor associated with polycythemia may allow it to interfere with the respiratory center as in the case of other rare neural lesions. The frequency of the association between hepatic tumors and polycythemia is second only to that of renal tumor. Testosterone and its analogues have a useful therapeutic effect in certain anemias because they increase erythropoietin production or activity. The occasional association of polycythemia with exogenous androgen administration or Cushing's disease and other androgen-secreting tumors probably relates to an effect of androgenic steroids in promoting erythropoietin secretion or activity.

B. Primary polycythemia (polycythemia vera)

An increased red cell mass occurs in both polycythemia vera (erythremia) and the various secondary polycythemias; however, the relatively advanced age of patients with polycythemia vera and the frequent increases in their leukocytes and platelets contrast with secondary polycythemias, which occur at any age and affect only the red cells. Polycythemia vera is one manifestation of the panmyelosis that characterizes the myeloproliferative disorders and is a disease of late middle life and beyond.

As noted in lecture 20, the myeloproliferative disorders are of unknown etiology. There is presumably neoplastic overproduction of one or more of the cell lines arising by differentiation of the marrow stem cell. The underlying defect is probably of the pluripotent stem cell. Consistent with this is the observation that when isoenzymes of G-6-PD were used as cell markers for the study of the cellular mosaicism as determined by the Lyon hypothesis (see lecture 15), it was shown that when females who are Gd^B/Gd^A heterozygotes get polycythemia, all blood cells (red cells, white cells, and platelets) contain one or the other form of G-6-PD. Marrow fibroblasts contain both markers. This implies that the three hematopoietic cell line cells have a clonal origin, as would be expected if initial pathogenesis were due to a rare oncogenic influence (e.g., somatic cell mutation in the hematopoietic stem cell). In additon to occasional chromosomal aberrations, such mutated stem cells have altered proliferative capacities in vitro. Recently stem cells from the marrow of a female G-6-PD heterozygote with polycythemia vera were shown to develop in culture the mutated type of erythroid colonies without the addition of erythropoietin. When erythropoietin was added, however, colonies of the normal erythroid clone appeared, and those of the abnormal clone increased.

1. Clinical features

Clinical symptoms are due to

- Increased red cell mass and blood volume (headache, plethoric appearance, pruritus, dyspnea, and hemorrhage)
- Increased blood viscosity (paresthesias, circulatory stagnation, and thrombosis);
- Hypermetabolism (night sweats, weight loss, and elevated basal metabolic rate). Hyperuricemia results from the increased nucleoprotein catabolism of hyperactive hematopoiesis. Attacks of gout occur infrequently.
- Splenomegaly is commonly present. It may not be apparent early but may become massive late in the disease.

Paradoxically, hemorrhage and thrombosis are common. Hemorrhage is promoted by (1) increased blood volume that distends veins and capillaries with results similar to the local effects of a venous tourniquet; (2) defective platelet function; and (3) defective clot formation because of masses of red cells entrapped in the clot. Activation of the intrinsic coagulation cascade occurs, but apparently vascular thrombosis is the result of increased blood viscosity with high platelet levels that predispose to platelet aggregation. In addition, the platelets are resistant to PGD_2, a platelet prostaglandin that opposes collagen-induced aggregation in vitro. Blood

Table 26.4
Features of Primary Polycythemia, Secondary (Hypoxic) Polycythemia, and Relative Erythrocytosis

Manifestations	Primary polycythemia	Secondary polycythemia	Relative erythrocytosis
Clinical features			
Cyanosis (warm)	Absent	Present	May be present
Heart or lung disease	Absent	Present	Absent
Splenomegaly	Present in 75%	Absent	Absent
Hepatomegaly	Present in 35%	Absent	Absent
Laboratory features			
Arterial oxygen saturation	Normal	Decreased	Normal
Red cell mass	Increased	Increased	Normal
White count	Increased in 80%	Normal	Normal
Platelet count	Increased in 50%	Normal	Normal
Nucleated red cells, poikilocytes	Often present	Absent	Absent
LAP	Elevated	Normal	Normal
Bone marrow	Hypercellular; increased erythropoiesis and myelopoiesis; increased megakaryocytes; fibrosis	Increased erythropoiesis	Normal
Serum erythropoietin	Decreased	Increased	Normal
Serum cobalamin	Elevated in 75%*	Normal	Normal

*Owing to an increase in transcobalamin III (see lecture 5).

studies reveal increases of granulocytes and platelets, as well as red cells in many patients with polycythemia vera even in early stages (table 26.4). Some, when first encountered, have only a high platelet count, derived, in contrast to those of reactive thrombocythemia, from strikingly polyploid megakaryocytes. In time they develop erythrocytosis and leukocytosis with a marked shift to the left and elevated LAP. Red cell morphology is normal early in the course unless iron deficiency is present. At this stage the bone marrow is hypercellular with increases of erythroid, granulocyte, and platelet precursors. In time nucleated red cells and irregularities in red cell size and shape ("teardrops") may become prominent in the blood as marrow fibrosis develops in a centrifugal direction. The picture is now that of myeloid metaplasia and myelofibrosis, the latter probably resulting from stimulation of stromal cells by platelet-derived growth factor. This phase in turn may give way to acute myelocytic leukemia, which occurs mainly in patients who have received therapeutic irradiation or myelosuppressive drugs.

Ferrokinetic studies with scanning over the enlarged spleen may provide an indication of the presence of extramedullary erythropoiesis there. Iron deficiency with microcytosis, hypochromia, and decreased marrow and serum iron develops in some patients as a result of (1) increased utilization of iron stores by excessive hemoglobin synthesis; (2) decreased intestinal iron absorption (in contrast to the increase occurring in anemia); and (3) loss by therapeutic blood removal or gastrointestinal bleeding, especially from peptic ulcer. With appropriate therapy median survival ranges from 10 to $14\frac{1}{2}$ years.

2. *Laboratory features*

Blood volume is increased by the amount of increase in red cell mass. Plasma volume remains normal. However, with massive splenomegaly, there may be either an anomalous increase in red cell mass or, more commonly, plasma volume. Blood oxygen saturation is normal. Blood viscosity is increased because of the increased hematocrit. Cardiac output is elevated by the increased venous return due to increased blood volume and lowered peripheral resistance. Clinical and laboratory features of polycythemia vera, secondary hypoxic polycythemia, and relative erythrocytosis are compared in table 26.4.

3. *Cytokinetics*

Early in polycythemia vera bone marrow culture reveals normal erythroid and granulocyte/macrophage committed stem cells. The size of the neoplastic stem cell pool is undefined, but with time the percentage of normal committed stem cells declines for both red cells and granulocytes, though at a different rate. Normal CFU-GMs begin to drop out of cycle, and with time normal granulocytes are no longer seen in the blood. Meanwhile an unknown mechanism (independent of erythropoietin) begins inhibiting the development of CFU-Es and BFU-Es so that normal red cells also disappear eventually from the circulation.

4. *Therapy*

The primary goal of therapy is reduction of blood viscosity. This can be achieved by repeated bleeding and/or by myelosuppressive drugs or radiation.

Bleeding at once reduces blood volume, but it decreases viscosity only after restoration of plasma volume from extravascular sources. It must not be done too rapidly since increased blood volume sustains the increased cardiac output essential for tissue oxygenation with viscous blood. For this reason dehydration is also dangerous, and plasma expanders may be desirable at the time of blood removal. In hypoxic polycythemia phlebotomy is judged beneficial if it increases the oxygen content of the mixed venous blood in the right atrium, which reflects the average tissue PO_2. Bleeding also leads to iron deficiency, which may further the goal of therapy by lowering the internal red cell viscosity and delaying erythropoiesis. Severe iron deficiency should be avoided. Rapid (or even slow) bleeding may lead to intolerable hemodynamic changes in some patients and unacceptable rises in the platelet count with increased risk of thrombosis.

Radiation, usually with ^{32}P, controls panmyelosis and extends life expectancy but may increase the frequency of late acute leukemia. Myelosuppressive cytoxic drugs (melphalan, chlorambucil, and hydroxyurea) control panmyelosis but they are also leukemogenic in a certain percentage of cases. This percentage was once thought to be low (around 5%) but recent studies have reported incidences up to 36%, especially in patients given multiple cytoxic drugs. Moreover, these drugs improve morbidity but not survival. Probably only scheduled phlebotomy should be employed, especially in younger patients, unless it is ineffective alone or too inconvenient.

Although increased erythropoietin secretion is not responsible for the erythrocytosis of polycythemia vera, it is of interest that erythropoietin levels do rise in these patients when anemic hypoxia occurs. Thus acute hemolysis or hemorrhage, including excessive therapeutic bleeding, elicits qualitatively normal erythropoietic responses. There is in vitro evidence that both a normal remnant of erythroid precursors and the abnormal anomalous clone respond to strong erythropoietic stimulation. In vivo the abnormal autonomous erythropoiesis proceeds despite the elevated hemoglobin level and decreased erythropoietin production typical of the polycythemic state.

SELECTED REFERENCES

Reviews

Anger, B., Haug, U., et al. Polycythemia vera. A clinical study of 141 patients. *Blut* 59(1989): 493–500.

Conley, C. L. Polycythemia vera. *JAMA* 263(1990): 2481–2483.

Egli, F., Wieczorek, A., et al. Polycythemia vera: clinical findings and course in 86 patients. *Schweiz. Med. Wochenschr.* 118(1988): 1969–1975.

Erslev, A. J. Relative polycythemia (erythrocytosis). In Williams, W. J., et al., eds. *Hematology*, 4th ed. New York: McGraw-Hill, 1990, pp. 715–717.

Erslev, A. J. Secondary polycythemia (erythrocytosis). In Williams, W. J., et al., eds. *Hematology*, 4th ed. New York: McGraw-Hill, 1990, pp. 705–715.

Najean, Y., Deschamps, A., et al. Acute leukemia and myelodysplasia in polycythemia vera. A clinical study with long-term follow-up. *Cancer* 61(1988): 89–95.

Shabbad, E., Cassel, A., et al. Effect of adherent cells on the regulation of BFU-E in patients with myeloproliferative disease. *Am. J. Hematol.* 33(1990): 225–229.

Swolin, B., Weinfeld, A., et al. A prospective long-term cytogenetic study in polycythemia vera in relation to treatment and clinical course. *Blood* 72(1988): 386–395.

Original articles

Cashman, J. D., Eaves, C. J., et al. Unregulated proliferation of primitive neoplastic progenitor cells in long-term polycythemia vera marrow cultures. *J. Clin. Invest.* 81(1988): 87–91.

Da Silva, J. L., Lacombe, C., et al. Tumor cells are the site of erythropoietin synthesis in human renal cancers associated with polycythemia. *Blood* 75(1990): 577–582.

Egli, F., Wieczorek, A., et al. Polycythemia vera: clinical findings and course in 86 patients. *Schweiz. Med. Wochenschr.* 118(1988): 1969–1975.

Juvonen, E., Partanen, S., et al. Megakaryocytic colony formation in polycythaemia vera and secondary erythrocytosis. *Br. J. Haematol.* 69(1988): 441–444.

Kaboth, U., Rumpf, K. W., et al. Treatment of polycythemia vera by isovolemic large-volume erythrocytapheresis. *Klin. Wochenschr.* 68(1990): 18–25.

Means, R. T., Jr., Krantz, S. B., et al. Erythropoietin receptors in polycythemia vera. *J. Clin. Invest.* 84(1989): 1340–1344.

Nand, S., Messmore, H., et al. Leukemic transformation in polycythemia vera: analysis of risk factors. *Am. J. Hematol.* 34(1990): 32–36.

Phillips, W., Wold, H., et al. Risk factors for thrombosis in polycythaemia vera. *Br. J. Haematol.* 69(1988): 422–422.

Reid, C. D., Fidler, J., et al. Endogenous erythroid clones (EEC) in polycythaemia and their relationship to diagnosis and the response to treatment. *Br. J. Haematol.* 68(1988): 395–400.

Shabbad, E., Cassel, A., et al. Effect of adherent cells on the regulation of BFU-E in patients with myeloproliferative disease. *Am. J. Hematol.* 33(1990): 225–229.

LECTURE 27

Hemorrhagic Disorders I. Protein Interactions in the Clotting Mechanism

Robert D. Rosenberg

EDITOR'S COMMENT

Under normal circumstances the only role of clotting is to halt bleeding. One of the most interesting self-regulatory systems in all of biology, clotting is obviously essential to the survival of animals. The fact that blood clots when shed is as remarkable as the fact that it does not normally clot within blood vessels. Here Dr. Rosenberg takes us on a grand tour of this mechanism, describing the remarkable interactions of the various plasma clotting factors and their protein precursors and emphasizing in rigorous detail the nature of the reactions occurring when each clotting factor is activated, as well as the web of factors that control these systems. This lecture, I believe, is not for the fainthearted. We urge readers to brave it carefully. Its rewards are considerable.

I. INTRODUCTION

The normal process of **hemostasis** begins when vascular endothelium is damaged. Exposed subendothelial structures attract platelets and induce their loose **aggregation**. These components in turn initiate the **generation of thrombin**, which aggregates platelets irreversibly and causes the laying down of **clot**, a platelet-fibrin network that is an effective barrier against further escape of blood and a scaffold for repair of vessel damage. Simultaneously, **limiting processes** are activated that confine hemostasis to the site of injury. Finally, **lysis** of the platelet-fibrin network occurs when vascular endothelium is regenerated.

Typical transformations of the hemostatic system are depicted in figure 27.1. An enzyme precursor, or **zymogen**, is normally present in the blood, but possesses essentially no biologic activity. The protein is transformed to a trypsin-like protease (i.e., it is activated) either by a **conformational change** or by scission of peptide bonds via action of a **converting enzyme**. The rate of this reaction may be accelerated by a nonenzymatic protein cofactor, which may act either by altering zymogen conformation (figure 27.1, type 1) or by binding converting enzyme and zymogen close together on a phospholipid surface (figure 27.1, type 2).

During evolution, homologous sets of cofactors and zymogens arose through gene duplication and mutation. This resulted in the development of a linked series of reactions in which a zymogen is converted to a **serine protease** (i.e., a protease that contains an essential serine residue at its active site) that then catalyzes a subsequent precursor-protease transition. In fact,

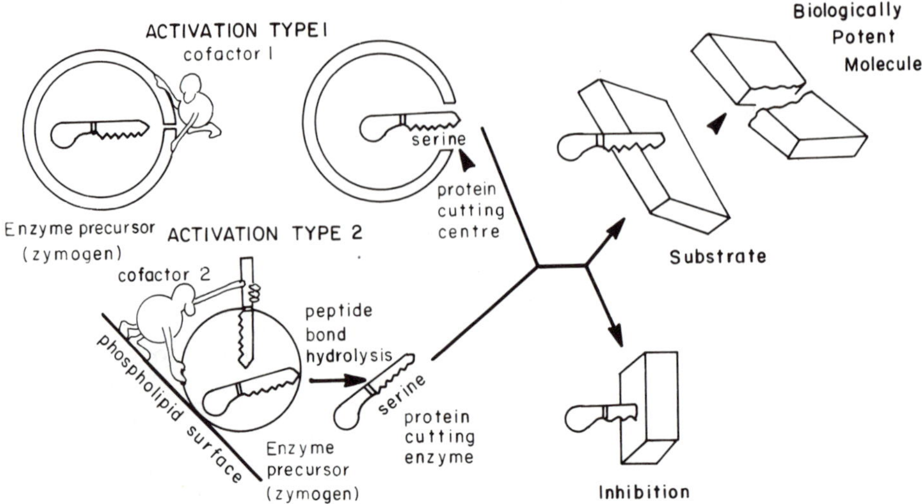

Fig. 27.1
Activation mechanisms for zymogens of the hemostatic reaction.

activation of zymogens in the initial stages of the hemostatic system is accomplished by conformational alteration induced by components (cofactors) that are exposed when vascular endothelium is damaged. But in later stages, activation occurs by proteolytic cleavage of the next zymogen in the sequence. Early reactions tend to occur on surfaces exposed by vascular injury; later reactions are thought to take place on phospholipid surfaces of aggregated platelets. This linked, multistage system permits both amplification and modulation of the initial stimulus that sets the hemostatic mechanism into action. (The soluble clotting factors are by international convention designated by Roman numerals, though various synonyms were used earlier. The factors and their several synonyms are summarized in table 27.1).

The hemostatic system consists essentially of two discrete series of proteolytic reactions. The first is the **clotting**, or **coagulation mechanism**, the end product of which is **thrombin**. The second is the **fibrinolytic mechanism**, the end product of which is **plasmin**. The major role of thrombin is to initiate formation of the fibrin clot by cleaving specific peptide bonds in the plasma protein **fibrinogen**. Plasmin breaks down the clot by hydrolyzing different peptide bonds in the fibrin molecule. These two serine proteases may also interact with plasma components that neutralize their enzymatic activities. These inhibitory species contain peptide sequences similar to those in fibrinogen and other natural substrates of the two enzymes. However, when thrombin or plasmin interacts with these inhibitors, bond hydrolysis is hindered and a stable complex is formed. Thus, similar biochemical mechanisms are responsible for the initiation and suppression of hemostatic system activity.

In this lecture, we shall summarize the biochemistry of these processes, especially the pathways for generation of thrombin, formation of the fibrin

Table 27.1
Glossary of Coagulation Factor Nomenclature

Coagulation factors (international nomenclature)	Synonyms
I	Fibrinogen
II	Prothrombin
III	Tissue factor, tissue thromboplastin
IV	Calcium (Ca^{2+})
V	Proaccelerin Labile factor Ac-globulin
VII	SPCA Convertin Stable factor
VIII	Antihemophilic globulin (AHG) Antihemophilic factor (AHF) Antihemophilic factor A
IX	Plasma thromboplastin component (PTC) Antihemophilic factor B
X	Stuart factor (Stuart-Prower)
XI	Plasma thromboplastin antecedent (PTA) Antihemophilic factor C
XII	Hageman factor Antihemophilic factor D
XIII	Fibrin stabilizing factor (FSF) Laki-Lorand factor
Prekallikrein	Fletcher factor
High-molecular-weight kininogen	Fitzgerald factor
Antithrombin	Antithrombin III
Lipoprotein-associated coagulation inhibitor (LACI)	Extrinsic pathway inhibitor (EPI)
Antiplasmin	
Plasminogen activator inhibitor	(PAI-1)
α_2-Macroglobulin	
Protein C	
Protein S	

Note: Not all coagulation factors have been given roman numerals. Roman numerals were assigned in order of discovery and do not imply place in sequence of reactions. There is no factor VI. This book follows the common practice of referring to factor I as fibrinogen, factor II as prothrombin, factor III as tissue factor, and factor IV as Ca^{2+}.

clot, mechanisms of fibrinolysis, and the several limiting reactions. The platelet and its role in hemostasis will be discussed separately in lecture 28.

II. GENERATION OF THROMBIN

The generation of thrombin can be subdivided into two major sets of reactions: (1) the **activation of factor X** and (2) the subsequent **conversion of prothrombin to thrombin**. These processes are precisely regulated by a series of complex interactions that include the **heparan sulfate–antithrombin** and **protein C–thrombomodulin** mechanisms.

A. Activation of factor X

Two distinct pathways exist for the conversion of the factor X zymogen to its corresponding serine protease, factor Xa (note that by convention the suffix "a" indicates that a factor is in "activated" form). These are the **intrinsic coagulation cascade** and the **extrinsic coagulation cascade**. Activation of each cascade is initiated when damaged vascular endothelium and blood come in contact with components that are normally hidden. Both pathways seem essential for the generation of adequate amounts of factor Xa in vivo.

1. Intrinsic coagulation cascade

a. ACTIVATION OF FACTOR XII

The activation of the intrinsic coagulation cascade is sparked when blood is exposed to collagen, basement membrane, or microfibrillar substance. Factor XII, a single polypeptide chain zymogen of mol. wt. 80,000, is normally present in plasma. It binds to these subendothelial structures and undergoes a conformational transition to factor XIIa, which contains an active serine center. Alternatively, factor XII can be converted to factor XIIa by proteolytic cleavages that produce a diverse spectrum of products of mol. wt. 25,000–75,000. Once formed, factor XIIa is able to hydrolyze prekallikrein and factor XI as well as plasminogen and thus activate the kinin-generating coagulation and fibrinolytic mechanisms (figure 27.2).

Prekallikrein is a single polypeptide chain zymogen of mol. wt. 85,000. It circulates in the blood as a 1 : 1 stoichiometric complex with a cofactor termed **high-molecular-weight kininogen** (mol. wt. 120,000). Factor XIIa can cleave the prekallikrein zymogen and convert it into the serine protease **kallikrein**, which has a heavy and a light polypeptide chain of mol. wt. 52,000 and 33,000, respectively. The presence of high-molecular-weight kininogen cofactor is essential for the rapid generation of kallikrein from prekallikrein. Once formed, kallikrein is able to cleave the single polypeptide chain of high-molecular-weight kininogen and release from the center of the molecule the decapeptide **bradykinin**, a potent substance that lowers

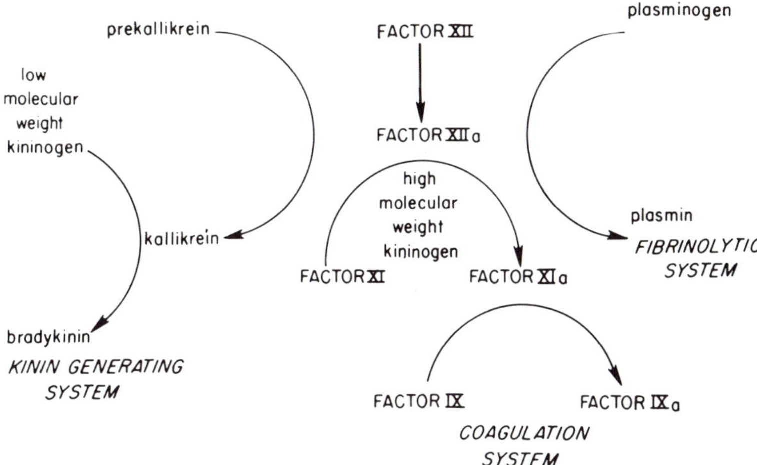

Fig. 27.2
Consequences of factor XII activation.

blood pressure, increases capillary permeability, and acts as a vasodilator. Kallikrein itself exhibits chemotactic activity for neutrophils and monocytes, recruiting them into sites of tissue injury.

b. ACTIVATION OF FACTOR XI

Factor XI is a zymogen formed by two identical polypeptide chains of mol. wt. 80,000 that are connected by disulfide (S–S) bonds. It circulates in plasma as a 1 : 1 stoichiometric complex with high-molecular-weight kininogen. Factor XIIa can convert the factor XI zymogen into the serine protease factor XIa by the scissioning of specific bonds within each of the polypeptide chains of the zymogen. This gives rise to two sets of fragments of mol. wt. 50,000 and 30,000 that are held together by disulfide bonds. Thus, factor XIa structurally is a two-headed dimeric enzyme. High-molecular-weight kininogen must be present if factor XIa is to be rapidly generated in significant quantities. Once formed, factor XIa initiates activation of the remainder of the intrinsic coagulation cascade with the eventual formation of factor Xa (figure 27.3).

Factor XIIa also activates **plasminogen**, a zymogen normally present in the blood, to form the serine protease **plasmin**, which can lyse the fibrin clot (see below). Since factor XIIa can convert plasminogen to plasmin, it can initiate systemic fibrinolysis. It is still unclear whether factor XIIa can directly activate plasminogen or whether this is accomplished indirectly via generation of kallikrein as well as factor XIa, both of which subsequently cleave the zymogen. It is of interest that kallikrein, plasmin, and factor XIa (all generated by factor XIIa) can produce in turn additional factor XIIa by proteolytic cleavage of the factor XII zymogen. **High-molecular-weight kininogen** is a critical cofactor in this process. These multiple path-

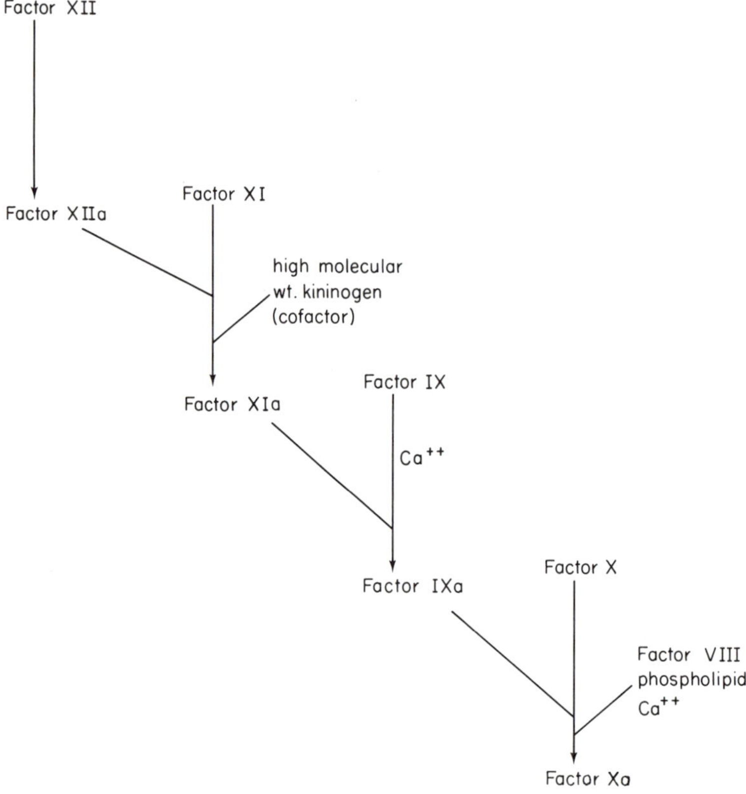

Fig. 27.3
The intrinsic coagulation cascade.

ways autocatalytically magnify the initial stimulus activating factor XII and thereby produce greater amounts of enzyme. However, the species generated is a low-molecular-weight form of factor XIIa, which cannot bind to surfaces and is relatively impotent in activating the coagulation mechanism. This type of factor XIIa is a powerful mobilizer of the fibrinolytic as well as the kinin-generating system. Thus the amplication process described previously orients the hemostatic mechanism toward clot resolution and kinin formation as opposed to fibrin deposition.

c. ACTIVATION OF FACTOR IX

Once generated, factor XIa can interact with a zymogen termed factor IX (a single polypeptide chain of mol. wt. 55,000) and convert it to the serine protease factor IXa (figure 27.4). The initial step in activation is scission of a specific bond within the zymogen to form an inactive two-chain disulfide-linked intermediate that has heavy and light chains of mol. wt. 38,000 and 16,000, respectively. In a later step, a polypeptide of mol. wt. 9000 is split from the newly formed N-terminal of the heavy chain. The product is the serine protease factor IXa.

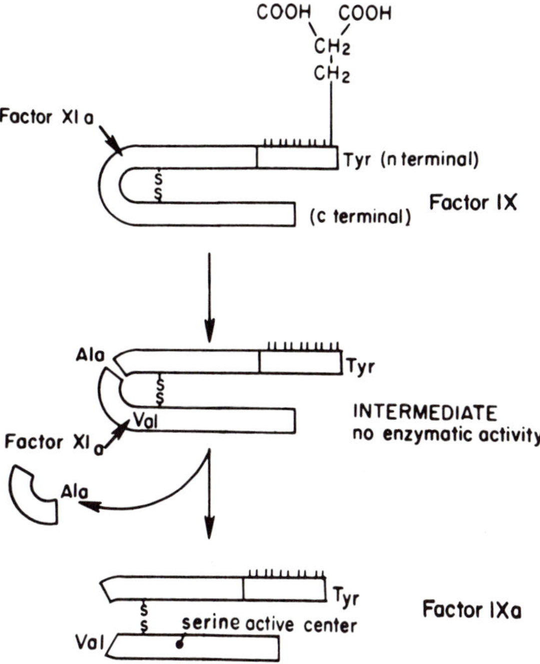

Fig. 27.4
The activation of factor IX.

Preservation of the original N-terminal region of the zymogen within the structure of factor IXa is a critical feature of the activation mechanism. This area contains a number of **γ-carboxyglutamic acid** residues (abbreviated Gla residues) whose presence is due to a vitamin K–dependent postribosomal modification in which preexisting specific glutamyl residues are γ-carboxylated.

The signal for carboxylation is located within the first 18 amino acid residues of the leader sequence of the zymogen which is eventually cleaved to form the mature protein. This region is involved in either translocating the zymogen to the site where carboxylation takes place or is directly involved in binding of the zymogen to the carboxylating enzyme. A similar set of interactions occur with the other vitamin K–dependent coagulation proteins (see below). These unique γ-carboxyglutamic acid residues are directly or indirectly responsible for the binding of factor IXa to phospholipid or platelet surfaces in association with Ca^{2+} ions. Therefore, these residues are essential for the subsequent surface-dependent activation of factor X. The maintenance of these γ-carboxyglutamic acid moieties within factor IXa parallels the situation occurring when prothrombin is transformed to thrombin. In the latter case, these residues are absent from the enzymatic end product. The γ-carboxyglutamic acid residues in factor IXa may localize this enzyme to the area of hemostatic injury and allow it to interact with factor X bound to the same surface. The absence of the same residues in thrombin facilitates diffusion of the enzyme from this locale and permits it to act upon platelets as well as fibrinogen at some distance from the site of hemostatic system activation.

d. ACTIVATION OF FACTOR X

When factor IXa is formed, it converts the factor X zymogen to the serine protease factor Xa. Factor X (mol. wt. 55,000) circulates in plasma as a two-chain species whose primary structure is homologous to that of the factor IX intermediate. The site at which the newly synthesized single-chain factor X is scissioned to form this two-chain zymogen is unknown. The mechanism of activation of this latter component is virtually identical to the second step of factor IX conversion depicted in figure 27.4 Additional scissions at the C-terminal of the heavy chain of factor Xa can occur when high levels of reactants are utilized, but this represents a biologically unimportant set of side reactions.

e. FACTOR VIII AND VON WILLEBRAND'S FACTOR

In vivo, the activation of factor X by factor IXa must occur at a rapid rate and yet be localized to the site of hemostatic injury. This is accomplished by the action of a cofactor termed **factor VIII** in association with Ca^{2+} ions and a phospholipid or platelet surface (see figure 27.3). Factor VIII is synthesized as a single polypeptide chain (mol. wt. 270,000). The primary structure of the cofactor reveals the presence of two different repeating homologous regions. One region occurs twice within the N-terminal domain, and once within the C-terminal domain, whereas the second region is represented twice within the C-terminal domain. The large central domain of the cofactor (about 90,000 daltons) is highly glycosylated. Either during biosynthesis or within the blood, factor VIII is scissioned near the C-terminal domain to generate a heavy chain of 200,000 daltons and a light chain of 80,000 daltons. The two-chain cofactor has minimal biologic activity until it is cleaved by thrombin or factor Xa at three separate sites. The activation process results in the loss of the central domain as two separate fragments, and the release of a 41 amino acid activation peptide from the light chain. The latter event initiates the dissociation of the cofactor from von Willebrand's factor (see below), allows the assembly of the newly formed heavy and light chains via complexing with calcium ions, and permits these two domains to separately bind factor IXa and factor X while interacting with a phospholipid surface. The acceleration of factor X activation is probably achieved by close approximation of enzyme and zymogen on platelet and endothelial cell phospholipids as well as by a conformation change in factor X that renders it more susceptible to attack by factor IXa. Localization of factor Xa generation is attained by formation of the multimolecular complex only at sites of injury and by the presence of γ-carboxyglutamic acid residues on the enzyme. These structures bind factor Xa to the phospholipid surface via Ca^{++} ions and prevent it from diffusing away from the locale.

Factor VIII, the cofactor required for rapid conversion of factor X, circulates bound to a related but distinct protein, **von Willebrand's factor**. This latter substance has a multimeric (polymeric) structure with molecular weights that range up to 5×10^6. Von Willebrand's factor is synthesized as a monomer of 320,000 daltons with cysteine-rich N-terminal and C-terminal nodular regions as well as a central flexible coil domain. The stable protomeric unit of this multimeric structure is a dimer which is disulfide bonded via the C-terminal nodular regions. The dimeric species is then able to slowly assemble via labile disulfide bridges between N-terminal nodular regions. The presence of the N-terminal propolypeptide of about 90,000 daltons is required to guide polymerization of dimers. Thereafter, this large propolypeptide domain is variably removed prior to secretion of the polymers into the blood.

Current data suggest that factor VIII is predominatly bound to the N-terminal nodular regions of the high-molecular-weight multimers of von Willebrand's factor. Given the relative concentrations of these two components, it is apparent that only 3% of the von Willebrand's factor molecules are able to be complexed with factor VIII. Von Willebrand's factor also interacts with the specific platelet receptor **glycoprotein Ib** as well as collagen and thereby mediates adhesion of platelets to the subendothelium. The specific binding sites for the platelet receptor and collagen are found within the central flexible coil domains of the protein. A similar interaction between this plasma protein and the platelet receptor glycoprotein Ib is required for the ristocetin-induced aggregation of these cellular elements. The larger multimeric forms of von Willebrand's factor are essential for its biologic action on platelets. This appears to be due to the high affinity of this form of the protein for the platelet receptor as well as its subsequent ability to bridge the distance between these cellular elements and induce platelet association. The lower molecular weight forms of von Willebrand's factor exhibit this ability to only a minimal extent.

Congenital abnormalities in the function of von Willebrand's factor are widespread and are caused by four major types of defects.

- Relatively common deletions of the gene, alterations in the regulatory domains of the gene, or specific mutations in the exons or introns of the gene may result in decreased levels of circulating protein.
- Relatively infrequent specific mutations within the coding region of the gene may permit proteolytic cleavage of the mature protein, which subsequently decreases the ability of the subunits to form biologically active high-molecular-weight polymers.
- Relatively infrequent specific mutations within the coding region of the gene may also generate high-molecular-weight polymers with an increased propensity to interact with the platelet glycoprotein Ib receptors as well as other components of the vascular tree. This abnormality leads

to decreased levels of the biologically active high molecular weight polymers as well as transient thrombocytopenia.

- Extremely rare mutations of the platelet glycoprotein Ib receptor might either augment interactions with von Willebrand's factor with a resulting reduction in the biologically active high-molecular-weight polymers in a fashion similar to that outlined above or could completely suppress complexing of the platelet receptor with the protein (see Chapter 28).

f. COMPARISON OF VON WILLEBRAND'S DISEASE AND FACTOR VIII DEFICIENCY

It is revealing to contrast the abnormalities noted in von Willebrand's disease with those in factor VIII deficiency. Patients with the former disorder suffer abnormalities in platelet function as well as reductions in factor VIII activity. Patients with the latter abnormality have normal platelet function but exhibit defects in the intrinsic coagulation cascade. These findings support the view that von Willebrand's factor is a carrier of factor VIII. This view is strengthened by the observation that transfusion of plasma from individuals with severe factor VIII deficiency into patients with von Willebrand's disease promptly restores the latter's factor VIII activity to normal. This is accomplished by providing a source of endogenous von Willebrand's factor that can associate with the endogenous factor VIII.

2. *Extrinsic coagulation cascade*

Factor X can also be activated by the addition to plasma of **tissue extracts** (figure 27.5). Two discrete components interact in this mechanism.

a. TISSUE FACTOR

The first is tissue factor, an integral membrane glycoprotein (mol. wt. 35,000) on the surfaces of various somatic cells, especially subendothelial structures such as smooth muscle cells and fibroblasts. Surfaces of cells that are normally in contact with plasma (e.g., endothelial cells, leukocytes) also possess tissue factor. However, the tissue factor present on these surfaces is usually inaccessible unless proteolytic enzymes or membrane damage exposes it.

b. FACTOR VII

The second required component is factor VII (mol. wt. 60,000). It comprises a single polypeptide chain and is structurally homologous to factor II (prothrombin), factor IX, and factor X. Damage to the vascular surface exposes tissue factor, which interacts with factor VII. The phospholipid

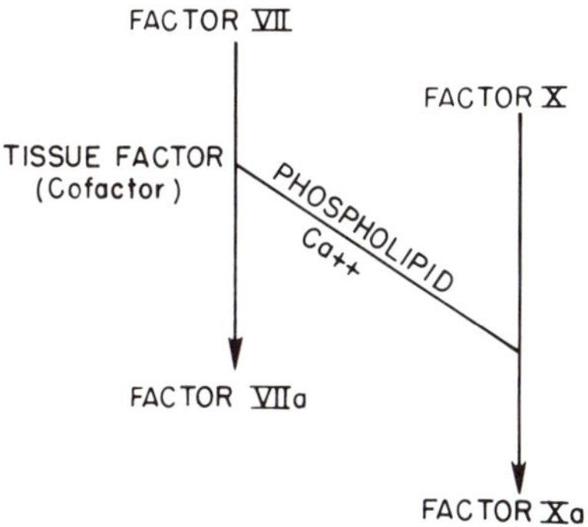

Fig. 27.5
The extrinsic coagulation cascade.

component of tissue factor appears critical for complex formation. When the complex has formed, factor VII is converted into an active serine protease, probably by conformational changes rather than peptide bond scission. However, this issue is being fiercely debated. Both factor VII and factor X are bound to the tissue factor complex via phospholipid-Ca^{2+}-γ-carboxyglutamic acid residues interactions similar to those described above. Factor X is then rapidly converted to factor Xa. The transformation process occurs via proteolytic cleavage identical to those occurring in the intrinsic activation of factor X.

c. CONTROL MECHANISMS

The extrinsic pathway exhibits both positive and negative control mechanisms. For example, generation of factor Xa results initially in the specific cleavage of factor VII to form a disulfide-linked two-chain molecule. This new molecular species binds more tightly to tissue factor and has ~80-fold greater potency with respect to factor X activation. As greater quantities of factor Xa are produced, additional peptide cleavage of the two-chain form of factor VII renders this species inactive.

B. Activation of prothrombin (the common pathway)

Prothrombin is a single chain zymogen (mol. wt. 65,000) with two triple-loop structures termed **kringles** (after a Danish pastry of similar configuration) within its N-terminal region (figure 27.5). The kringles divide this area of the prothrombin molecule into two semi-independent domains termed F_1 and F_2 regions. The F_1 region also contains ten unique γ-carboxyglutamic acid residues, of which six are present as three pairs. These moieties are also formed by a vitamin K–dependent postribosomal process. **Coumarin drugs** act as anticoagulants by opposing the action of vitamin K and preventing the process of γ-carboxylation from taking place. A similar result occurs with factors VII, IX, and X. **Warfarin** is a coumarin drug.

Once the intrinsic and extrinsic coagulation cascades have generated factor Xa in sufficient amounts, it can convert prothrombin to the disulfide-linked two-chain serine protease thrombin. This is accomplished by scissioning Arg_{273}–Thr_{274} and/or Arg_{155}–Ser_{156} and releasing the N-terminal polypeptides F_{1+2} or F_1 and F_2. In a subsequent step of the activation mechanism, factor Xa cleaves Arg_{322}–Ile_{323} in the remaining C-terminal region of prothrombin and generates a two-chain component with enzymatic activity. Release of a 12-amino acid polypeptide from the N-terminal of the latter species also occurs. Direct scission of the Arg_{322}–Ile_{323} bond within the zymogen may also take place to generate an enzymatically active form of thrombin without liberation of the N-terminal region. This short-circuited reaction sequence appears to occur to only a minimal extent under in vivo conditions.

In vitro thrombin generation via this sequence of events proceeds slowly, requiring many hours. In vivo, the process is dramatically accelerated by the action of the cofactor V in conjunction with Ca^{2+} and a phospholipid or platelet surface.

Factor V is synthesized as a single polypeptide chain (mol. wt. 270,000). The primary structure of the cofactor is highly homologous to that of factor VIII. However, factor V circulates as a free single-chain form within the blood. The single-chain cofactor has minimal biologic activity until it is cleaved by thrombin or factor Xa at four separate sites. The activation process results in the loss of the central domain as three separate fragments. This event allows the assembly of the newly formed heavy and light chains via complexing with calcium ions, and permits these two domains to separately bind factor Xa and prothrombin while interacting with a phospholipid surface.

Prothrombin has two specialized features within the N-terminal region that play an essential role in its conversion to thrombin (figure 27.6). First, the γ-carboxyglutamic acid residues of the F_1 region have great avidity for Ca^{2+} ions and are critical sites in the interaction of the zymogen with the phospholipid or platelet surface. During coumarin ingestion, prothrombin is synthesized without a full complement of these unique residues. Hence, the zymogen cannot bind tightly to appropriate surfaces and cannot be rapidly activated to thrombin. Similar functional defects are noted with factors VII, IX, and X synthesized during the same time period. Second, the F_2 region contains a factor V–binding site, which allows the cofactor to interact with the zymogen. Factor V can simultaneously complex with Factor Xa and the platelet phospholipid surface. The **factor V–factor Xa–prothrombin–platelet complex** brings prothrombin and factor Xa into close approximation and increases their chances for interaction. Furthermore, the binding of prothrombin to the factor V–platelet complex probably induces a conformational alteration in the zymogen that renders it more susceptible to proteolysis by factor Xa. The result of these multiple interactions is a 10,000- to 15,000-fold acceleration in the rate of conver-

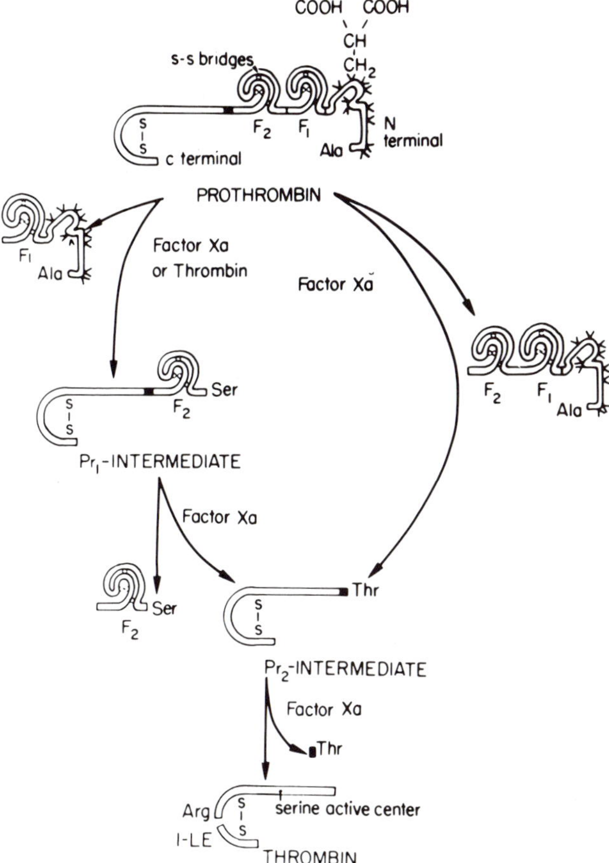

Fig. 27.6
The common pathway of thrombin generation.

sion of prothrombin to thrombin so that this process can take place in a matter of seconds (figure 27.6).

Two regulatory mechanisms may aid in the in vivo control of thrombin generation. On the one hand, thrombin proteolyzes factor V as outlined above and thereby renders it 50–100 times more potent. This favors an augmentation in thrombin production. On the other hand, thrombin generated within the multimolecular complex diffuses out into the blood and is eventually able to release the F_1 fragment from circulating prothrombin. This altered zymogen binds to the factor V–Ca^{2+}–phospholipid complex or to the factor V–factor Xa–platelet complex with lower affinity and can only be slowly converted to thrombin.

C. Relations among cascades and common pathway of thrombin generation

We have considered various control mechanisms that may operate *within* each of the three discrete elements of the hemostatic system. However, certain specific interactions *among* the intrinsic cascade, the extrinsic cascade, and the common pathway are also important in regulation.

1. Effect of thrombin on factor VIII

The first intersystem control mechanism is based on the ability of thrombin to increase dramatically the potency of factor VIII as outlined above. Indeed, without prior thrombin activation, this protein is unable to act as cofactor in the factor IXa–dependent conversion of factor X to factor Xa.

2. Interactions between factors VII and IX

The second intersystem control mechanism depends on the capacity of the factor VII–tissue factor complex to convert factor IX to factor IXa and subsequently factor X to factor Xa. This is accomplished at about the same rate of direct transformation of factor X to factor Xa under the conditions normally present in blood.

3. Interactions between factors Xa and IX

The third intersystem control mechanism involves the interaction between factor Xa and factor IX. Factor Xa can proteolyze factor IX and convert it into a serine protease. The capacity of the extrinsic cascade to bypass the earliest phases of the intrinsic cascade may explain the minimal hemorrhagic complications noted in factor XI deficiency.

These three intersystem control mechanisms allow the extrinsic cascade to activate the more complex and slower-acting intrinsic cascade. This would permit the intrinsic cascade to produce additional thrombin.

4. Interactions between factors XIIa and VII

A fourth intersystem control mechanism depends on the proteolysis of factor VII by factor XIIa. This results in the production of a disulfide-linked two-chain form of factor VII with increased affinity for tissue factor and an enhanced potency as an activator of factor X. Thus, activation of the intrinsic cascade can augment the thrombin-generating ability of the extrinsic cascade.

The existence of these multiple intersystem control mechanisms suggests that the intrinsic and extrinsic cascades are linked in a complex kinetic fashion. Indeed, such interactions are probably essential for the generation of adequate amounts of thrombin in vivo. This surmise is supported by the observation that patients with an isolated congenital defect in *either* cascade exhibit profound bleeding diatheses.

D. Protein C–thrombomodulin mechanism

Protein C is one of several vitamin K–dependent glycoproteins (other than the four classic ones). It consists of a heavy chain of mol. wt. 41,000 and a light chain of mol. wt. 21,000, which are joined by a single disulfide bridge. To perform its biologic function, protein C is converted to the serine protease **protein Ca** by thrombin. This process involves the scissioning of a single Arg_{12}–Leu_{13} bond at the N-terminal end of the heavy chain with release of an activation peptide of mol. wt. ~1400. Both protein C and protein Ca possess γ-carboxyglutamic acid residues on their light chains that are required for the binding of either protein to Ca^{2+} ions and cell membranes.

Thrombin is the only physiologic serine protease that can convert protein C to protein Ca. The rate of this reaction is quite slow then blood is allowed to clot under in vitro conditions. This observation raised questions about the biologic role of protein C within the body; however, perfusion of protein C and thrombin through the vascular tree of animals resulted in a 20,000-fold increase in the rate of conversion of zymogen to serine protease. Since this process can be saturated wth either excess protein C or thrombin, it seems likely that a receptor is present on the endothelium that can dramatically accelerate the reaction.

This hypothesis was substantiated by isolating the putative receptor termed **thrombomodulin** (mol. wt. 75,000) from rabbit lungs. The primary structure of thrombomodulin includes a highly charged N-terminal domain, six homologous epidermal growth factor-like domains, a highly glycosylated serine/threonine–rich domain, a membrane spanning domain, and a short cytoplasmic tail. The addition of thrombin to this receptor leads to the avid formation of a 1:1 stoichiometric complex of enzyme and cofactor that rapidly activates protein C in the presence of calcium ions. Thrombin and protein C assemble on the three epidermal growth factor-like domains that are close to the cell membrane. It should be noted that thrombin attached to thrombomodulin can be neutralized by antithrombin at a rate equivalent to that of free enzyme (see below). However, the thrombin-thrombomodulin complex exhibits a greatly diminished ability to clot fibrinogen, activate factor V, or trigger platelet activation.

Once evolved, protein Ca functions as a potent inhibitor of the cofactors factor Va and factor VIIIa (figure 27.7). Its first site of action is located at the surface of the platelet where factor Va bound to specific sites acts as a receptor for factor Xa. This multimolecular prothrombinase complex rapidly converts prothrombin to thrombin. Protein Ca functions as a naturally occurring anticoagulant by specifically scissioning the heavy chain of factor Va in the presence of a cofactor for this process termed **protein S** (see below). Thus protein Ca possesses the necessary specificity to prevent assembly of the so-called prothrombinase complex and thereby suppress production of thrombin.

This inhibitory effect of protein Ca is modulated by a variety of additional interactions. On the one hand a slow rate of cleavage of factor V–Va allows factor Xa to bind to the unaffected cofactor, thereby protecting this protein against any subsequent action of protein Ca. On the other hand various plasma proteins appear to be involved in the protein Ca-dependent destruction of factor Va on the platelet surface. For example, another

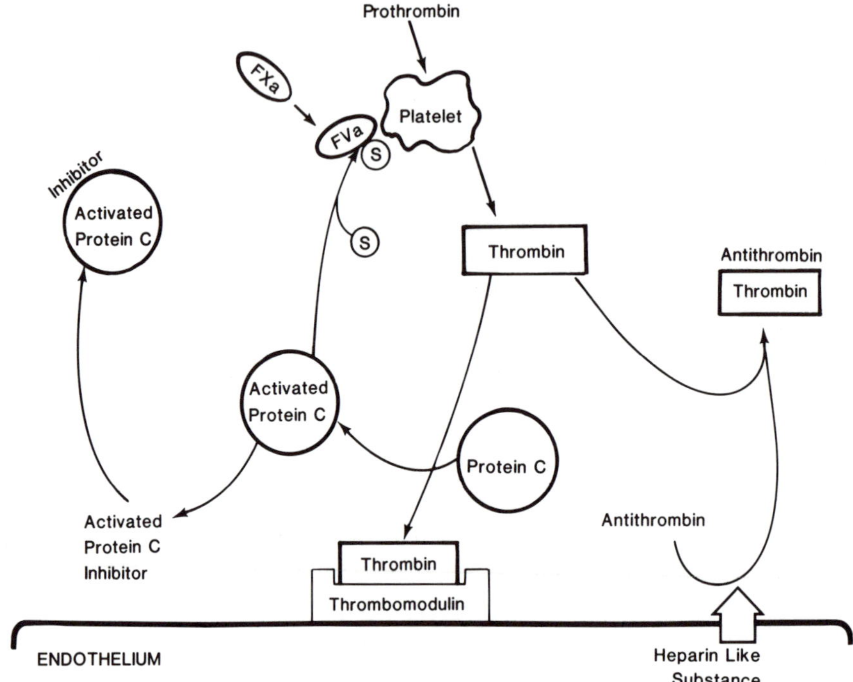

Fig. 27.7
Natural anticoagulant functions of the protein C–thrombomodulin and heparin-antithrombin systems.

vitamin K–dependent protein, **protein S**, enhances the binding of protein Ca to phospholipid-containing membranes and accelerates the cleavage of factor Va by this serine protease. The complement component, **C4b binding protein**, complexes with protein S and may be involved in regulating its function.

Thus several interactions are probably responsible for determining the rate of translocation of protein Ca from its site of production on the endothelium to the surface of the platelet. One might expect that small amounts of protein Ca remain bound to the endothelial cell surface by γ-carboxyglutamic acid residues on this serine protease. In this manner protein Ca could also regulate the factor Va-dependent thrombin generation, which is known to occur on the endothelial cell surface in a fashion analogous to that described for the platelet membrane.

The second site of action of protein Ca occurs at the platelet and endothelial cell surfaces where factor VIIIa regulates the interaction between factor IXa and factor X. The biochemical details of the protein Ca dependent cleavage of this activated cofactor are similar to those outlined for factor Va. This inhibitory process would limit the generation of factor Xa and thereby prevent production of thrombin.

Clinical observations indicate that the protein C-thrombomodulin mechanism functions under in vivo conditions to suppress hemostatic system activity. Many families have been described who have congenital reductions of about 50% in the antigenic levels of protein C and who exhibit repeated thrombotic episodes. In other kindreds individuals heterozygous for protein C deficiency have minimal symptoms, whereas those who are homozygous for this trait die in infacny with massive venous thrombosis and purpura fulminans. These data suggest that other factors such as the density of thrombomodulin on the endothelium, the levels of protein S within the blood, the amounts of Factor V–Va present of the platelet surface, and so forth, are likely to modulate the effects of protein C deficiency. Similar instances of thromboembolism have been noted in other families with congenital reductions of about 50% in the antigenic levels of protein S.

III. FORMATION OF FIBRIN CLOT

A. Structure of fibrinogen

Fibrinogen is a plasma protein (mol. wt. 340,000) composed of three pairs of polypeptide chains designated Aα, Bβ, and γ. The six chains are held together by numerous disulfide bridges. As shown in figure 27.8, the N-terminal regions of all chains are maintained by several disulfide bridges in a rigid, symmetrical configuration at one end of the molecule. This

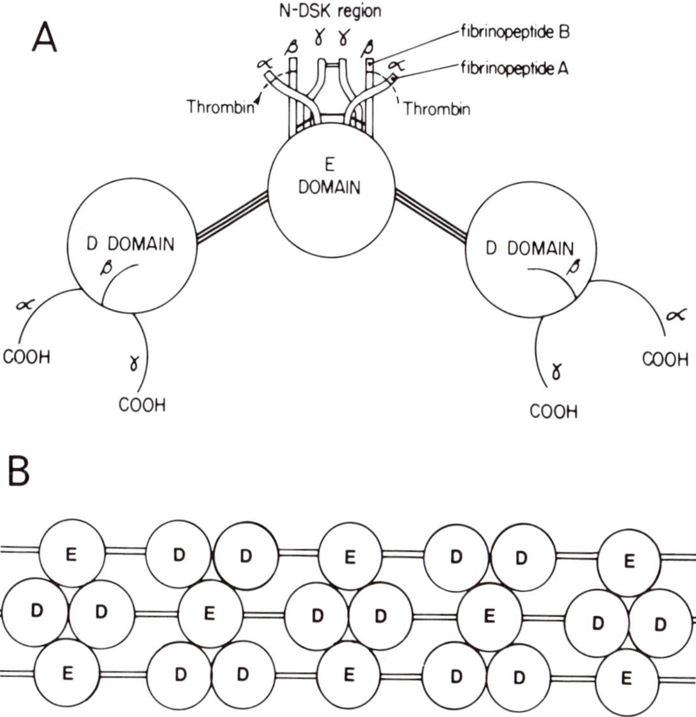

Fig. 27.8
Structures of fibrinogen (*A*) and fibrin clot (*B*).

region of the fibrinogen molecule is referred to as the N-terminal disulfide knot or **N-DSK region**. It is part of a larger nodular structure, termed the **E domain**, that is made up of intertwined polypeptide chains. The six chains emerge from this area of the molecule to form two lateral bundles of three each, each bundle containing single Aα, Bβ, and γ polypeptide chains. The C-terminal region of each of these bundles intertwines to form two separate nodular structures termed the **D domains**. The C-terminal regions of the Aα and γ chains are in a particularly exposed position within the D domain. The last 12 residues of the C-terminal segment of the γ chain constitute the major domain by which fibrinogen binds to the platelet membrane. The final phases of platelet aggregation require the interaction of divalent fibrinogen with exposed glycoprotein IIb/IIIa receptors of separate platelets in order to bridge the distance between these cellular elements (see lecture 28).

B. Conversion of fibrinogen to fibrin

Once thrombin is evolved, it cleaves the two sets of Aα and Bβ chains within the N-DSK region and thereby converts fibrinogen to fibrin (figure 27.8). Initially this enzyme clips a pair of **arginine-glycine** bonds in the Aα chains (Arg_{16}–Gly_{17}), with release of the highly acidic **fibrinopeptide A** (mol. wt. 1800) and conversion of fibrinogen to **fibrin I monomer**. Subsequently thrombin cleaves another set of arginine-glycine bonds within Bβ chains (Arg_{14}–Gly_{15}), liberating the highly acidic **fibrinopeptide B** (mol. wt. 1500) with concomitant generation of **fibrin II monomer**, which rapidly polymerizes to form a thrombus. Release of fibrinopeptide A from fibrinogen initiates **fibrin polymerization**. Indeed, snake venoms such as **reptilase** can liberate only fibrinopeptide A, but are still capable of generating a fibrin clot. Such venoms can be employed to assay for fibrinogen in the presence of heparin (see lecture 29) and to anticoagulate patients by lowering fibrinogen levels. Fibrinopeptide B release also promotes fibrin polymerization, but its function is unclear. Sensitive radioimmunoassays for both types of fibrinopeptides appear to be useful indicators of ongoing thrombosis and can be expected gradually to come into clinical use.

C. Polymerization of fibrin

Release of fibrinopeptides appears to unmask specific sites on α and γ chains within the D domains that are responsible for fibrin polymerization. This process may result from simple reduction in negative charge or from more complex molecular transformations induced by liberation of the fibrinopeptides. Once formed, fibrin may undergo two different fates.

1. Interaction of fibrin and fibrinogen: paracoagulation

On one hand, single molecules of fibrin (or low-molecular-weight fibrin polymers) may interact with fibrinogen to form **soluble fibrin-fibrinogen**

complexes or **SFC**. (These complexes also form when fibrin associates with certain plasmin-induced degradation products or fibrinogen.) This phenomenon is termed **paracoagulation**. Patients with hyperative coagulation systems exhibit elevated levels of SFC as assayed by a variety of techniques. Assay methods are of two types: (1) methods based on immunologic identification of soluble fibrinogen-like material at molecular weights that are multiples of 340,000 and (2) methods in which fibrin is discharged from SFC by disruption of hydrophobic and electrostatic bonds. This may be accomplished by addition of **protamine sulfate or ethanol** to plasma, or by **cryoprecipitation**. The discharged fibrin subsequently polymerizes into fine strands. Unfortunately, procedures for demonstrating paracoagulation are variable and thus not wholly satisfactory for detection of ongoing thrombosis or disseminated intravascular coagulation.

2. *Insolubilization of fibrin polymers*

On the other hand, fibrin polymers may gradually grow in size and become insoluble. The resulting fibrin clot is held together by hydrophobic as well as electrostatic interactions. Therefore, its gel structure can be disrupted by addition of denaturing agents such as **urea** and **monochloroacetic acid**. In the next step of the coagulation mechanism (discussed below), covalent cross-links are introduced between polymerized fibrin molecules. Disruption of the clot by denaturants is then no longer possible.

D. Activation of factor XIII: cross-linking of fibrin

The covalent cross-linking of fibrin is accomplished by a **transamidination** reaction catalyzed by **factor XIIIa**. Factor XIII, the precursor of this enzyme, is found in plasma, on platelet surfaces, and in other tissues. **Plasma factor XIII** is a **tetramer** composed of two pairs of identical subunits termed ***a*** and ***b*** (mol. wt. 80,000), **Platelet factor XIII** is a **dimer** comprised of two *a* subunits.

Once it is generated, thrombin hydrolyzes a specific arginine-glycine bond in the N-terminal segment of the *a* chain of both plasma and platelet factor XIII, with release of a peptide of mol. wt. 4500. In platelet factor XIII, this process generates enzymatic activity. In plasma factor XIII, a subsequent dissociation of *a* and *b* subunits that requires Ca^{2+} is required for exposure of an —SH group that is the active enzyme center. Either form of factor XIIIa can stitch neighboring fibrin polymers together by covalently joining the side chains of specific lysine residues with the side chains of certain glutamine acceptors. The critical areas cross-linked are within the C-terminal regions of the α and γ chains in the D domains of fibrin. As discussed above, these areas are brought into close proximity during fibrin polymerization. It is of interest that these regions are relatively inaccessible to factor XIIIa unless fibrinogen is transformed to fibrin. Thus thrombin must, in parallel, convert fibrinogen to fibrin as well as activate factor XIII if a stable clot is to be formed (figure 27.9).

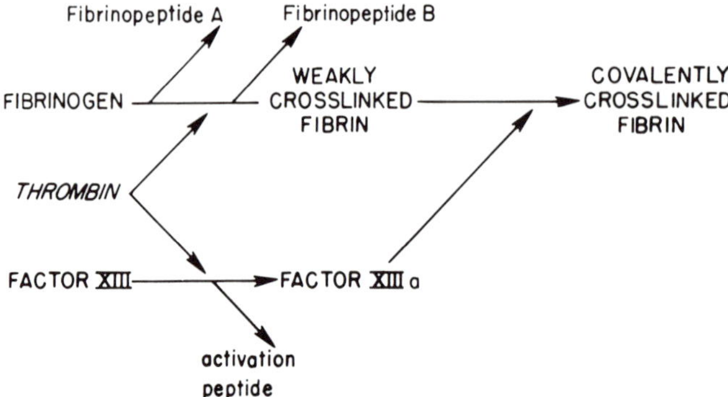

Fig. 27.9
Formation of the cross-linked fibrin clot.

The cross-linked clot is mechanically stronger and better able to withstand the brunt of collisional events within the vascular system. It is also less likely to be rapidly dissolved by the fibrinolytic mechanism. The physiologic importance of fibrin cross-linking is emphasized by the occurrence of bleeding diatheses in patients with defects in this mechanism.

IV. FIBRINOLYTIC SYSTEM

The **fibrinolytic system** is in part responsible for dissolution of the fibrin clot. In this section we shall discuss the manner in which this is accomplished and describe abnormalities in this mechanism that can lead to thrombosis.

A. Transformation of plasminogen to plasmin

A pivotal component of this mechanism is the zymogen **plasminogen** (mol. wt. 81,000). A scheme of its structure is shown in figure 27.10. A major section of the N-terminal region of this protein is composed of a series of five triple loop structures (kringles) resembling those found on the non-thrombin portion of prothrombin (see above). These unique features appear to represent specific binding sites on plasminogen that permit this zymogen to interact with and become concentrated within the fibrin meshwork. Furthermore, antifibrinolytic amino acids such as **ε-aminocaproic acid** bind to these areas of plasminogen. This interaction causes a marked conformational alteration in plasminogen that significantly limits the ability of this zymogen to be converted to active enzyme.

The central event in the fibrinolytic system is the transformation of the single-chain plasminogen to the enzymatically potent two-chain serine protease **plasmin**. This conversion is accomplished by scission of the zymogen at the Arg_{560}–Val_{561} bond as depicted in figure 27.10. The initial generation of plasmin frequently permits this enzyme to act upon plasminogen and induce several additional proteolytic cleavages within the zymo-

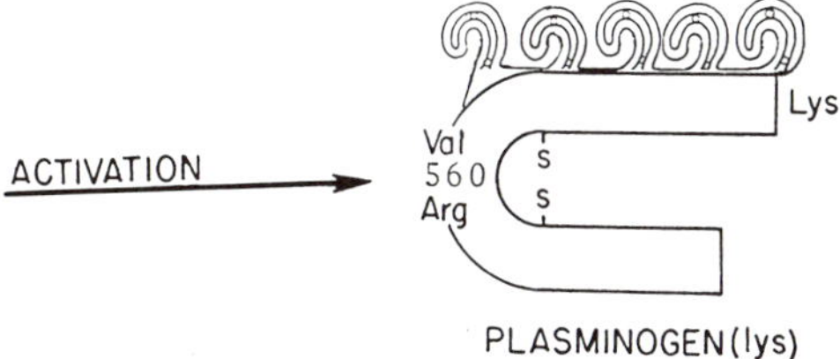

Fig. 27.10
Structure of plasminogen and its mechanism of activation.

gen at Lys_{77}–Lys_{78}, Arg_{68}–Met_{69}, and so forth, prior to its activation. These auxiliary scissions result in the release of a fragment of mol. wt. 10,000 that has been termed the **preactivation peptide**. However, this series of additional bond cleavages takes place to a minimal extent when plasminogen is converted to plasmin in the presence of protease inhibitors such as antiplasmin or antithrombin. Thus, the physiologically relevant pathway of plasminogen-to-plasmin conversion probably requires a scission of only the Arg_{560}–Val_{561} bond. The serine protease generated by this process still possesses the five kringle structures. These binding sites are critical for the interaction of plasmin with its natural substrate fibrin as well as for the rapid neutralization of this enzyme by antiplasmin (discussed below).

B. Plasminogen activators

Four types of naturally occurring substances can convert plasminogen to plasmin.

1. Endothelial cell activators: major activation pathway

The activation of plasminogen is initiated by the action of **tissue-type plasminogen activator (tPA)** or **urokinase**. Tissue-type plasminogen activator (mol. wt. 70,000) is an active proteolytic enzyme with a primary structure that contains several discrete functional modules, including a fibronectin-like finger domain, an epidermal growth factor-like domain, two kringle domains, and a serine protease-like catalytic triad of amino acid residues (figure 27.11). This enzyme has a high affinity for fibrin due to the presence of the finger and kringle domains, and employs fibrin as a cofactor to accelerate the conversion of plasminogen bound within the interstices of the clot.

Tissue-type plasminogen activator can also be cleaved at a single site by plasmin or other proteolytic enzymes to generate a two-chain species with greatly improved fluid-phase kinetic properties. It is of interest to note that the single-chain and two-chain forms of tPA have virtually identical behavior when bound to fibrin, suggesting that the single-chain species probably adopts the more kinetically favorable conformation of the two-chain

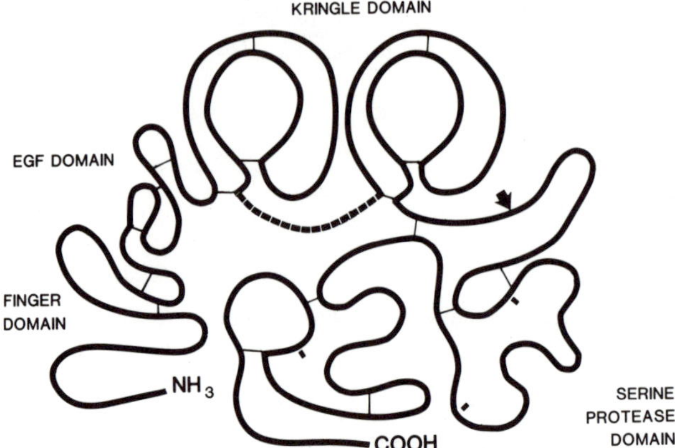

Fig. 27.11
Two-dimensional model of human tissue-type plasminogen activator. The arrow indicates the cleavage site to generate the two-chain form of the enzyme. The bars indicate the critical three amino acids within the serine protease domain.

species during interaction with fibrin. **Urokinase** (mol. wt. 54,000) has a primary structure that is quite homologous to tPA except that it lacks the finger domain as well as one of the kringle domains. The protein can be cleaved at two sites by plasmin or other proteolytic enzymes to generate a two-chain form. Single-chain urokinase exhibits rather low levels of proteolytic activity, whereas two-chain urokinase possesses high levels of enzymatic activity. As one might expect, neither form of the protein exhibits significant affinity for fibrin nor utilizes fibrin as a cofactor in the conversion of plasminogen to plasmin. It is suspected that the single-chain form of urokinase which is not inactivated by plasma protease inhibitors may function in concert with tPA to initiate lysis of the fibrin clot, and that its subsequent conversion to the two-chain form of urokinase may accelerate the process. The single- and two-chain forms of the protein may also be involved in fluid-phase generation of plasmin. Both tPA and urokinase are synthesized by a wide variety of cellular elements including microvascular and macrovascular endothelial cells.

Thrombin binds to endothelial cells, inhibits the synthesis of urokinase, and stimulates the production of tPA. The last effect may be mediated in part by the generation of protein Ca. Both plasminogen activators are readily released into the blood by **physiologic** stimuli such as exercise, **pharmacologic** stimuli such as nicotinic acid or hypoglycemic agents, and **pathologic** stimuli such as hypotensive shock. These macromolecules are partially responsible for keeping the microcirculation open and free of fibrin deposits.

2. *Factor XIIa: role in fibrinolysis*

Activation of factor XII not only triggers the coagulation cascade and kinin-generating mechanism, it also converts plasminogen to plasmin.

Thus the event that triggers clot formation by activation of factor XII also sets in motion a mechanism for its ultimate resolution.

3. *Poorly characterized activators*

A number of poorly characterized activators are found in the lysosomes of heart, kidney, and other organs. These substances are insoluble and have little physiologic significance; however, at times of extensive organ damage, these activators can be released into the blood. This phenomenon may be responsible for the frequent occurrence of systemic fibrinolysis in patients with widespread trauma.

4. *Streptokinase: use of fibrinolytic agents*

Streptokinase, a bacterial protein, has been administered to patients in an effort to dissolve established thrombi in coronary and pulmonary vessels. **Urokinase** has been employed for the same purpose. If used early enough, the infusion of streptokinase into the coronary artery may lyse existing thrombi and prevent myocardial infarction. The use of **tPA** has recently been advocated in place of streptokinase since it can be infused into a vein, would be expected to dissolve fibrin clots, but might not induce a systemic fibrinolytic state with potential hemorrhagic consequences (see below).

The cloning of tPA has made this form of therapy available in the last few years. Recent studies have indicated that the benefits of this protein, as compared to streptokinase, are not as great as expected. These findings might be due to the partial loss of fibrin selectivity at the relatively high levels of protein utilized, or to the normal role that continuous evolution of fibrin could play in maintaining vascular integrity.

C. Function of the fibrinolytic system

Under normal conditions, fibrinolysis is a precisely regulated process (figure 27.12). It is initiated by the incorporation of plasminogen into the fibrin clot as these polymers are deposited onto the vascular endothelium. This is due to the specific interaction of the kringle structures of the zymogen with the fibrin meshwork. In this locus, plasminogen is sequestered away from protease inhibitors normally present in the blood and in direct proximity to the fibrin substrate. Diffusion of plasminogen activators from the blood or endothelium into the clot transforms the zymogen into plasmin. The presence of plasminogen activator inhibitor bound within the clot regulates the generation of plasmin. The resultant enzyme remains bound to its substrate by interaction of the kringle structures with the fibrin strands and therefore can only be slowly neutralized by **antiplasmin**. In this manner, a gradual but effective lysis of the clot is started. The initial cleavage of fibrin by plasmin exposes new sites for interaction with plasminogen as well as plasminogen activators and thereby accelerates dissolution of the clot in an autocatalytic fashion. Leukocytes incorporated into the clot also elaborate proteases that may directly hydrolyze the fibrin mesh-

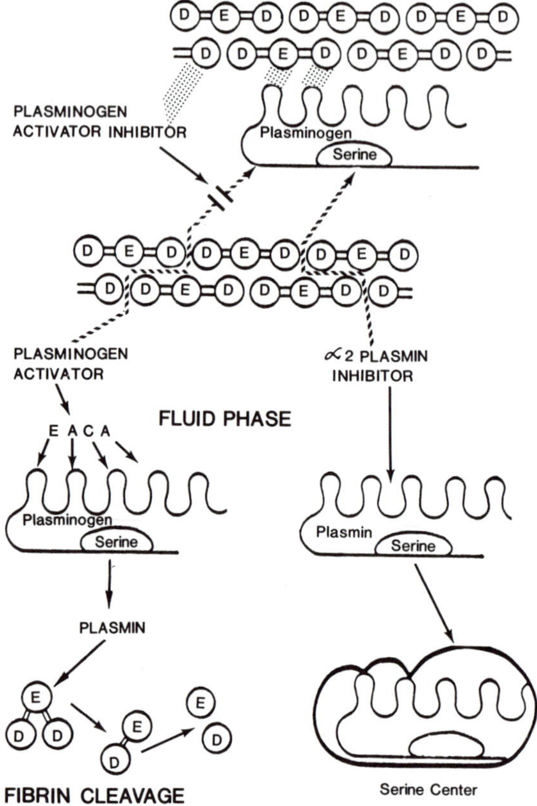

Fig. 27.12
Regulation of the fibrinolytic mechanism. The pharmacologic agent ε-aminocaproic acid is designated EACA.

work. Outside the area of the clot, activators of the fibrinolytic system are relatively impotent. This is due, in large measure, to the presence of antiplasmin, which can rapidly neutralize plasmin as it is formed. Thus fibrinolytic activity is restricted to the region of the resolving clot. However, in disease states, excessive release of activators occurs, and large amounts of plasmin are generated. This gradually overwhelms the capacity of antiplasmin to limit the fibrinolytic process, and free enzyme, as well as plasmin–α_2-macroglobulin complexes, is found within the circulation. These two entities induce systemic fibrinolysis with proteolysis as well as inactivation of proteins such as factor V, factor VIII, and fibrinogen.

D. Degradation of fibrinogen by plasmin

The effect of plasmin on the fibrinogen molecule has been extensively investigated. It is of interest because it is the basis for a variety of tests for detecting systemic fibrinolysis. Figure 27.13 shows the sequential proteoly-

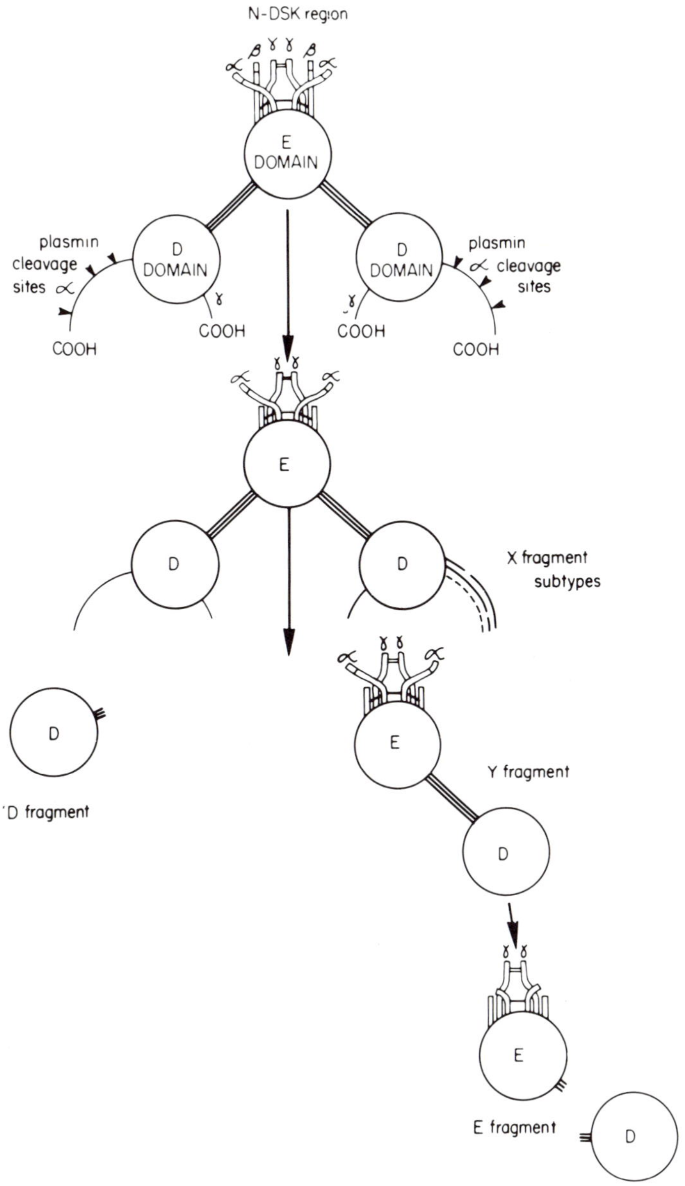

Fig. 27.13
Degradation of fibrinogen by plasmin.

sis of the fibrinogen molecule. The lysis of fibrin within the clot structure is thought to proceed similarly.

Exposed N-terminal regions of the Bβ chains of fibrinogen in the E domains as well as C-terminal regions of the Aα chains of fibrinogen in the D domains are cleaved initially. The remaining portion of the molecule is termed the **X fragment**. This limited degree of proteolysis appears to occur continuously in normal individuals since about 25% of circulating fibrinogen molecules are in this form. Next, plasmin cleaves one of the two bundles that connect the D and E domains with liberation of the D domain fragment and a binodular structure termed the **Y fragment**. Later, plasmin is able to clip the second of the two bundles connecting the D and E domains within the Y fragment and liberate these nodules as individual species called **D** and **E fragments** or **fibrinopeptides**.

The X, Y, D, and E fragments, called **fibrinogen split products**, have characteristic biologic properties. The X fragment partially retains its ability to be activated by thrombin to form fibrin. However, this happens more slowly than with normal fibrinogen. The Y, D, and E fragments cannot be clotted by thrombin and the thrombin-dependent conversion of fibrinogen to fibrin is slowed by these fragments. This effect may be due to direct inhibition of thrombin or to interference with normal fibrin polymerization. These fibrinogen split products also inhibit platelet aggregation. Thus, the X, Y, D, and E fragments are capable of suppressing the hemostatic mechanism at several loci.

Various other biologic actions are ascribed to the fragments X, Y, D, and E, including potentiation of the hypotensive effect of bradykinin, chemotactic properties with respect to monocytes as well as neutrophils, and an ability to impair the immune mechanism.

The clinical assays of fibrinogen split products include the **thrombin time**, which detects abnormalities in fibrin polymerization (and is most sensitive to X, Y, and D) as well as **immunologic tests**, which measure nonclottable fibrinogen-like material (mainly Y, D, and E).

E. Relations between coagulation and fibrinolytic systems

Three major links connect the coagulation and fibrinolytic systems:

- Activation of factor XII initiates transformation of plasminogen to plasmin.
- Plasmin can cleave factor XII and thus generate the activated form of the zymogen.
- Generation of activated protein C stimulates fibrinolysis by unknown mechanisms.

F. Defects in fibrinolytic system resulting in thrombosis

Multiple episodes of arterial and venous thrombotic disease have occurred in several families with congenital abnormalities of the fibrinolytic system (i.e., functional defects in the plasminogen molecule, reductions in the release of plasminogen activator, elevations in the levels of plasminogen activator inhibitor, and alterations in the structure of fibrinogen). Presumably, thrombotic phenomena in these patients are due to a reduced ability to lyse small fibrin clots and prevent extension. However, it has also been suggested that plasmin may serve as a natural anticoagulant.

Plasmin cleaves a set of Arg_{42}–Ala_{43} bonds within the Bβ chains of fibrin I monomer, releasing **Bβ 1–42** and thereby converting fibrin I monomer to fragment X, which is further degraded to form the soluble cleavage products mentioned previously.

Radioimmunoassays for fibrinopeptide A, fibrinopeptide B, and Bβ 1–42 have been used in studies of intravascular coagulation and venous thrombosis. These have shown in patients receiving hypertonic saline (to terminate pregnancy) that immediately after intrauterine infusion **fibrin I monomer** is generated by thrombin-mediated proteolysis of fibrinogen. Thereafter fibrin I monomer is either cleaved by thrombin to liberate fibrinopeptide B or proteolyzed by plasmin to release Bβ 1–42. Hence the relative rates at which thrombin and plasmin cleave the Bβ chain of fibrin I monomer could determine the occurrence of thrombosis. These techniques indicate that, compared to normal controls, individuals who develop venous thrombosis have levels of fibrinopeptide A that are considerably higher than the concentrations of Bβ 1–42 during the 4 days preceding the onset of thrombosis. These observations lend credence to the hypothesis that a sustained imbalance between the procoagulant effects of thrombin and the anticoagulant actions of plasmin upon fibrin I monomer may lead to thrombotic disorders in humans. The precise molecular defects responsible for these phenomena are still unknown but probably include abnormalities in the regulatory mechanisms governing the release of plasminogen activators of their inhibitors from cellular sites.

The blood levels of **low-density lipoproteins** (LDLs) also exert a profound effect upon fibrinolytic system function. The above macromolecular complex consists of a core of neutral lipids as well as the apolipoprotein B-100 molecule, which is linked to apolipoprotein (a) [Lp(a)] perhaps via an S–S bridge. Lp(a) is a highly glycosylated hydrophilic protein (mol. wt. ~500,000) with a primary structure consisting of about 37 kringles that are homologous to kringle 4 of plasminogen, as well as one kringle that is homologous to kringle 5 of plasminogen and a single serine protease domain that is highly homologous to that of plasminogen. Unlike plasminogen, Lp(a) cannot be converted to an active protease by tPA or urokinase because of a single amino acid substitution at the bond that must be cleaved to generate active enzyme. Numerous isoforms of Lp(a) exist within the population and indirect evidence suggests that this heterogeneity is related to varying numbers of kringle 4 repeats. The normal function of Lp(a) remains enigmatic but the levels of this lipoprotein including certain isotypes are highly inversely correlated with the frequency of myocardial infarction in patients with elevated levels of LDL, and represent an independent risk factor in the development of atherosclerotic vascular disease. Recent data indicate that the multiple kringle repeats within Lp(a) allow it to effectively compete with plasminogen for binding sites on fibrin, and thereby dramatically reduce fibrinolytic system activation. Thus this lipoprotein serves as a molecular link between thrombosis and atherosclerosis by favoring the development of coronary artery thrombosis in patients with high levels of LDL.

V. LIMITING REACTIONS

As we have seen, the hemostatic mechanism consists of a series of linked proteolytic reactions that sequentially generates various serine proteases. The kallikrein and complement mechanisms operate similarly. When these three mechanisms are activated at sites of injury, it is necessary to localize their actions in order to avoid propagation of their effects throughout the vascular system. If this were not the case, limited vascular damage would lead to widespread thrombosis, systemic fibrinolysis, and profound changes in vascular permeability. Nature has designed the following diverse mechanisms to localize activity and prevent such an explosive outcome.

A. Blood flow

Rapid movement of blood within vascular channels serves to dilute high concentrations of procoagulants or profibrinolytic components generated locally at sites of injury. Indeed, infusion of serine proteases of the coagulation system into experimental animals does not induce venous thrombosis unless blood flow is stopped within a vein segment during periods of induced hypercoagulability. Stasis alone does not produce a venous thrombosis. Thus, normal blood remains fluid in the face of some degree of hypercoagulability if it continues to flow freely.

B. Hepatic clearance of activated components

If coagulation system serine proteases or plasminogen activators are experimentally injected into the portal vein, the liver removes them before they reach the systemic venous circulation. This occurs via interactions of protease-protease inhibitor complexes with specific receptors on hepatic cell surfaces. The liver and RES also remove soluble fibrin complexes from the circulation. Liver disease (e.g., cirrhosis, viral hepatitis) can impair this clearance mechanism and may cause systemic fibrinolysis as well as widespread thrombosis.

C. Localization of enzyme generation

To activate hemostatic system zymogens at adequate rates, **multi-molecular complexes** must be sequentially formed between zymogens, cofactors, enzymes, Ca^{2+}, and an altered surface (that furnishes phospholipid). In the absence of these complexes, generation of serine proteases is minimal. In addition to dramatically accelerating enzyme production, these complexes also localize events to sites of vascular damage.

D. Specific destruction of cofactors or activated cofactors

The protein C-thrombomodulin mechanism suppresses the generation of thrombin by reducing the production of this enzyme by specific proteolysis of cofactors or activated cofactors (see discussion above).

E. Modulation of fibrin polymerization

The conversion of fibrin I to fibrin II by the action of thrombin results in thrombus formation. This transformation is avoided when fibrin I is converted to fragment X by the action of plasmin (see discussion above).

F. Plasma protease inhibitors

Several plasma proteins can dampen the activity of proteolytic enzymes generated in the coagulation, fibrinolytic, and kiningenerating systems. Molecular species that exert these effects and are reasonably well characterized include antithrombin (antithrombin III), heparin cofactor II, lipoprotein-associated coagulation inhibitor (LACI), activated protein C inhibitor, antiplasmin, plasminogen activator inhibitor (PAI-1), α 2-macroglobulin, α_1-antitrypsin, and C1 inactivator.

1. Deficiency states

Inherited deficiencies of four of these proteins are known to result in human disease:

- **Antithrombin deficiency** is found in patients with severe thrombotic disease.
- **Antiplasmin deficiency** has been observed in patients with a bleeding diathesis, presumably secondary to unrestricted local fibrinolysis.
- **C1 inactivator deficiency** is associated with hereditary angioneurotic edema.
- **α_1-antitrypsin deficiency** is present in patients with severe emphysema and liver disease.

To date, there have been reports of patients with elevated levels of PAI-1 in association with venous and arterial thrombotic disease as well as individuals with inherited reductions of α_2-macroglobulin and heparin cofactor II without overt clinical symptoms.

Based on the pathophysiologic consequences of inherited deficiencies as well as biochemical data, it appears that **antithrombin**, **LACI**, **antiplasmin**,

PAI-1, and **α_2-macroglobulin** constitute critical modulators of the hemostatic mechanism. The structure and function of these five components are discussed in the following sections. The physiologic importance of **heparin cofactor II** and **protein C inhibitor** is less certain and will only be briefly considered below. The remaining plasma proteins—**α_1-antitrypsin** and **C1 inactivator**—are of greater importance in the inhibition of complement kinin-generating, and leukocyte-derived serine proteases. However, these two species are capable of neutralizing proteolytic enzymes of the hemostatic system to some degree and may represent a second line of defense against activation of this physiologic mechanism. These latter protease inhibitors are not discussed further.

2. *Antithrombin: mechanism of action of heparin*

The major inhibitor of the coagulation cascade is antithrombin (mol. wt. 56,000). It is also the essential cofactor for the action of **heparin** (figure 27.14), a naturally occurring sulfated mucopolysaccharide of mol. wt. 5,000–50,000 that is employed clinically as an anticoagulant. This polymer is composed of alternating residues of hexosamine and hexuronic acid. The hexosamine residues are glucosamines that may be N-sulfated, N-acetylated, or ester-sulfated. Alternatively, they may have no substituents at one or more of these positions. The hexuronic acid residues can be glucuronic acid, iduronic acid, or ester-sulfated iduronic acid. Thus, a great variety of possible hexosamine-uronic acid sequences may exist within a heparin molecule. It is thought that the monosaccharide sequence iduronic acid–N-sulfated or N-acetyl glucosamine 6-0-sulfate–glucuronic acid–N-sulfated glucosamine 3,6-0-sulfate–iduronic acid 2-0-sulfate–N-sulfated glucosamine 6-0-sulfate represents the major antithrombin binding site on heparin. Heparin has been isolated from a variety of organs and is also found in mast cells and basophils. **Heparan sulfate**, a chemical relative with some anticoagulant properties, has recently been located on the surface of the vascular endothelium.

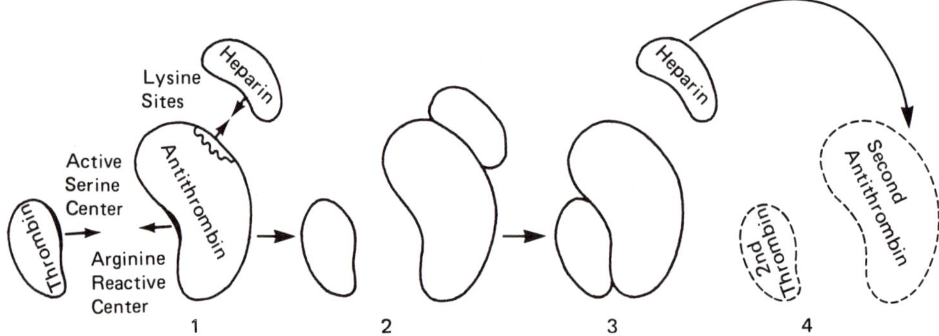

Fig. 27.14
Mechanism of heparin action.

In the absence of heparin, antithrombin neutralizes the activity of thrombin by slowly forming a 1:1 complex of enzyme and inhibitor. In the presence of the sulfated mucopolysaccharide, the rate of complex formation is increased 2000- to 10,000-fold, and neutralization of thrombin is virtually instantaneous. Formation of an enzyme inhibitor complex in the presence and absence of heparin is dependent on the active serine center of thrombin. If this residue is blocked, interaction between thrombin and antithrombin is inhibited. The reactive site of the inhibitor, which binds the active serine center of thrombin, contains an arginine residue. Modification of this group in antithrombin virtually eliminates the ability of the protein to inhibit thrombin in the presence or absence of heparin.

In view of the highly acidic nature of heparin, one would expect that positive groups on antithrombin (e.g., ε-aminolysyl residues) form the binding site for this negatively charged anticoagulant. Chemical alteration of these residues prevents binding of heparin to this protein and suppresses the acceleration of inhibitor action by the anticoagulant. However, the slow, progressive neutralization of thrombin by antithrombin is not appreciably affected. Furthermore, heparin functions as a catalyst in this reaction. Relatively small amounts dramatically accelerate the interaction of considerably large amounts of thrombin and antithrombin. This occurs because of the displacement of heparin from antithrombin during formation of the thrombin-antithrombin complex. Thus, the mucopolysaccharide is available to bind to free inhibitor and cyclically promote subsequent rounds of interactions.

In summary, antithrombin neutralizes the activity of thrombin by complex formation via a reactive site (arginine)–active center (serine) interaction. If small amounts of heparin are added to the system, it preferentially binds to the lysyl residues on antithrombin. The resulting heparin-antithrombin complex rapidly inactivates thrombin. This most probably is due to a heparin-dependent conformational alteration of the inhibitor, which renders the reactive site arginine more accessible to the active serine center of thrombin. Once thrombin-antithrombin complex formation has occurred, heparin is released and is again available for binding to free inhibitor. Thus, the mucopolysaccharide is capable of catalyzing numerous subsequent rounds of thrombin-antithrombin complex formation.

This mechanism of inhibitor action implies that antithrombin neutralizes all the serine proteases of the coagulation cascade and that heparin accelerates each of these interactions. This hypothesis has been shown to be valid with respect to factor IXa, factor Xa, factor XIa, and factor XIIa. The behavior of the remaining enzymes of the hemostatic system, that is, factor VIIa and protein C, are anomalous in this regard. The activities of these serine proteases are not affected by antithrombin in the presence or absence of heparin. Similarly designated enzymes generated in physiologic systems that are separate from but linked to the hemostatic mechanism (e.g., complement system, kallikrein system) are only minimally affected by this inhibitory process.

The availability of heparin-like substances on endothelium permits antithrombin to be selectively activated at blood-surface interfaces where enzymes of the hemostatic mechanism are generated. Thus the plasma protease inhibitor is critically placed to neutralize these enzymes and thereby protect natural surfaces against thrombus formation. Moreover the catalytic nature of heparin would ensure the continual regeneration of the nonthrombogenic properties of these natural surfaces. Once the antithrombin bound to vessel wall mucopolysaccharide complexes with enzyme, the enzyme-inhibitor complex would be liberated into circulation. The heparin-like material would again be available to recruit free antithrombin and thereby continually renew the ability of the surface to resist the attack of serine proteases of the hemostatic cascade.

It is noteworthy that the factor VII–tissue factor and protein C-thrombomodulin interactions operate virtually independently of the endogenous heparin-antithrombin mechanism. On the one hand this may permit the extrinsic pathway of thrombin generation to function as a "spark" to mobilize the intrinsic pathway of thrombin generation. On the other hand it may allow the protein C-thrombomodulin mechanism to utilize thrombin that escapes neutralization by the endogenous heparin-antithrombin mechanism to suppress thrombin production by specific destruction of cofactors or activated cofactors.

3. *Lipoprotein-associated coagulation inhibitor (LACI)*

The major inhibitor of the factor VII–tissue factor system is a plasma protein termed **LACI** (mol. wt. 35,000), which is loosely bound to plasma lipoproteins. LACI is synthesized by the liver as well as the endothelium and is also found within platelets. The primary sequence of this component contains three tandem repeated serine protease inhibitor binding domains that are homologous in structure to the Kunitz trypsin inhibitor and similar in function to the reactive site region of antithrombin. The suppression of the extrinsic pathway is accomplished by rapid formation of a quaternary interaction product between the factor VIIa–tissue factor and factor Xa. The inhibition of factor VIIa–tissue factor is wholly dependent on the presence of factor Xa, whereas factor Xa can be inhibited in the absence of factor VII–tissue factor. The first inhibitor domain of LACI is involved in the binding of factor VIIa–tissue factor, whereas the second inhibitor domain of the protein simultaneously complexes with factor Xa. The function of the third inhibitor domain remains enigmatic. Thus multifunctional LACI is designed to allow formation of factor VII–tissue factor as well as permit the production of factor VIIa–tissue factor by the generated factor Xa but would then suppress extrinsic pathway activity by simultaneously binding the two serine proteases within a quaternary complex. This novel multicomponent interaction would allow basal function of the factor VII–tissue factor pathway with subsequent suppression of the system after extensive generation of factor VIIa and factor Xa.

4. *Antiplasmin*

The first major inhibitor of the fibrinolytic mechanism is a plasma protein termed **antiplasmin** (mol. wt. 67,000). Two forms have been isolated with slightly different physiochemical properties, but the biologic significance of this microheterogeneity remains unclear. Plasmin is rapidly neutralized by antiplasmin by formation of 1 : 1 stoichiometric complex of enzyme and inhibitor. The mechanism appears to be similar to that discussed for the thrombin-antithrombin reaction and involves an interaction between the serine active center of plasmin and a reactive size on antiplasmin. However, accessory areas on the plasmin molecule such as the kringles are also critical for the rapid formation of enzyme-inhibitor complexes. The addition of low-molecular-weight ligands such as **ε-aminocaproic acid** (EACA) that bind to these regions of plasmin can reduce the rapid rate of this interaction 10- to 50-fold (see figure 27.11). Antiplasmin has also been observed to inactivate factors IXa and XIIa, albeit at a relatively slow rate. Thus it may be partially involved in suppressing plasminogen-to-plasmin conversion as well as opposing the action of the enzyme when formed.

Sufficient levels of antiplasmin are normally present to inactivate half the plasmin that can theoretically be generated wtihin the blood. Provided that this level of zymogen conversion is not exceeded in the fluid phase, plasmin neutralization is rapid, as well as complete, and systemic fibrinolysis is prevented. As noted, plasmin formed within the fibrin clot structure is sequestered from the action of protease inhibitors. This appears to be due to the interaction of the enzyme with the fibrin strands via its kringle structures. Under these conditions, plasmin can only be slowly neutralized by antiplasmin and is capable of gradually lysing the fibrin meshwork (see figure 27.11).

In pathologic states such as disseminated intravascular coagulation or during infusion of urokinase for therapeutic purposes, considerably more than half the circulating plasminogen may be converted to plasmin. Once the capacity of antiplasmin has been exceeded, excess proteolytic enzyme is bound to α_2-macroglobulin. Since a small percentage of the plasmin bound within this complex remains active, systemic fibrinolysis is able to take place. Thus antiplasmin appears to be the major barrier against the action of the fibrinolytic system.

5. *Plasminogen activator inhibitor-1 (PAI-1)*

The second major inhibitor of the fibrinolytic mechanism is a plasma protein called **PAI-1** (mol. wt. 50,000). Several other plasminogen activator inhibitors exist but are of lesser importance. PAI-1 is synthesized by various cell types including the liver as well as the endothelium, and the protein is also found within platelets. The normal plasma levels of PAI-1 are quite low, and its survival within the circulation is short because of a rapid conformational transition to a biologically inactive form unless stabilized by interactions with other specific components. The primary structure of this plasma protease inhibitor is quite homologous to antithrombin especially around the reactive site region. PAI-1 inhibits a wide spectrum of proteases including tPA, urokinase, plasmin, thrombin, activated protein C, factor XIa, factor XIIa, and kalleikrein via a mechanism similar to that previously described for antithrombin. However, the major physiologic role of PAI-1 is to suppress the function of tPA as well as urokinase and thus prevent the activation of the fibrinolytic mechanism. The above process is aided by the specific binding of PAI-1 to the fibrin clot in a manner analogous to plasminogen such that the protease inhibitor is positioned and maintained in an active state to capture plasminogen activators before they are able to generate plasmin. The importance of PAI-1 in regulating the fibrinolytic system is suggested by observations that elevated levels of the protease inhibitor are associated with deep vein thrombosis and myocardial infarction in certain patient populations.

6. α_2-Macroglobulin

The proteolytic inhibitor **α_2-macroglobulin** is capable of neutralizing a wide variety of proteolytic enzymes such as plasmin, trypsin, thrombin, kallikrein, elastase, collegenase, and cathepsins. However, the rates of inactivation are relatively modest compared with those of the other protease inhibitors.

This plasma protein is composed of two equivalent half-molecules of mol. wt. 360,000 that are held together by noncovalent interaction. Each half-molecule consists of two peptide chains of mol. wt. 180,000 that are linked by disulfide bridges. The various endopeptidases are inactivated by formation of either 1:1 or 2:1 stoichiometric complexes of enzyme and inhibitor. The initial phase of this process most probably requires an interaction between the active center of the protease and a reactive site on α_2-macroglobulin. Thereafter, a complex alteration in the spacing of the four subunits that make up the protease inhibitor is apparent. The latter event may be triggered by interactions between unique internal pyroglutamic acid moieties that are part of the structure of α_2-macroglobulin.

This latter transition has two major consequences. First, enzyme molecules trapped within α_2-macroglobulin are able to function in a limited fashion as proteases. Second, the endopeptidases bound to the α_2-macroglobulin are protected against the action of other circulating protease inhibitors that would completely inactivate these enzymes. The enzyme–α_2-macroglobulin complexes are cleared by the RES in 15–30 min.

The primary in vivo function of this inhibitor may be to preserve a portion of the biologic activity of bound enzyme within the circulatory system and allow this bound enzyme to express its activity for a specified period of time in the presence of other plasma inhibitors. For example, plasmin bound to α_2-macroglobulin may play a critical role in the normal process of fibrinolysis, whereas thrombin bound to this inhibitor may be important in activating small amounts of cofactors such as factor V or factor VIII. Thus these sequestered enzymes may be capable of maintaining coagulation-fibrinolytic system activity at some basal level and thereby keeping the hemostatic system poised and ready for action.

7. *Other inhibitors of the hemostatic system*

Two other protease inhibitors of the hemostatic system have been described and may be of physiologic importance. Activated **protein C inhibitor** (mol. wt. 57,000) slowly inactivates protein Ca generated within the blood but it is unclear whether alterations in the levels of this component modify the function of the protein C–thrombomodulin mechanism. **Heparin cofactor II** (mol. wt. 65,600) is homologous in structure to antithrombin and α_1-antitrypsin. This protease inhibitor neutralizes thrombin but no other enzyme of the coagulation system. Dermatan sulfate or heparin can bind to heparin cofactor II and accelerate the above reaction by 1000-fold. It has been suggested that the above plasma protein may serve as an inhibitor of thrombin in extravascular regions where dermatan sulfate is plentiful.

VI. SOURCES OF CLOTTING PROTEINS

A. Liver

The liver is the site for production of prothrombin, factor VII, factor IX, factor X, factor XI, factor XII, plasminogen and protease inhibitors such as antithrombin, LACI, antiplasmin, PAI-1, and α_2-macroglobulin. Factor V may also be synthesized in the liver.

1. *Role of vitamin K*

The biosynthesis of the five **homologous proteins** prothrombin, factor VII, factor IX, factor X, and protein C has a unique common feature. After these polypeptide chains are released from the ribosome, as suggested earlier, specific glutamic acid residues in the N-terminal region of these five proteins are γ-carboxylated. This process requires **vitamin K** as well as a poorly characterized microsomal enzyme carboxylating system. If these proteins are not so modified, they are functionally inactive.

2. *Coumadin (warfarin)*

Coumadin is a widely used coumarin anticoagulant that functions by interfering with the vitamin K–dependent γ-carboxylation process and thus prevents formation of functionally active prothrombin, factor VII, factor IX, factor X, and protein C.

B. Endothelial cells

Endothelial cells are the sites of production of von Willebrand's factor, tissue factor, thrombomodulin, heparin-like molecules, plasminogen activator inhibitor, plasminogen activator, and factor V.

C. Kidney

The kidney may be an auxiliary site for the synthesis of plasminogen.

SELECTED REFERENCES

Reviews

Bennett, J. S. The molecular biology of platelet membrane proteins. *Semin. Hematol.* 27(1990): 186–204.

Comp, P. C. Control of coagulation reactions. In Williams, W. J., et al., eds. *Hematology*, 4th ed. New York: McGraw-Hill, 1990, pp. 1304–1312.

Fajardo, L. F. The complexity of endothelial cells. A review. *Am. J. Clin. Pathol.* 92(1989): 241–250.

Furie, B., and Furie, B. C. Molecular basis of vitamin K-dependent gamma-carboxylation. *Blood* 75(1990): 1753–1762.

Gerlach, H., Esposito, C., et al. Modulation of endothelial hemostatic properties: an active role in the host response. *Annu. Rev. Med.* 41(1990): 15–24.

Nemerson, Y. Sequence of coagulation reactions. In Williams, W. J., et al., eds. *Hematology*, 4th ed. New York: McGraw-Hill, 1990, pp. 1295–1304.

Nemerson, Y., and Williams, W. J. Biochemistry of plasma coagulation factors. In Williams, W. J., et al., eds. *Hematology*, 4th ed. New York: McGraw-Hill, 1990, pp. 1267–1284.

Ratnoff, O. D. The evolution of hemostatic mechanisms. *Perspect. Biol. Med.* 31(1987): 4–33.

Rosenberg, R. D. Role of antithrombin III in coagulation disorders: state-of-the-art review. Introduction. *Am. J. Med.* 87 Suppl. 3B(1989): 1S-1S.

Rosenberg, R. D. Biochemistry of heparin antithrombin interactions, and the physiologic role of this natural anticoagulant mechanism. *Am. J. Med.* 87 Suppl. 3B(1989): 2S-9S.

Shearer, M. J. Vitamin K and vitamin K-dependent proteins. *Br. J. Haematol.* 75(1990): 156–162.

Original articles

Mann, K. G., Nesheim, M. E., et al. Surface-dependent reactions of the vitamin K-dependent enzyme complexes. *Blood* 76(1990): 1–16.

Rodgers, G. M. Hemostatic properties of normal and perturbed vascular cells. *FASEB. J.* 2(1988): 116–123.

LECTURE 28

Hemorrhagic Disorders II. Platelets

David J. Kuter

EDITOR'S COMMENT

We are now living through a renaissance of research interest in the platelet, its production, functional regulation, and metabolism. Platelets are involved in many normal and pathologic processes. They have beneficial roles in hemostasis, would healing, inflammation, and phagocytosis of foreign particles. But they also play deleterious roles in the pathogenesis of atherosclerosis and other occlusive vascular diseases, transplant rejection, vasculitis, and thrombotic thrombocytopenic purpura. In all of these roles, whether advantageous or harmful, platelets require activation. The platelet contains actin, myosin, and an abundance of ATP. It is an analogue of muscle cells, for its activation requires calcium. This lecture discusses this system and such recent advances in this burgeoning field as the relations of blood coagulation to endothelium and the important regulatory role of von Willebrand's factor.

I. INTRODUCTION

The **platelet** is a small anucleate cell which on Wright's stain appears as an irregularly shaped, refractile fragment of pale blue cytoplasm with a few azurophilic granules. Until the late nineteenth century this bit of stained material was considered debris derived from the degradation of other blood cells, or an unusual microorganism. This unremarkable appearance belies a highly developed secretory cell with a very complex internal architecture that cannot be fully appreciated with the light microscope. Platelets interact with the soluble coagulation factors and the endothelium, and perform several important functions:

- They adhere to injured blood vessel walls forming cellular **aggregates** (the **primary hemostatic plug**) that help stanch the flow of blood from damaged blood vessels.
- They provide a **surface** upon which soluble coagulation factors may become activated.
- They share **metabolic products** with the endothelium and in some poorly understood fashion promote the "integrity" of the endothelium.
- They release a wide variety of **mediators** that alter vascular tone, regulate inflammatory reactions, and initiate repair of the damaged vessel wall.

Bleeding disorders arise when there are too few platelets to perform these functions or when platelets are present but defective. Thrombotic disorders arise when pathologic processes promote platelet aggregation or when defective platelets clump excessively. Given this wide repertory of responses within the vasculature it is not surprising that platelets are considered to play a major role in the pathogenesis of atherosclerosis, coronary thrombosis, and tumor metastasis.

II. PLATELET STRUCTURE

A. Cell surface membrane

The platelet plasma membrane invaginates extensively into the platelet cytoplasm and forms the **open canalicular system** (figure 28.1). While massively expanding the surface area of the platelet, the open canalicular system also provides a close juxtaposition of the plasma membrane with the **dense tubular system**, a modified endoplasmic reticulum that stores calcium and is the site for cyclooxygenase activity. This close apposition allows surface membrane electrical potential changes during **platelet activation** to be communicated more efficiently to the major site of calcium storage within the platelet. A similar system is found in the transverse tubule system in skeletal muscle, where the sarcolemma invaginates deeply and lies adjacent to the sarcoplasmic reticulum, allowing for rapid communication of membrane potential changes to the sites of intracellular calcium storage.

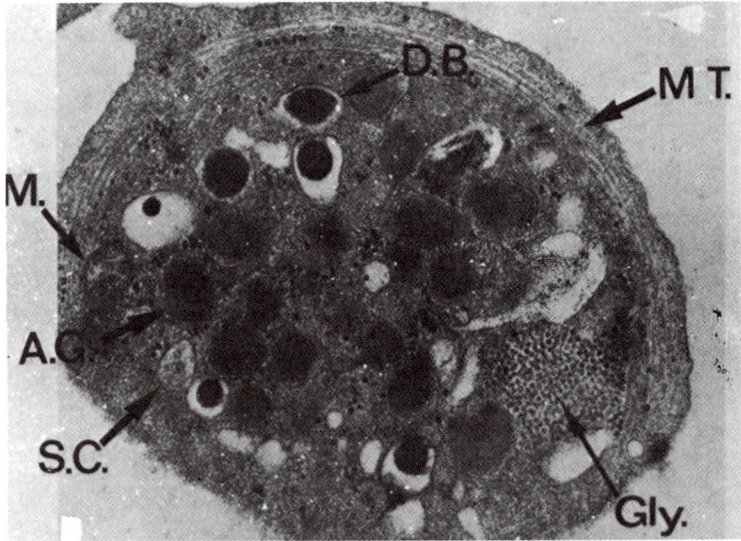

Fig. 28.1
Internal structure of a normal platelet as demonstrated by transmission electron micrograph (× 15,000). (MT, circumferential band of microtubules; BD, dense granule; AG, granule; M, mitochondrion, Gly, glycogen; SC, surface-connected open canalicular system.) (Reprinted with permission from J. A. White, in T. H. Spaet, ed., *Progress in Hemostasis and Thrombosis*, Vol. 2. New York: Grune & Stratton, 1974, p. 53.)

The platelet surface also contains a number of important glycoprotein antigens and receptors. Platelets contain ABO blood group antigens that are synthesized in platelet precursors and also are acquired in the circulation. Though platelets lack class II HLA antigens, they possess class I HLA antigens. In addition, platelets contain receptors for the Fc portion of immunoglobulin G which play a role in drug-mediated and AIDS-related thrombocytopenia. Receptors for collagen, epinephrine, thrombin, and ADP are present on the platelet surface and provide the mechanism by which these substances initiate **platelet activation**.

Several platelet receptors have been the source of extensive investigation. Platelet **glycoprotein 1b** (GPIb) is a heterodimer composed of GPIb *a* (mol. wt. 145,000) and GPIb *b* (mol. wt. 22,000) subunits linked by disulfide bonds (figure 28.2). This complex associates with two other membrane glycoproteins, GPV and GPIX, and is the primary binding site on the platelet for **von Willebrand's factor** (VWF). All of these glycoproteins are deficient in **Bernard-Soulier's syndrome**. Another surface protein complex, referred to as **glycoprotein IIb/IIIa** (GPIIb/IIIa), is a heterodimer in the integrin family of surface membrane adhesion protein receptors and consists of GPIIb (mol. wt. 140,000) and GPIIIa (mol. wt. 95,000) subunits (figure 28.2). This complex binds to fibrinogen, fibronectin, vitronectin, and von Willebrand's factor via their common R-G-D (arginine-glycine-aspartic acid) sequence. Upon platelet activation the GPIIb/IIIa complex undergoes a conformational change allowing the binding of fibrinogen, which serves as a molecular bridge between platelets, causing them to aggregate to each other. This complex is lost in **Glanzmann's thrombasthenia**. The GPIIb/IIIa complex contains epitopes with which most antisera from patients with idiopathic thrombocytopenic purpura (ITP) react and also contains other epitopes that constitute the major antigen system (PLA) of the platelet.

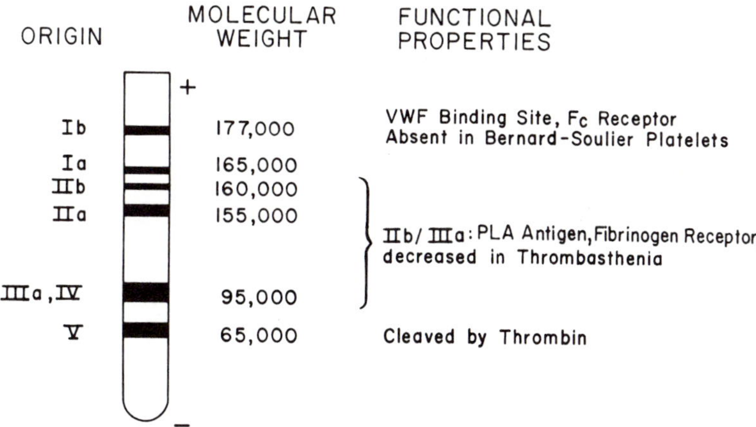

Fig. 28.2
SDS-polyacrylamide gel electrophoresis of platelet membrane glycoproteins.

B. Cytoskeleton

In the blood, the platelet has a discoid shape. This form is maintained by a circumferential ring of microtubules (see figure 28.1) just below the platelet surface. As in other contractile cells, there are also microfilaments and an active actin/myosin system. It has been estimated that 15% of the platelet mass is action. Upon platelet activation changes in calcium concentration alter these contractile elements and cause the platelet to send out pseudopodia (filopodia) and assume a spherical shape. At the same time the microtubular ring and the granules are moved toward the center of the platelet. Several of the aforementioned platelet glycoproteins are bound to the cytoskeleton: The cytoplasmic side of GPIb is bound to actin filaments in the resting and activated platelet, whereas the cytoplasmic side of the GPIIb/IIIa complex becomes bound to the cytoskeleton only upon platelet activation.

C. Granules

The platelet contains three different types of granules (table 28.1), which are released to varying degrees during platelet activation. Platelet **lysosomes** are like those in other tissues and contain a wide variety of hydrolytic enzymes. These may serve to mediate inflammatory processes in which

Table 28.1
Constituents of Alpha, Dense, and Lysosomal Granules in Platelets

α-Granules	Dense granules	Lysosomal granules
Plasma proteins	**Nucleotides**	**Hydrolytic enzymes**
α_1-Antitrypsin	ATP	Acid hydrolases
α_2-Macroglobulin	ADP	β-Galactosidase
C1-inhibitor	GTP	β-Glucuronidase
Coagulation proteins	**Other molecules**	Heparitinase
Factor XI (or XI-like)	Serotonin	Elastase
Factor V	Calcium	Collagenase
Fibrinogen		
von Willebrand's factor		
Heparin-binding proteins		
Thromboglobulin (LAPF-4, PBP)		
Platelet factor 4		
Other proteins		
Thrombospondin		
Fibronection		
Platelet activation-dependent granule external membrane (PADGEM)		
Growth factors		
Transforming growth factor β (TGF-β)		
Platelet-derived growth factor (PDGF)		
Epidermal growth factor (EGF)		

platelets participate. Of more specific interest are the **dense granules**, so called because they are physically dense and because they are osmiophilic when stained for electron microscopy. There are approximately ten of these granules per platelet and they contain ADP, ATP, and calcium as well as most of the serotonin and vasopressin in the blood. Release of ADP from these granules during platelet activation is necessary to recruit other platelets to form the primary hemostatic plug. There are, finally, approximately 100 **alpha granules** (α-granules) per platelet. These contain a wide range of proteins including fibrinogen, fibronectin, factor V, VWF as well as several platelet-specific proteins that bind heparin such as **platelet factor 4** and **β-thromboglobulin**. β-Thromboglobulin is a proteolytic derivative of **low-affinity platelet factor 4** (LAPF4), which is itself derived from **platelet basic protein** (PBP). A lectin-like protein called **thrombospondin** (mol. wt. 190,000) is released from α-granules by thrombin and appears to bind to fibrinogen on the platelet surface. Some of these proteins, such as fibrinogen, appear to be taken up from the plasma early in platelet formation, while others, such as VWF and platelet factor 4, are actually synthesized by the platelet precursor cells. Of considerable interest is the presence in the platelet of a number of important growth factors, including **transforming growth factor β** (TGF-β), **epidermal growth factor** (EGF), and **platelet-derived growth factor** (PDGF).

A unique component of the α-granule membrane has recently been described called PADGEM (**platelet activation-dependent granule external membrane**) or GMP-140 (**granule membrane protein**). This 140 kd protein is present on the internal surface of the α-granule membrane. Upon platelet activation the α-granule membrane fuses with the surface membrane and this protein is exposed on the platelet's outer surface, where it may serve as a marker of platelet activation.

III. PRODUCTION OF PLATELETS

A. Source of platelets

Platelets are produced from a bone marrow cell called the **megakaryocyte**. This unusual precursor cell has a number of characteristics:

- It is a relatively uncommon cell in the bone marrow, accounting for only 1 in 1000 cells.
- It is a massive cell with a diameter often of 50 μ (compared with 5 μ for the erythrocyte) and is capable of producing from 1000–2000 platelets per cell.
- It is a polyploid cell containing on the average 16 times the haploid amount (N) of DNA (i.e., 16N).

1. Source of megakaryocytes

Like all other differentiated bone marrow cells (see lecture 1), the megakaryocyte is derived from the pluripotent stem cell (figure 28.3; see figure

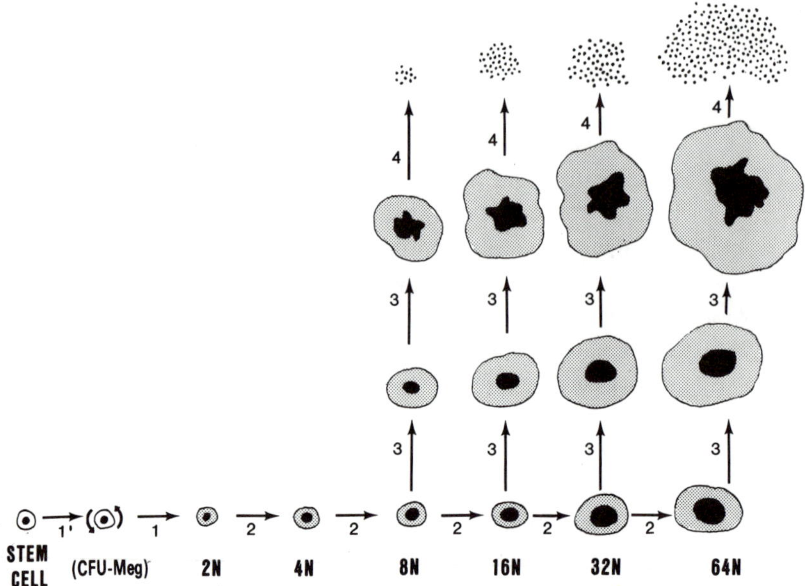

Fig. 28.3
Schematic diagram of the differentiation and maturation of megakaryocytes. (1′, "committment" of stem cell to megakaryocyte lineage; 1, CFU-Meg stops self-replication and expresses platelet-specific surface antigens; 2, megakaryocyte precursors undergo endomitosis; 3, cytoplasmic maturation follows the conclusion of endomitosis; 4, platelets are "shed" from megakaryocyte cytoplasm.) Shading denotes presence of platelet-specific surface and cytoplasmic markers.

1.1). This stem cell gives rise to progenitors committed to the megakaryocyte lineage called **CFU-Meg (colony forming units–megakaryocyte)** which undergo mitosis. At some stage, these committed megakaryocyte precursors cease cell division but continue to replicate their DNA by a process known as **endomitosis**, producing megakaryocytes with a geometric progression in ploidy from 4N to 64N. Once endomitosis is completed, **cytoplasmic maturation** ensues with the production of platelet-specific products like platelet factor 4 and the formation of α- and dense granules (figure 28.3). The surface membrane of the megakaryocyte undergoes deep invaginations to form demarcation membranes.

2. *Platelet formation*

Once matured, the megakaryocytes migrate toward the bone marrow sinusoids and platelets are formed. The exact mechanism for this is not well understood. It was initially thought that the demarcation membranes divided the megakaryocyte cytoplasm into platelet-sized domains and that the cytoplasm simply "shattered" into platelets. However, there is little evidence for this, and the demarcation membranes probably represent a means to store the large amount of membrane needed once platelets are formed from the megakaryocyte's cytoplasm. Recent electron microscope observations do little to clarify the mechanism but do show pseudopodia extending from the megakaryocyte into the bone marrow sinusoids, suggesting that platelets break off from these processes. However, the routine autopsy finding of megakaryocytes in pulmonary vessels lends support to a model whereby megakaryocytes or large fragments of megakaryocyte cytoplasm may break off and travel to the pulmonary circulation and there be converted into platelets.

3. Modifications of platelets in blood

Platelets have a rather complicated circulation as determined by kinetic studies. Once formed they migrate to the spleen and reside there for up to 8 hr. This "**nonexchangeable**" **platelet pool** subsequently reenters the circulation and survives for 8–9 days. This circulating pool of platelets consists of those in the blood stream as well as those (approximately 25–30% of the total) that are sequestered in the spleen ("**exchangeable**" **platelet pool**).

Circulating platelets are heterogenous with respect to their size and density. This heterogeneity is manifest at the time of their production from the megakaryocyte and presumably reflects the type (8N, 16N, or 32N) of the parent megakaryocyte. During their lifetime in the circulation, the average **size** and **density** of a cohort of platelets also declines. This presumably reflects the loss of platelet membrane and the loss of α-granules (the prime determinant of platelet density) with repetitive cycles of aggregation and disaggregation within the circulation. Unlike the megakaryocyte, platelets lack significant capability for protein synthesis. Once formed, platelet dense granules fill with serotonin and peptides like vasopressin from the plasma but they are are unable to replenish their membrane or granules. Consequently, younger platelets are large, have more granules, and are hemostatically more active than older platelets. This is at times clinically significant: In states of rapid platelet destruction (and consequent rapid platelet production) such as ITP, the very low levels of circulating platelets may provide almost normal hemostasis because the **megathrombocytes** are young, large, and more active.

The factors that determine the duration of platelet survival in the circulation are not understood. Clearly the platelet life span is not determined by the demands of forming a primary hemostatic plug since the number of platelets in the circulation far exceeds the number needed to maintain hemostasis (see below). Moreover, the survival of platelets is unaffected by enlargement of the spleen or its surgical removal. The presence in the circulation of small pieces of platelets ("platelet dust") suggests that platelets might simply self-destruct in the circulation and be cleared by the reticuloendothelial system.

B. Regulation of platelet production

Unlike the hematocrit, which shows a narrow range of variation within the normal population, the normal platelet count varies from 150,000–350,000 platelets/mm^3 of blood. However, for any one individual, the number of platelets is tightly regulated over the life span. It appears that the body regulates not the platelet count but the **platelet mass**. With enlargement of the spleen, for example, the number of platelets sequestered in the spleen ("exchangeable pool") increases and the platelet count measured in the blood stream decreases proportionately, but the body's total platelet number and mass remain constant.

When the platelet count (actually platelet mass) diminishes, as in ITP, a feedback loop is initiated that results in accelerated release of platelets from megakaryocytes in the bone marrow within 8 hr, followed by an increase in the average ploidy of the megakaryocytes in the bone marrow within 2 days, and then a rise in the number of megakaryocytes within 3–5 days. In experimental animal models in which the platelet count may be raised by transfusion, the opposite effects on the bone marrow are observed: Platelet release from megakaryocytes is slowed, the average ploidy and number of megakaryocytes decreases.

This feedback loop between the circulating platelet number (mass) and the bone marrow megakaryocyte is presumed to be mediated by a humoral factor or factors referred to as **thrombopoietin**. Proof that such a hormone is involved in platelet production is based on three lines of evidence. When plasma collected from patients with bone marrow suppression and thrombocytopenia due to ethanol ingestion was reinfused into these patients after bone marrow recovery, a rise in the platelet count was produced. More convincing is the evidence from animal models. Injection of selenomethionine-75 into animals results in incorporation of this label into platelet proteins and the extent of incorporation is related to the rate of platelet production. When plasma from thrombocytopenic animals is injected into such animals, the amount of ^{75}Se incorporated is increased. Finally, in cultures of bone marrow, the addition of plasma from thrombocytopenic animals was found to increase the average ploidy of megakaryocytes that grew, whereas plasma from thrombocytotic (increased platelet count) animals decreased the average ploidy of megakaryocytes that grew.

The mechanism by which this humoral factor(s) regulates platelet production is not well defined. Sufficient evidence exists to suggest that in states of increased or decreased demand for platelets there is no change in the number of stem cells being committed to the megakaryocyte lineage (CFU-Meg). The effects of humoral factors are therefore likely to be at later stages in megakaryocyte growth and would include:

- Increasing the number of megakaryocytes produced per CFU-Meg
- Increasing the rate of endomitosis and thus megakaryocyte ploidy
- Increasing the rate of cytoplasmic maturation and hence megakaryocyte size

While most experiments to date have considered that thrombopoietin acts as a **positive effector** on megakaryocytes just as erythropoietin acts on erythroblasts, an equally plausible model is that the "thrombopoietic activity" found in thrombocytopenic plasma actually reflects the lack of an inhibitor (**negative effector** model) normally present. Until this putative factor(s) is purified, the exact mechanism of action will remain in doubt.

IV. PLATELET FUNCTION

A. Overview

1. Evolutionary aspects

Though humans and other higher vertebrates possess a complicated hemostatic mechanism, hemostasis is also complex in some primitive animals. For example the arthropod *Limulus polyphemus*, the horseshoe crab, possesses a single blood cell, the **amebocyte**, which serves as a phagocyte, platelet, and source of coagulation proteins. When a particle of foreign matter enters the circulation, the wandering amebocytes are attracted to the area and adhere to the particle, forming cellular aggregates. The amebocyte also secretes a clottable protein, roughly similar to mammalian fibrinogen, which then immobilizes the invader and initiates repair of tissue damage.

These two functions—**formation of intercellular aggregates** and **production of coagulable proteins**—later became increasingly complex and were segregated into separate systems consisting of cellular elements (platelets) and soluble plasma proteins. Though evolutionarily separated, the hemostatic mechanism in the human must be considered as an integrated system consisting of platelets, soluble coagulation factors, and endothelial cells. While each of these elements is reviewed separately below, they are all interacting components with at times a bewildering array of functions.

2. Relation between platelets and soluble clotting factors

As in the amebocyte, there is a close relation between platelet function and coagulation protein function. There are many examples of this relationship. Various coagulation factors require the addition of **phospholipid**. While synthetic phospholipids can be used in vitro, the platelet is the major source in vivo. In vivo activated coagulation factors such as **factor Xa** bind to the platelet and carry out their coagulation reactions there rather than in the plasma, where they are much more readily subject to inactivation. In addition, certain coagulation proteins, such as **factor V**, are contained in the platelet as well as in the circulation and upon activation are released from the granule and become exposed on the platelet surface. Conversely, platelets need plasma proteins such as fibrinogen and VWF in order to function normally.

3. Relation between platelets and the endothelium

Platelets have long been thought to help in some manner to maintain the integrity of vascular endothelium. Usually when the platelet count is low, capillary permeability increases and blood cells spontanously pass between endothelial cells to the outside of the vascular lumen. Clinically this gives rise to **petechiae**, tiny, pinpoint hemorrhagic lesions that do not disappear when pressure is applied. Isolated organs also survive better when perfused with fluids containing a few platelets. Specifically, platelets supply the endothelium with arachidonic acid metabolites and may provide growth factors that enhance endothelial cell viability. Activated platelets may stimulate proliferation of arterial smooth muscle cells via the release of PDGF and TGF-β.

Though long known to be subject to platelet influences, the endothelial cell has recently gained prominence as having profound effects on the platelet and soluble coagulation factors. The endothelial cell is the major source of VWF. Moreover, it is the source of biologically active materials like **prostacyclin (PGI_2)**, a potent vasodilator and inhibitor of platelet function.

4. Relation between endothelial cells and soluble clotting factors

In additon to supplying the bulk of plasma VWF, endothelial cells produce **tissue factor** (a potent activator of factor VII [see 27]) and **tissue-type plasminogen activator**, a potent activator of the fibrinolytic system. Finally, the endothelial surface contains several molecules that function as anticoagulants. Surface **heparan sulfate** proteoglycan binds circulating antithrombin III and inhibits thrombin. Endothelial cell surface **thrombomodulin** binds thrombin and converts circulating **protein C** to an active form that is able (with protein S) to inactivate factor Va (and probably factor VIIIa) even on the platelet surface.

B. Formation of the primary hemostatic plug

In the circulation the platelet exists as a relatively inactive cell; it is discoid, not adherent, and contains its full complement of granules. When it encounters damaged endothelium or exposed subendothelium a rapid change (**platelet activation**) occurs and the platelet changes shape, becomes very adherent, and releases its granule contents. We will review this complex process first at the cellular level and then at the biochemical level.

1. Cellular aspects

Upon encountering exposed subendothelium, platelet activation begins with **adhesion** of the platelet to exposed collagen and is followed by a **change in shape** and release of α- and dense granules (**degranulation**, **release** or **secretion reaction**). The extent of granule release is related to the intensity of the stimulus and may be reversible in some situations. For any level of stimulus, dense granules are released preferentially followed by α- and then lysosomal granules. Lysosomal granules maximally release 60% of their contents, whereas the other granules maximally release 100%. The ADP released from dense granules leads to **recruitment** of other platelets in the circulation (not attached to exposed collagen) by causing them to become activated and in this way to undergo **aggregation** to form the growing

primary hemostatic plug (a process also referred to as **primary hemostasis** [see lecture 29]). In addition to collagen and ADP, another potent agonist, **thrombin**, is generated on the platelet surface by the plasma coagulation system, which is also activated on contact with exposed subendothelium. The synergistic effect of these potent platelet agonists promotes additonal degranulation and the generation of yet another potent aggregating agent and vasoconstrictor, **thromboxane A_2** (TXA_2). Important in the recruitment of platelets to the forming platelet aggregate is the presence of **fibrinogen**. With platelet activation the GPIIb/IIIa receptor undergoes conformational change and increases its affinity for fibrinogen, which links one activated platelet to another. Finally, as higher concentrations of thrombin are generated, fibrinogen in the plasma is converted to fibrin strands that solidify the platelet plug and form the **secondary hemostatic plug** (also referred to as **secondary hemostasis** [see lecture 29]).

A number of **limiting reactions** exist that normally prevent massive platelet deposition in the wake of trivial injury. These include:

- Continued **flow of blood** past the growing platelet plug, which removes loosely adherent platelets and dilutes the concentration of ADP and other mediators
- Actions of plasma and endothelial **ADPases** that degrade ADP to **adenosine**, a competitive inhibitor of platelet aggregation
- Production by endothelial cells of **prostacyclin (PGI_2)**, a potent platelet inhibitor

The balance between platelet thromboxane and endothelial prostacyclin production may be critical for normal hemostasis.

2. *Biochemical aspects*

The initial event in the formation of the hemostatic plug appears to be the binding of circulating platelets via their receptors for **exposed collagen**. This adhesion requires that the collagen be in a native fibrillar quaternary form, and multiple sites of interaction with the platelet may be present. The **initial adhesion reaction** is reversible and is critically dependent on the presence of (VWF), which seems to stabilize binding to collagen. Though VWF is present in the plasma, it is also a component of the subendothelium (formed by the endothelial cell) and this local presence may be the more critical factor for platelet binding. In the absence of VWF the initial adhesion reaction with collagen is transient (see lecture 27). Other mediators that cause platelet activation such as ADP, TXA_2, epinephrine, and thrombin also act via specific receptors on the platelet surface. Except for collagen and thrombin, most of these mediators require small amounts of ADP to potentiate their effect.

Upon binding to their receptors, all of these agonists cause alterations in the platelet membrane potential, ion fluxes, and the generation of a number of important **second messengers** including **calcium**, **1,2 diacylglycerol** (DAG), **inositol 1,4,5-triphosphate** (IP_3), **endoperoxides**, and **throm-**

boxane A_2 (TXA_2). While this multitude of second messengers are interacting and reinforcing virtually simultaneously, several important effects may be singled out (figure 28.4). Upon receptor binding, signal transduction at the membrane results in activation of **phospholipase C** (PLC), which cleaves **phosphatidylinositol 4,5-bisphosphate** (PIP_2) into DAG and IP_3. DAG activates **protein kinase C**, which in turn activates a number of proteins (including myosin light chain) by phosphorylation. IP_3 meanwhile promotes release of calcium from dense tubular system (DTS) stores.

The rise in $[Ca^{2+}]$ from 100 nM to 10 μM due to release from DTS stores and influx from extracellular stores has several consequences. Elevated calcium activates **phospholipase A**, which releases **arachidonate** (20:4) from phospholipids, which in turn activates platelet **cyclooxygenase**, generating the **endoperoxides PGG_2** and **PGH_2** (and a "burst" of O_2 consumption). These endoperoxides are converted by **thromboxane synthetase** into an unstable (half-life, 30 sec) intermediate, TXA_2. Elevation in intracellular TXA_2 causes alpha and dense granule release, inhibition of adenylate cyclase—and lowering of [cAMP] (see below)—and further release of cellular calcium. **Aspirin**, an irreversible acetylator of cyclooxygenase, is a potent inhibitor of TXA_2 production and prevents granule release. Elevated calcium alters the cytoskeleton by causing microfilaments to elongate producing pseudopodia and a spheroidal shape of the platelet. This corre-

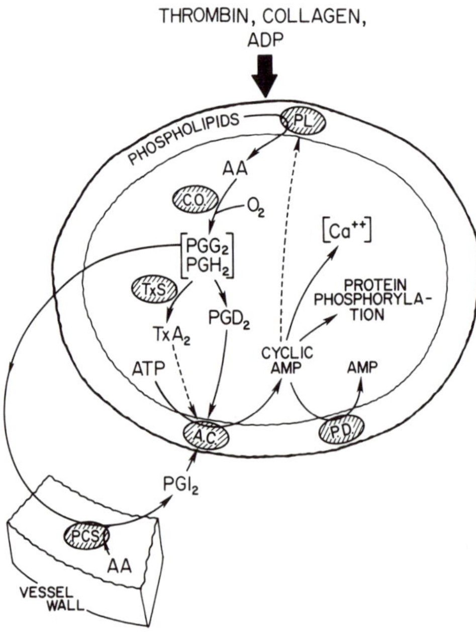

Fig. 28.4
Outline of biochemical mechanisms underlying platelet aggregation and release reaction. (PL, phospholipases; CO, cyclooxygenase; TXS, thromboxane synthetase; AC, adenylate cyclase; PD, phosphodiesterase; PCS, prostacyclin synthetase; AA, arachidonic acid.) Dashed lines denote inhibitory effect, solid lines denote stimulatory effect.

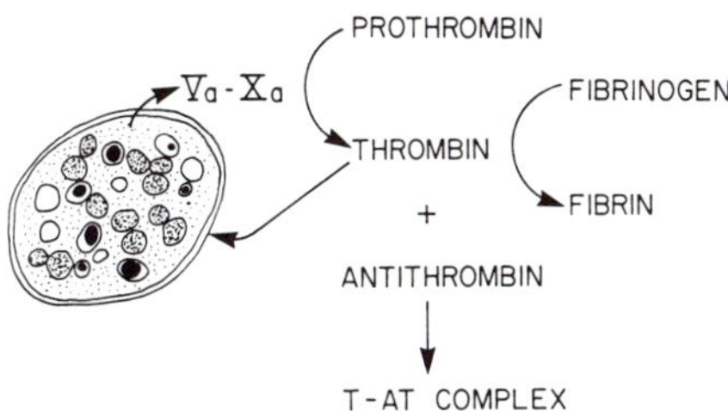

Fig. 28.5
Platelet binding of factors Va and Xa and prothrombin conversion.

lates with phosphorylation of the 20,000-dalton myosin light chain. The rise in intracellular calcium also results in changes of the platelet surface membrane:

- The **GPIIb/IIIa complex** binds to the cytoskeleton, is conformationally altered, and becomes an avid receptor for fibrinogen.
- Platelet **factor V** is released from α-granules and binds to the platelet surface where it becomes activated (figure 28.5).

ADP and TXA_2 are released together and bind to their receptors on locally circulating platelets (not bound to collagen) where they induce platelet activation and (in the presence of fibrinogen) attach to the growing hemostatic plug. Platelets lacking dense granules (**storage pool disease**) or unable to secrete their granules (**defective release mechanism**) or lacking the fibrinogen receptor (**Glanzmann's thrombasthenia)** are unable to recruit platelets and fail to aggregate sufficient platelets to form an adequate primary hemostatic plug.

These mechanisms promoting platelet activation are opposed by several mechanisms that **inhibit platelet activation** (see figure 28.4). Whereas in the platelet endoperoxides are converted into the potent platelet agonist TXA_2 in the endothelial cell they are converted into the potent antagonist PGI_2. The endothelial cell uses endogenous arachidonate or platelet-derived PGG_2 and PGH_2 to make PGI_2, which is secreted. PGI_2 binding to the platelet activates adenylate cyclase which raises levels of **3′,5′-adenosine monophosphate** (cAMP), which in turn promotes DTS sequestration of calcium and a reduction in $[Ca^{2+}]$ as well as decreased activity of phospholipase C and cyclo-oxygenase. The anti-platelet drug **dipyridamole (Persantine®)** promotes elevation of the cAMP level by inhibiting its degradation by phosphodiesterase. Other proposed inhibitory mechanisms include guanylate cyclase and IP_3 phosphatases. Activation of the former elevates cyclic GMP to inhibitory levels while increasing activity of the latter decreases IP_3 levels.

C. Platelet procoagulant activity

The long-recognized fact that platelets can accelerate certain coagulation reactions has been referred to as **platelet factor 3 activity**. This property is due to the binding of factor V from platelets or plasma to the platelet membrane. When activated, factor Va serves as a receptor for factor Xa, forming the **prothrombinase complex**, which converts prothrombin to thrombin on the platelet surface (figure 27.5). **Factor Xa** bound to the platelet is protected from the inhibitory effect of antithrombin and accelerates prothrombin conversion 300,000-fold. In addition, the binding of factor Xa to Va on the platelet protects factor Va from inactivation by **activated protein C** (and protein S). Platelets may play an important regulatory role in initiating coagulation reactions since platelets can release and bind factor Va without the production of thrombin (see lecture 27). The severity of bleeding in factor V deficiency has been related to intraplatelet factor V content, and patients have been described with a bleeding disorder who lack the platelet binding site (presumably factor Va) for factor Xa.

Most other factors (including XII, XI, IX) in the intrinsic coagulation system have markedly increased activity for their substrates when bound to activated (but not resting) platelets.

V. PLATELET DISORDERS

A. Quantitative disorders

Platelet disorders may be due to alterations in the number of platelets (quantitative disorders), alterations in the quality of platelets (qualitative disorders) or mixtures of both.

Quantitative platelet disorders are due to a reduction in the platelet count (**thrombocytopenia**) or an elevation in the platelet count (**thrombocytosis**). Diagnosis of these conditions depends on an accurate **platelet count**. The count can be roughly estimated in a good Wright's stained blood smear, each platelet in an oil immersion field representing approximately 10,000 platelets/mm^3 of blood. Platelets are counted more precisely in a hemacytometer with a phase microscope (see Appendix). However, this is accurate to only $\pm 10\%$ even when expertly performed. Thus minor changes in the platelet count are as likely to reflect technical factors as a true variation when performed in this way. Automated platelet counting using electrical (Coulter) or laser techniques are now routinely available and are accurate to $\pm 3\%$ at platelet counts from 1000–3,000,000/mm^3. These methods also report the distribution of the platelet volume and its mean value. However, the use of such automated platelet counting equipment is subject to occasional errors. Inappropriately low platelet counts ("spurious thrombocytopenia") are reported when platelets aggregate following blood collection, such as may occur with platelets that have a high rate of spontaneous aggregation or in the presence of EDTA anticoagulants and cold agglutinins. Aggregation of platelets about white blood cells ("platelet satellitism") also rarely produces spuriously low platelet counts. Inappropriately elevated platelet counts ("spurious thrombocytosis") are less common but occur when small particulate debris such as red and white cell fragments are counted as platelets. In evaluating quantitative platelet disorders, it is therefore mandatory to inspect the blood smear to exclude these entites. If quantitative platelet disorders are not spurious, then further evaluation may be aided by accurate information on spleen size and bone marrow morphology.

1. *Thrombocytopenia*

Thrombocytopenia is generally said to be present when the platelet count falls below 150,000 platelet/mm^3. However, the **bleeding time** is not usually prolonged (in the presence of qualitatively normal platelets) and hemostasis is usually normal until the count drops below 100,000 platelets/mm^3. Even at about 50,000 platelets/mm^3 ("moderate thrombocytopenia") surgical hemostasis is usually normal. Between 50,000 and 20,000 platelets/mm^3 there is some increase in hemorrhagic tendency. The incidence of bleeding increases dramatically below 5,000 platelets/mm^3 ("severe thrombocytopenia"). In any patient, the risk of bleeding is related not just to the platelet count but to the qualitative platelet function. For example, at a platelet count of 20,000/mm^3 a patient with ITP may have very young, hyperfunctional platelets and normal hemostasis, whereas a patient with leukemia may be experiencing severe hemorrhage.

Table 28.2
Classification of the Thrombocytopenias

Decreased production	
Hypoproliferation (see lecture 4)	Toxic agents (see table 4.1)
	Radiation, infection
	Constitutional disorders (e.g., Fanconi's anemia)
	Aplastic anemia
	Paroxysmal nocturnal hemoglobinuria
	Myelophthisis (e.g., tumor, fibrosis)
Ineffective thrombopoiesis	Megaloblastic anemia (see lectures 5, 6)
	Di Guglielmo's syndrome
Abnormal distribution	Congestive splenomegaly
	Myeloid metaplasia, lymphoma
	Gaucher's disease
Dilutional loss	Massive blood transfusion
Abnormal destruction	
Nonimmune mechanisms	Disseminated intravascular coagulation (DIC), vasculitis, thrombotic thrombocytopenic purpura (TTP), hemolytic-uremic syndrome (HUS), intravascular malignancy
Immune mechanisms	Idiopathic thrombocytopenic purpura (ITP)
	Drug-induced thrombocytopenia
	Chronic lymphocytic leukemia, lymphoma, LE
	Neonatal thrombocytopenia
	Post-transfusion purpura

Most cases of thrombocytopenia can be classified (as outlined in table 28.2) according to probable mechanism into

- Production defects
- Distribution defects
- Dilutional loss
- Abnormal destruction (nonimmune or immune)

Figure 28.6 is an algorithm for the evaluation of thrombocytopenia. It should be remembered that complex situations may occur in which multiple factors contribute to the low platelet count.

a. PRODUCTION DEFECTS

Reduction in platelet production accompanies a wide range of disorders of **bone marrow hypoproliferation** (see table 28.2). It can best be correlated with an absolute reduction in total megakaryocyte mass. However, mass is tedious to measure, requiring careful examinations of serial microscopic sections of marrow, and hence is not widely employed. Clinicians usually estimate megakaryocyte mass by inspection of a needle biopsy section or a bone marrow aspirate smear. A low-power (× 10) field of a needle biopsy section normally contains an average of five megakaryoctyes.

In additon to a reduction in the number of megakaryocytes, decreased platelet production is often associated with other bone marrow abnormalities. For example, thrombocytopenia due to aplastic anemia is associated with marrow hypocellularity that may involve all cell lines, and thrombocytopenia due to myelophthisis is associated with tumor cells, fibrosis, or leukemic cells (see lecture 4). Though often accompanied by bone marrow hypoplasia, some toxic ingestions may present with marked thrombocytopenia and a normal bone marrow biopsy. A common example of this is the moderate to severe thrombocytopenia associated with episodic ingestion of large quantities of ethanol.

In contrast with these hypoproliferative states, the mild thrombocytopenia associated with megaloblastic anemia is due to **ineffective thrombopoiesis** (see lecture 5). The marrow contains an increased number of megakaryocytes, often with megaloblastic morphology and megaloblastosis of other cell lines.

b. DISTRIBUTION DEFECTS

As noted in lecture 3, splenomegaly enlarges the splenic platelet pool and may thereby cause thrombocytopenia (figure 28.6). This redistribution does not cause severe thrombocytopenia or bleeding even in massive splenomegaly. In some myeloproliferative disorders (e.g., chronic myelocytic leukemia [CML]), platelet production in marrow can be great enough to produce thrombocytosis despite massive splenic enlargement. Interestingly, patients with myeloid metaplasia have a complex combination of

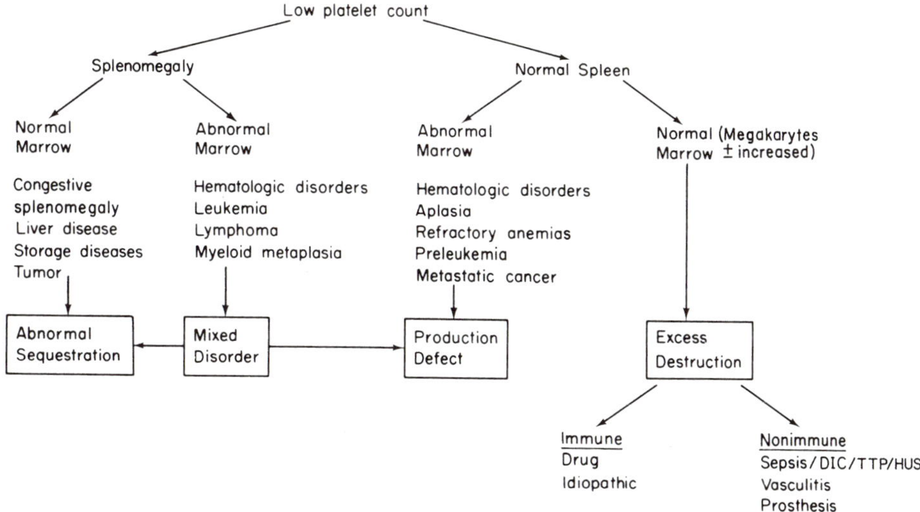

Fig. 28.6
A schematic approach to the clinical evaluation of patients with thrombocytopenia.

abnormal platelet production from dysplastic megakaryocytes, splenic sequestration, and production of platelets from extramedullary sites such as liver and spleen.

c. DILUTIONAL LOSS

Patients who receive many blood transfusions within a short time period may develop **dilutional thrombocytopenia** because infused blood does not contain viable platelets. As noted in lecture 17, platelets are no longer viable after blood is stored for more than a few hours at 4°C. Thrombocytopenia may persist for several days until the marrow syntehsizes a sufficient number of new platelets. If bleeding, these patients are treated by infusion of fresh platelets.

d. ABNORMAL DESTRUCTION

(1) Classification

As mentioned above, few platelets are consumed in the normal maintenance of hemostasis. However, platelets can be destroyed so rapidly that the marrow cannot compensate and thrombocytopenia develops. This occurs by **nonimmune mechanisms** such as disseminated intravacular coagulation (DIC) and by **immune mechanisms** such as ITP. The accelerated platelet destruction results in decreased ^{51}Cr platelet survival and in failure to respond to platelet transfusions. The feedback mechanism between the platelet and megakaryocyte becomes activated. Platelet production is accelerated and this is made manifest by the appearance on the blood smear of large platelets called **megathrombocytes**. While it would be useful to have a clinical index of young platelets that would illuminate platelet kinetics as the reticulocyte illuminates red cell kinetics, evaluation of the number of megathrombocytes in a blood smear is highly subjective and does not provide an adequate production index. The most striking megathrombocytes are seen in myeloproliferative disorders, megaloblastic anemia, severe thrombocytopenia ($<50{,}000/mm^3$), and in rare inherited platelet disorders such as the Bernard-Soulier syndrome (see below). In addition to the megathrombocyte, another response of the feedback mechanism to thrombocytopenia is an increase in the number and size of megakaryocytes seen on the bone marrow aspirate.

(2) Nonimmune thrombocytopenia

Many of the nonimmune causes of platelet destruction are readily apparent. **Acute** (e.g., secondary to sepsis) and **chronic** (e.g., secondary to malignancy) **DIC** may produce moderate to severe thrombocytopenia. The ongoing rapid consumption of coagulation factors causes concomitant platelet activation and trapping in the vasculature. A related but localized phenomenon occurs in the renal vasculature of transplanted kidneys undergoing acute rejection. In **thrombotic thrombocytopenic purpura** (TTP) the widespread formation of platelet thrombi in the vasculature occurs in the absence of activation of coagulation factors (PT, PTT, and fibrin split products are normal). Though often associated with a viral prodrome, the etiology is really unclear. The platelet thrombi cause regional tissue damage most marked in the CNS (obtundation and stroke), thrombocytopenia, and breakage of red blood cells into fragments called **schistocytes**. The infusion of fresh frozen plasma, plasma exchange and corticosteroids have all been felt to be of benefit. A related illness, **hemolytic-uremic syndrome** (HUS), is found mostly in children and is manifested by deposition of platelet thrombi in the renal vasculature resulting in thrombocytopenia, the formation of schistocytes, and reduced renal function. No specific interventions have been found to help, and many children recovery with aggressive support measures including dialysis.

Other alterations of the vascular bed such as by intravascular tumor, burns, or congenital hemangioma (**Kasabach-Merritt syndrome**) may shorten platelet survival and produce thrombocytopenia.

(3) Immune thrombocytopenia

Immune-mediated platelet destruction covers a wide range of disorders and may present a diagnostic challenge. Often the diagnosis is made by exclusion. In general, platelet surface antigens have not been studied and catalogued as extensively as those on the red blood cell. Platelets have several surface antigenic systems that are capable of reacting with antibody. As mentioned above, platelets have ABO and class I HLA antigens. Unlike for red blood cell transfusions, the ABO antigens are not very important since transfusion of ABO incompatible units of platelets show only a modest reduction in platelet survival. On the other hand, platelet HLA antigens usually result in sensitization following transfusion. This sensitization may be prevented by using platelet preparations depleted of lymphocytes and monocytes (which both contain class II antigens). In addition, the platelet has a unique PLA antigen system that plays a role in **neonatal** and **post-transfusion purpura**. The GPIIb/IIIa complex has been estimated to cover approximately 10% of the platelet surface and appears to be the major antigen in **ITF**. Platelets also contain receptors (probably on or near to the GPIb complex) for the Fc portion of immunoglobulin and can bind altered IgG or immune complexes such as occur in **drug-induced thrombocytopenia** and some cases of **AIDS-related thrombocytopenia**.

The most important pathophysiologic effect of Fab or Fc mediated binding of antibody to the platelet is to sensitize the platelet so that its subsequent clearance from the circulation and phagocytosis by macrophages is accelerated. If only a small amount of antibody is bound, platelets are usually cleared by the spleen, with larger amounts, clearance by the liver plays a greater role. However, certain platelet antibodies (e.g., HLA antibodies) elicited by chronic transfusions or multiple pregnancies fix complement and may cause direct platelet lysis. In addition, deposition of drug-antibody complexes onto the platelet can cause complement fixation and intrvascular platelet lysis. The relative importance of sensitization with IgG antibody alone, platelet opsonization with C3, or activation of the entire complement sequence varies with the type of antibody stimulus. It also changes with time in a single patient.

(i) Drug-induced thrombocytopenia

A large number of drugs can induce thrombocytopenia. A few are frequent offenders—for example, quinine, quinidine, sulfonamides, and antibiotics like cephalothin. Patients usually show a rapid fall in platelet count while they are taking the sensitizing medication. This may occur within 2–3 days of starting a drug that the patient has previously taken or may occur 7 or more days after starting a drug for the first time. There is then a prompt rise in platelet count within 7–10 days after drug withdrawal, though this time may be prolonged with drugs such as gold thiomalate or diphenylhydantoin (Dilantin®) that are metabolized and eliminated slowly.

Heparin has been implicated in an increasing number of cases of thrombocytopenia. The incidence varies from 3–25% of patients receiving heparin and may vary with the source of heparin or production lot. Some cases arise by an immune mechanism and others by a direct effect of certain heparin fractions on the platelet. **Heparin thrombocytopenia** is unique in that patients may develop **paradoxical thrombosis** that improves after heparin withdrawal.

The offending drug usually acts as a **hapten**, and the ensuing drug-antibody complex binds to the platelet, fixes complement, and causes intravascular lysis or subsequent removal by the reticuloendothelial system. **Quinidine-induced thrombocytopenia** has been studied most extensively. In this disorder, passive transfer of immune serum to a normal individual, followed by drug challenge, produces transient thrombocytopenia. This drug-dependent antibody can be detected by quantitative complement fixation techniques. Unlike the situation in drug-induced hemolysis (see lecture 14), drug-induced platelet antibodies are not usually directed against specific platelet antigens, nor do drugs coat platelets and then elicit and interact with circulating antibody.

A unique and significant case was reported several years ago in which a patient was sensitized to a metabolite of acetaminophen (Tylenol®) rather than to the drug itself. This case illustrates the difficulties of excluding a diagnosis of drug-induced thrombocytopenia in a given patient or of trying to make a laboratory diagnosis without strong suspicions of which drug or metabolite to test. The sudden onset of thrombocytopenia that remits shortly after discontinuing a particular drug remains the best clinical proof of drug-induced thrombocytopenia.

(ii) AIDS-related thrombocytopenia

Thrombocytopenia has been frequently noted in **HIV-seropositive individuals, narcotic addicts** and **hemophiliacs**. While this may be associated with the pancytopenia seen in patients with AIDS, it may also present as solitary thrombocytopenia indistinguishable from classic ITP and occur prior to the clinical development of AIDS in seropositive individuals. Unlike classic ITP which involves IgG directed toward platelet antigens, AIDS-related ITP is felt to be due to circulating immune complexes and C1, which bind to the platelet and shorten platelet survival. AIDS-related ITP responds to the usual therapies for classic ITP (see below) but also to the antiviral drug **3′ azido-2,3′ dideoxythymidine** (formerly called **azidothymidine** [AZT] and now **zidovudine** [Retrovir®]).

(iii) Neonatal isoimmune thrombocytopenia

Newborn infants often have abnormalities in the vitamin K–dependent synthesis of coagulation factors, but they usually have a normal platelet count. Most cases of thrombocytopenia arise in sick, premature infants with sepsis or DIC, but some infants are otherwise normal. In some of these cases, the mother's platelets lack the PLA-1 antigen, which is carried by 97% of the population. This produces a syndrome analagous to erythroblastosis fetalis (see lecture 17). The PLA-1-negative mother carrying the PLA-1-positive fetus develops antibody against this antigen that is transmitted through the placenta to the fetus, so that the child is born with temporary thrombocytopenia. The platelet count returns to normal in 13–28 days as the level of antiplatelet antibody (7S IgG) declines. The infant is susceptible to intracranial hemorrhage and requires temporary platelet infusions. The mother is the ideal platelet donor; her PLA-1-negative platelets, washed free of antibody-containing plasma, can be safely transfused to the child for several days.

(iv) Post-transfusion purpura

Since only 3% of the population lacks the PLA-1 antigen, PLA-1-negative individuals commonly become sensitized during preganancy or after blood transfusions. This has little effect on the PLA-1-negative recipient of an incompatible blood transfusion except for rapid destruction of the "mismatched" platelets. Rarely, PLA-1-negative individuals, usually multiparous females who have received blood containing PLA-1-positive platelets, develop profound thrombocytopenia 7–10 days after the transfusion. The mechanism of this **post-transfusion purpura** is not clear. Probably PLA-1 antigen in transfused blood is adsorbed onto PLA-1-negative platelets, which are then destroyed by antibody. In 10–14 days, the platelet count returns to normal as the patient clears the foreign antigen. The patient then continues to produce PLA-1-negative platelets that coexist with anti-PLA-1 antibody. Although rare, it has been fatal and is difficult to treat since all platelets are incompatible.

(v) Idiopathic thrombocytopenic purpura (ITP)

In the group of disorders termed **idiopathic thrombocytopenic purpura** (ITP), the cause of accelerated platelet destruction is more elusive than in the syndromes discussed above. In most cases an antibody is directed against platelets, although the actual stimulus for antibody production is usually not known. It was shown decades ago that some women with ITP deliver children with **transient neonatal thrombocytopenia**, which differs from **neonatal isoimmune thrombocytopenia** in that the mother does not lack PLA-1 antigen. This suggestion of transplacental passage of a causative humoral agent was bolstered by Harrington's demonstration that infusion of plasma from patients with ITP into normal individuals lowered the platelet count and that the active principle was a 7S IgG.

The majority of antibodies in patients with ITP are directed against determinants on GPIIIa. The epitopes are distinct from the PLA-1 antigen, which is also on GPIIIa. Despite the fact that fibrinogen binds to sites on GPIIIa, most antibodies do not inhibit fibrinogen binding or impair platelet aggregation. Tests for platelet antibody analogous to the red cell Coombs or direct antiglobulin test have been developed to measure platelet surface IgG, IgM, and C3. They reveal the presence of elevated quantities of **platelet-associated IgG, IgM,** or **C3** in most, but not all, patients with ITP. Unfortunately, the presence of significant overlap between normal and pathologic levels of platelet-associated antibody and the presence of elevated platelet-associated antibody in other disorders give this test low sensitivity and specificity.

ITP may present as an acute, transient disorder or as a chronic condition. **Acute ITP** is a self-limited condition that occurs mainly in children following a viral infection (e.g., rubella, cytomegalovirus, viral hepatitis, infectious mononucleosis). Thrombocytopenia, often severe (platelet counts $<10{,}000/mm^3$), may lead to mucosal bleeding and petechiae. However, mortality is low, and recovery usually occurs in 2–6 weeks. A viral antigen-antibody complex may be adsorbed onto platelet surfaces. Complete recovery follows clearance of these complexes. The few who do not recover in 6 months enter a chronic phase and resemble the patients described below.

Chronic ITP, a disorder of young and middle-aged women, is associated with an autoantibody against unknown platelet antigens. The patients may present with a long history of easy bruising and skin hemorrhage, or with a more acute picture. Some patients have other diseases, such as systemic lupus erythematosus, lymphoproliferative disorders (CLL or lymphoma), or immunohemolytic anemia (the combination being termed **Evans' syndrome**). The risk of intracranial hemorrhage and other serious complications is much higher in adults with chronic ITP than in children with acute ITP. Treatment usually consists of corticosteroids, splenectomy, or immunosuppressive drugs. Most patients who respond to corticosteroids will respond well to splenectomy, entering a long or permanent remission during which platelet counts are normal despite persistent antibody activity and accelerated platelet destruction. Splenectomy removes a major site of clearance of opsonized platelets (figure 28.7) and also a major site of production of anti-platelet IgG. **Danazol**, a synthetic attenuated androgen, has recently been found to decrease platelet destruction presumably by "down-regulating" the Fc receptor on macrophages. Nonresponders to these

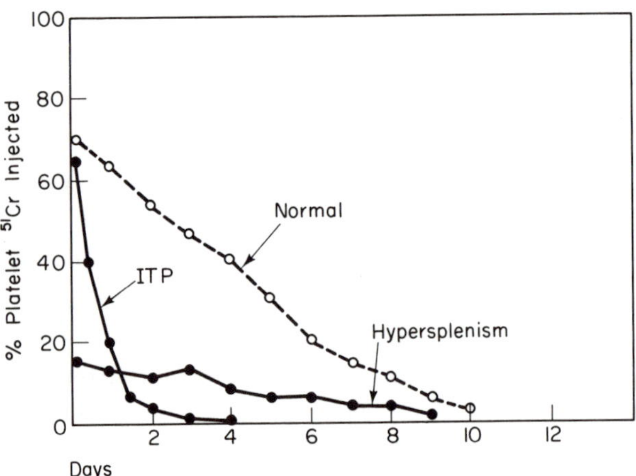

Fig. 28.7
Recovery and subsequent life span of isotopically labeled platelets infused into a normal individual and a patient with ITP. Note that platelet recovery is reduced in patients with splenomeglay (and hypersplenism), but platelet life span is normal. Patients with ITP have normal recovery and shortened life span. (Reprinted permission from R. Aster, in W. J. Williams et al., eds., *Hematology*. New York: McGraw-Hill, 1972, pp. 1159–1161.)

treatments may develop refractory thrombocytopenia and require immunosuppressive drugs such as vincristine, vinblastine, or cyclophosphamide.

Occasionally emergency situations (e.g., intra-abdominal hemorrhage) require the rapid correction of the thrombocytopenia. Intravenous IgG has been shown to block the reticuloendothelial system and may dramatically raise the platelet count over a few days. While use of intravenous IgG has been shown to be effective in most other disorders of immune destruction of platelets, its widespread use is limited by its considerable expense. Although platelets transfused into patients with ITP invariably have shortened survival, platelet transfusions may provide a transient rise in the platelet count and may be effective in treating severe bleeding episodes in these patients.

2. *Thrombocytosis*

Thrombocytosis is generally said to be present when the platelet count rises above 450,000 platelets/mm^3, but elevation of the platelet count even above 1,000,000/mm^3 is usually not associated with symptoms. However, thrombocytosis may produce thrombosis or, paradoxically, hemorrhage and the presence or absence of these symptoms is as much dependent on qualitative defects in the platelets as on the platelet count. Elevation of the platelet count may be **reactive** or may occur **autonomously**. In the former case it is termed **thrombocytosis**, in the latter, **thrombocythemia**.

a. REACTIVE

Platelet counts commonly up to 1,000,000 and on occasion reaching several million per cubic millimeter occur in association with malignancy, inflammation, bleeding, and iron deficiency. The platelets are functionally normal and the thrombocytosis is not related to excessive bleeding or thrombosis. In the few patients rigorously investigated, the total number of megakaryocytes was greatly increased but the average ploidy was decreased, suggesting that these "reactive" disorders are due to stimulation of CFU-Megs and concomitant "reflex" inhibition of ploidy development by the excessive number of platelets. In moderate iron deficiency platelet counts up to 1,000,000/mm^3 may be noted; if the iron deficiency becomes more severe, thrombocytopenia may then occur.

Following splenectomy the platelet count invariably rises and may approach several million/mm^3. This degree of thrombocytosis is out of proportion to that expected from eliminating the site in the circulation where 30% of the platelet mass is sequestered. It suggests that the spleen may play a more active role in the regulation of platelet production.

b. AUTONOMOUS

As noted (see lecture 20) platelet counts may be elevated in all the myeloproliferative syndromes (CML, polycythemia vera, myelofibrosis). In myeloproliferative syndromes where the platelet elevation is not associated with significant defects in the other lineages, the term **essential** or **autonomous thrombocythemia** is applied. In this entity and the other myeloproliferative syndromes showing thrombocythemia, the total number of megakaryocytes in the bone marrow may be increased up to tenfold along with a great increase in the average megakaryocyte ploidy. Platelet counts are commonly over $1{,}000{,}000/mm^3$ and may be asymptomatic or may cause either thrombosis or hemorrhage. The explanation for this variable presentation is that platelets produced in these myeloproliferative syndromes may have qualitative defects making them more or less likely to become activated. Defects in membrane glycoprotein content and loss of specific receptors and enzymes such as lipoxygenase have been described. Symptomatic patients require treatment aimed at lowering the platelet count and inhibiting excessive platelet activation if present.

B. Qualitative disorders

Patients with a normal platelet count and a clinical picture suggesting a platelet abnormality are said to have a **qualitative** or **functional platelet disorder**. As noted above, platelet functions may be subdivided into three major reactions—adhesion, release, and aggregation. Specific defects have been described in each reaction. Collectively, they comprise a major cause of easy bruising and minor bleeding tendency.

1. Tests of function

a. BLEEDING TIME

The overall reaction sequence mediated by platelets is simulated by the **bleeding time** (BT), a most useful test of platelet function. A small incision is made on the skin of the forearm and the time recorded that is required for cessation of blood flow. Mechanical aids such as a plastic template help standardize the incision and improve precision. Normal BT is $4\text{–}9\frac{1}{2}$ min. It should be remembered that the BT can be prolonged by quantitative and qualitative platelet disorders. A patient with a normal platelet count and a normal BT is unlikely to have a significant platelet abnormality. Since the BT does not become prolonged until the platelet count falls below $100{,}000/mm^3$, the presence of moderate thrombocytopenia and severely prolonged BT should suggest the possibility that a qualitative platelet disorder coexists with thrombocytopenia.

b. RELEASE REACTION TESTS

Released adenine nucleotides and **serotonin** (5-hydroxytryptamine) are convenient assay parameters for the platelet release reaction. In addition, it is possible by incubating platelets with ^{14}C-adenine to estimate the pool of adenine nucleotides in platelet granules. Granule-bound ADP and ATP, termed **storage pool ADP and ATP**, are to be distinguished from **metabolic pool ADP and ATP** in the cytoplasm. Since ^{14}C-adenine is readily converted to metabolic pool nucleotides and excluded from granules, relative sizes of the two pools can be estimated by measuring and comparing total and radioactive adenine nucleotides. As will be noted below, this procedure identifies patients in whom failure to achieve normal secondary aggregation is due to a reduced adenine nucleotide pool in the granules, rather than a defect in release per se. It is also possible to measure release of granule constituents using radioimmunoassays for platelet-specific proteins such as β-thromboglobulin or PF-4. This is of practical importance, since selective deficiencies of granule contents have been discovered. Such specific granule deficiencies may also be diagnosed morphologically by electron microscopy of platelets.

C. PLATELET AGGREGATION TESTS

Platelet plug formation is also studied in turbidimetric assays of the time course and extent of platelet aggregation following the addition to platelet-rich plasma of ADP, collagen or epinephrine, increased light transmittance through the cuvette indicating platelet aggregation (table 28.3). As shown in figure 28.8, when ADP (1 μM) is added, some platelets are activated and a few aggregates form (**first wave** or **primary aggregation**), which may then disaggregate. As [ADP] is increased, a point is reached (at about 1.5 μM) at which a **second wave** of aggregation (**secondary aggregation**) occurs. This second wave of aggregation coincides with the platelet granule release of ADP. A similar biphasic curve occurs on addition of epinephrine. However, incubation with collagen produces monophasic aggregation because collagen itself does not cause aggregation directly but requires release of endogenous ADP following adhesion of platelets to collagen fibrils. When the defunct antibiotic **ristocetin** is added, however, it promotes the binding of VWF to its platelet receptor resulting in aggregation. This direct effect is not mediated by granule release and is lacking in von Willebrand's disease and Bernard-Soulier's syndrome.

d. BIOCHEMICAL TESTS

Aggregation and release require normal membrane structure and intact protein metabolism. Functional platelet abnormalities can be correlated with metabolic defects sufficiently often to merit special testing of patients with platelet dysfunction. The glycoprotein electrophoretic pattern of platelet membranes is depicted in figure 28.2. Two specific membrane glycoprotein defects, **Glanzmann's thrombasthenia** and the **Bernard-Soulier syndrome**, may be assessed in this fashion. Furthermore, the adequacy of arachidonic acid metabolism can be assessed by (1) measuring the burst in oxygen consumption or production of TXA_2 by radioimmunoassay or

Table 28.3
Test Results in Qualitative Platelet Disorders

	Aggregation								
	ADP		Epinephrine						
Disorder*	1°	2°	1°	2°	Collagen	Ristocetin	5-HT uptake	Release of ADP, ATP, 5-HT	VWF:An
Adhesion									
von Willebrand's disease	N	N	N	N	N	↓	N	N	↓
Bernard-Soulier's syndrome	N	N	N	N	N	↓	N	N	N
Primary aggregation									
Thrombasthenia	↓	↓	↓	↓	↓	N	N	N	N
Secondary aggregation and release									
Aspirin(-like) defect	N	↓	N	↓	↓	N	N	↓	N
Storage pool disease	N	↓	N	↓	↓	N	↓	N/↓	N

Abbreviations: 1°, primary wave; 2°, secondary wave; N, normal; ↓, decreased; 5-HT, 5-hydroxytryptamine, serotonin; VWF:An, VWF antigen detected by immunoassay.

*The bleeding time is prolonged in all of the listed disorders.

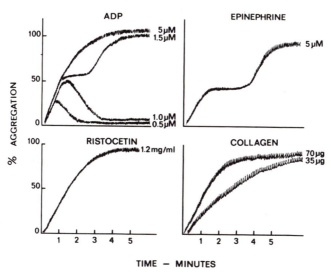

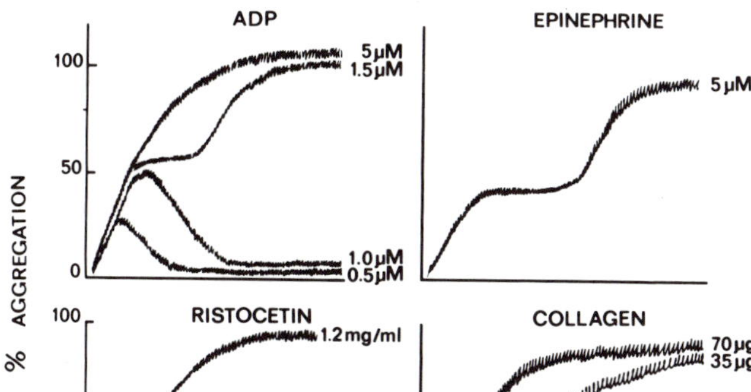

Fig. 28.8
Aggregation patterns of normal platelets after challenge with various aggregating agents. Note that a biphasic pattern can be obtained with certain concentrations of ADP and with epinephrine. The secondary wave, which corresponds to the platelet release action, is abolished by drugs such as aspirin.

radiochemical techniques following induction by aggregating agents or (2) measuring aggregation with arachidonic acid.

2. *Platelet defects*

a. ADHESION DEFECTS

(1) von Willebrand's disease

The most common cause of defective adhesion is **von Willebrand's disease**, usually an autosomal dominant disorder in which a plasma deficiency in VWF decreases platelet adhesion to vessel walls. Von Willebrand's disease and related syndromes have turned out to be common causes of minor and sometimes major bleeding. As discussed in lecture 27, VWF is a protein of 230,000 daltons that forms a series of polymers with molecular weights up to 20 million. The bulk of these polymers are produced by endothelial cells and released into the circulation. Megakaryocytes also produce VWF and store it in α-granules—since the content of the endothelial cell cannot be easily assessed, analysis of platelet VWF stores may reflect those in the endothelial cell. Normal plasma contains a heterogenous collection of these VWF polymers, which vary in size and biologic activity. The **higher-molecular-weight polymers (multimers)** promote platelet adhesion most effectively in vivo and in ristocetin-induced platelet aggregation. Polymers of all sizes have antigenic determinants and are detected in immunoassays quantifying the total amount of VWF. VWF of all sizes has binding sites for the antihemophiliac factor (factor VIII) and though produced by separate genes and separate tissues in the body, they associate and circulate together as a high-molecular-weight complex. In the formation of the primary hemostatic plug, high-molecular-weight multimers of VWF bind to the platelet receptor (GPIb) and to the subendothelium and thus serve to stabilize the initial binding of the platelet to collagen. In the absence of VWF, platelet adhesion is reduced and, because its half-life in the circulation is normally prolonged when bound to VWF, factor VIII levels fall. A moderate to severe bleeding problem ensues.

Patients with von Willebrand's disease report a life-long, though variable, history of mucosal bleeding, epistaxis, and bruising. Platelet aggregation and release are normal. They have a prolonged bleeding time and abnormalities in other tests which measure VWF function, such as aggregation in response to ristocetin [called **ristocetin cofactor activity** (VWF: RCo)]. They may also have **decreased amounts of VWF antigen** (VWF: An) measured by immunoassay and diminished amounts of **factor VIII activity** (VIII: c) measured by clotting assays.

In **classic** or **type I von Willebrand's disease** (VWD), the most common form, VWF is made in the endothelial cells and polymerizes normally but fails to be released. This results in greatly diminished total amount of VWF in the circulation but a normal distribution of multimer sizes. Tests for VWF antigen (VWF: An) and function (VWF: RCo) are diminished in parallel. The PTT is prolonged and factor VIII activity (VIII: c) is also diminished since Factor VIII is not stabilized in the circulation in the absence of VWF. If symptomatic, treatment consists of infusion of plasma or plasma fractions (such as **cryoprecipitate**) rich in VWF. The vasopressin analogue **1-deamino-8-D-arginine vasopressin** (DDAVP) promotes the release of VWF from endothelial cells and has proven useful in treating or preventing bleeding complications.

A number of variants of VWD have been described in which the amount of VWF protein and the level of factor VIII are usually normal but the ability to promote adhesion is deficient. These variants are collectively referred to as **type II VWD** and are due to the absence of large VWF multimers in the plasma. Type II subtypes are defined by differing plasma and endothelial cell (inferred from the platelet) multimeric patterns, unique functional characteristics of VWF, or structural abnormalities of VWF. In **type IIA** large VWF multimers are absent in both plasma and endothelial cells (platelets) owing to a failure of subunits to polymerize fully. In **type IIB** high molecular weight multimers are formed but have an abnormally increased affinity for the platelet, are bound to the platelets, and are cleared from the plasma. In **types IIC, IID, IIE,** and **IIF**, VWF is structurally defective and fails to polymeize. Type III is the most severe form of von Willebrand's disease and the most uncommon. Ristocetin cofactor activity

(VWF:RCo) and VWF antigen (VWF:An) are undetectable in plasma. This is felt to be due to a homozygous or doubly heterozygous deficiency.

Other von Willebrand's variants have been described, including patients with recessively inherited disorder and patients with a platelet VWF receptor defect (**pseudo-von Willebrand's disease**) that promotes VWF binding, depletes the plasma of high molecular weight multimers and mimics IIB disease. So-called **acquired von Willebrand's disease** may be due to an antibody that reacts with VWF.

(2) Bernard-Soulier's syndrome

Bernard-Soulier's syndrome is a rare, inherited disorder in which platelet adhesion is decreased and platelets do not respond to ristocetin despite normal plasma levels of VWF. The defect appears to be lack of the specific receptor protein (GPIb and associated proteins GPIX and GPV) on the platelet membrane that binds VWF. These patients are distinctive because they often also have mild thrombocytopenia and large platelets. Therapy requires infusion of normal platelets, not plasma.

b. RELEASE DEFECTS

Most patients with qualitative platelet disorders have **defects in release and in secondary aggregation**. A heterogeneous group of congenital and acquired platelet defects has been described. The consistent features are a prolonged BT accompanied by a normal primary response to exogenous ADP but absent secondary platelet aggregation with ADP and epinephrine, and a poor response to collagen. Patients typically show normal platelet aggregation with ristocetin as well as normal levels of VWF by immunoassay. The major groups of patients with this syndrome are those with an abnormality in the release mechanism itself and those with a deficiency in platelet storage pool nucleotides.

(1) Defective release mechanism—aspirin effect

The most common cause of this release defect is the ingestion of medications such as **aspirin (acetylsalicylic acid)**. Aspirin specifically acetylates the platelet cyclooxygenase system and thus decreases production of the prostaglandin endoperoxidase intermediates of TXA_2 that are necessary for release and aggregation. It should be emphasized that many **nonsteroidal anti-inflammatory drugs** (NSAID) such as **indomethacin** also inhibit cyclooxygenase but do so reversibly (recovery in 6 hr). Aspirin is particularly potent as a platelet inhibitor as it irreversibly inactivates the enzyme. Other cells recover from aspirin inhibition in 4–8 hr by synthesizing new enzyme but platelets lack the protein synthetic machinery to produce new enzyme and new platelets must be made over 6–8 days before recovery is complete. **Thromboxane synthetase inhibitors** such as **imidazole** produce a similar release defect and may be better anti-platelet agents than aspirin for they do not inhibit endothelial cell synthesis of PGI_2. A few patients have been reported with **inherited cyclooxygenase** or **thromboxane synthetase deficiencies** with similar functional platelet abnormalities.

(2) Storage pool disease

Patients who have a normal release mechanism but who lack granules or whose granules are present but lack important constituents such as ADP ("empty granules") have so-called **storage pool disease**. The defect can occur as an isolated autosomal dominant disorder or in association with a wide variety of conditions (e.g., leukemia, alcoholic intoxication). In the **Hermansky-Pudlak syndrome** oculocutaneous albinism is associated with a specific deficiency of only dense granules and a severe bleeding disorder. In additon to a long BT and defective secondary aggregation, these patients have

- Decrease in total platelet ADP and ATP
- Increase in specific labeling of the metabolic pool of platelet nucleotides
- Decreased uptake followed by excess leakage of radiolabelled serotonin

In the rare **gray platelet syndrome** only α-granules are reduced or lacking, giving the platelet an agranular or "gray" appearance on Wright's stain. There is a concomitant decrease in α-granule products such as PF-4 and PDGF. Patients also have modest thrombocytopenia, large platelets, and mild bleeding problems. Finally, many other storage pool disorders occur that show mild bleeding tendancies and deficiencies of both dense and α-granules.

C. AGGREGATION DEFECTS

Failure of the platelet to respond to an aggregating agent such as ADP occurs in a rare but serious autosomal recessive disorder called **Glanzmann's thrombasthenia** ("weak platelets"). The platelets show a disk-sphere transformation in response to aggregating stimuli and can undergo a release reaction; however, they do not aggregate and hence do not form normal hemostatic plugs. Though their genes contain no major deletions and the cells contain adequate amounts of the mRNA for these proteins, platelet membranes usually lack the GPIIb/IIIa complex. This complex contains the binding site for fibrinogen, which forms bridges between platelets and is critical for aggregate formation. A few thrombasthenic patients have been reported with detectable but probably dysfunctional GPIIb/IIIa.

d. OTHER ACQUIRED DEFECTS

Uremia commonly produces platelet dysfunction and an elevated BT. This is in part due to platelet sensitivity to unexcreted metabolites such as the

phenolic acids and **guanidinosuccinic acid**. In additon, there is evidence that uremic plasma stimulates the vascular wall to synthesize excess quantities of PGI_2. There may also be deficient cyclooxygenase activity and defective GPIb binding of VWF. With dialysis, there is some but not complete improvement in the BT. Recently the use of **cryoprecipitate infusions** or **DDAVP** have been found to improve the BT in uremic patients. This occurs despite the apparent absence of quantitative or functional deficiencies of VWF in uremic patients.

A number of other acquired conditions may produce platelet dysfunction. During **cardiac bypass**, platelet activation may produce platelets with decreased granules and an acquired storage pool disorder. Dysproteinemias may produce Fc-mediated binding and produce dysfunctional platelets with little effect on platelet survival. Similarly in ITP, antibody binding may produce a shortened platelet survival but also lead to qualitative platelet abnormalities.

The fact that many drugs interfere with platelet function has been exploited in the development of antithrombotic drugs such as **dipyridamole** (Persantine®) that act by inhibiting **platelet phosphodiesterase**. Correlation is still not good between the antithrombotic effect and antiplatelet effect, some drugs showing distinct antithrombotic effects but no discernible effects on hemostatic tests when given in usual doses. Thus while pharmacologic manipulation of platelet function is a desirable goal, means for testing the antithrombotic effect of drugs remain limited.

Novel approaches to manipulating platelet function have recently entered clinical trials. In one, **monoclonal antibodies to GPIb** havb been used to inactivate this VWF receptor, prevent adhesion, and mimic Bernard-Soulier's syndrome. In another **monoclonal antibodies to the GPIIb/IIIa complex** have been found to prevent fibrinogen binding, abrogate completely platelet aggregation and mimic Glanzmann's thrombasthenia. Finally, **fibrinopeptides** containing the R-G-D sequence have been synthesized that bind to the GPIIb/IIIa complex and prevent fibrinogen-mediated platelet aggregation. By preventing platelet adhesion or aggregation these approaches may be useful in promoting dissolution of platelet thrombi in coronary arteries or preventing their recurrance following fibrinolytic therapy.

SELECTED REFERENCES

Reviews

Bellucci, S., et al. Inherited platelet disorders. In E. B. Brown, ed., *Progress in Hematology*, Vol. 13. New York: Grune & Stratton, 1983, pp. 223–264.

Bennett, J. S. The molecular biology of platelet membrane proteins. *Semin. Hematol.* 27(1990): 186–204.

Berchtold, P., and McMillan, R. Therapy of chronic idiopathic thrombocytopenic purpura in adults. *Blood* 74(1989): 2309–2317.

Colman, R. W., Hirsh, J., et al., eds. *Hemostasis and Thrombosis: Basic Principles and Clinical Practice*, 2nd ed. Philadelphia: J. B. Lippincott, 1987.

Coughlin, S. R., Escobedo, J. A., et al. Role of phosphatidylinositol kinase in PDGF receptor signal transduction. *Science* 243(1989): 1191–1194.

George, J. N., and Aster, R. H. Thrombocytopenia due to diminished or defective platelet production. In Williams, W. J., et al., eds. *Hematology*, 4th ed. New York: McGraw-Hill, 1990, pp. 1343–1350.

George, J. N., Caen, J. P., et al. Glanzmann's thrombasthenia: the spectrum of clinical disease. *Blood* 75(1990): 1383–1395.

George, J. N., and Shattil, S. J. The clinical importance of acquired abnormalities of platelet function. *N. Engl. J. Med.* 324(1991): 27–39.

Gerlach, H., Esposito, C., et al. Modulation of endothelial hemostatic properties: an active role in the host response. *Annu. Rev. Med.* 41(1990): 15–24.

Harker, L. A., and Slichter, S. J. The bleeding time as a screening test for evaluation of platelet function. *N. Engl. J. Med.* 287(1972): 155–158.

Jones, S. D., Hall, D. J., et al. Platelet-derived growth factor generates at least two distinct intracellular signals that modulate gene expression. *Cold Spring Harbor Symp. Quant. Biol.* 53(1988): 531–536.

Karpatkin, S. Immunologic thrombocytopenic purpura in HIV-seropositive homosexuals, narcotic addicts and hemophiliacs. *Semin. Hematol.* 25(1988): 219–229.

Kelton, J. G. The measurement of platelet-bound immunoglobulin: an overview of the methods and the biological relevance of platelet-associated IgG. In E. B. Brown, ed. *Progress in Hematology*, Vol. 13. New York: Grune & Stratton, 1983, pp. 163–199.

Kroll, M. H., and Schafer, A. I. Biochemical mechanism of platelet activation. *Blood* 74(1989): 1181–1195.

Lopez-Fernandez, M. F., Batlle, J., et al. Secretion of von Willebrand factor from platelets. *Methods Enzymol.* 169(1989): 244–250.

Mannucci, P. M. Desmopressin: a nontransfusional hemostatic agent. *Annu. Rev. Med.* 41(1990): 55–64.

Mazur, E. M. Megakaryocytopoiesis and platelet production: a review. *Exp. Hematol.* 15(1987): 340–350.

Patrono, C. Aspirin and human platelets: from clinical trials to acetylation of cyclooxygenase and back. *TIPS* 10(1989): 453–458.

Ratner, L. Human immunodeficiency virus-associated autoimmune thrombocytopenic purpura: a review, *Am. J. Med.* 86(1989): 194–198.

Screiber, A. D., Chien, P., et al., Effect of danazol in immune thrombocytopenic purpura. *N. Engl. J. Med.* 316(1987): 503–508.

Sims, R. B., and Gewirtz, A. M. Human megakaryocytopoiesis. *Annu. Rev. Med.* 40(1989): 213–224.

Stenberg, P. E., and Levin, J. Mechanisms of platelet production. *Blood Cells* 15(1989): 23–47.

Warkentin, T. E., and Kelton, J. G. Heparin-induced thrombocytopenia. *Annu. Rev. Med.* 40(1989): 31–44.

Zucker, M. A., and Nachmias, V. T. Platelet activation. *Arteriosclerosis* 5(1985): 2–18.

Original articles

DiMichele, D. M., and Hathaway, W. E. Use of DDAVP in inherited and acquired platelet dysfunction. *Am. J. Hematol.* 33(1990): 39–45.

Finch, C. N., Miller, J. L., et al. Evidence that an abnormality in the glycoprotein Ib alpha gene is not the cause of abnormal platelet function in a family with classic Bernard-Soulier disease. *Blood* 75(1990): 2357–2362.

Harker, L. A., and Finch, C. A. Thrombokinetics in man. *J. Clin. Invest.* 48(1969): 963–974.

Harrington, W. J., Minnich, V., et al. Demonstration of a thrombocytopenic factor in the blood of patients with thrombocytopenic purpura. *J. Lab. Clin. Med.* 115(1990): 636–645.

Kuter, D. J., and Rosenberg, R. D. Regulation of megakaryocyte ploidy in vivo in the rat. *Blood* 75(1990): 74–81.

Ohlstein, E. H., Storer, B., et al. Endothelin and platelet function. *Thromb. Res.* 57(1990): 967–974.

Parise, L. V., Criss, A. B., et al. Glycoprotein IIIa is phosphorylated in intact human platelets. *Blood* 75(1990): 2363–2368.

Peake, I. R., Liddell, M. B., et al. Severe type III von Willebrand's disease caused by deletion of exon 42 of the von Willebrand factor gene: family studies that identify carriers of the condition and a compound heterozygous individual. *Blood* 75(1990): 654–661.

Tsai, H. -M., Nagel, R. L., et al. Multimeric composition of endothelial cell-derived von Willebrand factor. *Blood* 73(1989): 2074–2076.

LECTURE 29

Hemorrhagic Disorders III. Disorders of Hemostasis

David J. Kuter and Robert D. Rosenberg

EDITOR'S COMMENT

This lecture ties together the didactic material on clotting and platelets in the two previous lectures and presents a diagnostic schema for approaching patients with a suspected hemostatic defect. The classic screening tests remain the prothrombin time, partial thromboplastin time, platelet count, bleeding time, and plasma fibrinogen level, but new and important tests continue to be added, among them studies of platelet function, the lupus anticoagulant procedure, and many more. This lecture is organized in a functional way so that various diagnostic possibilities are considered according to the test pattern results. It also explores newer work on the hypercoagulable states. The most common cause of death is thromboembolism in one of its many clinical expressions—coronary thrombosis, peripheral vascular occlusion, and pulmonary embolus. Our greatest peril, therefore, is imbalance between adequate hemostasis and its regulatory mechanisms. This lecture (with its two predecessors) notes the remarkable orchestration of this system as revealed by recent work on fibrinolysis, fibrinolytic regulation, and coagulation control.

I. INTRODUCTION

Hemorrhagic disorders are common in both medicine and surgery. A major goal in the evaluation of clinical bleeding is to determine whether the bleeding is due to an **anatomic lesion** (e.g., a ruptured aneurysm) or to a defect in the **hemostatic system** (e.g., von Willebrand's disease). While these latter disorders of bleeding will be the subject of this lecture, it should be remembered that defects in the hemostatic system may commonly complicate bleeding from anatomic lesions (e.g., a prolonged PT and PTT in cirrhotic liver disease may exacerbate bleeding from varices).

In most cases the hemostatic problem can be localized to defects in **primary hemostasis** (platelets) or **secondary hemostasis** (coagulation proteins), but sometimes both systems are involved. In this lecture we will summarize the diagnostic approach to these disorders and their therapy. In addition, we will discuss several inherited disorders associated with thromboembolism. Since diagnosis of these hemostatic disorders is critically dependent on laboratory procedures, we will emphasize the relevant coagulation tests. In particular we will distinguish between information obtained from **screening tests** that are widely available and inexpensive

Table 29.1
Patient Charges for Hematologic Tests and Blood Product Transfusions

General hematology tests	
CBC	$8.55
Differential	4.95
Hematocrit	4.00
Hemoglobin	6.00
Red count	6.00
Reticulocyte count	6.60
Sedimentation rate	5.40
Bone marrow biopsy/aspirate	$75.00
Interpretation	75.00
Coagulation tests—screening	
Bleeding time	$34.50
Platelet count	6.85
PT	6.05
PTT	9.20
TT	43.50
Factor XIII screen	43.00
Coagulation tests—special	
Platelet aggregation	$112.75
With ristocetin	141.75
VWF:RCo	56.00
VWF:An	171.75
Lupus anticoagulant test	56.25
Fibrin degradation products	43.50
Antithrombin III level	68.75
Factors II, V, VII, VIII, IX, X, XI, XII, each	112.75
Reptilase time	61.00
Fibrinogen level	10.55
Blood product transfusions	
Type and cross-match	$43.00
Plasma—one unit	84.00
Platelets—one unit	105.00
Red blood cells—one unit	160.00

(Charges from Massachusetts General Hospital, Boston, MA as of May 19, 1989.)

(table 29.1) and that obtained by more definitve (and more expensive) **special tests** that may be available only in larger centers. As in all clinical evaluations, the appropriate selection of these tests is determined only after a thorough history and physical examination of the patient.

II. DISORDERS OF PRIMARY HEMOSTASIS: PRINCIPLES

A. Disagnostic features

As discussed in Lecture 28, platelets participate in blood coagulation by adhering to areas of vessel injury and forming cellular aggregates or hemostatic plugs. This is the process referred to as **primary hemostasis**. Patients can bleed because of a decrease in the number of circulating platelets or from a variety of congenital and acquired qualitative defects that prevent platelets from undergoing normal adhesion, aggregation, or release.

1. History

A careful history is often helpful to determine the type of platelet disorder since platelet disorders may be inherited or may be associated with a systemic disorder or drug ingestion. For example, patients with **oculocutaneous albinism** have an associated functional platelet defect; patients with **Wiskott-Aldrich syndrome** are usually thrombocytopenic. The family history may provide clues to the diagnosis since many platelet disorders are inherited as autosomal dominant traits, whereas the major coagulation protein disorders—deficiencies of factors VIII and IX—are sex-linked recessive abnormalities. Although inheritance is important, a negative family history does not exclude a platelet defect, for many patients with platelet dysfunction have acquired abnormalities due to metabolic disorders such as **uremia**. Moreover, since many drugs may alter platelet function a diligent review of prescription and nonprescription drug usage is mandatory.

2. Physical examination

On physical examination patients with defective primary hemostasis have a characteristic bleeding pattern (table 29.2). **Ecchymoses** (bruises) and **petechiae** appear on arms or things without antecedent trauma. These patients also bleed from mucous membranes and often have menorrhagia, gastrointestinal bleeding, repeated nosebleeds (**epistaxis**) and gingival bleeding following the brushing of teeth. This pattern, when part of the patient's evaluation, is to be contrasted with the joint, muscle, or retroperitoneal hemorrhage of insidious onset that occurs in patients with coagulation protein defects, that is, **defects of secondary hemostasis**. In addition to these findings, the physical examination is directed toward assessing **splenic size** and the presence of **enlarged lymph nodes**.

Table 29.2
Nature of Bleeding in Primary and Secondary Hemostatic Disorders

Parameter	Primary hemostatic disorders	Secondary hemostatic disorders
Bleeding source	Usually capillary	Usually small artery
Lesion	Cutaneous and mucosal petechiae and/or ecchymoses	Often intramuscular and deep hematomas
Preceding trauma	Unusual	Frequent, but delayed onset of bleeding
Complications of venepuncture	Superficial ecchymoses around venipuncture site	No superficial ecchymoses, but hemorrhage may occur if firm external pressure not maintained long enough

3. Laboratory tests

From the history and physical examination, it is usually possible to determine the presence of a platelet defect and predict its severity. Confirmation of this impression is aided by two simple screening tests—the **platelet count** and the **bleeding time** (BT).

As noted in lecture 28, further laboratory evaluation of the patient with a low platelet count will focus on the mechanism of **thrombocytopenia** by assessing the morphology of the platelet on the blood smear and the abundance of megakaryocytes on the bone marrow aspiration or biopsy. The patient with a normal platelet count and a prolonged BT should be tested in order to defined that nature of the **qualitative platelet defect**. This abnormality may be localized to one of more stages of th platelet activation mechanism—adhesion, aggregation, and release. A schematic approach to the patient with a prolonged BT is outlined in figure 29.1.

B. Classification and treatment

Disorders of primary hemostasis were summarized in lecture 28.

III. DISORDERS OF SECONDARY HEMOSTASIS

A. Introduction

Disorders of **secondary hemostasis** are due to alterations in the protein components of the coagulation system. The most important initial steps in diagnosing these abnormalities are a careful history, physical examination, and certain screening laboratory tests.

1. History

The history should take note of the age at onset of symptoms, their relationship to trauma (e.g., response to dental extractions or surgical

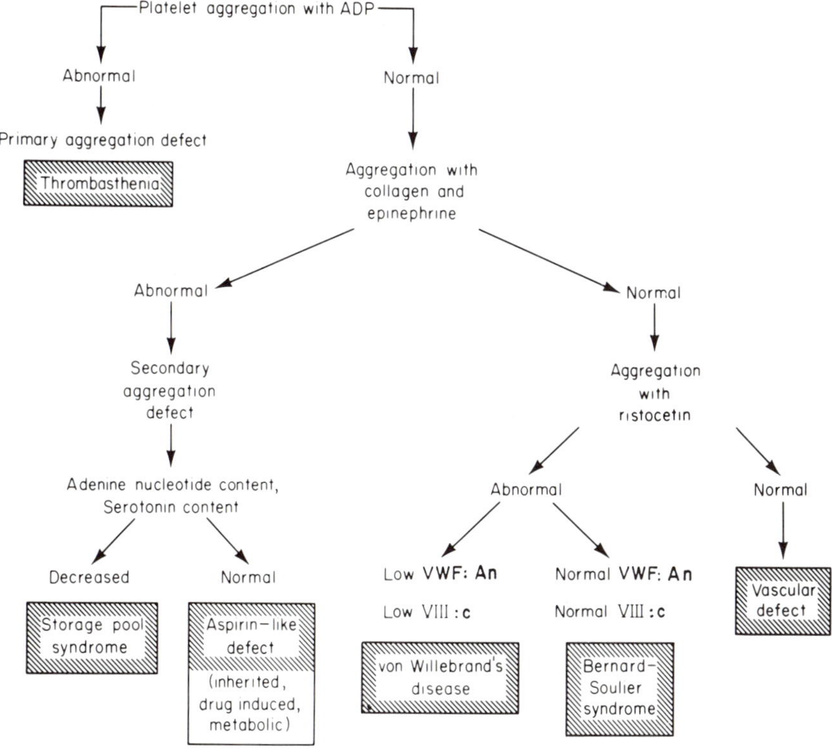

Fig. 29.1
Evaluation of a patient with a prolonged bleeding time and normal platelet count.

procedures, including circumcision), description of hemorrhagic phenomena, their association with other illnesses, genetic factors, dietary history, and recently ingested drugs. Table 29.2 summarizes some characteristics of bleeding in secondary hemostatic disorders and contrasts them with those in primary hemostatic abnormalities. Other features of these states (e.g., genetics, sex predilection, pattern of laboratory test results) will be outlined below.

2. *Physical examination*

The physical examination may show ecchymoses but rarely petechiae. Joints may be warm, swollen, and tender if subject to recent or recurrent bleeds. Fluctuant and tender subcutaneous or flank masses may be due to subcutaneous or retroperitoneal **hematomas** (localized collections of extravasated blood). Frank or occult blood may be present in urine or stool.

3. *Screening tests and special tests*

In most cases, four **screening tests** will identify the general locus of a hemostatic abnormality:

- Prothrombin time (PT)
- Parital thromboplastin time (PTT)

- Thrombin time (TT)
- Fibrin stability test

These tests are available in most hospitals and are simple to perform. They should be done before more specific tests—often termed **special tests**—are chosen to pinpoint the defect responsible for a particular bleeding disorder. Special tests which are widely available include assays of

- Plasma fibrinogen
- Fibrin(ogen) split products
- Various individual coagulation factors
- Specific inhibitors

Other even more specialized measurements (e.g., von Willebrand's factor electrophoresis) may be available only in research laboratories.

B. Major screening tests

In all of these tests, blood is collected with a calcium-chelating anticoagulant (usually **citrate**) and then centrifuged to remove the erythrocytes, leukocytes, and platelets. The remaining **platelet-poor plasma** (PPP) serves as the substrate for these tests. Dependig on the test, **phospholipid** is added to the PPP to substitute for platelets and an **activating agent** is added. The PPP is then recalcified and the time needed for a clot to form (**clotting time**) is measured. In most laboratories automated devices are now employed to make these additions and measure the time required for a clot to form.

1. Prothrombin time (PT)

The principle of the PT is outlined in figure 29.2. A commercial preparation of **phospholipid and tissue factor** (called **thromboplastin**) is added to an aliquot of the patient's citrated plasma. The mixture is recalcified and the stopwatch is started. The clotting time is determined and compared with results obtained with plasma from a normal subject. The normal PT is 11–13 seconds.

The PT is prolonged by deficiencies (usually <30% of normal levels) of the coagulant activity of **factors VII, X, II, V,** and **fibrinogen**. It is not affected by variations in factors VIII, IX, XI, XII, XIII, prekallikrein, high-molecular-weight kininogen, or platelets. While heparin therapy rarely prolongs the PT, treatment with **warfarin** produces deficiencies in factors II, VII, IX, X, and the PT is usually employed to monitor therapy.

2. Partial thromboplastin time (PTT)

The PTT is summarized in figure 29.3. **Kaolin** or **celite** is first incubated with an aliquot of patient's citrated plasma for 3–5 minutes to activate factor XII. Phospholipid is then added and the mixture is recalcified at time 0. Clotting time is noted and compared with results obtained with normal plasma. The normal PTT is 28–35 seconds.

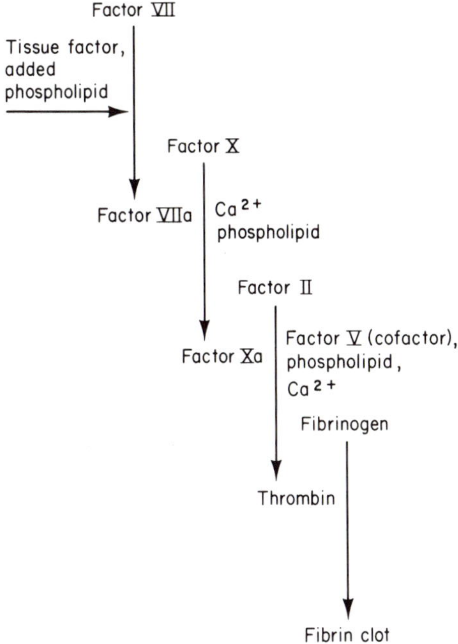

Fig. 29.2
Factors influencing the prothrombin time.

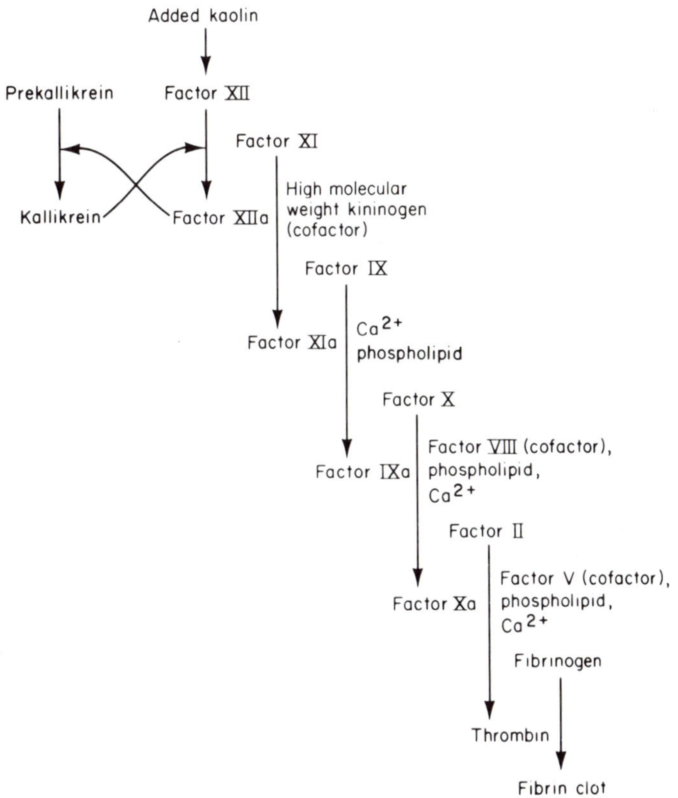

Fig. 29.3
Factors influencing the partial thromboplastin time.

The PTT is prolonged by deficiencies of the coagulant activity of **prekallekrein, high-molecular-weight kininogen, factors XII, XI, IX, VIII, X, V, II,** and **fibrinogen**. It is unaffected by variations in factors VII, XIII, and platelets. While the PTT is modestly prolonged in most patients on warfarin, **heparin** results in relatively greater prolongation of the PTT, and the PTT is commonly used to follow heparin treatment.

3. Thrombin time (TT)

Exogenous thrombin is added to an aliquot of patient's citrated plasma. The clotting time is measured and compared with the time obtained with normal plasma. The concentration of thrombin utilized is adjusted to give a normal clotting time of approximately 16–20 seconds. The TT measures the ability of thrombin to catalyze the transformation of fibrinogen to fibrin and the capacity of that fibrin to undergo polymerization. It is not affected by factors, II, V, VII, VIII, IX, X, XI, XII, XIII, prekallikrein, high-molecular-weight kininogen, or platelets. The thrombin time is prolonged in **hypofibrinogenemia** and in congenital or acquired **dysfibrinogenemias**, in which abnormal fibrinogen molecules may fail to be activated normally by thrombin or the fibrin generated may polymerize poorly. **Fibrin(ogen)-specific antibodies** and, more commonly, **fibrin(ogen) split products** prevent fibrin polymerization and prolong the TT.

Heparin in the patient's blood sample also prolongs the TT since it accelerates neutralization of exogenously added thrombin. It is surprising how often the physician is not aware that the patient has received heparin, for example, when it is being given intravenously in low doses to maintain patency of intravascular catheters or subcutaneously as prophylaxis for thrombophlebitis. Indeed, heparin in such low doses in the presence of conditions (such as renal or liver failure) that reduce its clearance may completely anticoagulate the patient. The presence of heparin in blood samples may be determined by neutralizing its effect on the TT with **protamine** or by performing a **reptilase time** (RT, see below). Since the RT is insensitive to the presence of heparin, a prolonged TT and a normal RT suggest the presence of heparin in the blood sample.

4. Fibrin stability test

Plasma from the patient is recalcified and allowed to clot. The clot is suspended in an excess of 5 M urea or 1% monochloracetic acid, which disrupts hydrophobic and electrostatic interactions. The normal clot does not dissolve rapidly because covalent peptide cross-links have been introduced between the fibrin molecules by factor XIII. An abnormal clot that is not fully cross-linked is rapidly solublized by these agents. This test provides a qualitative measure of **factor XIII** activity as well as the availability of fibrin cross-linking sites. This screening procedure is valuable because other tests fail to detect abnormalities in this phase of the hemostatic mechanism.

C. Special tests

1. Plasma fibrinogen

Fibrinogen is measured by

- Quantifying the greatest plasma dilution at which a clot is still produced by exogenous thrombin
- Assaying photometrically the amount of clottable protein
- Using specific antifibrinogen antisera in immunoassays

The normal fibrinogen level is 200–400 mg/dl. The first two methods are widely used but may provide erroneously low fibrinogen values in situations (e.g., dysfibrinogenemia, disseminated infravascular coagulation [DIC]) where clotting is impaired.

2. Fibrinogen or fibrin degradation products ("split products")

When fibrinogen or fibrin is exposed to plasmin, a number of proteolytic fragments are produced of which **fragments D** and **E** are the most abundant. These **fibrin degradation products** (FDP), also called **fibrin split products** (FSP), are not clottable upon exposure to fibrin and may actually inhibit fibrin polymerization and inactivate platelets. They are cleared by the liver and are elevated in **DIC, primary fibrinolysis**, and during the use of **thrombolytic agents** such as **urokinase, strepokinase**, and **tissue-type plasminogen activator**. FDP are measured by drawing blood into a tube containing soybean trypsin inhibitor and thrombin. The soybean trypsin inhibitor prevents further proteolysis of fibrin and fibrinogen in vitro while the thrombin causes the remaining fibrinogen (but not FDP) to clot. The non-clottable FDP (mostly fragments D and E) remaining in the serum may then be quantitated by specific antisera.

Unfortunately the presence of elevated amounts of FDP cannot distinguish plasmin's effect on fibrinogen from that on fibrin. In some clinical settings (e.g., thrombolytic therapy) it is important to distinguish the extent of **fibrinolysis** in the clot from **fibrinogenolysis** in the plasma. Advantage has recently been taken of the observation that adjacent fibrin monomers in clots are covalently cross-linked via their D domains by factor XIII. Plasmin proteolysis of such cross-linked fibrin (but not free uncross-linked fibrinogen) produces a unique product, a dimer composed to two D fragments (**D-dimer**), which may be measured by a specific monoclonal antibody.

3. Reptilase time

The thrombin-like venom of the American pit viper (*Bothrops atrox*), called **reptilase**, cleaves fibrinopeptide A, but not B, from fibrinogen and promotes clotting. Addition of reptilase to an aliquot of citrated plasma results in a normal **reptilase time** (RT) of 16–20 seconds. Though reptilase generation of fibrin is not inhibited by heparin, the RT is prolonged by **hypofibrinogenemia, dysfibrinogenemia**, or the presence of **inhibitors of**

fibrin polymerization such as **FDP** or **antibodies to fibrin(ogen)**. While the TT is prolonged to a greater degree than the RT in the presence of FDP, the RT is prolonged more than the TT in dysfibrinogenemias.

4. *Specific factor assays*

Specific factor assays are available for each of the coagulation proteins—factors II, V, VII, VIII, IX, X, XI, XII, XIII, prekallikrein, and high-molecular-weight kininogen. These tests are based on the ability of normal but not patient's plasma to correct results obtained with a plasma known to be deficient in the factor to be measured. The procedures themselves are similar to the PTT and PT assays.

D. Diagnostic approach

The four screening procedures described above permit classification of disorders of secondary hemostasis into the following six patterns or syndromes.

1. *Fibrin stabilization abnormal; other tests normal*

In this rare syndrome, all clotting tests are normal but one: The fibrin clot is soluble in agents such as urea or monochloracetic acid. Abnormal clot solubility is due to a reduction in the number of covalent cross-links between fibrin molecules. Underlying abnormalities may include

- Inherited factor XIII deficiency
- Antibodies that specifically inhibit factor XIII
- Structural alterations in the cross-linking sites within fibrinogen-fibrin
- Antibodies specifically directed against these cross-linking regions

Choice of therapy depends on the nature of the defect in a given patient. Further specialized techniques are necessary to delineate the defect.

2. *TT abnormal; PT and PTT often abnormal*

This constellation of test results is usually attributable to a number of abnormalities in the **conversion of fibrinogen to fibrin or its subsequent polymerization**.

a. NEUTRALIZATION OF THROMBIN

Heparin in the blood sample may neutralize exogenously added thrombin and prolong the TT (and the PTT).

b. QUANTITATIVE ALTERATIONS IN FIBRINOGEN LEVEL

Significant reductions in plasma fibrinogen usually prolong the TT. **Hypofibrinogenemia** may result from a rare inherited disorder (**congenital afibrinogenemia** or **hypofibrinogenemia**). More commonly, it is due to consumption of fibrinogen during **DIC**, which is discussed below. If plasma fibrinogen is sufficiently depressed, hemorrhage can occur. Paradoxically, **hyperfibrinogenemia** (seen in **pregnancy, inflammation**, and **infection**) may occasionally prolong the TT because fibrinogen in high concentrations can trap fibrin within soluble complexes and therapy inhibit fibrin polymerization. This abnormality occurs in vitro, has little pathophysiologic significance, and does not cause bleeding.

c. QUALITATIVE ABNORMALITIES OF FIBRINOGEN (DYSFIBRINOGENEMIA)

Qualitative abnormalities of fibrinogen (**dysfibrinogenemia**) may prolong the TT and cause bleeding. In some inherited cases, specific amino acid changes have been noted, while in others the defect appears to be in glycosylation of the fibrinogen. These changes may result in defective release of fibrinopeptides A and B or in normal fibrinopeptide release but defective polymerization. **Acquired dysfibrinogenemia** occurs in **liver disease** and is probably related to **abnormal fibrinogen glycosylation**. Diagnosis may require further specialized techniques but may be suspected when fibrinogen measured by clotting activity is diminished compared with normal values obtained by immunoassay. The RT is often prolonged to a greater extent than the TT.

d. INTERFERING SUBSTANCES

The presence of substances that interfere with fibrin polymerization can prolong the TT and cause bleeding. High concentrations of **fibrin split products** generated during intense fibrinolysis or DIC are common causes of this syndrome. Occasionally, high levels of a **monoclonal immunoglobulin** encountered in multiple myeloma interfere with fibrin polymerization (see lecture 25).

3. PTT abnormal; PT and other tests normal

Defects responsible for this syndrome are within the intrinsic cascade of the coagulation system. They may be divided clinically into two groups.

a. GROUP WITH NO BLEEDING

Patients in the first group do not bleed. These relatively rare patients may have deficiencies of **factor XII, prekallikrein (Fletcher factor),** or **high-molecular-weight kininogen (Fitzgerald factor, Flaujeac, Williams trait)**. Each of these states is identifiable by appropriate factor assays utilizing plasma from patients known to be deficient for the specific coagulation component. Each of these deficiencies appears to be heterogeneous. For example, prekallikrein-deficient patients include those with no detectable prekallikrein as well as those with up to 30% of the normal amount detectable by specific antisera. At present, it is unclear why these three deficiency states do not lead to hemorrhage. Perhaps low levels of these proteins are adequate for hemostasis in vivo but insufficient for artificial activation of coagulation during the PTT assay. More likely, activation of the coagulation system may occur in vivo at the factor XI level; the proteins under discussion may be physiologically important only with respect to kinin generation and fibrinolysis.

b. GROUP WITH SIGNIFICANT BLEEDING

Patients in the second group have significant bleeding and may be more common than patients in the first group. In general, whenever the PTT is abnormal, it should be assumed that the patient has a tendency to bleed until it has been proved otherwise. Underlying disorders include **von Willebrand's disease** and **deficiencies of factors VIII, IX,** or **XI**. Specific factor assays define the precise etiology. However, as noted below, diagnosis is aided by data on the mode of transmission, sex, BT, and other clinical findings. We briefly summarize the four major disorders in this group.

(1) von Willebrand's disease (VWD)

This is the most common coagulation disorder with an incidence of 1 in 10,000 in the general population. It is probably even more common than that since only the more severely affected patients are usually diagnosed. A recent study of Italian school children found a surprisingly high frequency of 6–11 in 1000 children. As noted in lecture 28, VWF circulates as a complex with factor VIII (which is why VWF was previously known as "factor VIII-related antigen"). In classic VWD, the decrease in VWF is accompanied by a decrease in factor VIII resulting in a prolonged BT and a prolonged PTT. Other variant forms of VWD exist in which VWF is present in normal to moderate amounts, and these are usually associated with normal factor VIII levels and a normal PTT. The evaluation and treatment of these disorders is discussed in further detail in lectures 27 and 28.

(2) Factor VIII deficiency

Deficiency of factor VIII (hemophilia A) is inherited as a sex-linked recessive trait. Incidence is approximately 1 in 10,000 of the population. Next to von Willebrand's disease it is the most common inherited coagulation disorder. The disorder is thought to be caused either by a defective factor VIII protein or impaired conversion of a precursor molecule to a species with full biologic activity. **Severe cases** (factor VIII level $<1\%$ of normal) often bleed in infancy (e.g., at circumcision) and have multiple episodes of **hemarthrosis**. **Moderately affected** individuals (factor VIII level 1–5% of normal) have occasional hemarthroses, but usually lack crippling deformities. **Mild cases** (factor VIII level 5–25% of normal) rarely suffer bleeding episodes and often are not diagnosed until they bleed after dental or surgical procedures. Efforts to detect the **carrier state** in clinically unaffected females by measurement of factor VIII activity have been unsuccessful owing to wide variations of factor VIII concentration in the general population. Many normal individuals have low levels of factor VIII (50–60%) similar to those in female carriers. Our ability to detect carriers has improved significantly with the developmemt in recent years of antisera that can quantify the factor VIII antigen (VIII:An). These new reagents have permitted accurate detection of carriers and the intrauterine prenatal diagnosis of hemophilia. These tests have also demonstrated that most patients with decreased factor VIII activity (VIII:c) have a parallel decrease in factor VIII antigen.

The availability of **factor VIII replacement therapy** has dramatically altered the care of patients with severe hemophilia A. Crude factor VIII concentrates (**cryoprecipitate**) and, more recently, **highly purified factor VIII** are widely available. They may be administered to the hospitalized patient to control acute bleeding episodes or to prepare for surgery. A major innovation has been the administration of factor VIII at home immediately following trauma or at the first sign of bleeding. This prophylactic approach has markedly reduced hospitalization and the incidence of crippling deformities. Unfortunately, the use of these factor VIII preparations may be associated with the development of **antibodies to factor VIII**, which complicates further factor replacement therapy. In addition, because these products are made from large pools of donor plasma, there has been a significant incidence of **viral hepatitis** and **HIV infection**. The use of viral antigen-negative and heat-treated factor VIII preparations may reduce but does not eliminate these infectious risks. The production of factor VIII by molecular biology tecnhiques promises to yield a safer factor VIII replacement product.

For **mild** and **moderately affected** hemophiliacs **1-deamino-β-D-arginine vasopressin** (DDAVP) is the treatment of choice for acute bleeding as well as prophylaxis for surgery. DDAVP acts by releasing previously formed factor VIII from storage sites and may raise levels two- to fourfold. Since **severely affected** hemophiliacs lack these stores of preformed factor VIII, DDAVP is not a treatment option.

(3) Factor IX deficiency

Deficiency of factor IX (**Christmas disease**, **hemophilia B**) is inherited as a sex-linked recessive trait. It resembles factor VIII deficiency with respect to mode of transmission and clinical manifestations. The incidence, however, is only 1.5 in 100,000 of the population. Affected individuals appear to have either normal levels of inactive protein or reduced levels of active zymogen. The carrier state is more often associated with reduced levels of factor IX activity than is the case with factor VIII deficiency. An immunoassay is available to aid in the classification of factor IX disease and in carrier detection. In addition, the factor IX gene has been cloned and a closely linked genetic polymorphism identified that may permit intrauterine diagnosis. Rarely, acquired factor IX deficiency is due to selective urinary loss of this protein in the **nephrotic syndrome**. Concentrates containing factors, II, VII, IX, and X are available for treatment of hemorrhagic episodes or preparation of patients for surgical procedures. These preparations must be used with care since they contain activated enzymes such as factor Xa or thrombin and can produce thrombotic phenomena. They can also transmit serum hepatitis and HIV infection.

(4) Factor XI deficiency

This deficiency is inherited as an autosomal recessive trait and is particularly prevalent among Jews of Eastern European descent. It is the fourth most common coagulation disorder following von Willebrand's disease and deficiencies of factors VIII and IX. Based on indirect immunoassays it appears to be associated with reduced levels of functional protein rather than the presence of an altered protein. For reasons that are unclear the hemorrhagic diathesis tends to be mild. Often, bleeding occurs late in life or after surgical or dental procedures. Factor XI concentrates are not available; in most instances, plasma infusion effectively controls hemorrhage.

4. PT ABNORMAL; PTT AND OTHER TESTS NORMAL

Defects responsible for this syndrome are located within the extrinsic limb of the coagulation system. **Tissue factor** is made and released by endothelial cells as well as by many other tissues and disorders due to its lack have not been described. Therefore, **factor VII deficiency** is a unique cause of this syndrome.

Inherited deficiency of factor VII is exceedingly rare (1 in 500,000 of the population). It is transmitted as a recessive autosomal trait. An acquired form of this syndrome can be observed in early **vitamin K deficiency**, at the **onset of coumadin therapy**, or in **mild liver disease**. This is explained by the fact that factor VII has the shortest half-life of all coagulation proteins (3–5 hr). Cessation in production of the vitamin K–dependent proteins (factors II, VII, IX, X) is manifested initially as factor VII deficiency.

5. PTT ABNORMAL; PT ABNORMAL; OTHER TESTS NORMAL

Defects responsible for this syndrome are of two types. The first includes **inherited** or **acquired deficiencies of the proteins of the common pathway**, that is, **factors II, V** or **X**. The inherited disorders are autosomal recessive disorders that appear to be due to the production of altered inactive forms of each protein species. The incidence is approximately 1 in 500,000–1,000,000 of the population and definitive diagnosis requires specific factor assays. Acquired deficiencies include:

- Antibodies to factors II, V, or X
- Antibodies to phospholipid (lupus anticoagulants—see below)
- Systemic amyloidosis in some patients when the amyloid fibrils bind factor X specifically

In the second group are **multiple defects of the coagulation mechanism**. These are relatively common and are caused by

- Vitamin K deficiency
- Transfusion of frozen plasma
- Liver disease

Vitamin K deficiency may be due to ingestion of coumadin, intestinal malabsorption of fat, chronic diarrhea, parenteral feedings without vitamin K supplementation, or antibiotic administration (which destroys the gastrointestinal flora that produce a significant portion of the vitamin K absorbed by the body). Lack of this vitamin results in reduced γ-carboxylation of specific glutamyl residues located on factors, II, VII, IX, and X (see lecture 27) with decreased biologic activity of these coagulation proteins. Parenteral administration to patients with normal liver function of as little as 1 mg of vitamin K restores normal hemostatic function promptly (in 4–18 hr).

While **freshly donated plasma** contains normal amounts of coagulation factors, storage for more than several hours results in reduced levels of factors V and VIII. In fresh frozen plasma, these factors decline more slowly over several weeks. However, when extensive blood replacement is needed such as with surgery or major trauma, transfusion with large amounts of fresh or frozen plasma that have been subject to long storage may result in inadequate levels of factors V and VIII.

Liver disease is associated with multiple defects, as discussed below.

3. Inhibitor syndrome

The hallmark of this syndrome is an abnormal PTT (or rarely an abnormal PT) that cannot be corrected in vitro by a 30-min incubation of patient plasma plus an equal volume of normal plasma (called a **1:1 mix test**). Since the PT and PTT are prolonged only when specific coagulation factors drop to below 30% of their normal levels, the failure of added normal plasma to correct the abnormality rules out a deficiency state and implicates a **circulating inhibitor**. Inhibitors are of two types.

a. INHIBITORS OF SPECIFIC COAGULATION PROTEINS

The first type of inhibitor is an **antibody directed against a specific coagulation protein**. The effects of these immunoglobulins are time-dependent and their most common target is **factor VIII**. Inhibitors of factor VIII are found in

- Five to ten percent of patients with factor VIII deficiency (these individuals may have no circulating factor VIII protein and transfusions of factor VIII may stimulate antibody production)
- Systemic lupus erythrematosus
- Women during the postpartum period
- Certain elderly individuals

Precise diagnosis requires specific inhibitor assays. Treatment depends on the inhibitor level. If the titer is low, massive infusion of factor VIII concentrate can promptly correct the abnormality. In many instances, however, infusion of factor VIII will have little effect. Various experimental procedures have been utilized to treat active bleeding in this situation, for example, transfusion of concentrates containing activated intermediates such as factor Xa to control the acute bleeding episode and immunosuppression to reduce antibody production.

b. INHIBITORS OF PHOSPHOLIPID FUNCTION

A second type of inhibitor includes those antibodies that bind to phospholipid and prevent the interaction of coagulation factors with the phospholipid. As described in lecture 28, many interactions in the coagulation cascade take place on the phospholipid surface of the platelet. In most coagulation test, platelets are removed and the platelet surface is replaced by added phospholipid. In systemic lupus eruthematosus and in some other unrelated disorders, polyclonal immunoglobulins (called **lupus anticoagulants**) are produced which bind to phospholipids in vitro and prolong the PTT (and the PT to a lesser extent). The extent of effect of these inhibitors on the PT and PTT in vitro is critically dependent on the (relatively small) amount of phospholipid added to the plasma which subsequently may be neutralized by antibody. In vivo, however, there is an excess of phospholipid and little effect of the antibody on the amount of phospholipid available. This may best be illustrated by replacing the phospholipid with platelets in the clotting reactions and demonstrating that the PTT and PT become normal. In general these lupus anticogulants cause no clinically apparent bleeding and are an in vitro phenomenon. Indeed, there is an association of the presence of lupus anticoagulants with excessive venous and arterial thrombosis. It is important, however, to be able to distinguish these lupus anticoagulants from the more clinically relevant inhibitors of the first type mentioned above.

IV. MIXED DISORDERS

Three major types of disorders exhibit dual defects that suppress the activity of both the primary and secondary hemostatic mechanisms.

A. von Willebrand's disease

The pathophysiology of this disease has been discussed earlier in this lecture as well as in lecture 27 and 28. As we have seen, it is due to a defect in platelet adhesion secondary to alteration in von Willebrand's factor quantity or functional competence. In some cases (type I von Willebrand's disease) there may also be a decrease in the level of **factor VIII coagulant activity** (VIII:c). If the concentration of factor VIII:c activity is only modestly reduced, the patient exhibits only platelet-related bleeding (e.g., ecchymoses, petechiae, and mucosal bleeding). If factor VIII:c activity is profoundly depressed, the patient may present with clinical symptoms similar to those of the patient with severe classic hemophilia A. In such situations, the prolonged BT will help confirm that the diagnosis is von Willebrand's disease, not hemophilia.

B. Disseminated intravascular coagulation (DIC)

We have seen that the sequential activation of coagulation factors and platelets is a response to localized vascular injury. Several limiting reactions dampen and restrict the activity of the hemostatic mechanism. These include

- Dilution by blood flow
- Hepatic clearance
- Adsorption of coagulation factors to the fibrin-platelet meshwork
- Circulating inhibitors such as antithrombin

The presence of activated coagulation factors in the circulation leads to a **hypercoagulable state** which, if unchecked, can produce **thrombosis**.

1. Causes

Patients with a number of serious illnesses often develop rapid and massive activation of the coagulation sequence that overwhelms the normal body defenses. As a result, they consume circulating platelets as well as coagulation proteins and develop a severe hemorrhagic disorder called **disseminated intravascular coagulation**, or DIC. DIC is not a specific disease but a disorder triggered by a number of factors (table 29.3) that can be grouped into four categories:

- Conditions that introduce tissue factor into the circulation (e.g., tissue necrosis)
- Damage to endothelial surfaces
- Stagnation of blood flow
- Infection of various types

These stimuli activate both limbs of the coagulation cascade so that thrombin is generated and fibrinogen is rapidly converted to fibrin. This leads to irreversible aggregation of many circulating platelets and production of **microthrombi**. Red cells are destroyed in the resulting fibrin meshwork with

Table 29.3
Pathogenesis of Disseminated Intravascular Coagulation

Causative factors	Examples
Liberation of tissue factor	Obstetric catastrophes
	Hemolysis
	Tissue damage
	Neoplasms
	Fat embolism
	Snake bite
Stagnant blood flow	Kasabach-Merritt syndrome
Endothelial damage	Heat stroke
	Aortic aneurysm
	Hemolytic-uremic syndrome
	Acute glomerulonephritis
	Microangiopathic hemolytic anemia
	Rocky Mountain spotted fever
Infection	Bacterial: staphylococcus, streptococcus, pneumococcus, meningococcus, gramnegative spesis
	Viral: arboviruses, varicella, variola, rubella
	Parasitic: malaria, kala-azar
	Mycotic: acute histoplasmosis

production of **microangiopathic hemolytic anemia** (see lecture 14). The major body defense is activation of the **fibrinolytic system** with resulting lysis of thrombi in the microcirculation. This leads to increased levels of **fibrin degradation products**. There may also be indiscriminate degradation of fibrinogen or other coagulation proteins along with fibrin debris. On occasion the fibrinolytic system may not degrade the thrombi and tissue necrosis ensues.

2. *Diagnosis*

Patients usually present with an identifiable serious illness that may be accompanied by hypotension, acidosis, and infection. There may be evidence of skin necrosis over the digits, nose, and genitals; diffuse ecchymoses and mucous membrane bleeding; or persistent oozing at sites of venepuncture. The laboratory diagnosis of DIC is uncomplicated: The blood smear shows microangiopathic red cell changes and variable degrees of thrombocytopenia; there is prolongation of the PT, PTT, TT, and low levels of fibrinogen. Fibrin degradation products detectable by immunologic assays are greatly elevated.

3. *Therapy*

Treatment of DIC should be directed at correcting the triggering event. Patients with no bleeding or thrombosis require careful observation. Patients with diffuse hemorrhage may need intensive support with plasma, platelets, and red cell transfusions. There is some controversy about the efficacy of heparin in treating this syndrome. While heparin will usually suppress the deposition of fibrin clot in DIC, regulation of the dose and the risk of heparin-induced hemorrhage may make therapy difficult. Most patients with DIC can be managed with plasma and platelets alone. Heparin can be life-saving in the occasional patient who presents with predominantly thrombotic manifestations of DIC, which can lead to tissue ischemia and gangrene.

C. Liver disease

Since the liver is involved in the synthesis and catabolism of hemostatic system components, it is not surprising that liver dysfunction is often associated with bleeding. Although the liver is a major source of coagulation proteins, it should be kept in mind that chronic liver failure induces a number of nonhematologic abnormalities that may contribute to bleeding. **Portal hypertension** causes abnormal vascular channels (**varices**) to develop in the stomach and esophagus that are fragile and easily ruptured. In addition, portal hypertension causes **splenomegaly** and concomitant thrombocytopenia that may exacerbate mechanical causes of bleeding.

1. Pathophysiology

It is established that factors II, V, VII, IX, and X are synthesized in the liver; factors XI and XII may be. Four of these proteins—factors II, VII, IX, and X—require vitamin K for normal activity. As we have noted, this vitamin is an essential cofactor for a unique carboxylation reaction in which a second carboxyl group is attached to a number of glutamic acid residues on these proteins. This postsynthetic modification permits the proteins to bind calcium and participate in coagulation reactions. Biliary tract obstruction and poor bile flow can lead to hemorrhage by **impairing vitamin K assimilation**. However, because of hepatic cell failure there is also **impaired synthesis and inadequate carboxylation of coagulation factors** in most patients with liver disease despite adequate vitamin K stores. The decreased synthetic rate of coagulation proteins in stable liver failure is reflected by a moderately prolonged PT and PTT that is improved only slightly by vitamin K. The liver also synthesizes the major inhibitors of coagulation proteins, α_2-macroglobulin and antithrombin. A marked **reduction in inhibitor levels** might increase the rate of coagulation reactions. Moderate thrombocytopenia (50,000–80,000 platelets/mm^3) is often due to associated splenomegaly. Liver disease can also **impair clearance of activated coagulation factors** and **fibrin degradation products** although the mechanisms and cell involved in the normal liver are not clearly defined. There is often **increased plasma fibrinolytic activity** because of failure to clear plasminogen activators secreted in the microcirculation. Thus laboratory studies may show a mild increase in plasma fibrinolytic activity or a slight elevation in the concentration of fibrin degradation products. However, intense fibrinolysis or overt DIC may occur with sudden prolongation in the PT and PTT as well as further fall in platelet count, fall in fibrinogen level, and increase in fibrin degradation products. These abnormalities exacerbate bleeding due to local mechanical effects by superimposing a systemic bleeding disorder.

In summary, patients with liver disease have a complex coagulation disorder that may be in constant flux, and there is precarious and limited hemostatic reserve.

2. *Therapy*

Treatment of bleeding in liver disease is complicated. Transfused platelets are sequestered in the spleen, and the large protein and salt loads that accompany plasma infusion are poorly tolerated. Prothrombin complex concentrates rich in factors II, VII, IX, and X that have become available recently are of limited value because they do not provide adequate replacement of other needed coagulation factors. Furthermore, these products carry an increased risk of viral hepatitis and may contain traces of activated forms of the coagulation factors that can trigger thrombosis. The use of heparin or other anticoagulants to suppress the hemostatic mechanism in patients with DIC secondary to liver disease is dangerous because these drugs may induce bleeding. The use of ε-aminocaproic acid to suppress fibrinolysis may promote hemostasis.

V. PRETHROMBOTIC OR HYPERCOAGULABLE STATES

There are no simple screening tests for identifying patients at increased risk for developing thrombosis; however, some promising clinical research procedures can defect the limited activation of the coagulation system associated with thromboembolism. These tests are immunoassays that measure released **platelet membrane** or **granule proteins** or **fibrinopeptides** released from coagulation factors or coagulation factor inhibitor complexes that are formed during thrombosis. For example, patients with deep venous thrombosis have increased circulating levels of fibrinopeptide A, prothrombin fragment 1 + 2, and thrombin-antithrombin complex as a consequence of thrombin generation and clot formation. These abnormalities revert to normal when suitable anticoagulant therapy is administered. Similar abnormalities have been noted in other patients with active thrombosis or embolism as well as in patients with so-called **prethrombotic states**, that is, patients who are currently asymptomatic but may develop thrombosis at a later date. Interestingly, these changes that reflect significant activation of the coagulation mechanism are not associated with any change in the usual screening tests of hemostasis (PT, PTT, TT, bleeding time, and platelet count).

Although the etiology of thrombosis is still uncertain in the vast majority of patients, the following well-defined genetic abnormalities qualify as prethrombotic or **hypercoagulable states**.

A. Antithrombin deficiency

The first is **antithrombin deficiency**, an autosomal dominant disorder that occurs once in 2,000 individuals. Affected patients have recurrent venous thrombosis and pulmonary emboli. They are usually symptomatic by the third decade of life and require prophylactic treatment at times of surgery or trauma and lifelong anticoagulation after the onset of symptoms. The diagnosis is made by demonstrating decreased immunologic or functional antithrombin in plasma. Although most patients have a mild to moderate decrease in the quantity of antithrombin, a few variants have been described in which defective heparin binding or activation by heparin has been noted.

B. Protein C and protein S deficiencies

A second group of genetic disorders that lead to venous thrombosis and embolism is represented by isolated deficiencies of protein C or protein S. A 50% reduction in the levels of either of these vitamin K–dependent proteins is inherited as an autosomal dominant trait. The rare occurrence of homozygous deficiency of protein C permits massive activation of the coagulation system, and fatal DIC in the neonatal period has been reported.

C. Abnormalities of the fibrinolytic mechanism

Several families have been described who have an **abnormal form of plasminogen** that cannot be readily activated to plasmin and a high incidence of venous thrombosis and embolism. The variant form of plasminogen has altered electrophoretic mobility and has been partially separated from the normal plasminogen molecule. There are also some less well characterized kindreds with venous thromboembolism or myocardial infarction who either fail to release **tissue-type plasminogen activator** from blood vessels after local ischemia or vigorous exercise or exhibit elevated levels of PAI-1. Finally, families have been identified with **abnormal fibrinogens** as judged by long thrombin times or reptilase times who exhibit thrombotic phenomena. It is thought that these abnormal molecules are relatively insensitive to the action of the fibrinolytic mechanism.

SELECTED REFERENCES

Reviews

Blanchard, R. A., Furie, B. C., et al. Acquired vitamin K-dependent carboxylation deficiency in liver disease. *New Engl. J. Med.* 305(1981): 242–248.

Brettler, D. B., and Levine, P. H. Factor concentrates for treatment of hemophilia: which one to choose. *Blood* 73(1989); 2067–2074.

Colman, R. W., Hirsh, J., et al., eds. *Hemostasis and Thrombosis: Basic Principles and Clinical Practice*, 2nd ed. Philadelphia: J. B. Lippincott, 1987.

Furie, B. Disorders of the vitamin-K dependent coagulation factors. In Williams, W. J., et al., eds. *Hematology*, 4th ed. New York: McGraw-Hill, 1990, pp. 1510–1513.

Gralnick, H. R. von Willibrand disease. In Williams, W. J., et al., eds. *Hematology*, 4th ed. New York: McGraw-Hill, 1990, pp. 1493–1509.

Hermans, J. and McDonagh, J. Fibrin: structure and interactions. *Semin. Thromb. Hemostas.* 8(1982): 11–24.

Mannucci, P. M. Desmopressin (DDAVP) for treatment of disorders of hemostasis. *Progress in Hemostasis and Thrombosis*. New York: Grune & Stratton, 1986, pp. 19–45.

Marder, V. J. Consumptive thrombohemorrhagic disorders. In Williams, W. J., et al., eds. *Hematology*, 4th ed. New York: McGraw-Hill, 1990, pp. 1522–1543.

Roberts, H. R., and Jones, M. R. Hemophilia and related conditions: congenital deficiencies of prothrombin (factor II), factor V, and factors VII to XII. In Williams, W. J., et al., eds. *Hematology*, 4th ed. New York: McGraw-Hill, 1990, pp. 1453–1473.

Sirridge, M. S. and Shannon, R. *Laboratory Evaluation of Hemostasis and Thrombosis*, 3rd ed. Philadelphia: Lea & Febiger, 1983.

Williams, W. J. Classification and clinical manifestations of disorders of hemostasis. In Williams, W. J., et al., eds. *Hematology*, 4th ed. New York: McGraw-Hill, 1990, pp. 1338–1342.

White, G, C., II, and Shoemaker, C. B. Factor VIII gene and hemophilia A. *Blood* 73(1989): 1–12.

Original articles

Antonarakis, S. E. Youssoufian, H., et al. Molecular genetics of hemophilia A in man. *Molec. Biol. Med.* 4(1987): 1–14.

Bauer, K. A., and Rosenberg, R. D. Congenital antithrombin III deficiency: insights into the pathogenesis of the hypercoagulable state and its management using markers of hemostatic system activation. *Am. J. Med.* 87 Suppl. 3B(1989): 39S–32S.

Devine, D. V., Kinney, T. R., et al. Fragment D-dimer levels: an objective marker of vaso-occlusive crisis and other complications of sickle cell disease. *Blood* 68 (1986): 317–319.

Funk, C., Gmur, J., et al., Reptilase-R—a new reagent in blood coagulation. *Br. J. Haematol.* 21(1971): 43–52.

Furie, B., Voo, L., et al., Mechanism of Factor X deficiency in systemic amyloidosis. *New Engl. J. Med.* 304(1981): 827–830.

Lijnen, H. R., Van Hoef, B., et al. On the molecular interactions between fibrin, tissue-type plasminogen activator and plasminogen. *Thromb. Res.* 57 Suppl. 10 (1990): 45–54.

Petri, M., Rheinschmidt, M., et al., The frequency of lupus anticoagulant in systemic lupus erythrematosus. *Ann. Intern. Med.* 106(1987): 524–531.

Saito, H., Goodnough, L. T., et al. Heterogeneity of human prekallikrein deficiency (Fletcher trait). *N. Engl. J. Med.* 305(1981): 910–914.

APPENDIX

Laboratory Methods in Hematology

Alice Weaver Flaherty

GENERAL METHODS

SPECIAL METHODS

EDITOR'S COMMENT

Students in the first- and second-year hematology courses at Harvard Medical School and the Harvard–MIT Division of Health Sciences and Technology have a laboratory experience in which they perform various basic hematologic tests. The fifth edition of *Hematology* includes for the first time a brief laboratory syllabus that replaces the handout issued separately in the past. Despite advances in automation, we believe students should perform these tests. They should know what normal and abnormal blood and bone marrow cells look like and they should get a feel for drawing blood and handling blood samples. The teaching of morphology to medical students remains a controversial topic, with wide disagreement on what to teach and how best to teach it. We are not teaching our students to be hematologists at this point, but we do want them to recognize the morphologic aspects of the major cell types and their disorders. Even this has been a daunting goal for teachers, given limited time and the inherent problem of sticky study-slide sets and Kodachromes. We greatly enhanced our ability to cover this material with *HEMAVID*, the computer program that accompanies this edition of *Hematology*. The program makes abundant reference to this book and we hope our readers will have access to it.

GENERAL METHODS

This appendix has two purposes: (1) to provide protocols to guide students in laboratory exercises and (2) to acquaint readers with the routine tests of clinical hematology. More specialized procedures may be found in references cited in bibliography.

Evaluating laboratory data

Physicians must be cautious and thoughtful in evaluating laboratory data. Each test result should be considered in several contexts:

- The inherent technical accuracy and precision of the assay procedure. Compared with most measurements of engineering and physics, many clinical laboratory methods are relatively inaccurate.
- The likelihood of false positives and false negatives in connection with a suspected diagnosis.
- The range of normal values displayed by the population of which the patient is a member. Even with an ideally accurate test, variation within a normal population is often wide.

All laboratorians are aware of the difficulties, both theoretical and practical, in establishing a biologically meaningful range of normal for a given test. Many factors contribute to data variance and disease is only one of them. Such factors in healthy individuals include:

- Genetic differences (e.g., sex, race, blood group)

- Long-term physiologic variations (e.g., age, pregnancy, obesity, diet, altitude of residence, smoking history)
- Short-term physiologic variations (e.g., hydration, timing of meals, circadian rhythms, recumbency, activity, stress, drugs)

The literature records data on variations associated with sex, race, age, pregnancy, and so on, but effects of most other variables are not well studied. **Normal values** are usually defined as those falling within two standard deviations of the mean of a normal reference population: 95% of truly normal results will lie within this range and 5% will fall outside of it. The wide spread of normal values, presumably a consequence of the factors listed, implies that, if they are treated as a normal distribution, the mean ± 2 standard deviations (SD) will have negative values at its lower limit. Some normal variations are so large they yield figures commonly judged to be pathologic.

It is difficult, if the truth be told, for laboratory directors to make rigorously useful determinations of a sufficiently large number of normal subjects in each of the countless reference classes—newborn infants, adults, old people, pregnant women, males, females, different racial and ethnic groups, and so forth. Moreover, one is never certain that an ostensibly normal subject is in fact normal. In our view, these circumstances should justify the practice, common in Europe, of establishing **reference classes** based on age and determining the statistical frequency of a finding in each class of the general population without reference to state of health. It is the clinician's task to interpret these ranges in light of the clinical picture.

In practice, one should remember both the mean normal value for various tests and the SD, which is usually expressed as a **range** of normal. Thus, the normal female hematocrit is 37–48% or 42 $\pm$ 4%. This means that 68% of normal women will have hematocrits between 38 and 46% (i.e., within one SD of the mean); 95% will have hematocrits between 34 and 50% (i.e., within 2 SD). Thus 5% of normal women will have hematocrits outside this range.

Whether or not an individual value is abnormal cannot be reliably inferred from normal distribution curves, especially when we recognize that a "normal" population includes may normal subpopulations. A woman with a hematocrit of 42% (the "normal") would be anemic if she lived in La Paz, Bolivia (altitude 14,000 feet). A pregnant woman with a hematocrit of 32% is probably showing the normal hemodilution of pregnancy rather than a decreased red cell mass. For these and other reasons, the probability that any single value is abnormal cannot be defined as the reciprocal of the normal distribution. Distributions often vary under different conditions (figure A.1). At best, then, a given laboratory value must be reviewed in terms of the **probability** that it is abnormal. Often this is difficult to do, even when a value is far from the mean.

The physician should also remember that not all frequency distributions are bell-shaped, gaussian curves. A mean and SD may not adequately

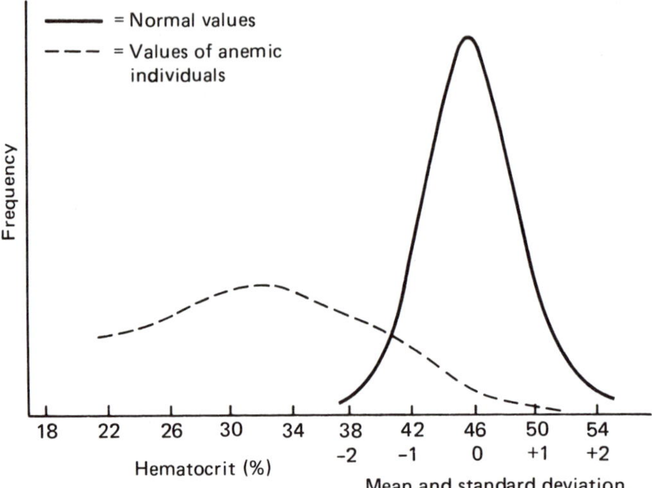

Fig. A.1
The gaussian frequency curve is typical for the random error seen in most laboratory techniques and for large population measurements such as height and I.Q. Normal value distributions that conform to this curve are usually reported as a mean and standard deviation. This is the hematocrit curve for normal men, age 18–40. A similar distribution for women will have a mean of 42 ± 5.0. Note the overlap of abnormal values.

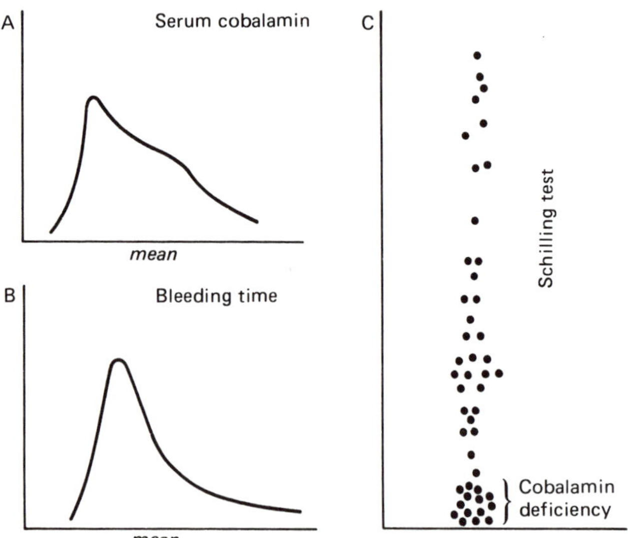

Fig. A.2
A, Range of normal for broad distributions with abnormal values both above and below the normal range. *B*, Mean and standard deviation or limit of normal. *C*, Range of normal for a distribution where abnormal values are restricted to one side of the normal range.

characterize a nongaussian distribution (figure A.2). In such cases, other expressions must be used. When distributions of normal values are broad, it is common to consider a limit of normal, beyond which certain investigations are warranted. This approach is used often when abnormal values tend to occur on only one side of the distribution, for instance, in Schilling test measurements of cobalamin absorption.

Normal hematologic values are listed in tables A.1 and A.2. These were established at the Massachusetts General Hospital and are taken from lists published triennially in the *New England Journal of Medicine*.

Collecting blood samples

Capillary blood by lancet

Capillary blood is collected with sterile disposable lancets when a small blood sample is required, or when venipuncture is not feasible. Usually blood is collected from the fingertip, or, in infants, the plantar surface of the heel. Clean the area to be punctured and pierce deeply enough to ensure

Table A.1
Blood Cell Values in a Normal Adult Population

		Men	Women
White cell count, $\times 10^9$/liter blood		7.8 (4.4–11.3)	
White cell differential			
Polys	47–63%		
Bands	0–4%		
Lymphocytes	24–40%		
Monocytes	4–9%		
Eosinophils	0–3%		
Basophils	0–2%		
Red cell count, $\times 10^{12}$/liter blood		5.21 (4.52–5.90)	4.60 (4.10–5.10)
Hemoglobin, g/dl blood		15.7 (14.0–17.5)	13.8 (12.3–15.3)*
Hematocrit, ratio		0.46 (0.42–0.50)	0.40 (0.36–0.45)
Mean corpuscular volume, fl/red cell		88.0 (80.0–96.1)	
Mean corpuscular hemoglobin, pg/red cell		30.4 (27.5–33.2)	
Mean corpuscular hemoglobin concentration, g/dl RBC		34.4 (33.4–35.5)	
Red cell distribution width, CV (%)		13.1 (11.5–14.5)	
Platelet count, $\times 10^9$/liter blood		311 (172–450)	

*The mean hemoglobin level of blacks of both sexes and all ages has been reported to be 0.5 to 1.0 g/dl below the mean for comparable whites.

Table A.2
Other Hematologic Values in Normal Adults

Determination	Men	Women
Clotting tests:		
Bleeding time	3–9 min	
Factor I (fibrinogen)	0.15–0.35 g/dl	
Factor II (prothrombin)	60–140%	
Factor V (accelerator globulin)	60–140%	
Factor VIII-X (proconvertion-Stuart)	70–130%	
Factor X (Stuart factor)	70–130%	
Factor VIII (antihemophilic globulin)	50–200%	
Factor IX (plasma thromboplastic cofactor)	60–140%	
Factor XI (plasma thromboplastic antecedent)	60–140%	
Factor XII (Hageman factor)	60–140%	
Partial thromboplastic time (activated)	25–40 sec	
Prothrombin time	Within 2 sec of control (12 sec)	
Thrombin time	Within 5 sec of control (16–20 sec)	
Cobalamin (serum)	200–850 pg/ml	
Erythrocyte sedimentation rate	1–13 mm/hr	1–20 mm/hr
Erythropoietin (serum)	2–5 mU/ml	
Ferritin (serum)	20–50 ng/ml	
Folate (serum)	6–20 ng/ml	
Hemoglobin A_2	<3% of hemoglobin	
Leukocyte alkaline phosphatase	33–188 U	30–160 U
Schilling test	>10% excretion/24 hr	

a spontaneous flow of blood. Avoid undue pressure which might cause dilution of blood with tissue fluids.

Venous blood by venipuncture

Venipuncture in normal adults is usually done in the antecubital vein. Place a tourniquet around the upper arm, tight enough to distend the veins of the forearm, and thoroughly clean the puncture site. It is convenient to use a 21-gauge double-ended needle and vacuum tubes containing appropriate anticoagulants.

- **EDTA** (ethylenediaminetetraacetic acid) and **sodium citrate** act as anticoagulants by chelating ionic calcium. EDTA is preferred for most hematologic tests because it has little effect on blood cell morphology. Thus smears can be safely made from venous blood drawn into EDTA. In general, it is preferable to make smears from capillary blood.
- **Citrate** anticoagulation is preferred for clotting tests.
- **Heparin** inhibits coagulation by acting as an antithrombin and antithromboplastin (see lecture 27). It produces the least hemolysis of any of the anticoagulants and has the least effect on red cell size. However, it is costly.

Most commercially available vacuum tubes are nonsterile. If blood backflows from tube to vein, it may introduce bacteria into the bloodstream. The following maneuvers may help to avoid such backflow:

- Remove the tourniquet before blood flow into the tube has stopped.
- Keep the patient's arm motionless.
- Do not exert pressure on the stopper end of the tube.

Blood drawn is usually submitted for a complete blood count (CBC) and additional tests if indicated.

Complete blood count (CBC)

The most commonly performed medical screening test, the CBC, includes measurements of hemoglobin (Hb), hematocrit (Hct), white cell count, red cell count, white cell differential count, and inspection of the blood smear. The platelet count is often (but not always) considered part of the CBC. Expect for the differential count, the CBC is now widely done by Coulter counters and other electronic devices. Although the traditional methods are less precise, they remain important, because (1) they are still used in the field; (2) they are often needed when the Coulter is down or unavailable, or when a quick answer is needed; and (3) they are essential for cell counts in body fluids other than the blood (e.g., pleural fluid, spinal fluid).

Normal values appear in table A.1. Abnormal values obviously signal the need for further investigations.

Hematocrit (microhematocrit method)

The hematocrit is the volume of packed red blood cells expressed as a percentage of blood volume. It can be performed on venous or freely flowing capillary blood. EDTA is the preferred anticoagulant becase it has no effect on red cell volume. Note that Coulter counters do not rely on centrifugation.

A decreased hematocrit is a sign of anemia or increased plasma volume. An elevated hematocrit suggests erythrocytosis or decreased plasma volume.

PROCEDURE

1. Draw venous blood without stasis. Avoid prolonged tourniquet obstruction of peripheral veins which may elevate the hematocrit by 1–3%. Be sure to release the tourniquet before the needle is withdrawn to avoid spurting. Anticoagulate the blood in an EDTA Vacutainer (purple top) and carefully mix by inverting. Avoid foaming. A mechanical rotator should be used if available.
2. When the blood is adequately mixed, dip the unmarked end of a uniform-bore glass capillary tube into the blood and allow it to fill to approximately three-quarters of its length by capillary action. Remove the tube from the blood, plug one end with modeling clay, wipe off excess blood, and place the tube in microhematocrit centrifuge with the clay-filled end

against the rubber gasket (away from the rotor). Do each determination in duplicate.

3. Running the laboratory centrifuge for 10 minutes at top speed separates blood cells from plasma, packing the red cells at the bottom of the tube and leaving a thin band (<1%) of white cells and platelets (the **buffy coat**) at the plasma interface. An abnormally thick buffy coat is a sign of leukocytosis or thrombocytosis.
4. To determine the percent of whole venous blood represented by packed cells, obtain a distance ratio along the capillary tube on a microhematocrit reader. First, set the reader's 100% line to correspond with the distance from the clay–red cell interface to the top of the plasma. Then, by shifting the ruled scale to the red cell–white cell interface, read the percent hematocrit directly.

SOURCES OF ERROR

For any single blood sample, this assay should be reproducible to within ±1% (hematocrit units). However, errors introduced by tourniquet stasis and plasma volume variations may increase this error to ±2%, as can be shown by replicate analysis of individual samples or of different samples from a single patient. Thus, consecutive hematocrits that change by up to 4% may not necessarily reflect a meaningful difference.

Hemoglobin (cyanmethemoglobin method)

The following protocol measures total hemoglobin, including oxyhemoglobin, carboxyhemoglobin, and methemoglobin. The reagent, Drabkin's solution, contains potassium cyanide, potassium ferricyanide, and sodium bicarbonate. Ferricyanide oxidizes hemoglobin iron from the ferrous to the ferric state, forming methemoglobin. Cyanide then combines with methemoglobin to produce the stable pigment cyanmethemoglobin. The two reactions are rapid and stoichiometric. Absorbance of the solution is measured spectrophotometrically at 540 nm.

PROCEDURE

1. Dilute blood 1:250 with Drabkin's reagent. For a small-diameter cuvette, this may be done conveniently and automatically by adding 13 μl of blood in a capillary tube to 3.25 ml Drabkin's reagent in a Unopette (figure A.3). Rinse the capillary with the reagent. Mix blood and reagent by inversion.
2. Transfer blood and reagent to a cuvette and allow it to stand for 10 minutes.
3. Measure absorbance at 540 nm. Using Drabkin's solution as a blank, set the spectrophotometer to show zero absorbance. Convert absorbance of the test solution to g/dl using an appropriate calibration curve or hemoglobin standard for that instrument.

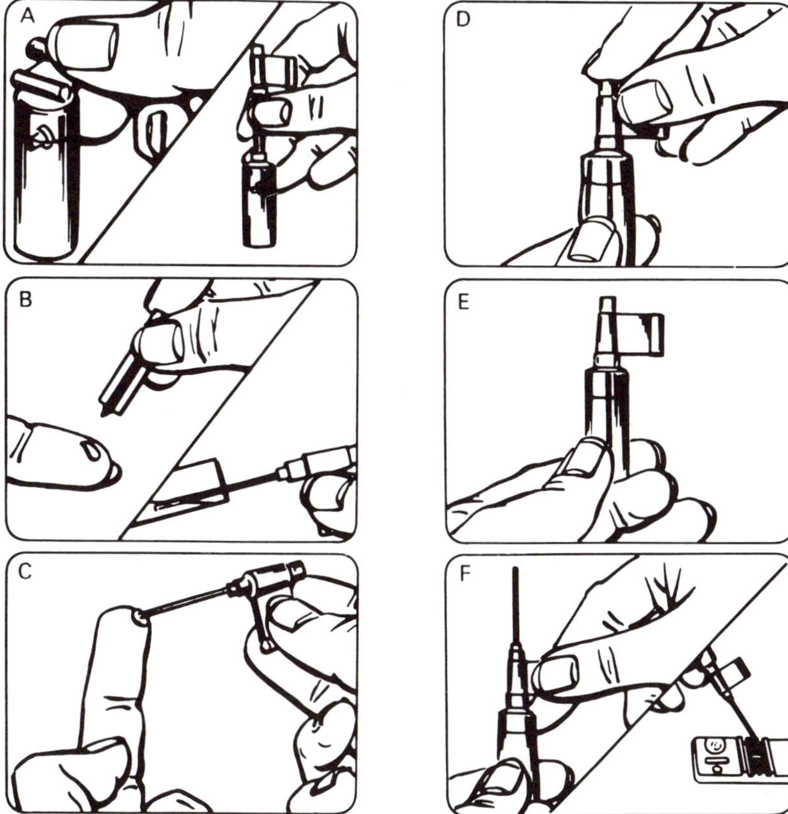

Fig. A.3
Use of Unopette in hemoglobinometry and cell counting (Courtesy of Becton, Dickinson & Co.).

A, Using flag of capillary holder, firmly depress plug on top of plastic reservoir. Use tip of capillary shield to push plug into reservoir, where it will serve as a "mixing pellet."

B, Remove protective shield covering capillary. Obtain blood sample from free-flowing finger puncture (or use well mixed venous blood sample).

C, Holding capillary nearly horizontal, touch tip to blood drop as shown. Capillary action fills tube and blood collection stops automatically. Wipe blood from outside of capillary, making sure that blood is not drawn from inside of the capillary tube.

D, Squeeze reservoir slightly. Cover upper opening of overflow chamber with finger and seat holder in reservoir neck. Release pressure on reservoir and remove finger from overflow chamber opening. Suction draws blood into diluent.

E, Squeeze reservoir gently two or three times to rinse capillary tube, thus forcing diluent into (but not out of) overflow chamber. Release pressure to return diluent to reservoir. Correct blood dilution has now been made automatically with premeasured volume of diluent (Drabkin's solution for hemoglobinometry, glacial acetic acid for white counting, Gower's solution for red counting). Close upper opening with finger and invert unit a few times to mix blood sample and diluent.

F, If Unopette is designed for white or red cell counting, charge the hemocytometer as shown.

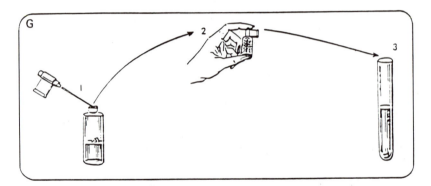

Fig. A.3 (continued)
G, If Unopette is designed for hemoglobinometry, add contents to cuvette and assay spectrometrically.

PROCEDURAL NOTES

Red cells which contain certain abnormal hemoglobins (Hb S, Hb C, and others) do not hemolyze completely in Drabkin's solution, and the solution may remain cloudy. Turbidity should therefore be reported, as it suggests a hemoglobinopathy. Turbid solutions are unsuitable for spectrophotometric determination, but the hemoglobin analysis can be completed by adding a drop of Redout/B to the cuvette. The agent hemolyzes all of the cells responsible for the cloudy solution. The absorbance of the solution can then be measured.

Blood cell counts

The manual counting of blood cells and platelets includes three steps:

- Accurately diluting a blood sample with an appropriate diluent
- Filling a counting chamber of known volume and allowing the cells to settle
- Viewing the chamber under a microscope and counting the cells within a defined area (or volume) of the counting chamber.

The counting area (or volume) is defined by an engraved grid at the bottom of the chamber (figure A.4). The volume of blood represented in the counted areas and a dilution factor are then used in a calculation that coverts the number of cells counted to the number of cells per cubic millimeter of blood. The techniques for counting red cells, white cells, and platelets differ in the diluent used and in the area of the grid over which cells are counted. Manual counts of white cells and platelets are reasonably accurate and reproducible. Manual red counts are inherently lacking in precision.

For manual cell counting, special glass pipettes facilitate the dilution of the blood sample (figure A.5). The red cell pipette (also used for platelets) dilutes the blood 1:200; the white cell pipette dilutes blood 1:20.

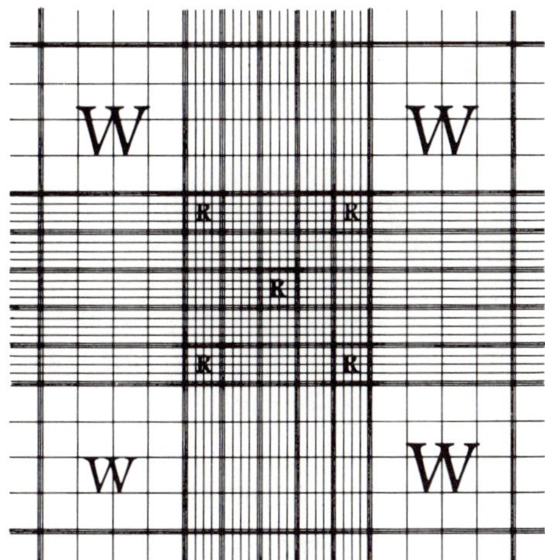

Fig. A.4
The hemocytometer chamber. Its depth is 0.1 mm. The area of the entire ruled area is 9 mm^2. Its volume is 0.9 mm^3. **To count white cells**, use the low power objective (10 ×) and count all cells in the four 1-mm^2 squares (marked W). Multiply the total number of cells counted by 50. **To count red cells**, use the high power objective (40 ×) and count all the cells in five of the 25 0.2 mm^2 squares (marked R). Multiply the total number of cells counted by 10,000. **To count platelets**, charge the counting chamber and allow platelets to settle for 10–15 minutes. Using the high power phase objective (40 ×), count all the cells in the central 1-mm^2 square. Multiply the cells counted by 1000. (From M. L. Turgeon, *Clinical Hematology*. Boston: Little, Brown, 1988.)

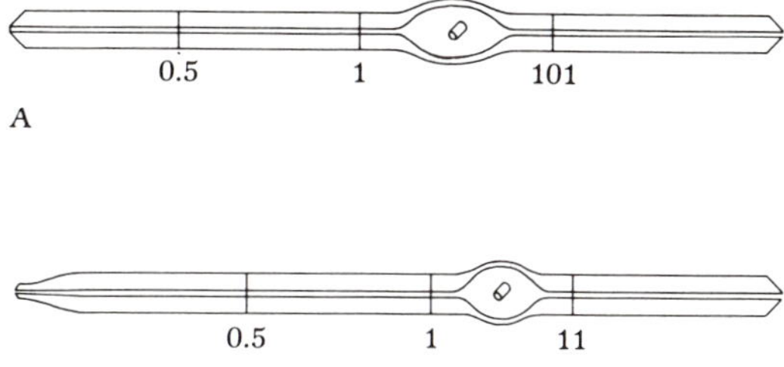

Fig. A.5
A, Erythrocyte (red cell) pipette. *B*, Leukocyte (white cell) pipette. (From M. L. Turgeon, *Clinical Hematology*. Boston: Little, Brown, 1988.)

PRELIMINARY PROCEDURE

Sampling, dilution, and filling the chamber are done as follows for all three types of cell counts.

1. Mix the vial of blood by carefully inverting it ten times. Shaking it generates foam, which should be avoided.
2. Draw blood into the appropriate pipette to exactly the lower mark. Wipe excess blood from the pipette. Hold the pipette almost horizontal while drawing up the column of blood. If the mark is slightly overshot, one can remove the excess from the tip by touching it to gauze or paper. If a large excess has been drawn up, the procedure is abandoned. Clean the pipette before using it again.
3. Draw the appropriate diluent into the pipette until the total volume in the pipette reaches the mark above the bulb.
4. Mix blood and diluent on a mechanical shaker or by hand for 3 minutes. The motion should be at right angles to the long axis of the pipette.
5. Before charging the counting chamber of the hemocytometer, discard the first 6–10 drops of fluid from the end of the pipette.
6. Cover the counting chamber with its special coverslip and fill it with fluid from the pipette. Hold the pipette at about a 30° angle, with the tip resting at the outer opening between coverslip and chamber bottom. The chamber will fill by capillary action. Allow entering fluid to spread slowly and evenly. Stop the addition when the chamber is full. Keep fluid from spilling into the gutters of the hemocytometer. Carefully blot excess fluid from the mouth of the chamber.
7. Allow the chamber to stand for a few minutes to permit the cells to settle. Platelets should be allowed to settle for 10–20 minutes, no more or less. Keep the chamber moist if the white or red count cannot be done immediately.
8. Count cells in the appropriate area (see below). Count any cell touching any of the lines on the left-hand or top borders; exclude any cells touching the right-hand or bottom borders. To decrease sampling error, make two cell counts, with two pipettes and two chambers. Use the following equation to calculate the number of cells per cubic millimeter. Remeber that the height of the volume counted in the chamber is 0.1 mm. Therefore, the chamber volume counted equals 0.1 × its area counted.

$$\text{Cell counts/mm}^3 = \frac{\text{cells counted} \times \text{dilution}}{\text{chamber volume counted}}$$

WHITE CELL COUNT

An acidic diluent is used in order to lyse red cells and leave white cells (and nucleated red cell precursors) intact.

1. Make the 1:20 blood sample dilution in 2% acetic acid. If the count is above 50,000/mm^3, repeat the count with a higher blood dilution.
2. Count white cells in the four 1-mm^2 squares labeled **W** in figure A.4. The total area counted is 4 mm^2. The total volume counted is 0.4 mm^3.
3. White cells/mm^3 blood = leukocytes counted in four squares × 50.
4. Results are erroneous if nucleated red cells are counted as white cells.

RED CELL COUNT

Red cells are diluted with an isotonic fluid that preserves their structure. White cells are not destroyed by this fluid, but they are relatively few in number and thus can be identified and excluded from the count.

1. Dilute a blood sample 1:200 in Gower's solution (12.5 g sodium sulfate and 33 ml glacial acetic acid in 200 ml of water).
2. Count red cells in the five 0.04 mm^2 squares labeled **B** in figure A.6. The total area counted is 0.2 mm^2. The total volume counted is 0.02 mm^3.
3. Red cells/mm^3 blood = red cells counted × 10,000.

PLATELET COUNT

The diluent for platelet counting must contain an anticoagulant. In addition, it is necessary to use a special thin hemocytometer chamber that can accomodate the phase contrast microcope.

1. Dilute a blood sample 1:200 in 1% ammonium oxalate that was filtered just before use.
2. Fill the chamber in the usual way. Let it stand in a Petri dish with a wet wick for 10–20 minutes.
3. Count platelets using a medium-dark phase contrast lens in the large central 1-mm^3 square (which includes 25 small 0.4-mm^2 squares) in the center of the chamber. Repeat the count on the other side of the chamber. Total area counted is thus 2 mm^2. Therefore, total volume counted is 0.2 mm^3. Platelets are seen as round or oval purple bodies that sometimes show dendritic processes. Dirt particles are refractile; platelets are not.
4. Platelets/mm^3 blood = platelets counted × 1000.
5. If a platelet count is low, repeat it using a 1:20 dilution in a white cell pipette. Count the platelets in the large central square (25 small squares). Multiply the platelets counted by 200 to calculate platelets/mm^3.

Red cell indexes (see lecture 2)

The red cell indexes characterize the average red cell in a number of useful ways by calculating relationships between hematocrit, hemoglobin, and red cell count. For example, the mean corpuscular volume (MCV) distinguishes macrocytic, normocytic, and microcytic anemias. The mean corpuscular hemoglobin concentration (MCHC) identifies normochromic and hypochromic red cell populations. Unlike the three direct measurements from which they are calculated, the indices are independent of changes in plasma volume. Table A.1. summarizes the ranges of normal values.

MEAN CORPUSCULAR VOLUME (MCV)

The MCV is the calculated volume of the average red cell by dividing the hematocrit, expressed as the total red cell volume per volume of blood, by the number of red cells in the same volume. It is expressed in units of volume (μm^3).

$$\mathrm{MCV} = \frac{\text{volume (in ml) of packed RBC/l}}{\text{red count/mm}^3\text{ (in millions)}} \quad \text{or} \quad \frac{\text{hematocrit (\%)} \times 10}{\text{red count/mm}^3\text{ (in millions)}}$$

MEAN CORPUSCULAR HEMOGLOBIN CONCENTRATION (MCHC)

The MCHC is the concentration of hemoglobin in the average red cell. It is expressed as a percentage.

$$\mathrm{MCHC} = \frac{\text{hemoglobin (g/dl)} \times 100}{\text{hematocrit (\%)}}$$

MEAN CORPUSCULAR HEMOGLOBIN (MCH)

The MCH is the calculated mass of hemoglobin per average red cell. It is expressed in units of mass (pg). Because hemoglobin levels are usually expressed per deciliter and the red cell counts in cells per cubic millimeter ($1\ mm^3 = 1\ \mu l$), the resulting quotient must be multiplied by 10.

$$\mathrm{MCH} = \frac{\text{hemoglobin (g/dl)} \times 10}{\text{red count/l} (\times 10^{-12})} \quad \text{or} \quad \frac{\text{hemoglobin (g/dl)} \times 10}{\text{red count/mm}^3}$$

Examination of the blood smear

Careful examination of stained blood smears reveals

- The types and relative numbers of white cells present (the white cell differential)
- Morphologic abnormalities of all three blood cell types
- Rough evidence of the white cell and platelet counts

Unfortunately, this examination, which direclty views a small sample of patient tissue (unlike an x-ray or ECG), is usually relegated to technicians unaware of the clinical problem.

PREPARATION OF SMEAR

Of the two common procedures for making blood smears—coverslip and slides—the coverslip method more reliably preserves red cell morphology and more evenly distributes cells. Both may be performed with blood from a fresh EDTA sample of venous blood or from a "finger stick."

Coverslip method

Place a drop of blood about 2 mm in diameter on the center of a coverslip held in one hand. Immediately place a second coverslip over the first, with its corners rotated 45° so that they may readily be grasped by the fingers of the free hand (figure A.6). The blood will spread between the coverslips. When it stops, separate them with a sliding motion. If there is no lifting motion, there will be an even film of blood on each coverslip. Both may be stained and then mounted, smear side down.

Slide method

Place a drop of blood 3–4 mm in diameter near one end of a glass slide. Using the edge of a second slide, push the drop down the length of the slide with a smooth motion (figure A.7). The thickness of the smear may be varied by changing the angle of the applicator slide and the speed of the push.

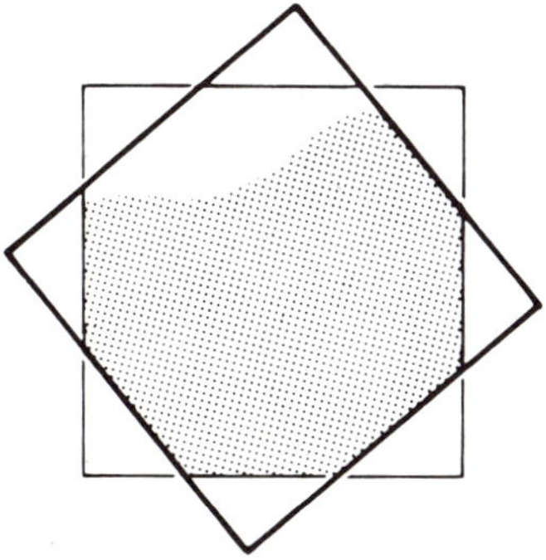

Fig. A.6
Coverglass method of making a blood smear. (From B. A. Brown, *Hematology: Principles and Procedures*, 3rd ed. Philadelphia: Lea & Febiger, 1980.)

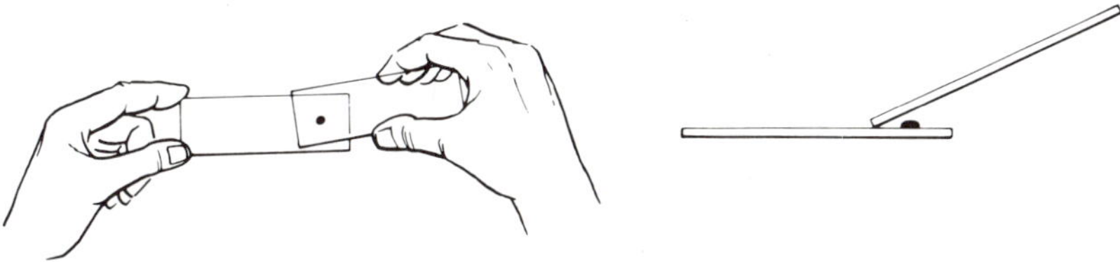

Fig. A.7
Method of holding slides of preparation of blood smear. (From B. A. Brown, *Hematology: Principles and Procedures*, 3rd ed. Philadelphia: Lea & Febiger, 1980.)

STAINING

The coverslip or slide is stained with Wright's stain, a mixture of methylene blue (or azure) and eosin. Methylene blue gives a blue-violet color to acidic cell components, such as nucleic acids. Eosin gives a red color to relatively basic components, such as hemoglobin.

1. Place the air-dried coverslip or slide, smear up, in a staining tray. Flood it with Wright's stain. After 3 minutes, slowly add water to the slide until a metallic green sheen appears on the surface of the liquid. Wait 5 minutes, pour off the stain and rinse the slide, air-dry it, and mount it or coverslip it with methacrylate sealer. The optimal times for stain and buffer will vary for each batch of dye, and must be determined by trial and error. Once stained, smears can be stored indefinitely.
2. Red cells in properly stained smears have a pinkish color. If they are blue or if nuclei are too deeply stained, the cause may be overlong staining, inadequate washing, or excessively alkaline stain or diluent. If the red cells are excessively red and nuclei poorly stained, the cause may be inadequate staining, excessive washing, or excessively acid stain or diluent.

INSPECTION OF SLIDES

Microscopic inspection of slide smears should be limited to the thin portion of the smear. Under low power, choos an area of the slide where red cells are not overlapping. This is important. An area is not ideally satisfactory unless the majority of red cells appear as biconcave disks. Now switch to the oil immersion objective.

WHITE CELL DIFFERENTIAL

Normal values for the white cell differential are given in table A.1.

1. Under oil, move the slide to successive fields from the extreme upper edge of the smear to the extreme lower edge. Count and classify each white cell in the successive fields. When that column of fields is finished, move the slide sideways one field, and begin again. Continue until the required number of cells have been counted.
2. The number of white cells to be counted depends on the total white cell count, as well as the degree of accuracy desired. When the white count is normal, 100 to 200 cells should be counted. When it is between 20,000 and 50,000, count 300 cells; when it is above 50,000, count 500 cells. On smears of bone marrow aspirates at least 500 cells should be counted.

BLOOD CELL MORPHOLOGY

White mounting, carefully note red cell and white cell morphology, and the morphology and number of platelets. Figure A.8 lists some common morphologic abnormalities of red cells and the stains needed to reveal them.

REPORTING RESULTS

Written reports of examinations of blood smears should include the following information.

- **White cell differential count**. Unless otherwise noted, it is assumed that the differential count was based on an examination of 100 cells. If cells were observed that could not be classified, the differential should include the percentage of unclassified cells. If such cells were seen rarely but not among the 100 cells counted, the report should note "occasional unclassified cells."
- **Description of red cells**. If abnormalities were noted, the report should grade them on a scale of 1–4+, e.g., anisocytosis 2+, poikilocytosis 3+, hypochromia 1+, polychromatophilia 2+, rouleaux 3+, and so no. Inclusion bodies should be mentioned as well as other morphologic abnormalities, such as spur cells, burr cells, schistocytes, and the like (see Table A.3).
- **Estimated platelet count** (normal, decreased 1–4+, or increased 1–4+) with notes on platelet morphology (e.g., megathrombocytes, megakaryocyte fragments).
- Any **other observations** of note, such as malarial parasites in red cells, white cell vacuolation, endothelial cells, "hairy" cells, and so forth.

Figure A.9 is an actual report of a recent normal blood study. The differential count on the top lines was performed by an automated differential counting apparatus, which is used only for screening purposes at the Massachusetts General Hospital. The differential under "Blood smear" was performed by a microscopist. Blood counts were performed by a Coulter counter. The ESR (sedimentation rate) and reticulocyte count were done by conventional methods.

Reticulocyte count

Reticulocytes are red cell precursors that still contain mitochondria and ribosomes. When these organelles are clumped or precipitated into a "reticulum" by exposure to the alcoholic component of vital (wet) dyes and stained, they acquire the artefactual structure for which they are named. Reticulocytes do not display a reticulum in an ordinary blood smear, which is dry when stain is applied. There they appear as **polychromes**, or **polychromatophilia**—cells that are slightly larger than mature red cells with a uniform bluish-gray color. An experienced observer veiwing a Wright's stained smear can often estimate the reticulocyte count by estimating the degree of polychromatophilia.

The reticulocyte count is often a valuable index of the rate of effective red cell production. It is not infallible, however. For example, the high reticulocyte count typically seen in hemolytic anemia may eventually de-

Fig. A.8
Inclusions and other abnormalities of red cells in peripheral blood.

Morphology	Abnormality	Special stain	Diagnostic significance
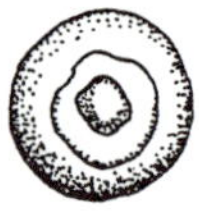	Target cells	No	Decreased osmotic fragility Liver disease (especially obstructive jaundice) Hemoglobinopathies (CC, SC, S-thal, C-thal, SS) Thalassemia (β-thal major) Postsplenectomy LCAT deficiency Iron deficiency
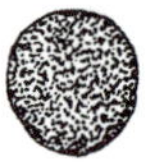	Spherocytes	No	Increased osmotic fragility Hereditary spherocytosis Immunohemolytic anemia Microangiopathic hemolytic anemia (occ) Oxidant hemolysis (G-6-PD deficiency)
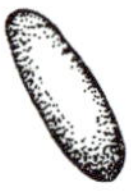	Elliptocytes	No	Hereditary elliptocytosis
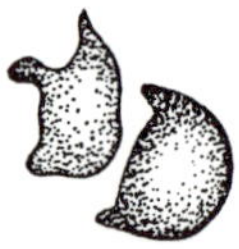	Schistocytes	No	Microangiopathic hemolytic anemia DIC (gram-negative sepsis, malignancy) Thrombotic thrombocytopenic purpura Aortic valve prosthesis Hemolytic-uremic syndrome
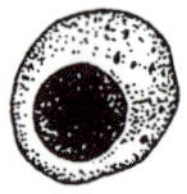	Normoblasts	No	Leukoerythroblastic anemia (myelophthisis) Cancer metastatic to bone marrow Miliary tuberculosis Myelofibrosis Thalassemia major Severe hemolysis Postsplenectomy
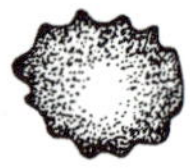	Burr cells (echinocytes)	No	Artifact Uremia
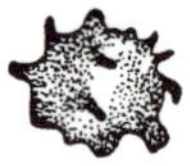	Spur cells (acanthocytes)	No	Severe liver disease (occ) Abetalipoproteinemia
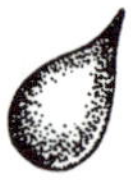	Teardrop cells	No	Myelofibrosis Leukoerythroblastic anemia Thalassemia major Severe iron deficiency
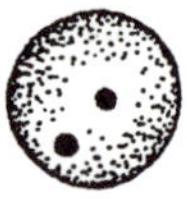	Howell-Jolly bodies	No	Small number present in normals Postsplenectomy Sickle cell anemia Myelodysplasia

Fig. A.8 (cont.)

Morphology	Abnormality	Special stain	Diagnostic significance
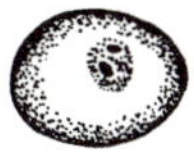	Siderocytes	Prussian blue	Postsplenectomy Severe hemolysis
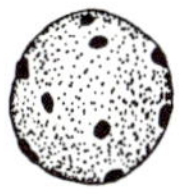	Heinz bodies	Supravital stain (e.g., crystal violet)	Small number present in normals G-6-PD deficiency Other defects of HMP shunt Congenital hemolytic anemias Unstable hemoglobin variants Thalassemia (α-thal, hemoglobin H)
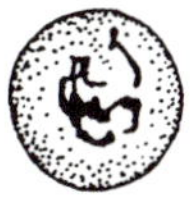	Reticulocytes	Supravital stain (e.g., new methylene blue)	Normal blood Increased in hemolytic anemia, hemorrhage
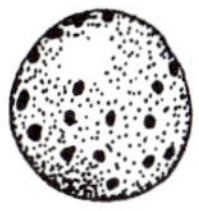	Basophilic stippling	No	Many bone marrow disorders Lead poisoning
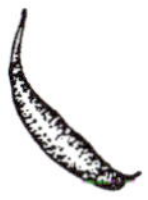	Sickle cells	No	Sickle cell anemia

DATE	(COMMENT)	HCT	WBC	RBC	HGB	MCV	MCH	MCHC	POLY	LYMP	MONO	PLT
03/05		44.5	4.2	5.12	14.7	87	28.7	33.0	66	24	10	197

****

DATE	PT (PAT/STD)	PTT	TT (PAT/STD)	ESR	RETIC
03/05				6	2.4

****BLOOD SMEAR****

03/05 WBC: 4.2
WHITE CELLS: POLYS 72% LYMPHS 18% MONOS 7% EOS 1%
META 2%
RED CELLS: RED CELL MORPHOLOGY NORMAL ON SMEAR
PLATELETS: PLATELET EST NORMAL

Fig. A.9
Report of a normal blood study (see text for description).

crease as a result of supervening folate deficiency. Many such examples could be cited.

In the following procedure, called the **new methylene blue method**, blood is mixed with fluid stain and then smeared and counted.

PROCEDURE (NEW METHYLENE BLUE METHOD)

1. Mix equal parts of anticoagulated blood and 0.5% new methylene blue in a test tube or the bottom of a centrifuge tube. Alternatively, fill a microcapillary pipette half full of blood and fill the remainder with new methylene blue. Allow the mixture to stand for 10 minutes.
2. Smear the blood-dye mixture onto a slide, allow it to dry, and mount a coverslip.
3. Carefully examine 1000 red cells and count how many of them are reticulocytes. Count all erythroid cells with *any* reticulum, however small or dotlike.
4. Results are expressed in percentage terms, but conversion to absolute numbers per cubic millimeter is sometimes more informative.

PROCEDURAL NOTES

If red cells with **basophilic stippling** are inadvertently counted as reticulocytes, it may be useful to count such cells—in effect, to do a "reticulocyte" count—on a control blood smear stained with Wright's stain. Then subtract this number from the number on a smear stained with new methylene blue.

Erythrocyte sedimentation rate

The erythrocyte sedimentation rate (ESR or "sed rate") is a nonspecific screening test that has been performed for many years in three settings.

- It is a screening test for a variety of illnesses and should trigger further studies in patients with ill-defined complaints.
- It is useful in monitoring the clinical course of fluctuating disorders ordinarily associated with elevated ESR during active phases (e.g., rheumatoid arthritis, temporal arteritis, polymyalgia rheumatica).
- It is often useful in detecting relapses of Hodgkin's disease, lymphoma, and hyperglobulinemic disorders, such as multiple myeloma.

In principle, the procedure is an indirect method of quantifying red cell agglomeration or rouleaux formation. Even in normal anticoagulated blood, red cells form loose agglomerations or aggregations. According to Stokes' law, which governs the rate of fall of spherical bodies in a fluid medium, the sedimentation rate of these agglomerants increases as their diameter increases. For that reason, the time course of the red cell sedimentation, if carefully observed, has a slow phase followed by a more rapid phase. This is true even in normal blood. When the red cell agglomeration is increased—as it is by increased levels of a variety of plasma proteins, especially immunoglobulins or fibrinogen—sedimentation is accelerated. Fibrinogen is a notably effective red cell agglomerant because it is fibrous rather than globular in shape. Many plasma proteins rise in a nonspecific manner as phase reactants in a variety of diseases.

Since the sedimentation rate of red cell agglomerations is decreased by increasing **plasma viscosity**, situations may arise (as in severe IgM hyperglobulinemia) in which viscosity has become so high, the ESR begins to slow.

PROCEDURE

Many procedures have been used over the years. The one decribed here employs the disposable Westergren tube called Dispette.

1. Pipette saline into the reservoir up to the line with a Pasteur pipette. This requires 0.24 ml of saline.
2. Add mixed whole blood into the reservoir up to the second line. This requires 0.96 ml of blood.
3. Insert the pipette tube to the bottom of the reservoir and adjust the blood level to the zero mark.
4. Allow the blood to sediment. At 60 minutes, note the distance in mm between the plasma meniscus and the top of the red cell column.
5. Normal values are given in table A.2.

SPECIAL METHODS

Heinz body stain

Heinz bodies represent denatured hemoglobin and are seen in hemoglobinopathies associated with unstable hemoglobins (e.g., Hb Zurich) as well as in G-6-PD deficiency and related disorders in th presence of oxidant drugs (e.g., primaquine). A few are seen in splenectomized patients and a very few in normal red cells.

Heinz bodies are not visible with ordinary polychrome stains, such as Wright's and Giemsa's. On phase microscopy of wet preparations they may be visible as rounded, refractile inclusions. The particles vary in size from less than 1 μm to half the size of the cells, tend to lie in proximity to cell membrane, and when in a wet cell suspension are subject to brownian movements. However, a properly stained smear is a better method of detecting and roughly quantifying Heinz bodies.

PROCEDURE

1. Mix equal volumes of blood and of 0.5% crystal violet or methyl violet in 0.85% sodium chloride in a test tube.
2. After 10–15 minutes, place 1 or 2 drops of the mixture on a glass slide and cover with a glass coverslip, which is then gently blotted with a sheet of filter paper.

PROCEDURAL NOTES

Heinz bodies are deep purple, whereas Howell-Jolly bodies and siderocytes are blue-black. The reticulum of a reticulocyte is pale blue. Heinz bodies may be single or multiple. As a control, Heinz bodies may be produced in a normal blood sample by adding a small amount of acetylphenylhydrazine and examining the cells after the sample turns brown.

If drug-induced hemolysis is suspected, tests for Heinz bodies should be carried out as soon as possible, since the cells in which hemoglobin has been denatured disappear from the circulation within hours to days after the toxic event.

Osmotic fragility test

The osmotic fragility test is a rough index of red cell surface-to-volume ratio. When red cells are introduced into hypotonic solutions, they imbibe water and swell until they are spherical. When a critical volume is reached, they rupture. The spherical shape obviously has the maximum volume for the surface area of the cell, and thus the lowest possible surface-to-volume ratio. Any further water influx causes them to rupture. A cell that is already spherical, as in hereditary spherocytosis, displays increased osmotic fragility, for it can swell to only a small extent before rupturing. Flat cells, such as target cells, have decreased osmotic fragility.

When red cells rupture, they release hemoglobin into the medium. The average osmotic fragility of the red cells in a blood sample is measured by adding blood to a series of increasingly hypotonic solutions, and noting the amount of hemoglobin present in the supernatant fraction after centrifugation of each mixture.

PROCEDURE FOR SCREENING TEST

The following protocol is a practical screening test for the detection of increased osmotic fragility, and uses only two concentrations of sodium chloride.

1. Prepare two test tubes containing 2 ml each of 0.85 snd 0.50 g/dl NaCl.
2. Add samples of 0.1 ml of venous blood to each of the two tubes, mix, and centrifuge.
3. If a pink color appears in the 0.50 g/dl solution and not in physiologic saline (0.85 g/dl), the osmotic fragility of red cells is probably increased.

STANDARD PROCEDURE

A more precise method of determining osmotic fragility measures hemolysis in a series of solutions ranging from isotonic saline to water as follows. Note that control of temperature and pH are important.

1. Place 1.0 ml of each of the following saline solutions in a small test tube (75 × 100 mm):

1. 1.20%	7. 0.70%	13. 0.55%	19. 0.40%
2. 1.00%	8. 0.675%	14. 0.525%	20. 0.35%
3. 0.90%	9. 0.65%	15. 0.50%	21. 0.30%
4. 0.85%	10. 0.625%	16. 0.475%	22. 0.20%
5. 0.80%	11. 0.60%	17. 0.45%	23. 0.10%
6. 0.75%	12. 0.575%	18. 0.425%	24. 0.00%

   Tube 24 contains 2.0 ml of distilled water. Use a separate pipette for each saline concentraion.
2. Add 0.1 ml defibrinated blood to each tube. With a single pipette, start by adding to the highest concentration and work down the scale, mixing by aspirating up and down three times and blowing out the last drop. Be sure to wipe exterior of pipette before placing it in the solution.
3. Centrifuge tubes for 10 minutes at 2000 rpm.
4. Using a separate disposible pipette with bulb for each sample, transfer supernatant fractions to clean tubes.
5. Determine percent hemolysis in each supernatant sample by mixing 0.4 ml supernatant with 6 ml Drabkin's solution. Measure absorbance at 540 nm using 6 ml Drabkin's solution as blank.
6. Calculation: Absorbance of water sample represents 100% hemolysis.

$$\text{Percent hemolysis of each sample} = \frac{A_{540}}{A_{540} \text{ of } 100\% \text{ hemolysis}} \times 100$$

   Calculate percent increments of hemolysis as follows:

$$\frac{A_{540} \text{ difference between two consecutive readings}}{A_{540} \text{ of } 100\% \text{ hemolysis}} \times 100$$

Table A.3
Normal Values for Osmotic Fragility

NaCl concentration (%)	Percent hemolysis: Before Incubation	Percent hemolysis: After Incubation
0.85	0	0
0.75	0	0–2
0.65	0	0–19
0.60	0	0–40
0.55	0	5–70
0.50	0–5	36–88
0.45	0–45	54–96
0.40	50–90	65–100
0.35	90–99	72–100
0.30	97–100	80–100
0.20	100	91–100
0.10	100	100

Plot the percent increments of hemolysis against the saline concentrations (see figure 14.5).

7. The osmotic fragility of blood incubated 24 hr is determined in the same manner as outlined above.
8. A normal control should be run along with the test specimen.
9. Normal values are listed in table A.3.

Demonstration of sickle cells

Red cells containing a high percentage of hemoglobin S sickle when the hemoglobin is in the deoxy- form. This can be demonstrated in the laboratory by lowering oxygen tension (i.e., by sealing fresh blood under a coverslip), or by adding a reducing substance such as sodium metabisulfite, as demonstrated by Daland and Castle.

PROCEDURE

1. Prepare a fresh aqueous solution of sodium metabisulfite ($Na_2S_2O_5$), 2 g/dl.
2. Add 2 drops of this solution to 1 drop of blood on a slide. Mix it at the corner of a coverslip, and then cover it with the coverslip. Gently press the coverslip with a piece of filter paper, to express excess blood. It is not necessary to seal the preparation.
3. Make a control slide using a drop of isotonic saline in place of reducing agent.
4. Observe red cell morphology immediately and 15–30 minutes after preparation. The presence of sickled cells signifies a positive test. Positive tests are reliable. Negative tests, however, are not, due to the instability of the reducing agent. Negative tests should therefore be repeated with fresh reagent if suspicion is high. Negatives may also occur if the concentration of hemoglobin S in the red cells is less than 7 g/dl.
5. The saline control is useful in differentiating elliptocytosis and poikilocytosis from sickled cells, especially in thalassemia. Sickled cells are easily distinguished from crenated cells, which are round and have short spinelike projections.
6. Sickle-cell homozygotes cannot be distinguished from heterozygotes or from the other hemoglobin S syndromes by this test. Blood from infants with hemoglobin disorders may not sickle until several months of age due to the presence of hemoglobin.

Red cell inclusions and abnormal forms

Careful study of red cell morphology often suggests useful diagnostic possibilities. The major inclusions and abnormalities of shape are summarized in figure A.8. Note that special stains are required to demonstrate certain inclusion bodies. The other abnormalities can be seen in routine Wright's-stained smears.

Examination of the bone marrow

Bone marrow is examined under the clinical circumstances summarized in table 1.5. As noted earlier (see figure 1.5), aspirated marrow samples are smeared out on coverslips. Hence, architecture is distorted. However, the Wright's stained preparations reveal cell morphology in striking detail. Biopsy samples preserve architecture, but display cell morphology less vividly.

It is usual today to employ a Jamshidi needle which permits aspiration of a marrow sample and then, after the needle is inserted another centimeter or two, the removal of a core biopsy.

Bone marrow aspiration and biopsy are best performed in the posterior iliac crest. The following procedure is recommended.

PROCEDURE

1. After scrubbing the area, infiltrate skin and periosteum with lidocaine and slit the skin with a Bard-Parker no. 12 scalpel blade. Inert the needle and press it through the outer table of bone with a boring motion. Entry into the marrow is usually signalled by a sudden diminution of resistance and momentary pain from endosteal nerve fibers.
2. Only about 0.5 ml of aspirated marrow is needed for smears. It should be handled quickly to avoid clotting. The marrow is squirted from the syringe onto coverslips, and the excess is allowed to flow off by touching the edge to gauze before applying a top coverslip and pulling the smear. It is also possible to place marrow directly onto a slide or watch-glass and then pick off selected spicules, which are smeared in the usual way.
3. Excess aspirate ("the clot") is placed in a separate fixative bottle and submitted for sectioning and pathologic study along with the biopsy. Often, sectioning of a clot may reveal adequate marrow tissue for proper biopsy. However, a core biopsy is a more reliable specimen.
4. Next take a biopsy sample and place it immediately in fixative. The sample is promptly sent for sectioing and pathologic examination.
5. Fix aspirate smears with 95% methanol and stain them with Wright's stain. After washing, they may be counterstained with Giemsa's stain by flooding the slide with water, adding two to three drops of Giemsa's stain, and allowing 5 minutes for staining. Air-dry the slides and mount them with methacrylate.
6. Examinations of both aspirate and biopsy usually includes examination of iron-stained preparations (see below).
7. Inspect smears of marrow aspirate under the microscope and look for the following:

Table A.4
Normal Values for Marrow Differential Cell Count According to Several Authors

Type of cell	Infants 1 month	Adults
Myeloblast	—	0.4 (0–1)
Promyelocyte	0.76 ± 0.65	1.4 (0–3)
Myelocyte	2.50 ± 1.48	4.2 (0–12)
Neutrophilic		
Eosinophilic		
Basophilic		
Metamyelocyte	11.34 ± 3.59	6.5 (3–10)
Band form	14.10 ± 4.63	24 (17–33)
Segmented		
Neutrophil	3.64 ± 2.97	15 (5–25)
Eosinophil	2.61 ± 1.40	2 (0–4)
Basophil	0.07 ± 0.16	0.2 (0–5)
Lymphocyte	47.05 ± 9.24	14 (3–25)
Monocyte	1.01 ± 0.89	2 (0–4)
Plasma cell	0.02 ± 0.06	—
Pronormoblast	0.10 ± 0.14	0.2 (0–1)
Normoblast		
Basophilic	0.34 ± 0.33	2 (0–4)
Polychromatophilic	6.90 ± 4.45	6 (4–8)
Orthochromatic	0.54 ± 1.88	3 (1–5)
Megakaryocyte	0.05 ± 0.09	—
E/M ratio	1:4.4	1:3.6 (1:2–1:8)

- Adequacy of marrow specimen.
- Megakaryocyte numbers.
- Presence of abnormal cells—tumor cells, plasma cells, etc.
- Abnormal red cell maturation—e.g., nuclear maturation defect (megaloblastosis), cytoplasmic maturation defect (hypochromia), nuclear dysplasia.
- Abnormal white cell maturation—megaloblastosis, leukemic transformation, etc.
- Estimate the E/M ratio (see lecture 2).
- Do a differential count. The normal bone marrow cell differential count is summarized in table A.4.

Iron stain

The Prussian blue iron stain is used on bone marrow aspirates and biopsies to detect **sideroblasts** (normal and "ringed") and to evaluate **iron stores** in reticulum cells (macrophages). In the Prussian blue reaction, ionic iron reacts with acidic potassium ferrocyanide to give a blue color.

Sideroblasts are normoblasts containing stainable granules of **ferritin**. In normal adults, 30–50% of the normoblasts are sideroblasts. The number is decreased in iron deficiency. Estimating the number of sideroblasts is useful in distinguishing iron deficiency anemia from defective iron re-utilization (the anemia of chronic disease). In the latter, conditioned iron stores in marrow are increased. **Ringed sideroblasts**, described below, are seen in the various sideroblastic anemias.

PROCEDURE

1. Place coverslip smears of blood or marrow in iron-free Coplin jars and fix them in methanol for 4–24 hr.
2. Mix equal parts of 2% HCl and 2% KCN and heat for 1–2 minutes at 56°C. This yields fresh Prussian blue stain.
3. Incubate the fixed smears in this stain for 10 minutes at 56°C.
4. Stop the staining reaction by exhaustively washing smear in tap water.
5. Counterstain smears with 0.1% safranin for 10 seconds. Wash, dry, and mount coverslips with methacrylate.
6. Examine a portion of the smear in which marrow cells are well-separated.

PROCEDURAL NOTES

Sideroblasts appear as pinkish (hemoglobinized) nucleated cells containing tiny blue cytoplasmic granules less than 1 μm in diameter. When the granules are larger and surround the nucleus, the cell is called a ringed sideroblast. These are not ferritin granules, but iron-laden mitochondria, which are typical of sideroblastic anemia. Iron stores are judged by examination of reticulum cells (macrophages). Normal iron stores appear as scattered blue granules. Increased iron stores appear as dense agglomerates.

Occasionally smears of peripheral blood are stained with Prussian blue to demonstrate **siderocytes**, which bear to red cells the same relation that sideroblasts bear to normoblasts. Siderocytes are rare in normal blood, but are common after splenectomy, in the hemoglobinopathies, and in lead poisoning.

Urinary sediments are also stained for iron. Hemosiderin is typically present as free granules or within tubule cells in patients with acute or chronic intravascular hemolysis and occasionally in hemochromatosis.

SELECTED REFERENCES

Reviews

Brown, B. A. *Hematology: Principles and Procedures*, 3rd ed. Philadelphia: Lea & Febiger, 1980.

Desforges, J. F., and Merritt, J. A. *Diagnostic Procedures in Hematology*. Chicago: Year Book, 1971.

Maslow, W. C., Beutler, E., et al. *Practical Diagnosis: Hematologic Disease*. Boston: Houghton Mifflin, 1980.

Miale, J. B. *Laboratory Medicine: Hematology*, 6th ed. St. Louis: Mosby, 1982.

Multiple authors. Laboratory techniques (Appendix). In Williams, W. J., Beutler, E., et al. *Hematology*, 4th ed. New York: McGraw-Hill, pp. 1693–1784.

Schmidt, R. M., ed. *CRC Handbook Series in Clinical Laboratory Science. Section I: Hematology. Vol. 2*. Boca Raton, FL: CRC Press, 1980.

Simmons, A. *Technical Hematology*. Philadelphia: Lippincott, 1976.

INDEX